Functional Occlusion:
From TMJ
to Smile Design

Functional Occlusion
From TMJ
to Smile Design

Peter E. Dawson, DDS

Founder & Director
The Dawson Center for Advanced Dental Study
St. Petersburg, Florida

with 1269 illustrations

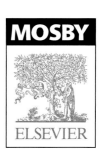
MOSBY

ELSEVIER

11830 Westline Industrial Drive
St. Louis, Missouri 63146

Functional Occlusion: From TMJ to Smile Design

ISBN-13: 978-0-323-03371-8
ISBN-10: 0-323-03371-7

Notice

Knowledge and best practice in this field are constantly changing. As new research and experience broaden our knowledge, changes in practice, treatment and drug therapy may become necessary or appropriate. Readers are advised to check the most current information provided (i) on procedures featured or (ii) by the manufacturer of each product to be administered, to verify the recommended dose or formula, the method and duration of administration, and contraindications. It is the responsibility of the practitioner, relying on their own experience and knowledge of the patient, to make diagnoses, to determine dosages and the best treatment for each individual patient, and to take all appropriate safety precautions. To the fullest extent of the law, neither the Publisher nor the Author assumes any liability for any injury and/or damage to persons or property arising out or related to any use of the material contained in this book.

The Publisher

ISBN-13: 978-0-323-03371-8
ISBN-10: 0-323-03371-7

Publishing Director: Linda Duncan
Acquisitions Editor: John Dolan
Developmental Editor: Julie Nebel
Publishing Services Manager: Pat Joiner
Senior Project Manager: Rachel E. Dowell
Interior Design: Paula Ruckenbrod
Cover Design Direction: Mark Oberkrom

Printed in Canada

Last digit is the print number: 9 8 7 6 5

Working together to grow
libraries in developing countries

www.elsevier.com | www.bookaid.org | www.sabre.org

ELSEVIER   BOOK AID International   Sabre Foundation

As the years pass, the values that really matter come into sharper focus.
It is to these great incentives in my life that I dedicate this book.

To My God

The designer of the masticatory system who programmed a complete set of instructions into every living cell using the alphabet of DNA. It is only because an element of love was integrated into that design that the masticatory system is also the organ of speech, expression, and beauty that is reflected in our smiles.

To My Family

To Jodie, my helper, supporter, best friend, and mom to our four wonderful children, Mark, Anne, Kelly, and Cary. I can't imagine how I could have the contentment I enjoy without such a loving family. This dedication also extends to the future of eight very special grandchildren.

To My Profession

Especially to those in it whose primary motivation is to care enough about every patient that they continue to study and improve their knowledge and skills. It is for those true professionals that this book was written.

Foreword

The form, function, and pathofunction of the dynamic masticatory system comprises one of the most fascinating, basic, and important areas of study in dentistry. The explosion of technological and procedural advances coupled with improved materials and the general public's awareness of the importance of quality oral health and its role in quality overall health herald a new age in dentistry. Additionally, the amalgamation of evolving science with the art of dentistry has fostered a true clinician-scientist model of dental practice in the quest to provide "complete dentistry" for patients. The goals of complete dentistry include optimal oral health, anatomic harmony, functional harmony, orthopedic stability, and natural esthetics. It is clear that to achieve these goals, today's dentist must become a physician of the masticatory system and beyond. Over the years, Dr. Dawson has advocated such a concept. Importantly, the keys to predictable treatment outcomes that have been espoused in his prior works stress that enhanced form (esthetics) does not have to come at the sacrifice of optimal function. In this book, he brings to the forefront basic principles of complete dentistry that can be applied to every dental discipline regardless of the practitioner's level of education and expertise.

Diagnosis is the key to successful treatment outcomes. Unless one understands the system in health, it will be difficult at best to accurately recognize pathology and to develop a case-specific, principle-centered plan of care. Dr. Dawson has done a masterful job of organizing the book in an easy-to-follow, logical flow, beginning with the complete examination. Each chapter is organized in a manner that will enhance one's understanding of how the interrelated components of the entire masticatory system function in health. With the aid of excellent drawings and photographs, the reader can attain a clear understanding of important anatomic relationships and gain a greater appreciation for basic orthopedic principles. The text clearly explains how pathology/dysfunction of one component may impact on the entire system.

The sequelae related to maladaptive occlusion are multifaceted. Compromise may occur at one or more of the occlusal interfaces to include: the tooth to tooth interface, the tooth to supporting structure interface, the neuromuscular interface, and/or the temporomandibular joint (TMJ) interface. It is well understood that the primary manner in which orthopedic systems are compromised is due to mechanical stress or overload. Once disequilibrium develops in the masticatory system the patient may develop one or more of a number of pathologic conditions representative of temporomandibular disorders (TMDs). To develop an individualized treatment plan the practitioner must be specific regarding the diagnosis, recognizing that TMD represents a number of arthrogenous and myogenous conditions. The symptoms associated with these conditions frequently provide a complex diagnostic dilemma for the dentist and physician. Even when the causative factors are apparent, implementation of appropriate therapeutic measures may be difficult. Important additions to this text are:

1. A scheme for the classification of occlusion
2. A classification system for TMJ pathology
3. Detailed discussion of myogenous forms of TMD
4. Diagnosis-specific treatment based on detailed assessment of all aspects of the stomatognathic system
5. Recognition of other potential causes, co-morbid conditions, maintaining factors as related or unrelated to TMD
6. A review of imaging of the TMJs in health and pathologic states

By providing these means of individualizing diagnosis, the reader is provided with important anatomic, physiologic, and neurologic perspectives that will certainly enhance problem-solving skills.

A highlight of the book is a detailed discussion of cases representative of commonly presenting restorative challenges. Each of these is presented with a detailed description of the problem list, appropriate diagnostics, and treatment considerations. Importantly, the potential pitfalls that might arise in the treatment of these cases are discussed. Postoperative care is delineated on a case-specific basis. Dr. Dawson has also provided objective measures that delineate specific criteria for success.

Dr. Dawson once said "If you are going to quote me, date me." It is clear that this text is the crowning jewel of a true pioneer in dentistry and clearly illustrates his commitment to being a perpetual student. Rare is the individual who excels at teaching a subject and writing about the subject, and who can perform to the level of excellence promoted by his teachings/writings. In this book he shares the wisdom, knowledge, and skill he has acquired during his illustrious career. He is to be commended for the logical sequencing of chapters, the detailed discussion of each concept in conformity with our present-day knowledge, and the reader-friendly style. This text will surely serve as an important reference to those who desire to better recognize orthopedic instability, develop and implement a treatment plan that will re-establish orthopedic stability, and help their patients attain and maintain their stomatognathic system in maximum comfort, function, health, and esthetics.

Henry A. Gremillion, DDS
Professor, Department of Orthodontics
Director, Parker E. Mahan Facial Pain Center
University of Florida College of Dentistry
Gainesville, Florida

Preface

There is a primary tenet that embraces the entire subject of occlusion from the TMJs to smile design. It is that the teeth are but one part of the masticatory system, and if the teeth are not in equilibrium with all the other parts of the total system, something is likely to break down. This means that to be a truly competent "teeth doctor" one must be a "masticatory system doctor." No specialty in dentistry can be effectively practiced at the highest level of competence without an understanding of how the teeth relate to the rest of the masticatory system, including the TMJs.

A reader of this text should have the following expectations:

- A clear picture of how the masticatory system functions in maintainable harmony.
- A detailed understanding of how to tell what is wrong when any part of the system is not functioning in complete comfort and long-term stability.
- A specific process for developing a complete treatment plan for every type of occlusal disorder from the simplest to the most complex.
- An understandable proficiency in diagnosis and treatment of orofacial pain, including management of TMDs. Every dentist should know this.
- Elimination of all guesswork in design of the most functional and esthetically pleasing smiles regardless of the initial starting condition.
- Reliable background information regarding how to analyze touted clinical concepts and procedures that violate principles of functional harmony and that can lead to problems of instability, discomfort, dysfunction, or patient dissatisfaction.

Dr. L.D. Pankey wrote that only 2% of dentists ever reach the status of "master." A master dentist can interview, diagnose, plan treatment, and motivate patients to proceed with a comprehensive treatment plan . . . but most important of all *he or she can execute the services needed with a very high level of predictive success.*

The primary motivation for writing this text was to provide a framework by which any dentist could develop into a master dentist. In my role as a restorative dentist, I have had the opportunity to treat thousands of complex occlusal problems and TMJ disorders. As a passionate student of the literature I have had the opportunity to evaluate research efforts for more than 50 years to see if the literature was true to clinical reality. In many cases it has opened new doors to our understanding, whereas in too much of the literature, conclusions have been based on false presumptions. The most prevalent misconceptions in the literature have been in the discipline of occlusion and the relationship of occlusion to the TMJs and orofacial pain. It is my goal to clarify those misconceptions and show

dentists that there need not be a big mystery about the cause or treatment of TMDs. This mindset is absolutely required if one is to be successful in treating problems of occlusion because all occlusal analysis starts at the TMJs. Not a single type of TMD cannot be understood and specifically classified today; it can be done by general practitioners and it must be done by any dentist who aspires to the level of master dentist. In this age of the "esthetic revolution" and the "extreme makeover," failure to relate "smile design" to the rest of the factors that control occlusal stability is an invitation to ultimate disharmony that can in time result in dysfunction and breakdown at the weakest part of the system. Most often that weakest part is the teeth or the TMJs, or both.

Dentists who ignore the TMJs can never be competent in smile design or in diagnosing or treating occlusions. Dentists who ignore occlusion can never be competent in diagnosing or treating problems of the TMJs. Dentists who ignore the relationship of the occlusion to the position and condition of the TMJs can only guess at diagnosing a myriad of problems that are seen in every general practice . . . problems such as excessive tooth wear, sore teeth, fractured restorations, loose teeth, masticatory muscle pain, and a variety of other orofacial pain problems. But understanding what it takes to keep the total masticatory system in harmony has positive consequences beyond achieving the goal of a peaceful neuromusculature. It is the absolute key to determining many of the most important decisions regarding esthetics and tooth alignment, including the *precise* positioning and contour of anterior teeth.

My goal is to take the guesswork out of everything the dental team must do to be successful in clinical practice. If you will study the pages that follow, and commit to the time-tested principles, you will eliminate the number one source of frustration and burnout in dental practice: a lack of predictability. Achieving that *high level of predicable success* that Dr. Pankey wrote about is not pie in the sky. It is the ultimate goal of the master dentist, and it is my fervent passion to help you achieve it.

It is easy to misinterpret clinical results because just relieving symptoms may not mean a problem has been corrected. We have learned through long-term observation that symptoms may sometimes be relieved at the expense of permitting worse problems to progress.

I have tried to expose my own clinical observations to the test of time as well as the invited scrutiny of a wide variety of special expertise. At the Dawson Center for Advanced Dental Study we have developed a multidisciplinary "think tank" to evaluate not only our own concepts but also the concepts of anyone with an opposing viewpoint. For more than 25 years we have been inviting an international array of clinicians, researchers, and specialists of many different persuasions to meet with us for the purpose of evaluating all the pros and cons of their ideas plus our own. In addition, all our treatment results are open for inspection to our entire practicing faculty, and criticism of results is invited. Many notable advancements have resulted from this effort and it has had a profound effect on the development of quality controls that start at the examination and carry through all phases of treatment through dentist-laboratory controls to post-op maintenance. These advancements in principles and clinical protocols are presented in this text.

One of the most notable results from this "think tank" environment is the formulation of specific, measurable *criteria for success* (see Chapter 47). I recommend an early reading of this chapter. It will enable you to start your study of this text with the end in mind.

Acknowledgments

I am grateful that there have been so many great minds in our profession who were willing to share so generously. I was particularly blessed to have come into the profession at a time when great changes were taking place. The journey has been one of constant excitement.

My eyes were opened to the importance of occlusion by Dr. Sigurd Ramfjord early in my practice years and we continued a close relationship until his death. Through Sig, I met and developed a wonderful friendship with Dr. Henry Beyron, from Sweden, considered by many to be the "father of occlusion." He was always a strong supporter of my recommended changes in centric relation and anterior guidance and he was a great encourager as well as a thoughtful critic.

One of the greatest influences in my life was Dr. L.D. Pankey. I was so fortunate in meeting him during my first year in practice and he soon became my role model and one of my closest friends. Through L.D. I was introduced to Drs. Clyde Schuyler, John Anderson, Henry Tanner, Harold Wirth, and many other super stars of that era who invited me to be a part of their excitement in elevating the status of dentistry. Dr. Pankey was a leaders' leader. His contributions to restorative dentistry, occlusion, and practice management were mixed with a philosophy of life that still affects the way I live. I am truly grateful. The L.D. Pankey Institute stands as tangible proof that many others feel the same gratitude that I do.

Dr. Clyde Schuyler gave dentistry the first sound principles of occlusion, and many of the thoughts and concepts in this book started with seeds that were sown by Dr. Clyde. I was privileged to have him as a friend, and his visits to my office that extended into long evenings are treasured memories.

Early in my career, I spent uncountable hours in learning about gnathology, particularly from Dr. Charles Stuart but also with Drs. Peter K. Thomas, Harvey Paine, Earnest Granger, and others. Dr. Niles Guichet and I developed a close personal relationship along with Dr. Frank Celenza that endures to this day. I am grateful to them for all the times we spent gelling our own conclusions about so many facets of occlusion.

On many occasions, arriving at the best treatment plan involves varying degrees of orthodontics. My mentor in my early years was Dr. Clair McCreary and I still use the many concepts I learned from him plus all the additional help received from Dr. Gerry Francatti.

Regarding analysis and treatment of TMJ disorders, all of dentistry should be grateful for the contributions of Dr. Mark Piper. Mark is a brilliant surgeon and the best diagnostician I have known. His innovative approaches to repair complex TMJ deformations is only one facet of his genius. His classification system is the gold standard for TMJ disorders and it is a privilege to present it in this text. Mark's expertise is tremendously enhanced by his thorough understanding and adherence to the principles of occlusion explained in this text. I have enjoyed his friendship and a close working relationship that has been the stimulus for many "think tank" discussions. I have looked through his microscope during his impeccable surgeries and I can testify to the integrity of his reporting of exceptional results.

Dr. Parker Mahan deserves special acknowledgment for all he has contributed to the profession and to my understanding of anatomy, physiology, neurology, and pharmacology in a clinical context. He has been one of my closest friends and a treasured ally. His contributions in diagnosis and treatment of orofacial pain are recognized internationally.

A special measure of appreciation goes to Vernon (Buddy) Shafer, CDT for his constant support and for his contributions to the doctor-technician interface. He has been a dynamo, incorporating solid principles of complete dentistry into the laboratory, and his influence has affected countless dentists as well as technicians.

Lee Culp, CDT has also been a resource of tremendous value to me and to the profession. A master teacher and innovator, Lee is one of the most respected leaders in all of dentistry. I am grateful for all the updated information he provides to me, and I thank him for the special contribution he makes to this text.

I have called on a number of special clinicians to provide the most current clinical updates for this text. Dr. Glenn DuPont, senior partner in my former practice, has been a tremendous resource and contributor. As Director of Faculty at the Dawson Center, he has developed an exceptional "hands-on" curriculum for teaching some of the most important concepts and techniques. He is a meticulous restorative dentist who excels in functional esthetics, so his contributions are much appreciated. Dr. DeWitt Wilkerson has also been a great source of current information and is a contributor to the text. Witt has taught thousands of dentists the fundamentals of occlusion and how to achieve a perfect centric relation. He directs classes at the Dawson Center that always achieve rave critiques. I treasure his friendship and his many contributions to the profession. I am also particularly proud of Dr. John Cranham, who has developed an international reputation as a clinician. I appreciate his continued support of our teaching efforts as well as his loyal friendship. Special thanks also for notable contributions to furthering the goals expressed in the text go to Dr. Jeff Scott, Dr. Michael Sesemann, Dr. Ken Grundset, and Dr. Kim Daxon. Many thanks also to technicians Rick Sonntag, CDT, Nancy Franceschi, CDT, Karl Wundermann, CDT, and Harold Yates for their continuing source of current technologic expertise. Robert Jackson, MDT has also been a steady source of support in many different ways. I would be remiss if I did not acknowledge Dr. Pete Roach for all the past great years of sharing ideas as my partner in practice. They were joyful years.

This text is in large part a compilation of the principles and procedures I have taught to more than 30,000 dentists and technicians at seminars and in classroom sessions at the Dawson Center for Advanced Dental Study. I owe a huge debt of gratitude to the very special staff that makes the curriculum run so efficiently and in such a happy, warm manner. A special thanks to Joan Forrest, the Executive Director, for her outstanding leadership. Deep appreciation also to Sallie Bussey, Mary Lynn Coppins, Jody Booth, Greg Sitek, and to my special assistant, Esther McCrackin. I also have the joy of working with my daughter Anne Dawson, who for 20 years has been a major source of help as my Seminar Coordinator. Dee Mortellaro was also an indispensable help in preparing the manuscript.

And finally, a very appreciative "thank you" to the excellent editorial staff at Elsevier/Mosby publishers. Julie Nebel has been great to work with and I have been grateful for the help from Publisher Penny Rudolph and Senior Editor John Dolan, as well as artist Don O'Connor. Thanks to all of you.

Peter E. Dawson, DDS

Contents

Functional Occlusion:
From TMJ
to Smile Design

PART I

Functional Harmony

Chapter 1

The Concept of Complete Dentistry

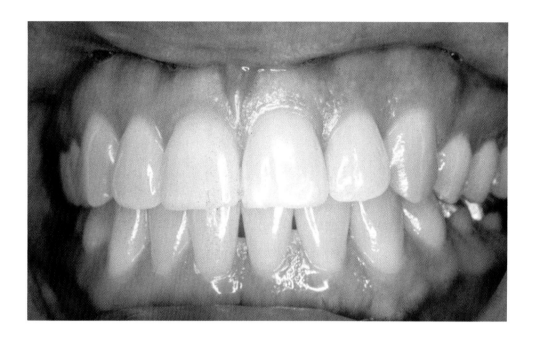

PRINCIPLE

The ultimate goal for every patient should be maintainable health for the total masticatory system.

COMPLETE DENTISTRY

The defining philosophy that underlies an honest concern for patients can be summarized in one word: *complete.*

Embracing the concept of complete dentistry always puts the patient first. It says that every patient is entitled to a complete examination and a clear understanding of every problem that should be treated. It recognizes that almost every dental disorder is, in all probability, a *progressive* disorder that will cause increased problems if not detected and treated in a reasonable time frame.

It is axiomatic that patients cannot perceive a need for treatment if they do not clearly understand what problems are present. That is the primary purpose of the complete examination. But think about this: patients cannot make a truly informed decision about treatment unless they also understand the *implications* of not treating each problem within a reasonable time frame. Practitioners cannot reliably predict implications if they don't have a working knowledge of the total masticatory system, which includes the interrelationships of the teeth, the temporomandibular joints (TMJs), the muscles, and the supporting tissues, in addition to a clear picture of the causes and effects of occlusal disease.

Examining With an "Implication Mindset"

A key question in every complete dental examination is fundamental to the integrity of the doctor-patient relationship: *"Are all the components of the masticatory system maintainably healthy?"* This requires analysis to determine the implications of not treating any parts that are disordered or diseased. Answering these questions is the foundational basis for the complete examination. It is also the guiding principle for formulating what treatment should be started, what could be deferred, and what may not be required to save teeth but might be desired for improved esthetics.

Understanding the short- and long-term implications of each type of dental disorder is the basis for establishing priorities of treatment and is the essential information that is used to establish "phased" treatment for patients who cannot proceed right away with an extensive treatment plan in its entirety.

Types of Implications

Every dentist needs to develop a clear picture of what a stable, maintainably healthy masticatory system looks like . . . not just teeth, but all parts of the system. In a complete examination, each part of the system should be analyzed to see if there are any signs or symptoms that indicate disease, disorder, or dysfunction. If any departure from health is noted in any structure, the key to both diagnosis and treatment recommendations will be directly related to the implications of not treating that disorder in a timely manner. Those implications can be classified into three types:

Immediate implications. These consist of problems that are in an active stage of progressive disease or deformation, or disorders that are a causative factor for pain or discomfort. If disorders in this category are not treated as priority, the implication is that delaying treatment will result in a greater, more complex problem, or an increase of pain, or will require more extensive, more complicated, or more expensive solutions with a possibility that delayed treatment results will not be as good as what could be achieved with immediate attention. Such decisions cannot rely only on what a patient perceives as "wants." It requires searching for signs, of which patients are often not aware, because signs of damage typically occur before symptoms are noticed.

Deferrable implications. These consist of problems that will need to be treated but could be deferred without causing more complex problems, and delaying treatment for a reasonable time period would not result in a less successful treatment outcome. Some problems with immediate implications can be made deferrable by conservative intervention that stops or slows the progression of the disorder so it can be effectively treated at a later time.

Implications for optional treatment. These are indications for treatment that would be nice to have but are not problems that will lead to progressive damage if left untreated. Cosmetic restorations that are done solely for the purpose of improving esthetics fall into this category. Careful observation for signs of stability versus instability is a critical part of the decision process before informing a patient that treatment is not necessary for long-term health. This does not imply that treatment done solely for esthetics is inappropriate, and experience has shown that being honest with patients about what is optional versus what is necessary will rarely deter a patient from accepting esthetic treatment for improving appearance.

GOALS FOR COMPLETE DENTISTRY

A dental examination is complete if it identifies all factors that are capable of causing or contributing to deterioration of oral health or function. It is *in*complete if it does not expose every sign of active deterioration within the masticatory system. A complete examination does not rely solely on symptoms because signs almost always precede symptoms. It is the responsibility of the examiner to observe signs of deterioration before they cause symptoms. In doing so, it is possible to develop treatment plans that are aimed at optimum maintainability of the teeth and their supporting structures. Seven specific goals should be the objective for patient care:

1. Freedom from disease in all masticatory system structures
2. Maintainably healthy periodontium
3. Stable TMJs
4. Stable occlusion

5. Maintainably healthy teeth
6. Comfortable function
7. Optimum esthetics

The establishment of these goals is the foundation for complete dentistry. If a goal is clear enough, it can be visualized and in fact *must* be visualized. A good rule is to avoid starting any treatment until the desired result can be clearly visualized. Until the practitioner has a clear picture of how each type of tissue looks and acts when it is optimally healthy, there will be no frame of reference for knowing whether treatment is needed or if it is successful when rendered. Clearly defined goals give purpose to treatment planning and make it possible to be highly objective. When the goals listed above are fulfilled, the consequence will be fulfillment of a further goal that is essential for long-term stability and comfort. That is the goal of a *peaceful neuromusculature*.

When the entire masticatory system is healthy and there is harmony of form and function, and the relationships are stable, the treatment can be said to be *complete*. Furthermore, esthetic requirements, including the highest level of functional smile design, can also be fulfilled because all of the guidelines for a naturally beautiful smile are dependent on the same harmony of form that is necessary for harmony of function.

In the analysis of any oral diagnosis, each of the above goals should be evaluated for fulfillment. This evaluation will fall short unless the *reasons* for form and function relationships are understood along with the cause-and-effect nature of health versus disease. This type of analysis eliminates dependency on empiric treatment or making patients fit averages. There are many stable healthy dentitions that do not fit the averages, that are not Class I occlusions, and that violate customary guidelines for normalcy. Attempts to "correct" these dentitions often end in failure, and existing harmony of form and function may be disturbed by the treatment. Such mistakes can be prevented, and a high degree of predictability can be developed if the goals of treatment are based on a foundation of "why" rather than "how."

There is an understandable reason for every position, contour, and alignment of every part of the gnathostomatic system. There is always a reason for every incisal edge position, every labial contour, every lingual contour, and every cusp tip position. There is always a reason why some teeth get loose, and others wear away. There is a reason why TMJs hurt, why masticatory muscles become tender, and why teeth get sensitive. There is a reason why certain occlusions remain stable and others do not. Treating the effect without treating the cause is rarely a satisfactory outcome, and is almost never necessary.

Every diagnostic or treatment decision should be made on the basis of understanding the reasons for the problem, and the reasons for the treatment. All treatment should be consistent with the goal of providing *and maintaining* the highest degree of oral health possible for each patient. Total elimination of all causative factors to the point of complete reversal of deterioration is not always possible. The problems of some patients are too severe, or have gone on too long to expect a complete return to ideal health. But the degree to which we can eliminate the *causes* of deterioration will directly relate to our degree of success in changing unhealthy mouths to healthy ones.

Causes of Deterioration

Dental disease rarely results from a single entity. It is almost always the result of a combination of factors. The same causative insult can produce a variety of responses because of differences in host resistance. The response can also be altered by variations in intensity or duration of the insult, sometimes to such an extent that a completely different set of symptoms may result from increased intensity of the same causative factor.

Because similar symptoms may result from different causes, and a variety of symptoms may result from the same causative factor, treating *symptoms* alone is generally short-sighted therapy. It is always advantageous to determine the cause of both signs and symptoms. If the causative insult can be completely eliminated (such as occlusal overload on a painful, loose tooth with a "high" restoration), the normal adaptive response of the body should activate a return to comfort and reduced hypermobility when the overload on the tooth is eliminated. Of course it may still be necessary to repair damaged tissues, but this can then be done with a greater chance of a long-term successful treatment outcome.

Much of the confusion about cause-and-effect relationships results from failure to differentiate between *causative* factors and *contributing* factors. A contributing factor does not by itself cause disease. Rather it lowers the resistance of the host to the causative factor, or increases the intensity of function or tension. Contributing factors may lower host resistance biochemically or increase intensity biomechanically. The resistance may be lowered in a specific tissue or in an entire system. Generally the weakest link breaks down. The greatest susceptibility to disease occurs when a causative factor is present in a host with increased stress and lowered resistance. Both causative and contributing factors must be considered when deciding on a path of treatment, but the most effective approach is to give the highest priority to *direct* causative factors. Attempts at increasing host resistance and decreasing stress levels should be kept in proper perspective as adjunctive therapy.

Let's use a simple illustration to show how a single direct causative factor can produce a variety of signs and symptoms, depending on variations in how different patients respond:

In a healthy patient with a perfect dentition, note the variety of responses that can occur if a single high restoration with deflective incline interference is placed on a second molar. There are many different ways that patients might respond to the same, specific causative factor (Figure 1-1):

1. The tooth may become sensitive to hot or cold, or it may ache
2. The tooth may become tender to biting on it
3. The tooth may become loose

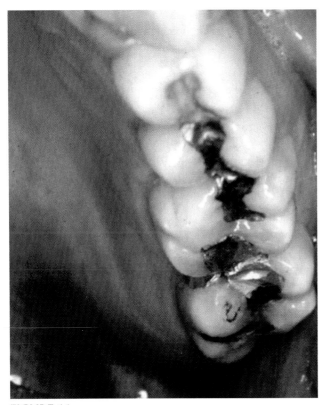

FIGURE 1-1   A deflective incline interference on a second molar can be the primary causative factor that results in many different signs and symptoms in the masticatory system.

4. The tooth may wear excessively
5. The mandible may be deflected around the interference into other teeth that become loosened
6. Other teeth can be abraded as the mandible is deflected forward
7. Other teeth can become sore as they are traumatized at the end of the slide
8. Forced deviation of the mandible can cause masticatory muscles to become painfully hyperactive, or even become spastic
9. Trismus may result from the spastic musculature
10. Muscle tension headaches may develop
11. The combination of sore teeth, sore muscles, and headaches may cause stress and tension
12. Constant tension and stress may lead to depression
13. The combination of the uncoordinated musculature and the deflected mandible may contribute to a condyle/disk derangement
14. Eventual displacement of the disk by uncoordinated masticatory muscle hyperactivity may initiate painful compression of retrodiskal tissues
15. Degenerative arthritic changes in the TMJ may follow disk displacement and subsequent perforation of the retrodiskal tissues
16. All of the above
17. None of the above

All of the signs and symptoms listed above can be a direct result of the same *causative* factor, the occlusal inter-

ference on the second molar. None of the *contributing* factors that altered the response actually *caused* the problem. If the causative insult (the deflective occlusal contact) had been corrected before irreversible damage occurred, all symptoms would have disappeared without any changes being made in host resistance or emotional stress levels.

Host resistance is not the only variable. Variations in intensity of function can dramatically alter the response. The same type of occlusal interference may go completely unnoticed by a very relaxed patient who has no tendency to clench or brux. The mouth breather or the person who sleeps with the mouth open will have fewer, if any, of the above symptoms because no stress or tooth damage results in the absence of tooth contact. The same person under duress may begin to clench or brux, activating the muscles into occlusal overload and an avoidance pattern that produces symptoms in the teeth, muscles, and possibly the joints.

Despite the complexity of the multicausality concept, it is still possible to simplify our approach to diagnosis and treatment planning if we understand how the masticatory system was designed to function. In the chapters that follow, you will learn how all parts of the system are interrelated in a functional design that is so logical, it will be apparent when there is destructive disequilibrium. By knowing how the system works, it will be obvious what is wrong when it isn't working properly, causing stressful forces to build up within the system. It is not possible to completely eliminate stress, but treatment planning should always be directed at reducing stress to a level that is not destructive. Ensuring that the total system is in equilibrium is a goal of complete dentistry.

It is a very popular concept to blame *emotional* stress for many of the disorders that are, in fact, caused by structural disequilibrium. None of the patient responses listed above would have occurred if the deflective incline on the "high" tooth were not present, regardless of the patient's emotional state. This is not to say that emotional stress cannot result in pain or discomfort. What is important is that it is possible and practical to isolate structural causes for pain or dysfunction and correct those causative factors. If treatment is limited to covering up symptoms with medications, the structural disharmony is allowed to continue its progressive deformation of teeth, joints, or supporting tissues. Experience has also shown that when pain or dysfunction is eliminated, emotional stress is relieved in many patients. It appears that psychosocial stress is often a result of, rather than a cause of, orofacial pain.

Patients lose their teeth in two ways: either the teeth break down, or the supporting structures break down. As simplistic as it may sound, if we exclude neoplastic disorders and specific pathological conditions, almost every deteriorating effect on the teeth or supporting structures is a direct result of one or both of two causative factors:

1. Stress from microtrauma or physical injury (macrotrauma)
2. Microorganisms including gingival diseases of specific bacterial, viral, or fungal origin

Stress from microtrauma results from repeated occlusal overload. Diagnosis and treatment of occlusal disharmony will be discussed in detail throughout the remaining chapters. As factors of occlusal overload are better understood and the destructive evidence of occlusal disease is better recognized, there is sometimes a tendency to downplay other equally important causes of deterioration. The role of microorganisms must always be given a high priority in every dental examination and treatment protocol.

The Role of Microorganisms

There is no doubt that the elimination of bacterial plaque and the thorough cleaning of gingival sulci are essential for maintenance of oral health. Acidic microbial waste products not only cause caries through decalcification of the tooth surface, but they are inflammatory to soft tissues and destructive to the bony support. Dentistry cannot be called "complete" if it fails to address the elimination of this important causative factor.

> Any condition that prevents thorough cleaning of any tooth surface or any portion of the sulcus should be considered a causative factor that can lead to loss of teeth.

There is no such thing as a "healthy" mouth that has long-standing deposits of bacterial plaque. As long as organized masses of microorganisms are present, progressive breakdown of the supporting tissues is almost inevitable. The only variable is the *rate* of deterioration, which may vary from patient to patient or even from tooth to tooth in the same mouth. The tissue response to the noxious products of the microbial colonies depends both on the general resistance of the host and the resistance of the specific areas that are being subjected to the microbial toxins.

Even in a dentition that is uniformly coated with plaque, the destructive effects may not be uniform. Periodontal destruction around some teeth may be severe, whereas other teeth may retain all or most of their bony support. Since the intensity of the microbial attack is about the same around all teeth, there must be a tooth by tooth difference in resistance to the microbial toxins. The difference in resistance from one tooth to the next is often directly related to differences in intensity of occlusal stress. It is a common clinical finding that the degree of bone breakdown is in direct proportion to the intensity and direction of occlusal overload on each tooth.

Although there does appear to be a clinical relationship between occlusal stress and the amount of microbial damage, occlusal stress is not a necessary factor in periodontal damage. Severe periodontal disease can occur in an environment of occlusal perfection. It is important to understand that even the best occlusal treatment cannot prevent deterioration of supporting structures if inflammation is present. Occlusal therapy without control of plaque is incomplete dentistry. On the other hand, soft-tissue management, even with exceptional control of plaque, falls short of the long-term maintainability that can be achieved when excessive occlusal forces are reduced.

Short-term improvements can be misleading. The dramatic results that can be achieved by *either* occlusal therapy or plaque elimination can be impressive, but years of careful observation almost always present a different picture of progressive breakdown if either treatment approach is ignored when a combination of periodontal and occlusal factors is present.

A concentrated mouth hygiene program may transform bleeding, edematous gingiva into healthy-appearing tissue. In addition, occlusal correction may greatly improve the comfort of the teeth, and even eliminate hypermobility. But such noticeable improvement can be misleading if, underneath the healthy-looking tissue, an untreated intrabony lesion remains. No matter how healthy the gingiva appears, deterioration of the alveolar bone and periodontal structures will continue if the entire sulcus is not cleanable. The healthy appearance on the outside merely produces a false sense of security while deterioration continues at the depth of the lesion.

No matter how thorough the plaque control, even if combined with perfected occlusal therapy, it is incomplete dentistry if there remain deep lesions that are capable of continued deterioration.

Occlusal Trauma and Pocket Formation

Despite the extreme mobility patterns that can be caused by occlusal disharmony, it is doubtful that occlusal trauma can cause an increase in pocket depth unless inflammation is present within the sulcus. If the gingival attachment is intact, and there is a sufficient level of supporting bone remaining, even severely mobile teeth can usually be returned to normal firmness and health by correcting the occlusion. With meticulous hygiene to keep the sulcus free of plaque, inflammation can be prevented. Lindhe and Nyman[1] have shown rather conclusively that occlusal trauma of the jiggling type, even with greatly reduced periodontal support, will not cause further destruction of the attachment apparatus once the plaque-induced periodontitis has been eliminated. However, the combination of plaque-induced periodontitis and occlusal trauma causes a more progressive loss of connective tissue attachment than in nontraumatized teeth.[2]

Recent clinical observations and scientific data have given added credibility to the relationship of occlusal overloads to periodontal damage.[3] Comparative studies to determine if there is an association between occlusal trauma and periodontitis[4] show that there appears to be a definite link. Teeth with a combination of functional mobility and widened periodontal ligament space were found to have deeper probing depth, more clinical attachment loss, and less radiographic bone support than nonmobile teeth. While this relationship between occlusally induced tooth hypermobility and increased levels of periodontitis has been a common clinical finding for years, the actual mechanism for the bone loss was not fully understood. Recent investigations have provided an explanation.

Interleukin-1 beta is a potent stimulator of bone resorption and a known key mediator involved in periodontal disease. It has now been determined that interleukin-1 beta is produced by human periodontal ligament cells *in response to mechanical stress.*[5] It has also been shown that older periodontal ligament cells produce an increased amount of interleukin-1 beta in response to mechanical force, and may well be positively related to the acceleration of alveolar bone resorption.[6]

Some authorities have argued that occlusal factors play *no* role in periodontal breakdown because inflammation is the essential causative factor for increased pocket depth. This opinion presents a limited viewpoint of what causes periodontal disease. A total picture of periodontal health, and the goal of complete dentistry, involves *all* of the structures that support the teeth, not just the gingival attachment. The way in which bone is destroyed can be learned from careful clinical observation. The reason why teeth in hyperfunction loosen is because the bone around the roots breaks down. The bone breakdown follows a specific pattern in which bone resorption directly relates to the direction of compressive forces by the root against the bone. The pressure stimulation results in thrombosis, hemorrhage, and destruction of collagen in concert with the activation of interleukins that have been shown to convert fibroblasts into osteoclasts. The osteoclastic activity, in turn, destroys bone in direct proportion to the intensity and direction of the pressures exerted. This means then, that intra-alveolar bone breakdown follows a pattern that is definitely related to occlusal stress patterns.[7] Careful clinical observation repeatedly confirms this relationship, which can occur even when the gingival attachment apparatus is intact.

If the occlusion is corrected to negate directional overloads on the teeth before inflammation or injury deepens the sulcus to create a communication through the gingival attachment into the area of bone resorption, osteoblastic activity will repair the osteoclastic destruction and bone will fill back in to its original level. The loose tooth will tighten and can return to normal health and function.

If the occlusal correction is delayed, our clinical experience has shown that in time, the sulcus depth very often deepens to eventually communicate with the bone loss area to form a deeper intrabony lesion. Understand that the increase in pocket depth requires inflammation or injury to penetrate the gingival attachment, so it theoretically can be prevented on selective patients who are willing to follow meticulous hygiene procedures under increased professional supervision. Although possible, successful maintenance on an overloaded, hypermobile tooth is unpredictable at best.

Bone resorption often is worst in furcation areas that are hardest to clean and where communication with the sulcus or pocket is most likely to occur. Once there is any breakthrough between the sulcus and the area of bone breakdown, the pocket is immediately deepened to the extent of the total intra-alveolar defect. More intensive periodontal treatment is then required, but even with that, the bone level will not be returned to its original contour. That opportunity is lost whenever occlusal correction is delayed too long.

The repair of intraosseous defects is more predictable when the teeth are firm. From almost every viewpoint of treatment, it is more difficult to keep the supporting tissues healthy around a loose tooth than it is around a firm one. Occlusal stress must be considered as a primary cause of supporting structure breakdown around the teeth. Correction of misdirected or excessive forces against the teeth is one of the essential considerations in maintaining optimum health of a dentition, and it also has the added benefit of making the patient more comfortable.

Anatomic Harmony

The most common shortcoming in analyzing or treating occlusal relationships is failure to consider *all* parts of the masticatory system. We are prone to many mistakes if our understanding of occlusion is limited solely to occlusal contacts. The teeth are just *part* of the total system, and frankly there is no way to evaluate occlusal relationships until we have ascertained that the temporomandibular articulation is in harmony. There is no such thing as a perfect occlusion with a displaced TMJ. That means both the position and the condition of the TMJs must be considered in relation to the maximum intercuspation of the teeth. The peaceful function of the masticatory musculature depends on a harmonious relationship between the occlusion and the TMJs, so this relationship is always of critical concern in diagnosis and treatment planning. There will always be some price to pay when any part of the masticatory system is at war with muscle. That includes the lips, tongue, and cheek musculature.

Harmony of form is a prerequisite for harmony of function, and it is necessary to have a working knowledge of how the two interrelate. Every aspect of each tooth's position and contour can be determined on the basis of its harmony with functional requirements. As examples, the upper anterior teeth must relate to the closing path of the lower lip as it moves up to seal contact with the upper lip during every swallow. The upper incisal edges must relate to a consistent alignment with the lower lip contour for proper phonetics. The upper lingual contours must relate to the functional pathways of the lower anterior teeth as they move along a repetitious pattern referred to as the *envelope of function*. Both upper and lower anterior teeth are subject to positioning within a zone of neutrality between the outward forces of the tongue versus the inward forces of the lips. There are other functional relationships that must be understood to achieve consistently predictable results in occlusal treatment, but the important point to grasp at this time is that every part of the masticatory system has an understandable reason for its position, contour, and alignment. Learning these reasons will take the guesswork out of everything from smile design to treatment of orofacial pain. Not knowing these interrelationships reduces too many diagnosis and treatment decisions to guesswork.

If any anatomic component is not in harmony with the rest of the masticatory system, some part or all of the system must adapt to regain equilibrium. Adaptive changes should be evaluated as responses to imbalance. Such adaptation is not always a problem. Whether the system's attempts at correcting imbalance are beneficial or destructive is dependent on the response of the altered tissue or part. Astute diagnosticians must know the norm and must be able to determine when an imbalance exists and whether the tissue or parts have successfully adapted to the altered balance.

There are many so-called "physiologic malocclusions" that are stable and function well. They do so because the cumulative effects of different dynamic factors produce a stable result, even though it does not fit the Class I stereotype of a classically correct occlusion. When we get into the section on treatment planning of different types of occlusal problems, it will be apparent how important it is to understand the dynamics of functional and anatomic harmony. It is not possible to adequately evaluate cause and effect influences in the dentition or the TMJs without knowledge of functional interdependencies, because if we don't know what *causes* a malrelationship we will probably fail in our treatment. We may subject our patients to unnecessary overtreatment or inadequate undertreatment if we attempt to treat signs or symptoms without knowing what caused them.

Teeth do not simply move out of alignment, become loose, or wear away without a specific underlying cause (or causes). The primary cause may be at the beginning of a chain reaction that is started by a structural disharmony. Regardless of how and when the process was initiated, treatment will not be successful unless all currently active causes for disharmony or deformation are corrected.

The goal of functional harmony is a peaceful neuromuscular system. The masticatory system is capable of high-capacity demands. The system must be free to function to its anatomic limit without mechanical interference, but must not be restricted to function solely at that limit. It must function to the limit when required. It must be at peace when functional demands are reduced. Achieving such functional harmony in an environment of optimally healthy teeth, joints, periodontium, and musculature, and in combination with the best possible esthetic result, is the essence of complete dentistry.

References

1. Lindhe J, Nyman S: The role of periodontal disease and the biologic rationale for splinting in treatment of periodontitis. *Oral Sci Rev* 10:11-13, 1972.
2. McGuire MR, Nunn ME: Prognosis versus actual outcome III. The effectiveness of clinical parameters in accurately predicting tooth survival. *J Periodontal* 67:666-674, 1996.
3. Nunn ME, Harrel SK: The effect of occlusal discrepancies on periodontitis. I. Relationship of initial occlusal discrepancies to initial clinical parameters. *J Periodontal* 72:485-494, 2001.
4. Harrell SK, Nunn ME: The effect of occlusal discrepancies on periodontitis II. Relationship of occlusal treatment to the progression of periodontal disease. *J Periodontal* 72:495-505, 2001.
5. Hallmon WW: Occlusal trauma: effect and impact on periodontium. *Ann Periodontal* 4(1):102-108, 1999.
6. Shemizu N, Gaseki T, Yamaguchi M, et al: In vitro cellular aging stimulates interleukin. 1 beta production in stretched human periodontal ligament derived cells. *J Dent Res* 76(7):1367-1375, 1997.
7. Pikhstrom BL, Anderson KA, Aeppli D, et al: Association between signs of trauma from occlusion and periodontitis. *J Periodontal* 57 (1):1-6, 1986.
8. Waerhaug J. The infrabony pocket and its relationship to trauma from occlusion and subgingival plaque. *J Periodontal* 50:355-365, 1979.

Chapter 2

Perspectives on Occlusion and "Everyday Dentistry"

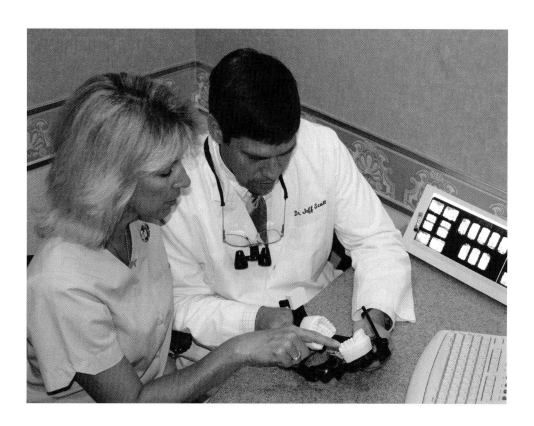

PRINCIPLE

Whether general practitioner or specialist, practicing without a comprehensive understanding of occlusal principles exacts a costly penalty in missed diagnoses, unpredictable treatment results, and lost production time.

OCCLUSAL PRINCIPLES AT EVERY LEVEL OF PRACTICE

At every level of general practice, a dentist routinely faces problems of sore teeth, excessive wear, loose teeth, temporomandibular joint (TMJ) disorders, and orofacial pain. Patients want correct answers. They want to know if they need orthodontic treatment, or an occlusal splint, or why a joint clicks, or why anterior veneers chip or crack. A dentist who does not have a working knowledge of occlusal principles must resort to guesswork and time-wasting trial-and-error attempts to solve problems that could be confidently solved by understanding cause-and-effect responses to occlusal disharmony. Even achieving predictable function and beauty of smile design is dependent on incorporation of sound occlusal principles. Those principles are not just for complete mouth prosthetics. When principles of occlusal harmony are understood, the entire approach to examination, treatment, and problem solving takes on a new perspective. It is a perspective that pays huge dividends of predictability and increased productivity, regardless of the type of practice.

There are good reasons why general practitioners should learn principles of occlusal harmony, and develop skills required to recognize and treat typical problems associated with occlusal disharmony. Descriptions of some of the benefits follow.

Patient Comfort

Many problems of discomfort are related to occlusal disharmony.[1-3] Teeth that are sensitive to hot or cold after a restoration is placed are frequently symptomatic because of a deflective incline interference or a vertical overload from a new restoration. Indiscriminate grinding to relieve the interfering tooth can trigger new and bigger problems in other teeth and/or the masticatory musculature, and even the TMJs. Not understanding occlusal principles is a barrier to solving such everyday problems, and it puts a practitioner in jeopardy of actually causing problems that are sometimes worse than the original complaint.

Restoration Longevity

Cracks, fractures, and excessive wear on restorations are all signs of occlusal disharmony. Such problems are rare in perfected occlusions.

Occlusal Stability

Post-treatment shifting of teeth, opening up of contacts, or creating unesthetic misalignment are common problems of occlusal mistakes. The use of long-term retainers to maintain post-orthodontic tooth alignment could be dramatically reduced if occlusal principles were better understood. Fremitus is almost always an early sign of a correctable occlusal disharmony.

More Accurate Treatment Planning

Most of the problems that lead to compromised treatment results could be avoided if requirements for occlusal stability were adhered to in the treatment planning stage. *Programmed treatment planning* (see Chapter 29) is based on selection of the best treatment options for fulfilling each requirement. Successful treatment planning pays huge dividends regardless of the type or level of practice.

Improved Esthetics

The very best, most naturally beautiful esthetics does not require guesswork if the relationship between anatomic harmony and functional harmony is understood. The best smile design is automatically achieved when the anterior teeth are in harmony with all of the guidelines for occlusal function and stability. Furthermore, these guidelines provide a precise framework for a step-by-step process.

Increased Productivity

Just imagine how much more productive a practitioner can be if all restorations could be placed without need for "grinding in" high or uncomfortable occlusions, or remaking restorations that are not correctable. How much time could be put to better use than trying to reshape anterior restorations that are too thick on the lingual. How much wasted time could be saved if incisal edges weren't too far out, too long, too short? These are the typical everyday problems that must be faced if principles of occlusal harmony are not understood and used to plan and execute treatment.

It is unrealistic to expect that *every* restoration could be placed without any need for some occlusal correction. But it should be unnecessary to do more than minimal corrections if the rules for occlusal harmony are faithfully practiced.

Decreased Stress

From interviews with more than 200 dentists, it appears that a major cause of burnout is a *lack of predictability* when attempting to satisfy the needs and desires of patients. This lack of predictability is especially noted in restorative and prosthodontic treatment and in attempts to solve issues of discomfort. When time is being wasted attempting to solve a bite problem by trial and error, the next patient is kept waiting, and an already full schedule gets further jammed up because of "working in" patients to redo or rework dentistry that isn't quite comfortable. The result is increased stress on the entire office team. Some of these problems are caused by inadequate quality- control procedures, including dentist-technician communication shortcomings. But the major cause of unacceptable treatment results is failure to visualize a clear correct goal for the treatment. This is usually accompanied by inadequate treatment planning. The problem is that unless the requirements for occlusal harmony are understood, there can't be a clear vision for a desired end result . . . and without a clearly defined goal, trying to arrive at a logical treatment sequence is folly. It is a problem that can only be solved by a clear understanding of requirements for a stable, comfortable, maintainably healthy masticatory system.

RELEVANCE OF OCCLUSION TO "EVERYDAY DENTISTRY"

Even though an understanding of occlusal principles has value to every level of dental practice, there is a pervasive misconception that concepts of dental occlusion are not relevant to "everyday dentistry." It is important to understand how such a viewpoint was ever germinated, and why it has influenced so many dentists and educators to regard principles of occlusal harmony with skepticism.

To a large extent, a negative viewpoint regarding the importance of occlusion has been by misguided assumptions that disorders of the TMJs and muscles represent the only focus for occlusion in dentistry.[4] A negative view of the occlusion-TMJ relationship has permeated the teaching of occlusion and has resulted in a profuse amount of literature that downplays the role of occlusal therapy[5-8] in general practice. A conceptual belief that occlusion is unimportant or is too difficult to teach at the dental school level has influenced a whole cadre of dentists who are ill equipped to properly diagnose or treat a broad spectrum of occlusal problems that are routinely faced in every dental practice.[9] The failure to embrace sound occlusal principles has also led to a plethora of fringe-type treatment modalities, unnecessary overtreatment, and denials of responsibility for problems that are a direct result of occlusal mismanagement.

The disparagement of occlusion as an important part of daily practice has become so pervasive that the National Institutes of Health (NIH) and the National Institute of Dental and Craniofacial Research (NIDCR) published a pamphlet[10] to advise the public that occlusal adjustment or any other irreversible occlusal treatment for temporomandibular disorders (TMDs) is "of little value and may make the problem worse." Further admonitions that "recent research disputes the view that a bad bite (malocclusion) can trigger TMD" provokes distrust of all forms of occlusal therapy. A profuse amount of seriously flawed literature supports this viewpoint and denounces all alterations of occlusions as an unacceptable choice of treatment.

Limiting judgment of occlusal principles on such a narrow focus as its effect on "TMD" distorts the true value of occlusal harmony as a realistic treatment goal for many different problems, in addition to its indisputable value in treating *certain types* of TMDs,[11] including masticatory muscle pain, by far the most common type of TMD.

The NIH admonishment that occlusal treatment "is of little value and may make a TMD problem worse" may be true if it refers to *inappropriate* occlusal changes that are representative of the lowest common denominator of treatment. But such a negative view of occlusal treatment is a misrepresentation of what knowledgeable clinicians consider appropriate treatment for specifically diagnosed disorders.

Trying to arrive at sensible answers about the importance of occlusion in daily practice requires some insight into evaluation of the literature. With the growing dependence on "evidence-based" reporting, the rules for judging research studies and even clinically based opinions have made it easier to evaluate differing dogmas.[12] Evidence-based research on occlusion may not provide final answers to every question, but it points out when there are serious enough flaws in any research study to invalidate its conclusions. Since so much of the negative literature proposes a nonrelationship of occlusion to "TMD," an analysis of that literature is in order.

When the NIH position states that "research refutes the view that a bad bite (malocclusion) can trigger TMD," the statement fails the test for a scientifically accurate conclusion. A truly scientific study must ask, *"What kind of TMD?"* TMD is not a single disorder. It is not even a single multifactorial disorder.

TMD is an all-inclusive term that includes many different types of disorders, any of which may be multifactorial. A cardinal rule for evidence-based research requires *homogeneity* of the disorder being studied. This means that for a proper study of the relationship between occlusion and TMD, the specific type of TMD must be isolated and defined. An evaluation of the literature illustrates that this is rarely done.[13-15] This error creates a glaring source of misinformation because there are many different disorders of the masticatory system that are typically included in the TMD category. These different disorders have many different etiologies, require different treatment strategies, and can result in different treatment outcomes. A proper choice of treatment demands specific classification of the type and stage of the disorder to be treated before treatment is selected. Any reported clinical studies that use the term *TMD* without specifically classifying the exact type of TMD being studied are too seriously flawed to be considered valid. This error is found almost universally throughout the literature on both sides of the occlusion-TMD debate.

Scientific analysis also demands a much-improved explanation that more clearly defines "a bad bite" and requires characterization of "malocclusion" in more descriptive terms.[16,17] The use of *Angle's Classification of Malocclusion*[18] to describe arch-to-arch relationships or to define "malocclusion" is perhaps the most consistent and serious flaw in the literature that disparages the idea of a relationship between occlusion and TMD. The cause of confusion is self-evident because Angle's classification does not relate maximum occlusal contact to either the position or condition of the TMJs. Use of a classification system that ignores any relationship between occlusion and the TMJs can hardly be considered an analytical model for studying the relationship between occlusion and the TMJs. A search of the literature confirms that this serious flaw has been consistent in a profuse amount of reported studies that are cited to discredit the value of occlusal harmony as a treatment objective.

Ruling out all rationales for occlusal changes in patients with TMD is an indefensible position in light of extensive clinical experience with conservative occlusal treatment that is close to 100 percent predictable when performed by properly skilled clinicians on properly selected patients. There is extensive clinical evidence to support the relationship between deflective occlusal interferences and masticatory muscle symptoms. There is also a proven scientific rationale for establishing occlusal harmony with the TMJs. The rationales for treatment are practical, learnable, and appropriate for general practitioners as well as specialists. Attempting to restore an occlusion, correct a bite problem, or even to reshape a high restoration without knowing the precisely correct maxillo-mandibular relationship, can be a time-wasting, frustrating, and unnecessary experience.

Diagnosis of Orofacial Pain in General Practice

The dentist of today must become a physician of the total masticatory system. A frequent focus of head, neck, and orofacial pain is within structures that comprise the masticatory system. Analysis of such pain requires a working knowledge of masticatory system structure and function, including the intraoral and collateral effects of dysfunction. The variety and vagaries of pain from dental origins are complex enough, but interrelationships between the TMJs, the teeth, and the masticatory musculature require special expertise to evaluate the diversity of signs and symptoms that can result from structural disorder within the system.

Dentists are the only health professionals who are trained (or should be) to diagnose problems of the teeth or to understand *masticatory system function* as a baseline for relating orofacial symptoms to variations of dysfunction. This means that the general dentist practitioner is regularly put into the position of "gatekeeper," responsible for determining if a dental or masticatory system disorder is or is not a factor in head, neck, or orofacial pain. Physicians and other health professionals who do not have the training to determine if a dental or masticatory system disorder is or is not a factor in head, neck, or orofacial pain must be able to rely on this expertise. Dentists must accept this responsibility and must develop the competence to fulfill it.

Pain from dental origins can combine with sources of pain from outside the masticatory system to produce confusing patterns of symptoms, so unraveling specific sources of overlapping or referred pain sometimes requires expertise from different specialists. For such a multidisciplinary effort to succeed, each specialist must separate out potentials for pain in the specific structures that fall within his or her specialty. This puts a serious responsibility on the dentist to be a reliable resource, capable of determining whether all of the pain, some of the pain, or none of the pain has its source within masticatory system structures. This is why it is so important for dentists to be able to *rule out* masticatory system structures as sources of pain, and to develop sufficient expertise to select appropriate medical specialists for evaluation of signs or symptoms that are not within dentistry's field of expertise.

It is a serious mistake for any dentist to minimize the importance of understanding the interrelationships of the teeth with the rest of the masticatory system structures. It is impossible to understand occlusion without understanding the relationship of the teeth to the TMJs, the musculature, and the functional patterns of jaw movement. It is equally impossible to have a realistic understanding of orofacial pain or TMD without a total masticatory system perspective. Failure to understand these perspectives is the primary reason why treatment of so many TMD pain patients is limited to medications for controlling *symptoms* while ignoring *signs* of progressive structural damage. Dentistry can do better than that.

Accepting the role of the dentist as a "masticatory system physician" puts the practitioner on a higher level of observation. Looking for signs of structural deformation while the cause of the problem is still correctable will enlighten any dentist to needs that too often go undiagnosed. The destructive factor, that in the opinion of many clinicians, causes more damage, more lost teeth, more discomfort, and more need for extensive dentistry than any other causative factor is *occlusal disease*.[19] Every practitioner should be able to recognize it, treat it, and when detected early enough, prevent it from destroying a dentition. Any dentist who does not feel competent to render adequate treatment should, at the very least, be able to recognize occlusal disease in its various forms. Patients should be informed of the problem and should be referred when a need for treatment is evident.

Occlusal disease can be detected in many forms. The next chapter describes its signs and symptoms.

References

1. Barber DK: Occlusal interferences and temporomandibular dysfunction. *General Dentistry* Jan Feb; 56, 2004.
2. Ramfjord SP: Dysfunctional temporomandibular joint and muscle pain. *J Prosthet Dent* 11:353-374, 2004.
3. Kirveskari P, LeBell Y, Salonen M, et al: Effect of elimination of occlusal interferences on signs and symptoms of craniomandibular disorder in young adults. *J Oral Rehabil* 16:21-26, 1989.
4. Ash MM, Ramfjord SP: *Occlusion,* ed 4, Philadelphia, 1995, WB Saunders.
5. Trolka P, Morris RW, Preiskel HW: Occlusal adjustment therapy for craniomandibular disorders; a clinical assessment by a double blind method. *J Prosthet Dent* 68:957-964, 1992.
6. McNamara JA, Seligman DA, Okeson JP: Occlusion, orthodontic treatment, and temporomandibular disorders; A review. *J Orofacial Pain* 9:73-90, 1995.
7. National Institutes of Health Technology Assessment Conference Statement: Management of temporomandibular disorders. *J Am Dent Assoc* 127:1595-1603, 1996.
8. Mohl ND, Ohrbach R: The dilemma of scientific knowledge versus clinical management of temporomandibular disorders. *J Prosthet Dent* 67:113-120, 1992.
9. Ash MM, Ramfjord SP: *Occlusion,* ed 4, Philadelphia, 1995, WB Saunders.
10. NIH #94-3497: *TMD Temporomandibular Disorders,* 1996.
11. Dawson PE: Position paper regarding diagnosis, management and treatment of temporomandibular disorders. *J Prosthet Dent* 81:174-178, 1999.

12. Sackett DL, Straus SE, Richarson WS, et al: *Evidence-based medicine: How to practice and teach EGM,* ed 2, New York, 2000, Churchill Livingstone.
13. Greene CS: Orthodontics and temporomandibular disorders. *Dent Clin North Am* 32:529-538, 1988.
14. Dworkin SF, Huggins KH, LaResche L, et al: Epidemiology of signs and symptoms in temporomandibular disorders: clinical signs in cases and controls. *J Am Dent Assoc* 120:273-281, 1999.
15. Goodman P, Greene CD, Laskin DM: Response of patients with pain-dysfunction syndrome to mock equilibration. *J Am Dent Assoc* 92:755-758, 1976.
16. Dawson PE: New definition for relating occlusion to varying conditions of the temporomandibular joint. *J Prosthet Dent* 74:619-627, 1995.
17. Dawson PE: A classification system for occlusions that relates maximal intercuspation to the position and condition of the temporomandibular joints. *J Prosthet Dent* 75:60-66, 1996.
18. Angle EH: *Classification of malocclusion of the teeth,* ed 7, Philadelphia, 1907, SS White Dental Mfg Co, pp 35-59.
19. Lytle JD: The clinician's index of occlusal disease; definition, recognition, and management. *Int J Periodont Rest Dent* 10:102-123, 1990.

Occlusal Disease

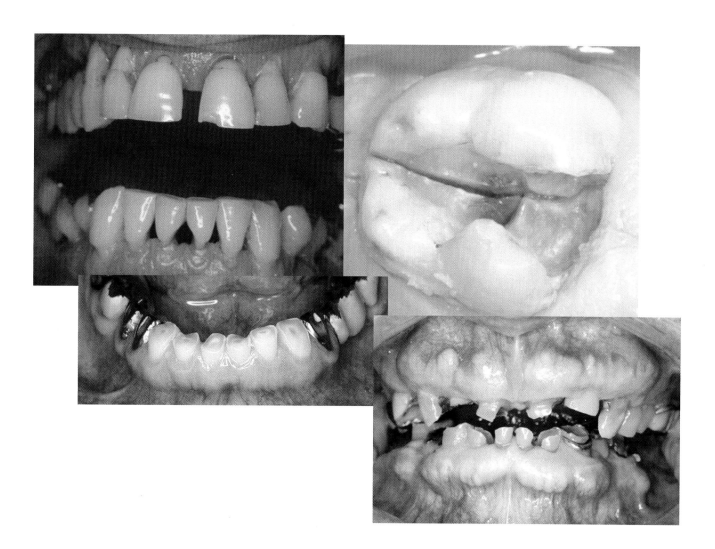

dis•ease *n*, the failure of the adaptive mechanisms of an organism to counteract adequately the stimuli or stresses to which it is subjected, resulting in a disturbance in function or structure of any part, organ or system of the body

—Gould Medical Dictionary

SIGNS AND SYMPTOMS

It is a puzzling observation that the most prevalent evidence of damage to teeth is so routinely ignored, both in clinical practice and in the dental curricula. It is still more bewildering if one recognizes that *signs* of occlusal disease are so easily observed even at the earliest stages when progression of the damage can usually be intercepted. *Symptoms* of occlusal disease may not be as obvious, but to an astute diagnostician, both signs and symptoms are readily recognized and typically respond to treatment at a high level of predictability. If therapy is not delayed until the damage is severe, the complexity and cost of treatment can be dramatically reduced.

Attention to occlusion would be elevated to a much higher priority if the following observations were more universally noticed and analyzed.

Occlusal disease is:

- The #1 most common destructive dental disorder.
- The #1 contributing factor to eventual loss of teeth.
- The #1 reason for needing extensive restorative dentistry.
- The #1 factor associated with discomfort within masticatory system structures. This includes pain/discomfort in the musculature, the teeth, and the region of the temporomandibular joints (TMJs).
- The #1 factor in instability of orthodontic treatment.
- The #1 reason for tooth soreness and hypersensitivity.
- The #1 most commonly missed diagnosis leading to unnecessary endodontics.
- The #1 most undiagnosed dental disorder until severe damage becomes too obvious to ignore.

The above observations have not, at this date, been confirmed by formal evidence-based protocols, but they are consistent with many years of careful observation of thousands of patients. Attention to periodontal disease and control of caries have become more consistent in most dental practices, but a complete evaluation of occlusal disease is incomplete in too many examinations.

Lytle[1] was the first to introduce the term *occlusal disease*. At that time, he defined it as "the process resulting in the noticeable loss or destruction of the occluding surfaces of the teeth." He postulated that the disease is primarily but not necessarily precipitated by bruxism or parafunction.

Abrahamsen[2] added greatly to our understanding of occlusal disease by defining different causes for destruction of tooth structure, and he showed specific pathognomonic characteristics for each different etiology. He did not diminish the role of bruxism or parafunction. He did show how combined mechanisms of chemical effects could interact with occlusal overloads to intensify destruction of tooth surfaces.

BASIC MECHANISMS FOR TOOTH SURFACE DEFORMATION

According to Grippo et al, it is now apparent that deformation of tooth structure results from three basic physical and chemical mechanisms that can act alone or in combination[3]:

1. *Stress* results in compression, flexure, and tension. It can produce microfracture and abfraction as a dental manifestation.
2. *Friction* includes *abrasion* from exogenous material and *attrition*, which is endogenous and results from empty mouth bruxing and parafunction. The end point of both is wear of tooth surfaces.
3. *Corrosion* is the result of chemical or electrochemical degradation.

These three basic mechanisms often overlap and interact to accelerate structural damage to the teeth. Thus much of the structural deformation of teeth must be considered as multifactorial. It does appear, however, that occlusal overload is almost always the dominant factor that must be addressed in treatment planning for severely damaged tooth structure.

Clarification of Terminology

Grippo, Simring, and Schreiners' classic work[3] should be studied in detail. It is a scholarly analysis of the many different causes of tooth surface lesions, and it includes their clarification of terminology. At this time however, there are conflicting concepts that should also be analyzed in every detail. The extensive effort by Abrahamsen[2] to clear up confusion regarding tooth surface lesions is based on an unmatched number of clinical case studies and results in some differences in terminology as well as causes and effects. In presenting my current viewpoint, I make no pretext of certainty. This debate will go on for a long time and will require critical analysis, research, and an open mind. Nevertheless, none of the disagreements regarding terminology or etiology diminishes the importance of recognizing and treating tooth surface damage.

Attrition

Attrition is wear due to tooth-to-tooth friction. This is the kind of wear that results from bruxism and empty mouth parafunction. The implication is that enamel is the hardest structure in the body. When wear penetrates enamel into softer dentin, wear increases seven times faster.

Abrasion

Abrasion is wear due to friction between a tooth and an exogenous agent. This is the kind of wear that comes from chewing on a food bolus or from tobacco chewing. It can also come from overzealous toothbrushing or improper use of dental floss, toothpicks, pencils, or any foreign object.

Erosion

Erosion is tooth surface loss due to chemical or electrochemical action. It can be endogenous or exogenous. By definition, it does not include association with bacterial activity.

Grippo and Simring have decried the use of this term. They suggest that erosion refers to loss of material from the action of fluids against a structure, as in beach erosion from water, and that no such mechanism exists in the mouth.[4] So, it is inappropriate terminology, and the term *erosion* should be discarded from the dental literature. Abrahamsen[2] and others disagree, and properly point out that Webster defines erosion as a "wearing away as acid erodes metal." *Gould Medical Dictionary* defines it as "superficial destruction of a surface area by inflammation or trauma." Gould also describes dental erosion as "loss of tooth surface due to a chemical process." Dental erosion is distinguished as a separate cause that excludes bacterial action.

Endogenous erosion. This can result from bulimia and is recognizable by a unique pattern of enamel loss on the palatal surfaces of the upper anterior teeth from forceful projection of vomitus.

Gastroesophageal reflux disease (GERD). This condition produces hydrochloric acid and the proteolytic enzyme pepsin from gastric juices. Erosion may occur wherever the acid reflux juice is permitted to pool. Erosion on the lingual of molars is diagnostic. Referral to a gastroenterologist is in order when signs of GERD are observed.

Gingival crevicular fluid. This has an acidic pH and can be erosive in combination with non-carious cervical lesions.[5]

Exogenous erosion. Any food or liquid with a pH of less than 5.5 can demineralize teeth. The tremendous increase in sale and consumption of soft drinks is taking its toll on patients who bathe their teeth in citric acid solutions on a daily basis. The "Coke swishers" and "fruit mullers" described by Abrahamsen[2] are classic examples of exogenous exposure to acidic products. Other examples are chewable vitamin C tablets, aspirin, and other acidic drugs.

Abfractions

The role of occlusal overload on non-carious cervical lesions has not been as incontrovertible as many have assumed. What Grippo[6] labeled as *abfractions* were first described by Lee and Eakle[7] as the *possible* consequence of tensile stresses through bending of teeth under occlusal overload. McCoy[8] added to the controversy by defining *McCoy's notches* as the result of what he labeled "dental compression syndrome." When Grippo put the abfraction label on his concept of stress-induced non-carious cervical lesions, it was almost universally accepted as a common form of occlusal disease. Numerous investigators have claimed that occlusal loading forces do in fact cause flexure of teeth that produce microfractures and structural loss in the cervical area. Further studies[9-12] indicated that acid penetrates the microcracks and undermines tooth surfaces that are then more susceptible to mechanical deformation.

I must admit that I was one clinician who accepted the validity of abfractions as a result of occlusal overload. I have had to rethink that position in light of some convincing data to the contrary. Abrahamsen[13] has demonstrated several inconsistencies to the occlusal overload theory. Since I consider Abrahamsen to be the foremost authority on occlusal wear, and recognize that he is a prosthodontist with an in-depth understanding of occlusion, I feel his analysis is worthy of my consideration. It is also consistent with the current research done by Dzakovich,[14] which leaves little doubt that the so-called abfraction lesions are not the result of occlusal overload, but rather are caused by toothbrushing with toothpaste.

The heretofore accepted characteristic of abfractions as wedge-shaped lesions with sharp line angles is actually characteristic of toothpaste abrasion, according to Dzakovich. His research using standardized brushing machine action on extracted teeth also showed that brushing without toothpaste does not cause any wear problem. The addition of toothpaste results in deep lesions with sharp line angles. The type of toothpaste has little effect on the resulting wear patterns. At this writing, it appears that almost all toothpastes are abrasive, and that the pattern and intensity of the brushing strokes account for the varied contours of the lesions.[14]

It is interesting that Miller described the same abrasive effects of toothpastes and powders in an extensive three-part series in 1907.[15] Miller's insights into the wasting of tooth tissue from various causes is as up-to-date today as it was in 1907. In repeating Miller's toothbrushing research, Dzakovich has verified that the original conclusions were correct. What we have been calling *abfraction* lesions are really the result of toothpaste abuse.

If there is an occlusal overload component to the cause of abfractions, it needs to be confirmed with convincing scientific data. It does appear that occlusal forces can definitely bend and torque teeth. If that is a co-factor in creating non-carious gingival lesions, more evidence is needed at this writing. Until this is confirmed, it is a certainty that deep, angular cervical lesions can be caused by toothpaste abrasion.

Admittedly, it is hard to give up a concept that appears so logical and is so solidly accepted into so much of the dental literature, including the *Glossary of Prosthodontic Terms*. There are many reasons to suspect that abfractions are the result of occlusal overload. While the current research seems to argue against that concept, the best advice is to keep an open mind while examining all the data. At this writing, one clinical observation that seems evident is that teeth with deep non-carious cervical lesions are more likely to produce signs and symptoms when subjected to occlusal overload.[14]

Confining occlusal disease to destruction of occluding tooth surfaces falls short of the true extent of occlusal overload. My partner in practice, Dr. R. R. (Pete) Roach, demonstrated on numerous occasions a view through a clinical microscope that showed carious lesions forming precisely in vertical cracks in the center of proximal surfaces. Such cracks were invariably on posterior teeth with wear facets on inner inclines of cusps in occlusal interference to lateral jaw movements, or were deflective inclines in interference to centric relation. The consistency of these findings and the rarity of proximal caries on non-stressed teeth in the same mouth suggest the possibility that occlusal overload can be a co-factor in the etiology of proximal caries on posterior teeth.

The stimuli and stresses from occlusal overload and misdirected forces are not limited to teeth. As noted in the definition of *disease,* a disturbance in function and structure extends into other structures in the masticatory system.

To appreciate the full scope of occlusal disease, it is necessary to understand how interdependent all parts of the masticatory system are. Any disharmony between the teeth, the muscles, and the TMJs is sufficient to cause stress, deformation, or dysfunction on any or all of the other parts in the system. With that understanding in mind, a redefinition of occlusal disease is in order:

> Occlusal *disease* is deformation or disturbance of function of any structures within the masticatory system that are in disequilibrium with a harmonious interrelationship between the TMJs, the masticatory musculature, and the occluding surfaces of the teeth.

EXAMPLES OF OCCLUSAL DISEASE

Attritional wear

This type of wear on the lower anterior teeth is one of the most common untreated problems. It is also a typical sign of two prevalent causes for such wear. The first place to look is at the posterior teeth where deflective incline interferences to centric relation are so often the cause of a forward slide of the mandible during closure to maximum intercuspation. This forces the lower anterior teeth forward into a collision with the upper anterior teeth. The muscles respond by attempting to erase the colliding tooth surfaces through bruxing or parafunctional rubbing (**A**). Destruction of lower incisal edges should never be allowed to progress to such a severe degree because the implications point to more complex treatment requirements if not corrected early.

The second most common cause for this type of wear is direct interference of the anterior teeth to complete closure in centric relation (**B**). This will virtually always be the result of improper restorations on the anterior teeth or improper positioning of the anterior teeth. Interference to the mandibular envelope of function is also a potent trigger for attritional wear. Correct diagnosis and treatment selection for this or any other example of attritional wear requires a complete understanding of occlusal principles.

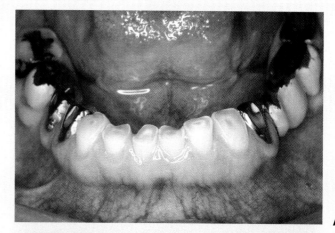

A

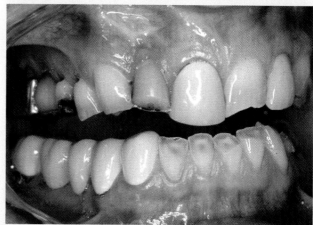

B

Erosion of enamel

A combination of acid from fruit, abrasion from mulling fruit between end-to-end anterior contacts, and attrition from bruxing produces invagination of incisal enamel. Evidence of erosion is obvious because cupped-out dentin areas cannot be contacted by opposing teeth.

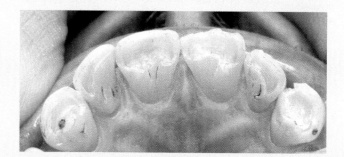

Splayed teeth

The same type of mandibular deflection that causes wear problems can, in a different patient, force the upper anterior teeth forward. Splaying of teeth is a common sign of occlusal disease that should be diagnosed and treated early by eliminating the deflective interferences that force the mandible forward.

Other signs of the same problem are fremitus and soreness of the anterior teeth in the early stages. Improperly contoured restorations that are too thick on the lingual of the upper anterior teeth or overcontoured lower restorations are common causes of splaying.

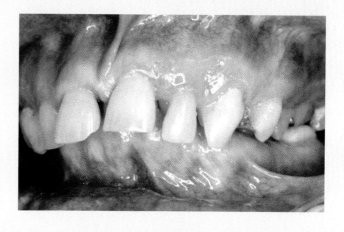

Destroyed Dentition

This is the result of not intercepting occlusal disease early. Signs of severe wear, fractured maxillary (**A**) and mandibular (**B**) teeth, and elongated alveolar processes are typical when treatment of delta-stage bruxism is delayed. This is one of the most demanding occlusal problems to treat even if diagnosed early. When such patients are "watched" until the problem becomes this severe, all aspects of treatment are made more complex and results are compromised.

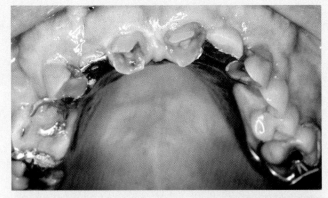

A

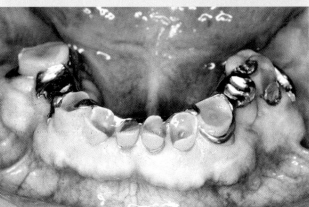

B

Advanced occlusal disease

This disease results from a combination of attritional wear and moved teeth. This is occlusal disease left undiagnosed and untreated until the late stage of progressive damage has occurred. In my practice, I treated hundreds of patients with severely advanced occlusal disease, and it was the rare patient who had ever been warned about the implications of allowing the damage to progress without treatment.

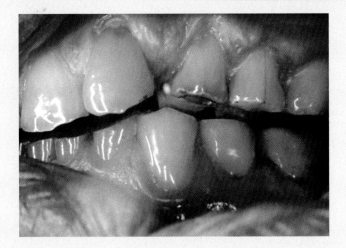

Anterior guidance attrition

This occurs when anterior teeth that either interfere with centric relation closure or interfere with functional jaw movement patterns (envelope of function) develop early signs of attritional wear of the lingual enamel on upper anterior teeth (**A**). This type of occlusal disease too often goes undiagnosed until the incisal edges become so thin they start to chip and fracture (**B**). Patients are rarely aware of the problem until major damage has been done.

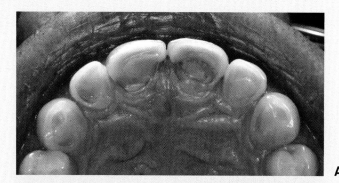

A

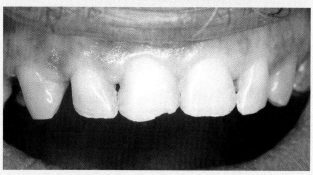

B

Sensitive teeth

One of the most missed diagnoses is failure to recognize that a common cause of hypersensitivity is occlusal overload. A tooth subjected to occlusal pounding or wiggling can become extremely sensitive even though the pulp is vital. The sensitivity can result from pulpal hyperemia or from the effects of non-carious cervical cracks. Coleman et al.[16] showed that sensitivity to a measured puff of air at cervical lesions was completely eliminated when occlusal equilibration corrected the occlusal overload. This is consistent with our experience.

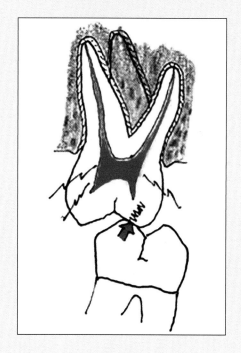

Sore teeth

Compression of periodontal ligaments can be combined with pulpal hyperemia to cause considerable soreness or pain on biting. If empty mouth clenching causes any discomfort in a tooth, it is an indication that the sore tooth is in occlusal interference. It does not rule out other possible causes for pain, but it is a definite indication that occlusal interference is a factor.

Note: The simple clench test to determine if occlusion is a cause of hypersensitivity or soreness in a tooth will eliminate a misdiagnosed need for endodontic treatment in a surprisingly large number of teeth that do not have radiographic evidence of pathology.

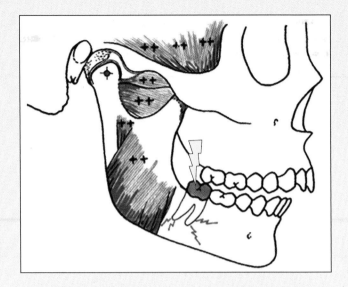

Hypermobility

An early sign of occlusal disease is tooth hypermobility. It can result in widened periodontal space and greater susceptibility to periodontal disease. Patients are rarely aware of mobility in teeth until later stages of bone loss, so every examination should include checking every tooth for signs of mobility. All loose teeth should be evaluated to see if a deflective contact or occlusal overload is a factor.

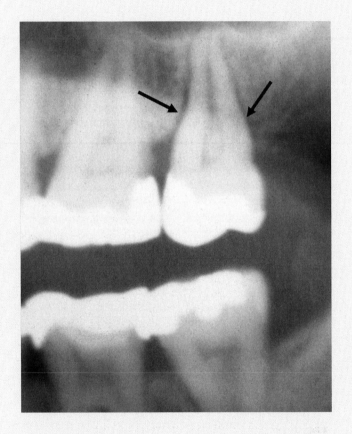

Split teeth and fractured cusps

A, Note the fracture lines that routinely develop when a cusp incline interferes with strong occlusal forces *(arrows)*. This is a typical sign of occlusal disease that precedes cusp fracture or split tooth **(B).**

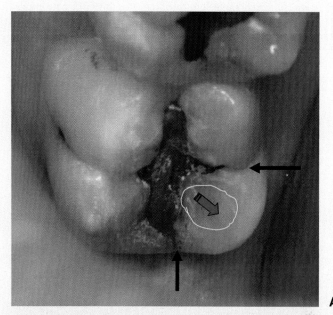

A

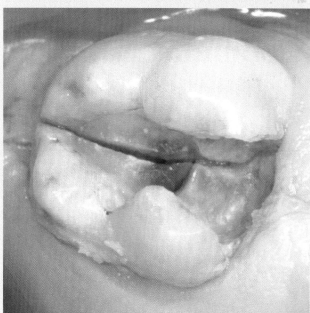

B

Painful musculature

A common symptom of occlusal disease results from disharmony between the occlusion and the TMJs. Deflective occlusal interferences that require the jaw joints to displace to achieve maximum intercuspation are a potent cause for painful masticatory musculature. The term for this is *occluso-muscle disorder.* Posterior teeth that are in interference also are subject to occlusal overload that can cause excessive wear, hypermobility, fractured cusps, and hypersensitivity. Observing and resolving this condition early can often prevent major problems of occlusal disease from developing.

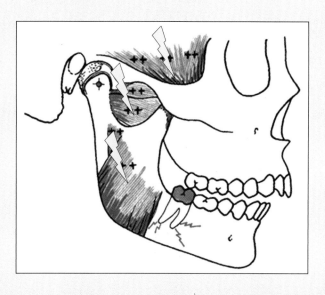

Other types of occlusal disease will be defined and discussed in the chapters that follow. It is important to understand that diagnosis and treatment of all forms of occlusal disharmony are dependent on the clinician's knowledge of total masticatory system design and function.

An all-too-common mistake is to overplay the role of psychosocial stress as the primary factor in bruxism and parafunction. Even if emotional factors are a dominant influence, teeth must be in interference to jaw movements to create attritional wear or tooth bending. Regardless of the emotional state of the patient or the intensity of bruxism, occlusal harmony must be established as a treatment goal. The chapters that follow are dedicated to explaining how this is accomplished.

References

1. Lytle JD: Clinician's index of occlusal disease: definition, recognition, and management. *Int J Periodontics Restorative Dent* 10(2):102-123, 1990.
2. Abrahamsen TC: Occlusal attrition—pathognomonic patterns of abrasion and erosion. Presented at the American Academy of Restorative Dentistry, Chicago, February 1992.
3. Grippo JO, Simring M, Schreiner S: Attrition, abrasion, corrosion and abfraction revisited: a new perspective on tooth surface lesions. *J Am Dent Assoc* 135(8):1109-1118, 2004.
4. Grippo JO, Simring M: Dental "erosion" revisited. *J Am Dent Assoc* 126(5):619-630, 1995.
5. Bodecker CF: Local acidity: a cause of dental erosion-abrasion. *Ann Dent* 4(1):50-55, 1945.
6. Grippo JO: Abfractions: a new classification of hard tissue lesions of teeth. *J Esthet Dent* 3(1):14-19, 1991.
7. Lee WC, Eakle WS: Possible role of tensile stress in the etiology of cervical erosive lesions of teeth. *J Prosthet Dent* 52(3):374-380, 1984.
8. McCoy G: On the longevity of teeth. *J Oral Implantology* 11(2):248-267, 1983.
9. Grippo JO, Masi JV: The role of biodental engineering factors (BEF) in the etiology of root caries. *J Esthet Dent* 39(2):71-76, 1991.
10. Khan F, Young WG, Shahabi S, et al: Dental cervical lesions associated with occlusal erosion and attrition. *Aust Dent J* 44(3):176-186, 1999.
11. Whitehead SA, Wilson NF, Watts DC: Development of noncarious cervical notch lesions in vitro. *J Esthet Dent* 11(6):332-337, 1999.
12. Palamara D, Palamara J, Tyas MJ, et al: Effect of stress on acid dissolution of enamel. *Dent Mater* 17(2):109-115, 2001.
13. Abrahamsen TC: The worn dentition—pathognomonic patterns of abrasion and erosion. *Int Dent J* (4):268-276, 2005.
14. Dzakovich JJ: In vitro reproduction of the non-carious cervical lesion. *Am Acad Rest Dent* February 2006 (in press).
15. Miller WD: Experiments and observations on the wasting of tooth tissue variously designated as erosion, abrasion, chemical abrasion, denudation, etc. *Dental Cosmos* Jan, Feb, March (3 parts), XLIX:1-23, 1907.
16. Coleman TA, Grippo JO, Kinderknecht KE: Cervical dentin hypersensitivity. Part III: resolution following occlusal equilibration. *Quintessence Int* 34(6):427-434, 2003.

The Determinants of Occlusion

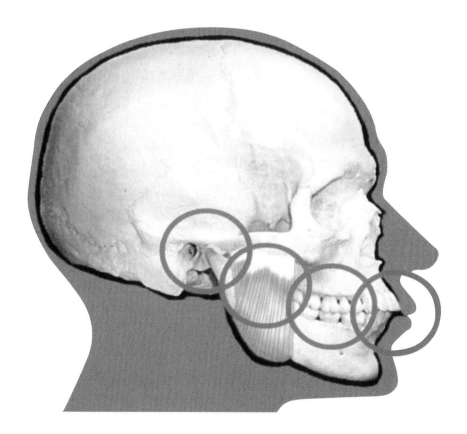

There are 10 factors that determine if an occlusion will function comfortably and remain stable. Recognizing that a goal of all occlusal therapy is a peaceful neuromusculature, the key to achieving it is to have the teeth in a relationship that is in harmony with all of those factors. Establishing equilibrium between the teeth and the neuromusculature is critical because whenever there is disequilibrium, the muscles will always attempt to regain it. When there is a war between the muscles and the teeth, the teeth lose. The evidence of this is excessive wear, fracture, tooth hypermobility, or movement of teeth that are in the way of jaw movements controlled by the musculature.

The best way to understand the relationship between the teeth and the rest of the masticatory system structures is to start by understanding some of the fundamental aspects of how the total masticatory system was designed.

DESIGN OF THE MASTICATORY SYSTEM

Every part of the masticatory system was designed for a specific purpose. Using a process of synthesis, we can dismantle the system and then reassemble it part by part to show why it was designed as it was. Only when we know how the system works will we know what is wrong when it isn't working properly.

Understanding the design also expands one's diagnostic intuition and ability to see the interrelationship of all parts of the masticatory system as a functional unit (Figure 4-1). Then, the relationship to other functional units such as the cervical complex can be evaluated more realistically.

Following the *synthesis* concept, what is the thought process that went into the design of the masticatory system, remembering that its purpose is for masticating and swallowing food? If you were designing it, where would you start?

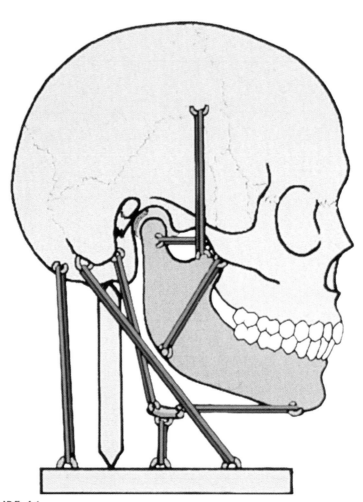

FIGURE 4-1 The design of the masticatory system requires balanced equilibrium of all its parts.

You would start with a socket in a fixed base. The design of this socket is critical and will be discussed later.

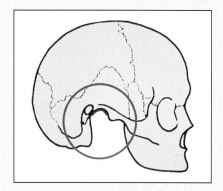

Then, you'd add a lever arm with a fulcrum so the mandible could hinge open and closed.

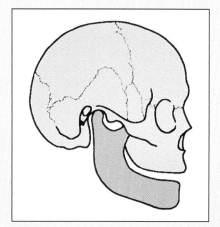

But now you have a design problem to overcome because the spinal column had to be moved forward so we can walk upright. If we stay on a fixed hinge when we open, we'd compress our airway and our alimentary canal.

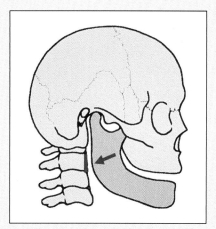

So you would have to make the fulcrum movable so it can slide forward while hingeing. This requires a complex disk to serve as a movable socket.

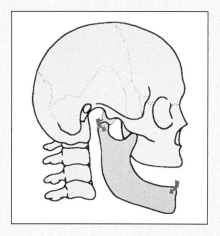

Next, you would have to limit movement of the jaw. You'd use ligaments to do this. You'd also attach the disk with ligaments so it couldn't displace.

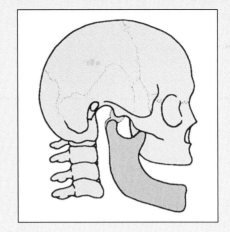

Now you could complete all the structures within the capsule that surrounds and encloses the temporomandibular joint (TMJ).

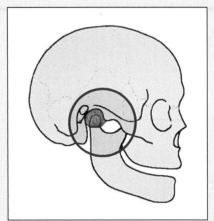

Now you have the mechanical parts in place, but you have no way to make the jaw function until you add the muscles.

Now please note a very important fact: The last thing that fits into the design is the teeth so . . .

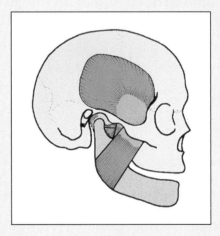

Now . . . align the teeth.

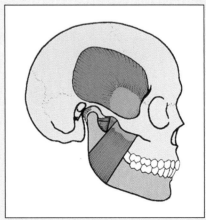

Do not miss this extremely important key understanding regarding the relationship of the teeth to the rest of the masticatory structures. Remember that the teeth did not come in until the jaw-to-jaw relationship was established. The teeth have to fit into that pre-established maxillo-mandibular relationship.

PRINCIPLE

Determination of the correct physiologic jaw relationship must always be determined *before* we can determine the correct alignment and occlusal relationship of the teeth.

The teeth must fit into the harmony of the jaw relationship—not vice versa. That is why we will go into detail on how to establish a correct jaw relationship before we attempt to analyze, diagnose, or prescribe any occlusal relationship.

That is also why we mount casts in centric relation on an articulator . . . (Figure 4-2)

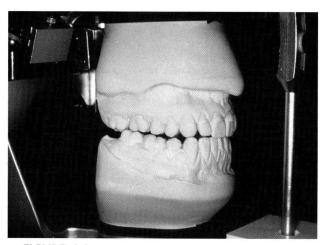

FIGURE 4-2 Cast mounted in centric relation on an articulator.

. . . so we can see the correct mandible-to-maxilla relationship regardless of how the dental arches align.

With this three-dimensional view, we can then determine the best treatment options for reshaping, repositioning, or restoring the teeth to put them in harmony with the correct jaw-to-jaw relationship. Remember that the correct jaw-to-jaw relationship is established by first determining the correct relationship of the TMJs, so let's concentrate on understanding what you must know about the TMJs and why the position and condition of the TMJs is the first concern in analysis of any occlusion. To put this into an understandable perspective, we'll relate the TMJs to the three primary requirements for successful occlusal therapy. All of the other factors are dependent on these three requirements.

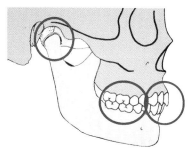

FIGURE 4-3 Each requirement for successful occlusal therapy *(circles)* is dependent upon the others.

PRIMARY REQUIREMENTS FOR SUCCESSFUL OCCLUSAL THERAPY (FIGURE 4-3)

1. *Comfortable and stable TMJs* . . . all occlusal analysis starts with the TMJs. The jaw joints must be able to function and accept loading forces with no discomfort. This is always the starting point for any dental treatment that involves the occlusal surfaces of the teeth.
2. *Anterior teeth in harmony with the envelope of function* . . . and in proper relationship with the lips, the tongue, and the occlusal plane.
3. *Non-interfering posterior teeth* . . . posterior occlusal contacts should not interfere with either the comfortable TMJs in the back or the anterior guidance in the front.

The complexities of occlusion can be simplified if each of the above requirements is understood along with its interrelationship to the other requirements. We will discuss each requirement separately. The ten extremely important factors of occlusion are all interrelated. When each of these factors is understood, confusion about occlusion will be eliminated. Remember that the goal is a peaceful neuromusculature because anything that causes muscle to become imbalanced in function creates a source of disruptive forces, so let's look first at the dynamics of equilibrium.

THE DYNAMICS OF EQUILIBRIUM

The reason we put so much emphasis on harmony between the TMJs, the anterior guidance, and the posterior teeth (*circles* in Figure 4-4, *A*) is because even the slightest disharmony can cause severe hyperactivity and incoordination of masticatory muscle function. So it is the fourth circle (muscle) shown in Figure 4-4, *B* that is affected positively or negatively by how the structures in the other three circles work together.

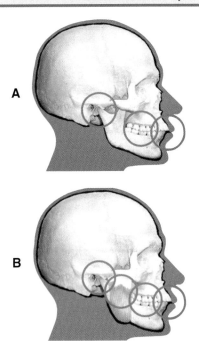

FIGURE 4-4 **A,** Three primary requirements for successful occlusal therapy. **B,** Masticatory muscle function is affected by the other structures.

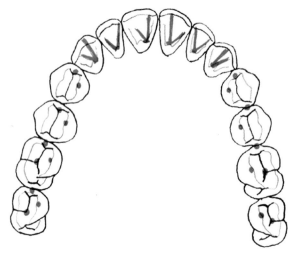

FIGURE 4-5 Formula for a perfected occlusion: dots in back, lines in front.

FORMULA FOR A PERFECTED OCCLUSION

We're going to jump ahead of a lot of necessary explanations about how occlusion relates to the masticatory musculature in order to first create a visualization of a perfected occlusion. Once Figure 4-5 is in your mind, the explanations that follow will have more meaning.

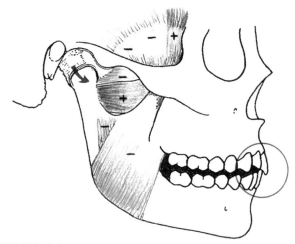

FIGURE 4-6 Posterior separation and resulting reduction of forces on TMJs *(arrow)* and anterior teeth *(circle)*.

The first step is to have simultaneous equal intensity contacts on all teeth when the condyle-disk assemblies are completely seated up in their respective sockets. The contact on the posterior teeth is on cusp tips (represented by dots.) The lines on the anterior teeth represent continuous contact from centric relation to incisal edges as the mandible moves forward and laterally.

The formula "dots in back, lines in front" is what the pattern of marks looks like if firm closing contact is followed by grinding the teeth together with marking ribbon placed between the arches of a perfected occlusion.

This formula represents contact in centric relation, and disclusion of all posterior teeth the moment the mandible moves from centric relation. The anterior teeth (the anterior guidance) assume the responsibility, along with the condylar path, of separating the back teeth during all excursions. The reason for this posterior separation is because at the moment of posterior separation almost all of the elevator muscles shut off . . . thereby dramatically reducing the forces on both the TMJs and the anterior teeth (Figure 4-6).

In addition to the effect of creating a peaceful neuromusculature, note also that it is impossible to overload or wear the posterior teeth during excursive movements, even if the patient bruxes. This holds true as long as the anterior guidance remains stable and the TMJs stay healthy. This is the goal of a perfected occlusion.

It also explains why it is so important to understand how both the TMJs and the anterior guidance function and what keeps these two determinants in a healthy state.

With this preliminary overview in mind, a more in-depth understanding of the TMJs is in order.

Chapter 5

The Temporomandibular Joint

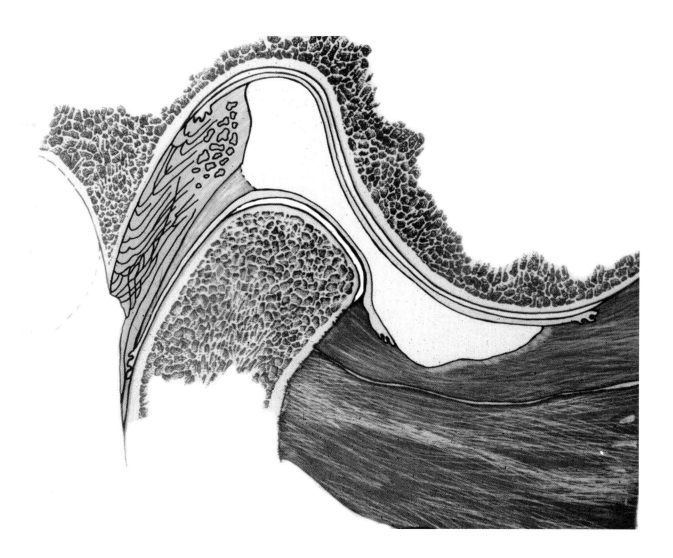

PRINCIPLE

All occlusal analysis starts at the temporomandibular joints (TMJs).

THE FIRST REQUIREMENT

It is impossible to comprehend the fine points of occlusion without an in depth awareness of the anatomy, physiology, and biomechanics of the temporomandibular joint (TMJ). The first requirement for successful occlusal treatment is stable, comfortable TMJs. The jaw joints must be able to accept maximum loading by the elevator muscles with no sign of discomfort.

> One of the most important rules to follow in dental practice is that if the TMJs cannot accept firm compressive loading with complete comfort, always find out why before proceeding with any irreversible occlusal treatment.

It is only through an understanding of how the normal, healthy TMJ functions that we can make sense out of what is wrong when it isn't functioning comfortably. This understanding of the TMJs is foundational to diagnosis and treatment of almost everything a dentist does (Figure 5-1).

Some of the most obvious aspects of the TMJ are often missed, even though they are extremely important. In fact, some of the most popular techniques for treating temporomandibular disorders (TMDs) are based on misconceptions of how the joint functions, and many of the procedures that are advocated for restorative or orthodontic treatment are either unnecessary or detrimental to long-term stability. To relate each aspect of form to function, it is helpful to separate the various components of the joint into understandable segments, starting with the passive structures of articulation and then progressing to an understanding of how the active elements make the system function.

THE ARTICULATING SURFACES

If we examine a dry skull, it is apparent that the articulating surfaces of the condyle and its reciprocal socket merely *allow* movement to occur. The condyle is often described as a universal joint, but that description does not apply because each condyle imposes limitations of movement on the other. One condyle cannot move in any manner without reciprocal movement on the opposite side. In opening-closing movements, the two condyles form a common axis and so, in effect, act as one hinge joint. Despite the fact that the condyles

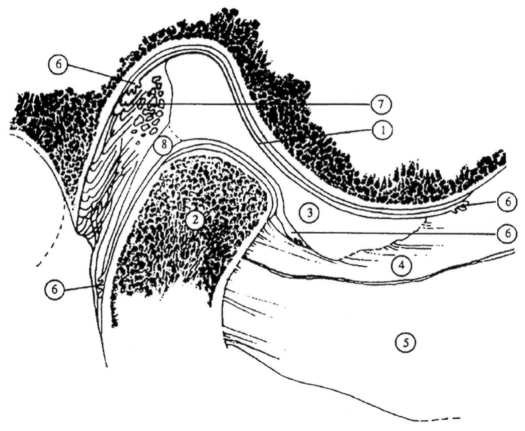

FIGURE 5-1 Lateral view of cross-section through the TMJ. *1*, Posterior slope of the eminentia (notice typical convex contour); *2*, condyle; *3*, disk (notice biconcave shape to fit both convex condyle and convex eminentia); *4*, superior lateral pterygoid muscle; *5*, inferior lateral pterygoid muscle; *6*, synovial tissue; *7*, retrodiskal tissue including posterior attachment of disk to temporal bone; *8*, posterior ligamentous attachment of disk to the condyle. *Note:* Every dentist should be able to draw this view from memory. A clear visualization of the anatomy of the TMJs is essential for analysis of problematical joints. Correct reading of the radiographs and other imaging is dependent on this ability.

are rarely symmetric, the axial rotation occurs around a true hinge that is on a fixed axis when the condyles are fully seated. Rotation around a *fixed* horizontal axis seems improbable because of the angulation of the condyles in relation to the horizontal axis. Each condyle is normally at about a 90-degree angulation with the plane of the mandibular ramus, which places their alignment at an obtuse angle to each other. To understand how the condyles with different alignments can rotate around a fixed common axis, we must look to the contour of the *medial poles* and their relation to the articular fossae. Because of the different angles and the asymmetry of the condyles, the medial pole is the only logical

common rotation point that would permit a true rotation to occur on a fixed axis. (Figures 5-2 and 5-3)

For the medial pole to serve as a point of rotation, the articular fossa must be contoured to receive it. Its triangular shape (Figure 5-4) serves this mechanical function very well, and in addition the medial part of the fossa is reinforced with thick bone so it can also serve as a stop for the upward force of the elevator muscles and the inward force of the medial pterygoid muscles (Figure 5-5).

Other than the strongly braced medial portion,[1] the roof of the fossa is always quite thin. Hold a skull up to the light and you will see that the bone in the roof of the fossa is quite

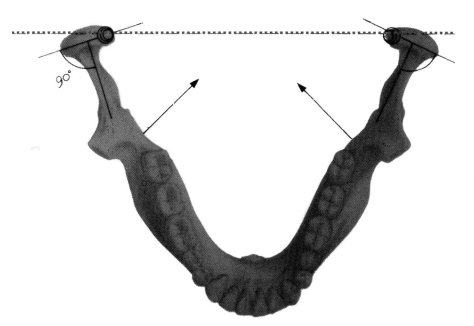

FIGURE 5-2 The medial poles of the condyles are the only rotation points that would permit a fixed axis of rotation because the condyles are not parallel to the horizontal axis. This means that the lateral poles of the condyles must translate, even if the medial poles are rotating around a fixed axis (as occurs in centric relation).

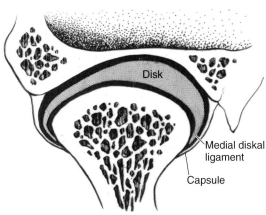

FIGURE 5-3 The condyle-disk assemblies are braced at the midmost, uppermost position by compression of the medial third of the condyle-disk assembly against the medial apex of each triangular fossa. To resist the inward, upward pressure from the internal pterygoid muscles, the fossae are heavily buttressed with bone in line with the direction of load. The anterior surface of each condyle is simultaneously compressed against the posterior slope of the eminentia.

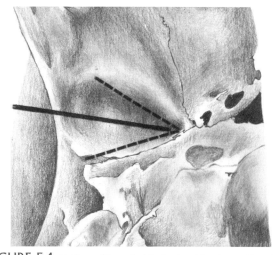

FIGURE 5-4 Further evidence that the horizontal axis runs through the medial poles of the condyles is found in the triangular fossae with the apex related to the medial pole. A horizontal axis through any part of the condyle other than the medial pole would result in translatory movements of the medial pole during a fixed rotational axis, and this would be incompatible with the V shape of the fossa.

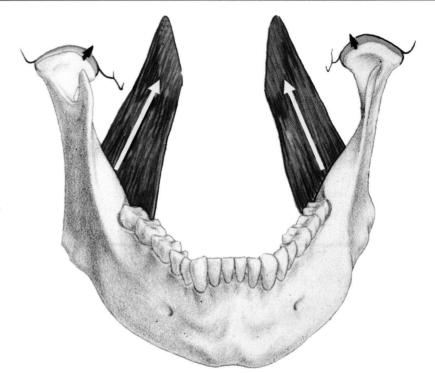

FIGURE 5-5 Medial pole bracing in line with internal pterygoid muscle contraction establishes the midmost position at centric relation. This braced position is consistently simultaneous with the uppermost position. This medial pole stop also prevents the lower posterior teeth from moving horizontally toward the midline, an essential anatomic design that makes a normal curve of occlusion possible. It also explains why an immediate side shift is not possible from the fully seated position of the condyles (centric relation).

translucent, but notice the density of the medial portion of the fossa and relate that difference to the relation of form to function. The TMJ is designed as a load-bearing joint[1] and must be capable of resisting forces that measure into hundreds of pounds. The condyles serve as a bilateral fulcrum for the mandible, and so the joints are always subjected to compressive force whenever the powerful elevator muscles contract. The specific areas of reinforcement of the fossa conform to the bearing areas for the upward, forward, and inward forces of the musculature.

The *articular eminence* forms the anterior part of the articular fossa. Because of the slightly forward pull of the elevator muscles, the condyles are always held firmly against the eminence (with the disk interposed). Of great importance is the strongly convex contour of the eminence. Since the anterior aspect of the condyle is also convex, one can see the purpose and the importance of the biconcave articular disk that fits between the two convex surfaces. Because of its position between the condyle and the temporal bones, the disk divides the joint into an upper and a lower compartment. The lower compartment serves as the socket in which the condyle rotates, whereas the upper compartment allows the socket to slide up and down the eminence. Thus the mandible can hinge freely as either one or both condyles translate forward.

Since each condyle serves as a fulcrum and is subjected to a predominantly upward force from the elevator muscles, it is provided with a definite stop to resist those forces. The condyle-disk assembly is able to slide up the eminence until the medial pole is stopped by the reinforced medial part of the fossa. This occurs at the highest point to which the properly aligned condyle-disk assembly can move. It occurs si-

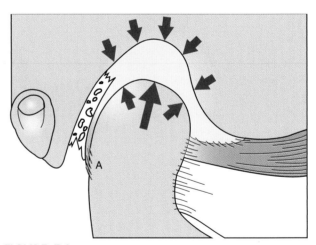

FIGURE 5-6 An intact, undamaged condyle disk assembly has a self-centering effect on the disk. Contrary to a popular belief that the condyle will slip off the posterior border of the disk if the TMJ is not supported by teeth, it is impossible for the disk to displace if its ligaments are intact and its biconcave shape has not been deformed. In addition to the self-centering shape of the disk, the posterior ligament extends from the disk and attaches to the back of the condyle (at *A*). It serves as an inelastic tether to prevent the disk from displacing anteriorly.

multaneously with contact still maintained against the eminence. The uppermost position is also the position at which the medial pole is braced against the medial articular lip (with disk interposed). This relationship stabilizes the midmost position of the mandible in centric relation and prevents any lateral translation from occurring while the condyle-disk assembly is in the uppermost position (Figure 5-6). Sicher[2] has stated that "only the fracture of the internal lip or its destruction could permit a medial displacement of the condyle. The presence of the medial articular lip also prevents a lateral displacement of the condyle, since this could occur only under simultaneous medial displacement of the other condyle."

As further evidence that this is a stress-bearing joint, all of the articular surfaces of the condyle, the fossa, and the eminence are covered with avascular layers of dense fibrous connective tissue. The absence of blood vessels is a sure sign that those specific areas are designed to receive considerable pressure. The avascular areas are also devoid of innervation, and this includes the bearing areas of the disk; so if the condyle and the disk are in proper alignment in the fossa, they can receive great pressure with no sign of discomfort, since there are no sensory nerves in the bearing areas to report discomfort.

The disk itself is a classic example of design for function. It is composed of layers of collagen fibers oriented in different directions to resist the shearing effect that might occur in a sliding joint. The bearing area is avascular, and so it is nourished by synovial fluids that also lubricate the joint for smooth gliding function. The reason for using collagen fibers instead of hyaline cartilage in the TMJ is that the stiffer cartilage that works well in most other joints would not be pliable enough to change shape as it conforms to the contours of the convex eminence in the sliding movements.

The disk is firmly attached to the medial and lateral poles of the condyle, and such attachment is the reason it moves in unison with the condyle. The diskal ligaments, which bind the disk to the poles, allow it to rotate from the front of the condyle to the top and vice versa. In normal function, the disk is always positioned so that pressure from the condyle is directed through its central bearing area. Positioning of the disk is controlled by the combination of elastic fibers attached to the back of the disk, which keep it under tension against the action of the superior lateral pterygoid muscle that is attached to the front of the disk. So while the diskal ligaments pull the disk along as the condyle moves, its rotation on the condyle is determined by the degree of contraction or release of the superior lateral pterygoid muscle.[3,4]

Many of the misconceptions about the disk have resulted from its depiction in illustrations as a little round cap that sits on top of the condyle. It actually wraps around the condyle to the points of attachment medially and laterally, and its posterior border is quite thick. The steeper the slope of the eminentia, the thicker the distal lip of the disk becomes, a feature that seems to indicate the importance of the disk as one of the structures that combine to determine the uppermost position of the condyle. The functional positioning of the disk is a critical factor in mandibular movements, and several disorders can result from its discoordination.

UNDERSTANDING CONDYLE
DISK ALIGNMENT

Medial and lateral diskal ligaments

The disk is designed to rotate on the condyle like a bucket handle that attaches to the medial and lateral poles of the condyle (collateral ligaments). This allows the disk to rotate from the top of the condyle to the front and back so it can stay aligned with the direction of force as the condyle moves up and down the curved eminentia.

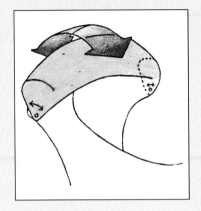

Posterior ligament

The disk is tethered to the back of the condyle by an inelastic band of collagen fibers. This prevents the disk from rotating too far forward. It also prevents the disk from being displaced anteriorly. The disk cannot displace anteriorly if the posterior ligament is intact. It must be stretched or torn to permit any forward displacement.

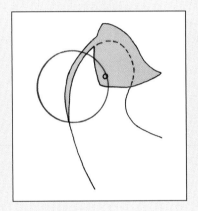

Superior elastic stratum

Elastic fibers bind the disk to the temporal bone behind it, and maintain constant tension on the disk toward the distal.

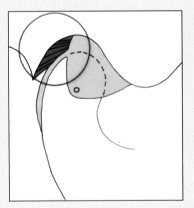

Superior lateral pterygoid muscle

If all the connective tissue attachments to the disk are designed to *prevent the disk from anterior displacement,* how does a disk become anteriorly displaced? The only forward pulling force that could anteriorly displace the disk is the muscle that attaches to the front of the disk. It is this muscle that in combination with the elastic fibers behind the disk controls the position of the disk on the condyle so it is always aligned with the direction of force as the condyle moves down the slope of the eminentia.

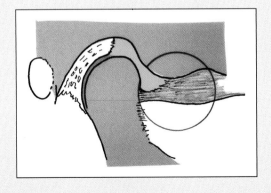

HOW MUSCLE CONTROLS DISK ALIGNMENT

Opening

If the condyle disk assembly is fully seated in centric relation, the disk is positioned at the most forward position (on top of the condyle) that the posterior ligament allows. At this position, the forces from condylar loading are directed up through the medial third of the disk and forward through the anterior surface of the condyle against the steepest part of the eminentia. As the *inferior* lateral pterygoid muscle (+) starts to pull the condyle forward, the *superior* lateral pterygoid muscle (−) releases contraction to allow the elastic fibers to start pulling the disk more to the top of the condyle.

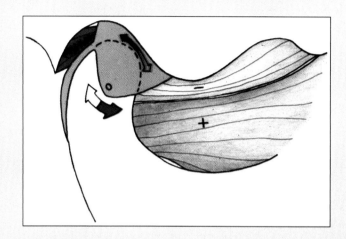

Maximum opening

When the condyle reaches the crest of the eminence, the disk should be directly on top of the condyle as forces are directed upwardly against the flattest part of the articular eminence. At this point, the elastic fibers have rotated the disk back because the superior lateral pterygoid muscle is in a controlled release. Note how the posterior ligament *(PL)* (which is not elastic) becomes more lax as the disk moves back.

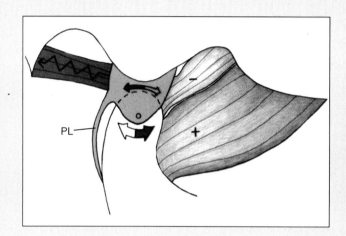

Closing

As the jaw closes, the condyle starts to move back and up the steeper slope of the articular eminence, so the disk must be pulled back to the front of the condyle. To accomplish this, the *superior* lateral pterygoid muscle (+) starts its contraction as the inferior lateral pterygoid muscle (−) releases the condyle to the elevator muscles that pull it back.

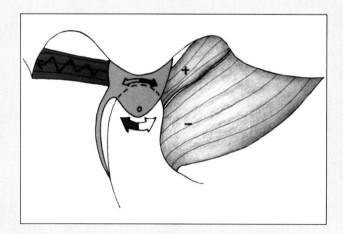

Closed

When the condyle reaches centric relation, the disk has been pulled as far forward as the posterior ligament will allow. If the ligament is intact and has not been stretched or torn, the disk is stopped in perfect alignment with the direction of loading through the condyle. In the absence of occlusal interferences to centric relation, the inferior lateral pterygoid muscle will stay passive, even if the patient clenches. The superior belly holds its contraction to maintain the disk in its correct alignment.

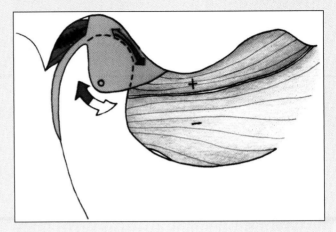

Note how the superior lateral pterygoid muscle attaches to both the disk and the neck of the condyle. This tethers the front of the disk with muscle fibers that can elongate to permit the disk to rotate to the top of the condyle, but can contract to pull the disk back when the condyle is fully seated.

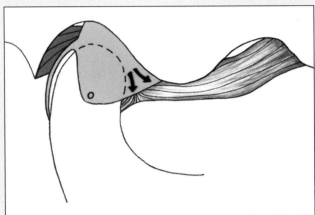

As the disk rotates to the top of the condyle as it approaches the crest of the eminentia, the inelastic posterior ligament folds. The functional aligning of the disk is an example of the importance of the coordinated contraction and release of the neuromusculature system in harmony with mandibular function.

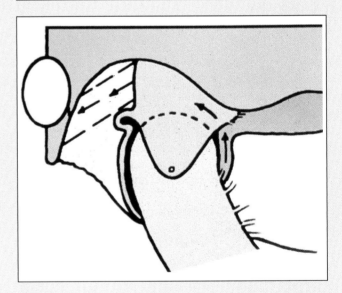

THE TEMPOROMANDIBULAR LIGAMENT

The temporomandibular ligament of the joint does not come into function until the jaw opens to 20 mm or more. At that point the ligament reaches its limit of length and stops the mandible from opening further in centric relation. The attachment of the ligament to the posterior side of the neck of the condyle stops the fixed hinge rotation and becomes a fulcrum that forces the condyle to translate forward as the jaw opens further. The designed purpose of this arrangement is to force the mandible to move forward as it opens wider so the floor of the mouth doesn't interfere with the airway when the jaw opens wide.

The temporomandibular ligament is *not* a factor in centric relation as it is not at its full length when the condyle disk assemblies are fully seated (unless the jaw opens 20 mm or more). Up to the point at which the ligament becomes fully extended, the condyle can rotate on a fixed axis at centric relation (Figure 5-7).

Misconception About Joint Physiology and Anatomy

Some authorities have claimed that centric relation is not a physiologic position because "it is a border position in which joints do not normally function." This concept is based on a misconception about joint physiology and anatomy as well as a lack of understanding of centric relation.

All joints, including the TMJs, function in a fully seated position in their sockets. Just as the joints in our leg are fully loaded at an end point of compression, the condyles are similarly loaded in centric relation by the elevator muscles. The misconception comes from confusion about a "fully packed" position at the end point of ligament length. Centric relation is *not* a ligament braced position, but rather it is the physiologic end point that is achieved by coordinated muscle function during jaw closure. The condyles must be forced distally down the posterior slope of the fossae for several millimeters from centric relation to reach their end point of ligament bracing.

THE ARTERIOVENOUS SHUNT

As each condyle disk assembly moves down the eminence, it evacuates the space up in the fossa. Nature cannot have a vacuum, so the retrodiskal tissue must expand to fill the space evacuated by the condyle and disk. It does this by a rush of blood into a network of vessels that are spread through the spongy retrodiskal tissues (Figure 5-8). Blood vessel walls are elastic, and the expansion of the vessels fills

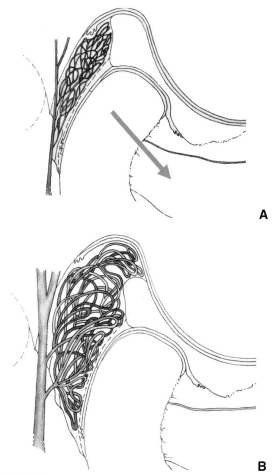

FIGURE 5-8 The space behind the condyle changes rapidly as the condyle moves forward and back. A network of blood vessels (**A**) with elastic walls allows blood to rush in to fill the space with the expanded vessels as the condyle moves forward (**B**). As the condyle moves back, the blood is shunted out the vessels. This shunting system is called the vascular knee.

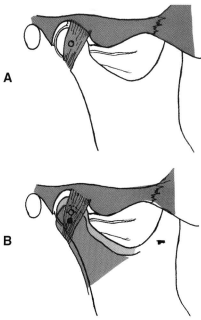

FIGURE 5-7 A, The ligament is lax in centric relation. It plays no role as a determinant of centric relation. **B,** The condyle can be forced distally from centric relation for several millimeters before the ligament reaches its full length.

the space. When the condyle and disk return to centric relation, the blood flows out and the vessels contract in size.

This arteriovenous shunt (also referred to as the vascular knee) is an important part of the intracapsular structure. It makes the retrodiskal tissue highly vascular and richly innervated. If the disk is displaced anteriorly, the condyle loads onto this tissue and causes pain. Inflammation and edema in these tissues are always considerations when the joint is traumatically loaded.

ARTICULATION

Most of the confusion about occlusion, centric relation, and TMDs is the result of wrong information about the structure of the TMJ articulation. The most prevalent misconception concerns the capacity of the TMJs to accept compressive loading. A typical example of the erroneous viewpoint is taken directly from the orthodontic literature, but it expresses a belief shared by many:

> Compression upon the TMJ intracapsular components is not well tolerated.

This erroneous depiction of the TMJs represents one of the most prevalent causes for confusion. Everything about the design of the TMJs points to a capacity to accept compressive loading as the fulcrum for the mandibular lever. All of the load-bearing structures of the TMJ are built to accept the loading forces as long as the condyle and disk are properly aligned for the forces to be directed through their load-bearing zone. Sicher[2] described the character of these tissues as anatomic and histologic evidence that the TMJs were made to be load bearing. Further evidence of this is the lack of blood vessels or nerves in any of the tissues in the load-bearing zone. Extensive studies by Hylander[4] have proven conclusively that loading forces are directed through the condylar fulcrum during all functional jaw movements.

Another misconception is that the articulation of the TMJs is very compressible, akin to a rubbery foundation that prevents the condyles from having a stable, definite stopping point in their sockets. A quote from the literature expresses this viewpoint:

> The natural condyle fossa relationship has 2.0 to 4.0 mm of superior joint space. Under the forces of the masseters, temporalis and medial pterygoids, this space can be over-powered and compressed.

This quote expresses one of the most popular and most seriously wrong misconceptions about the articulation of the TMJs. This viewpoint leads to attempts to "protect" the TMJs from loading forces by putting the forces on the teeth in order to stop the upward compression of the joints. This concept fails the test of clinical accuracy in two ways. First, it fails to recognize that the stopping surface for upward movement of the condyle-disk assembly is hard bone, not a spongy soft tissue. The disk that is interposed between the condyle and the bone stop is dense, strong, fibrous tissue with no blood vessels in its bearing surface, and no clinically observable compressibility. When the condyles are completely seated (centric relation), the inferior lateral pterygoid muscle is completely released and is inactive even during clenching if there are no deflective tooth inclines to interfere with complete seating of the joints. This removes all resistance to the upward loading effect of the elevator muscles to elevate the condyle disk assemblies as high as they can go against the bone at the medial part of each fossa. Mahan[6] has described this relationship as "unyielding" to upward movement when the condyles are in centric relation.

Nakazazawa et al[7] describe the uppermost, forward position of the condyles in the glenoid fossae as "a very stable position even under considerable stress. It is obvious that the compressive force at the joint produced by the masticatory muscles is not harmful. Since the disk is composed of extremely tough collagenous tissue and has no nerves or blood vessels in its central area, it can bear stresses that could cause traumatic inflammation in general soft tissue."

It is this understanding that explains why centric relation is at such a precisely repeatable endpoint (the apex of force position). It is this precise end point for the condyle disk assemblies that enables us to record centric relation with needlepoint accuracy.[7] It is for this reason that correctly mounted casts on an articulator are an absolutely reliable duplication of the patient's correct jaw-to-jaw relationship.

There is a second reason why forces should not be put on the teeth to prevent complete seating of the condyle-disk assemblies. This has the effect of putting the teeth *in interference* with the completely seated joints, requiring the condyles to displace down and forward from their seated position every time the teeth come together. This is a potent activator of incoordinated hyperactivity of the masticatory muscles and a prime causative factor in occluso-muscle pain.[8]

As you will learn in future chapters, one of the major goals in treatment planning is determining the best way to "get the posterior teeth out of the way" so the condyles can completely seat and the anterior teeth can contact without having to displace the condyles from centric relation. The goal of a perfected occlusion is to have equal intensity, simultaneous contact on the posterior teeth when the condyles are completely seated at their uppermost bone-stopping place. Anterior teeth should also contact at this same jaw position so the anterior guidance can do its job of discluding the posterior teeth the moment the mandible starts its excursive movements.

> If the TMJs are not stable, the occlusion will not be stable, so it is a risky proposition to undertake occlusal changes without knowing the condition of the TMJs.

It is also critically important that the TMJs be in a maintainably stable condition whenever any changes are contemplated to the occlusion. Thus the analysis of the TMJs is an important part of the examination process. Diagnosis and classification of the condition of the intracapsular structures should *precede* permanent changes to the occlusion. The details of proper examination and classification procedures are explained in Part II.

References

1. Zola A: Morphologic limiting factors in the temporomandibular joint, *J Prosthet Dent* 13:732-740, 1963.
2. Sicher H: The temporomandibular joint. In Sarnat B, ed: *The temporomandibular joint,* ed 2, Springfield, Ill, 1964, Charles C Thomas, Publisher.
3. Mahan PE, Gibbs CH, Mauderli A: Superior and inferior lateral pterygoid EMG activity, *J Dent Res* 61:272 (Abstract), 1982.
4. Gibbs CH, Mahan PE, Wilkinson TM, et al: EMG activity of the superior belly of the lateral pterygoid muscle in relation to other jaw muscles. *J Prosthet Dent* 51:691-702, 1984.
5. Hylander W: The human mandible: lever or link. *Am J Phys Anthropol* 43:227, 1975.
6. Mahan PE: Anatomic, histologic, and physiologic features of TMJ. In Irby WB, ed: *Current advances in oral surgery,* vol 3, St Louis, 1990, Mosby.
7. Nakazazawa K, Hong T, Tatashi J: The anatomic importance of centric relation. *Anatomic Atlas of the Temporomandibular Joint,* Tokyo, Quintessence, 1991.
8. Nelson S, Ash MM: *Wheeler's dental anatomy, physiology, and occlusion,* ed 8, St Louis, 2003, WB Saunders.

Chapter 6

The Masticatory Musculature

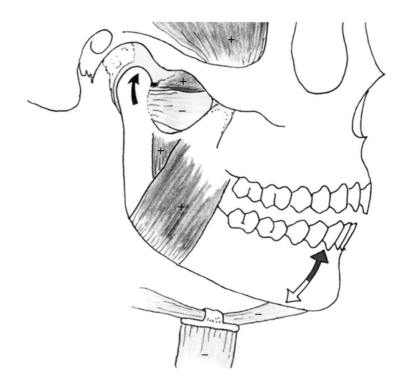

PRINCIPLE

The purpose of all occlusal therapy is a peaceful neuromusculature.

When bone and muscle war, muscle never loses.

—*Harry Sicher*

When teeth and muscle war, muscle never loses.

—*Peter E. Dawson*

THE DOMINANT DETERMINANT

We cannot keep teeth in a stable position where muscle does not want them to be. Muscle is the dominant determinant of both the horizontal and vertical position of the teeth. The compressive force of the jaw-closing musculature has been measured at up to 975 lbs. per square inch.[1] The devastation that aberrant muscle forces can wreak on the masticatory system goes beyond teeth. Incoordinated, hyperactive musculature can, over time, displace the disk from a condyle and cause a variety of structural deformations to the temporomandibular joints (TMJs). Muscle is the primary focus in vertical dimension, the neutral zone, arch form, occlusal disease, orofacial pain, and even smile design. If muscle is not a prime consideration in treatment planning for prosthodontics, restorative dentistry, implants, orthodontics, or maxillofacial surgery, predictability of treatment results will be reduced to guessing.

Research into how the masticatory musculature functions and dysfunctions has clarified much of our clinical thinking.[2-5] Sophisticated EMG studies have expanded our knowledge from gross muscle activity all the way down to the function of single motor units within different sections of individual muscles.[6,7] These elegant muscle studies have been further enhanced by research into the *neuro* part of the neuromusculature[8,9] to expand our understanding of the exquisite influence of mechanoreceptors within the periodontal ligaments, and the even more sensitive odontoblastic sensory units within the teeth.[10]

What we know today is that communication between the teeth and the musculature is far more exquisite in its sensitivity than was realized in the past. By matching this information up with extensive clinical observations, it explains why there has been so much controversy regarding the many different approaches to treatment of occlusal problems and TMJ-related disorders. The good news is that there are solid, dependable answers. Today there is little reason for confusion about diagnosis or treatment of occlusal problems, TMJ disorders, or pain within the masticatory system.

Let's start with a basic understanding of what is meant by *coordinated* muscle activity, because it is an essential goal for all occlusal treatment.

Coordinated muscle function during jaw opening

Coordinated muscle function refers to the timely release of a muscle or group of muscles as contraction of antagonistic muscles takes place. As the jaw opens, the depressor muscles contract while the elevator muscles release their contraction. The inferior lateral pterygoid muscle contracts during opening.

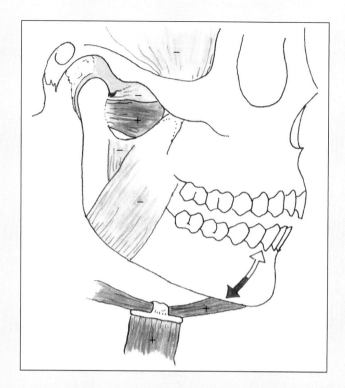

Coordinated muscle function during jaw closure

As the jaw closes, the elevator muscles contract while the depressor muscles release contraction. Note that during jaw closure the inferior lateral pterygoid muscle releases its contraction and is passive. In the absence of deflective occlusal interferences, it stays passive even during firm clenching.[11]

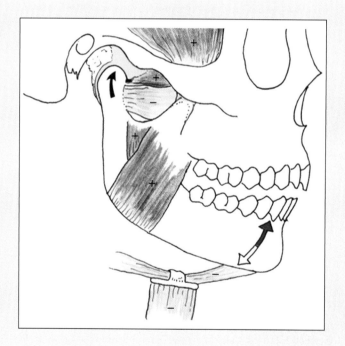

Coordinated muscle function at maximum intercuspation

Release of the inferior lateral pterygoid muscle during elevator muscle contraction is the goal of occlusal harmony. Such coordinated muscle function is only possible if the condyle-disk assemblies can completely seat up into their respective fossae during closure into maximum intercuspation. The superior belly of the lateral pterygoid muscle is active to hold the disk in alignment with contact against the posterior slope of the eminentia.

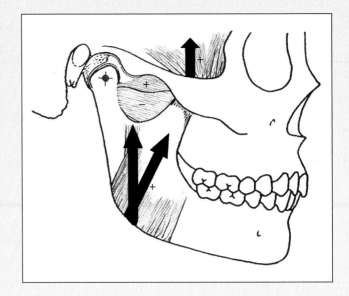

Disharmony between the occlusion and the TMJs

If the condyles must be displaced from centric relation to achieve maximum intercuspation, the inferior lateral pterygoid muscle *must contract* to move the mandible to the position of maximum intercuspation. Note that the condyles must be pulled *down* as they are pulled forward. What appears to be an ideal Class I occlusal relationship is actually a cause of muscle incoordination with a potential for occlusal disease, muscle pain, or disorders in the intracapsular structures of the TMJ.

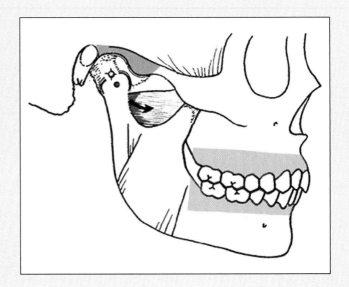

Incoordinated muscle function

If the TMJs must displace to achieve maximum intercuspation, the inferior lateral pterygoid muscles must actively contract to hold the condyles down on a slippery incline in direct opposition to contraction of all the elevator muscles every time the teeth are brought into maximum contact. The effect of having to displace the condyles to make the teeth fit is always directed at muscle. EMG studies have shown that muscle hyperactivity and incoordination are the result of such occlusal disharmony.[11-15]

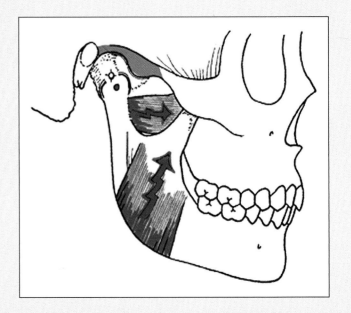

Undesired Features

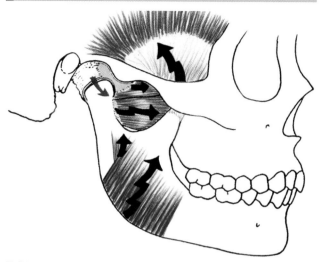

FIGURE 6-1 Displacement of the TMJs is one of the most predictably correctable causes of pain in the masticatory system.

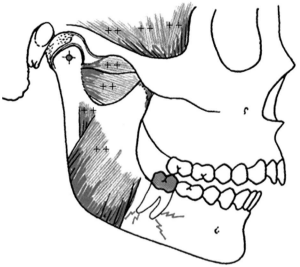

FIGURE 6-2 An occlusal interference such as a high crown or deflective tooth incline activates muscle hyperactivity. Pain is often focused in the masticatory muscles to give the impression of a TMJ disorder. A high percentage of misdiagnosed TMJ disorders are occluso-muscle disorders that are readily resolvable by occlusal correction.

Occlusal interferences that require displacement of the TMJs to achieve maximum intercuspation of the teeth can cause incoordination of all the masticatory neuromusculature (Figure 6-1). This is called *occluso-muscle pain.*[16,17] It is one of the most common masticatory system disorders, and is the cause of most of the so-called "TMD" pain. It is also one of the most predictably correctable causes for pain in the masticatory system. Occlusal equilibration is more often than not the choice of treatment, but only after careful diagnosis and determination that equilibration is the *best* choice of five treatment options.

Muscle Response to Occlusal Interference

When an occlusal interference such as a high restoration is introduced into a comfortable mouth, it typically evokes a response of hyperactivity and incoordinated contraction in all the muscles that are prevented from functioning in a co-ordinated pattern of contraction versus release of opposing muscles (Figure 6-2). It is also common for the interfering tooth to become sensitive and sore. Because of the prolonged hyperactivity of the temporal muscles, tension headaches in that region often occur in combination with pain in the masseter muscles and in the pterygoid complex.

There is no more convincing evidence of the relationship of occlusal interferences to masticatory muscle pain than the response achievable by separating the interfering tooth from contact. Placement of a simple flat interocclusal device on the anterior teeth separates the posterior teeth and allows the TMJs to completely seat up into centric relation. This permits the lateral pterygoid muscles to release contraction and results in a return to coordinated muscle function. The relief of all symptoms is almost immediate unless there is an intracapsular structural disorder (Figure 6-3). It is also an indication that the same relief could be achieved by direct correction of the occlusal interferences.

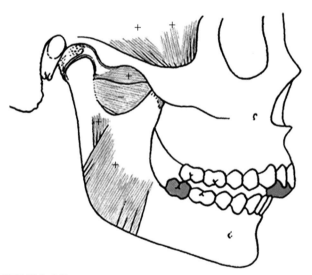

FIGURE 6-3 A permissive (smooth) anterior splint separates the interfering molar from contact, thus permitting the condyle disk assemblies to seat up into centric relation. This eliminates the trigger for muscle activity and allows the inferior lateral pterygoid muscle to release. Peaceful, comfortable muscle activity resumes quickly.

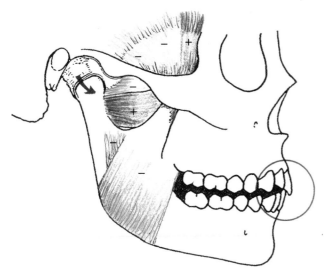

FIGURE 6-4 Posterior disclusion: When the posterior teeth are separated in all eccentric jaw movements by the combination of anterior guidance in the front and condylar guidance in the back, more than two-thirds of the elevator muscle force is shut off.

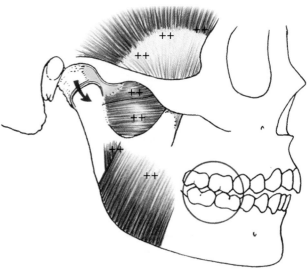

FIGURE 6-5 Posterior occlusal interference: When any posterior tooth interferes with the anterior guidance in eccentric movement, the lateral pterygoid muscles are activated and the elevator muscles are hyperactivated. This results in *incoordinated* muscle hyperfunction. It also puts the posterior teeth in jeopardy of horizontal overload, and subjects them to excessive attritional wear, fractures, and hypermobility.

Muscle Response to Posterior Disclusion

Irrefutable evidence for the role of occlusal interferences has been provided by Williamson,[12] Mahan et al.,[11] and many other investigators. The comparison of muscle hyperactivity versus peaceful coordination is easily demonstrated by what happens within the masticatory muscle complex when the posterior teeth are separated during protrusive and lateral excursions of the mandible (Figures 6-4 and 6-5). At the moment of separation of the posterior teeth, almost all of the elevator muscles shut off. This has three beneficial effects:

1. It greatly reduces the horizontal forces against the anterior teeth, which are the only teeth in contact during excursions.
2. It reduces the compressive loading forces on the TMJs.
3. It makes it impossible to overload or wear the posterior teeth, even if the patient bruxes.

Important Terms to Understand as They Relate to Muscle

Fulcrum: The pressure point of support on which a lever rotates. Because all upward force is applied behind the teeth, between the fulcrum and the teeth, the fulcrum is always under pressure (compression) when the elevator muscles contract. This is a very important fact to understand, as it affects both the TMJs and the teeth.

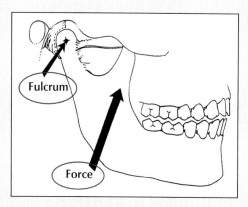

Force: Exertion of power that starts or stops movement. Can result in *compression* (loading) . . . or *tension.*

Loading: The pressure a structure bears from a compressive force.

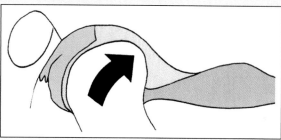

Tension: A pulling force against resistance.

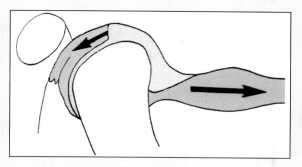

Strain: Distortion or change of shape as a result of compressive or tensive force.

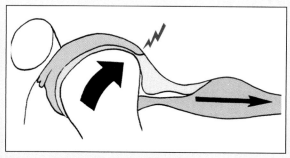

Muscle Incoordination as a Causative Factor in Disk Derangements

In a healthy, intact TMJ, the disk is not only self-centering, its posterior ligament is a band of inelastic collagen fibers that tethers the disk to the back of the condyle so it cannot displace anteriorly. The disk is also attached to the medial and lateral poles of the condyle. Incoordinated muscle activity pulls the disk forward while the elevator muscles pull the condyle up and back, applying tensive force to the posterior ligament of the disk.

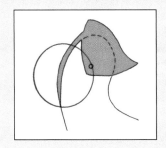

This tensive force is essential to cause displacement of the disk because it is impossible to displace the disk if its ligaments are intact.

One of three things must occur to allow the disk to displace:

1. The ligament must be stretched

or

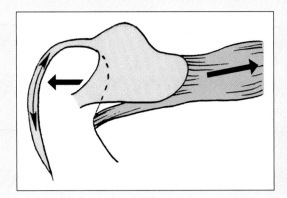

2. The ligament must be torn

or

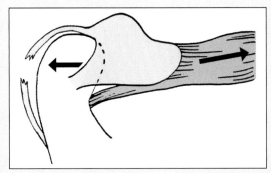

3. The attachment of the ligament must migrate.

For any of these deformations (strains) to occur, there must be a *tensive force* pulling the disk forward while the condyle is pulled or held back in resistance. The only source of tensive force on the disk is the superior lateral pterygoid muscle. Even if the condyle is forced back by a trauma to the jaw, the ligament cannot be stretched unless the distalizing force through the condyle is resisted by forward pull of the muscle that attaches to the disk.

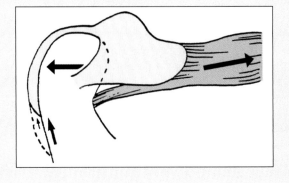

If one studies the structure and arrangement of the temporomandibular articulation, it should become apparent that the joint should be able to hinge freely and resist very strong pressure with complete comfort if all the parts are healthy and are in correct alignment. This is so because all the bearing areas are reinforced for strength and receive all functional pressures on avascular, noninnervated surfaces. But this occurs only if all of the passive parts are in balance with the active forces of the musculature. It has been my consistent clinical finding that whenever I find discomfort or dysfunction, I will also find muscle incoordination. Since muscle incoordination can so easily start a chain reaction of structural deformation, it is necessary to determine whether muscle incoordination is the cause or the result of the structural malrelationship. In my clinical experience, it is an extreme rarity to find masticatory muscle incoordination without a definite structural disharmony as the activating trigger for the muscle hyperactivity and incoordination. It is also my clinical experience that removal or correction of the structural disharmony results in a return to normal muscle function and comfort.

THE MASTICATORY MUSCLES

It is helpful to divide the muscles of mastication into the positioner muscles and the elevator muscles. The *positioner muscles* are responsible for the horizontal movements of the mandible from centric relation. The inferior lateral pterygoid muscles pull the condyles down and forward; and the elevator muscles pull the mandible back and up. The superior lateral pterygoid muscle is responsible for keeping the disk properly aligned with the condyle during function.

The elevator muscles are all positioned distal to the teeth so that they elevate the condyles and hold them firmly against the eminence while hinging the jaw. The masseter, the internal pterygoid, and the major part of the temporal muscle are responsible for elevation.

In the normal resting position of the mandible, the elevator muscles and their antagonistic depressor muscles are in a resting state of postural contraction. The mandible is balanced between them. To open the jaw from the resting position requires the contraction of the depressor muscles and the simultaneous release of the elevator muscles. As the jaw continues to open, the temporomandibular ligament reaches its restricting length at the neck of the condyle to stop the pure hinge rotation of the condyle. At this point, the condyle must translate forward. As the inferior belly of the lateral pterygoid muscle contracts, it pulls the condyle forward down the convex eminentia, and the disk is pulled along with the condyle. As the condyle-disk assembly moves down the steep incline and onto the crest of the eminence, the elastic fibers behind the disk keep tension on it to rotate it onto the top of the condyle so that the disk will be maintained in line with the direction of force. To permit the retrodiskal elastic fibers to rotate the disk to the top of the condyle, the muscle attached to the front of the disk must re-

lease contraction, and so the superior belly of the lateral pterygoid is in a controlled release upon opening or protrusive movements of the mandible.

The superior stratum of the bilaminar zone is responsible for the positioning of the disk in protrusive movements. The inferior stratum is attached to the condyle, so as the disk rotates back, tension is reduced in those fibers. Increasing tension in the superior stratum occurs as the condyle moves forward.

As the mandible starts its closure, the middle and posterior fibers of the temporal muscle contract to pull the mandible back while the inferior lateral pterygoid releases its protrusive action. The depressor muscles also release as the elevator muscles start their contraction. The combined contraction of the elevator muscles pulls the condyle up the lubricated incline until it is stopped by the bracing of the medial pole. The forwardly directed muscle contraction holds the condyle against the eminence.

The disk, being firmly attached to the poles of the condyle, is pulled up the incline with the condyle, but during that movement it must be rotated from the top of the condyle back to the more anterior relationship; so upon closure, the superior pterygoid becomes active to counteract the pull of the retrodiskal elastic fibers and, through controlled contraction, holds the disk so that it is rotated to the front of the condyle as it moves back up the incline.

It is obvious that much of the structural complexity of the TMJ is necessary to maintain coordinated function between the condyle and the disk. The past few years have brought new insight into condyle-disk function and pathofunction. It has become apparent that condyle-disk discoordination does not occur without the involvement of muscle. One must determine whether incoordination of muscle is the cause of the disk misalignment and, if so, the chain of muscle responses must be traced back until the originating stimulus for the muscle disharmony is determined. If structural alterations have occurred in the joint, it must be determined whether correction of the alignment will allow healing of the affected part, or whether the patient can function at a tolerable comfort level with the damaged part. If the damage is too severe and reparative surgery is the choice, it must be accompanied by a return to structural and functional balance of the entire system or the surgery will probably fail.

THE IMPORTANCE OF OCCLUSAL HARMONY

Ideal mandibular function results from a harmonious interrelationship of all the muscles that move the jaw. Muscle becomes fatigued if it is not allowed to rest. Muscle should not be forced into prolonged activity with no chance to rest. When teeth are added to the stomatognathic system, they can exert a unique influence on the entire interbalance of the system because if the intercuspation of the teeth is not in harmony with the joint-ligament-muscle balance, a stressful and tiresome protective role is forced onto the muscles.

When the muscles elevate the mandible in the absence of any deviating interferences, the closing muscles pull the condyle-disk assembly up until it is stopped by bone at the medial pole. If tooth inclines interfere with this uppermost position, the lateral pterygoid muscle is forced into positioning the mandible to accommodate to the teeth. The mandible is thus realigned to make the teeth intercuspate, even though to do so the lateral pterygoid muscles must take over the bracing function normally assigned to the bone.

The lateral pterygoid muscles are capable of holding the condyles during protrusive function, but in the presence of an occlusal interference they can never be relieved of this function without allowing the malaligned teeth to be stressed.

The mechanism that forces this prolonged contraction onto the lateral pterygoid muscles is the exquisitely sensitive protective reflex system that guards the teeth and their supporting structures against excessive stress. Mechanoreceptor nerve endings scattered through the periodontal ligaments are sensitive to even minute pressures on individual teeth. The mechanoreceptor system is designed like a glove of periodontal receptors capable of evaluating the direction and intensity of stresses on the teeth and designed to program the lateral pterygoid muscles to position the jaw so that the elevator muscles can close directly into maximum occlusal contact. If tooth interferences cause the mandible to move left, the right lateral pterygoid must contract to pull that condyle forward. Contraction of the left pterygoid moves the jaw to the right. Contraction of both pterygoids moves the jaw forward. There are unlimited variations of timing and degree of muscle contraction to precisely position the mandible for maximum intercuspation of the teeth, but the lateral pterygoid muscles are always involved in any deviation from centric relation.

This unique relationship between the lateral pterygoid muscles and the mechanoreceptor periodontal receptors is so definite that it even overrides the normal tendency of the muscle to rest when it becomes fatigued. The muscles cannot relax the protective bracing contraction as long as the occlusal interference is present.

The pattern of deviation is reinforced every time contact is made, and it is retained in the brain's memory bank so that muscular closure into the deviated jaw relationship becomes automatic. One important facet of the mechanoreceptor memory, however, is that it fades rapidly if continual reinforcement of the pattern ceases. Elimination of interfering contacts permits an almost immediate return to normal muscle function. The deviation pattern is forgotten as soon as it is no longer needed.

In the past few years, new research has shown that the effect of occlusal harmony or disharmony is more definitive than had been realized. Many investigators have documented the cause-and-effect relationship between occlusal interferences and muscle incoordination, but the work of Williamson[12] and Mahan[11] gave perspective to the importance of precise occlusal harmony and its relationship to physiologic condyle positioning.

Williamson demonstrated the precise effect of occlusal interferences on muscle coordination and normal muscle activity. Using electromyographic procedures, he showed that interfering contacts on posterior teeth in any eccentric position caused hyperactivity of the elevator muscles. But if the anterior guidance was allowed to disclude all posterior teeth from any contact other than centric relation, the elevator muscles either stopped active contraction or noticeably reduced it the moment the posterior teeth were discluded. If heavy contact on any posterior tooth in any eccentric position causes a response of muscle hyperactivity, it has the effect of loading the tooth or teeth with the occlusal interferences, but the elevator muscle hypercontraction also loads the joint with the same hyperactivity.

Williamson's research has particular meaning to the principles of occlusion outlined in this text because of his agreement with the description of centric relation and his meticulous attention to its precise recording.[12] This is the type of research that has been needed because it relates electromyographic results to a specifically described centric relation position that was verified and documented.

The noticeable reduction in elevator muscle activity at the precise moment of disclusion is one of the most important and clinically useful findings in many years.

An incoordinated musculature rarely exists without causing some form of adaptive structural change. Because of their tendency to wear, become loose, or move, the teeth are the usual focus for structural alteration. The TMJ has generally been regarded as the most stable component of the masticatory system, but remodeling can change the shape of the disk or the condyles. Mongini[18,19] has shown that a direct relationship exists between the shape of the condyle after remodeling and the attrition patterns on the teeth. His findings give support to the concept that remodeling of the joint can be considered, to a certain extent, a functional adaptation to occlusal disharmony.

The apex of force positioning of the condyle seems to relate rather consistently with Mongini's findings regarding the relationship between the type of displacement and condylar shape caused by remodeling. He showed that flattening and flaring of the anterior surface are the most common changes in condylar shape and are accompanied in most cases by anterior condylar displacement. Remodeling of the posterior surface of the condyle, leading to flattening or concavities, is common in posterior displacement.

When all the notable, related research of the past few years is analyzed, it is apparent that the occlusal interface must involve the articulating surfaces of the TMJs with equal importance to the occlusal surfaces of the teeth. All active and passive elements of this interrelationship must be carefully evaluated to make certain that a harmony of parts exists. Signs and symptoms of temporomandibular disorders are the effects that occur when some part of this interrelationship goes awry.

The new insights that so much of the recent research has given us has confirmed what many other clinicians and I have observed clinically: successful occlusal treatment is dependent on complete harmony of all the passive and active components of a very precise and complex system. It is not possible to have an adequate understanding of occlusion outside of the framework of the total stomatognathic system.

As we proceed to discuss the factors that determine whether an occlusion is stable, comfortable, and esthetic, further details regarding the role of muscle will be explained.

References

1. Gibbs CH: University of Florida School of Dentistry. Personal communication.
2. Lundeen HC, Gibbs CH: *The function of teeth,* Gainesville, Florida, 2005, L and G Publishers.
3. Dubner R, Sessle BJ, Storey AT: The neural basis of oral and facial function. New York, 1978, Plenum Press.
4. Williamson E: Anterior guidance: its effect on electromyographic activity of the temporal and masseter muscles. *J Prosthet Dent* 49:816-823, 1983.
5. Lerman MD. A revised view of the dynamics, physiology, and treatment of occlusion: a new paradigm. *J Craniomandib Pract* 22:50-63, 2004.
6. Murray GM, Phanachet I, Uchida S: The role of the human lateral pterygoid muscle in the control of horizontal jaw movements. *J Orofacial Pain* 15:279-291, 2001.
7. Phanachet I, Whittle T, Wanigaratne K, et al: Functional properties of single motor units in the inferior head of the human lateral pterygoid muscle: task firing rates. *J Neurophysiol* 88:751-760, 2002.
8. Herring SW: The role of the lateral pterygoid muscle in the control of horizontal jaw movements. *J Orofacial Pain* 15:292-295, 2001.
9. McMillan AS: The role of the lateral pterygoid muscle in the control of horizontal jaw movements. *J Orofacial Pain* 15:295-298, 2001.
10. Jacobs R, van Steenberghe D: Role of periodontal ligament receptors in the tactile function of teeth: a review. *J Periodont Res* 29:153-167, 1994.
11. Mahan PE, Wilkinson TM, Gibbs CH, et al: Superior and inferior bellies of the lateral pterygoid muscle EMG activity at basic jaw positions. *J Prosthet Dent* 50:710-718, 1983.
12. Williamson EH, Lundquist DO: Anterior guidance: its effect on electromyographic activity of the temporal and masseter muscles. *J Prosthet Dent* 49:816-823, 1983.
13. Bakke M, Moller E: Distortion of maximum elevator activity by unilateral premature tooth contact. *Scand J Dent Res* 88(1):67-75, 1980.
14. Schaerer P, Stallard RE, Zander HA: Occlusal interferences and mastication: an electromyographic study. *J Prosthet Dent* 17(5):438-449, 1967.
15. Riise C, Sheikholeslam A: The influence of experimental occlusal contacts on the postural activity of the anterior temporal and masseter muscles in young adults. *J Oral Rehabil* 9(5):419-425, 1982.
16. Ramfjord SP: Dysfunctional temporomandibular joint and muscle pain. *J Prosthet Dent* 11:353-374, 1961.
17. Dawson PE: Occluso-muscle pain. In: *Concepts of complete dentistry: Seminar one manual.* St. Petersburg, Florida, 1990, 2003, Center for Advanced Dental Study.
18. Mongini F: Remodeling of the mandibular condyle in the adult and relationhip to the condition of the dental arches. *Acta Anat* 82:437-453, 1972.
19. Mongini F: Dental abrasion as a factor in remodeling the mandibular condyle. *Acta Anat* 92:292-300, 1975.

Centric Relation

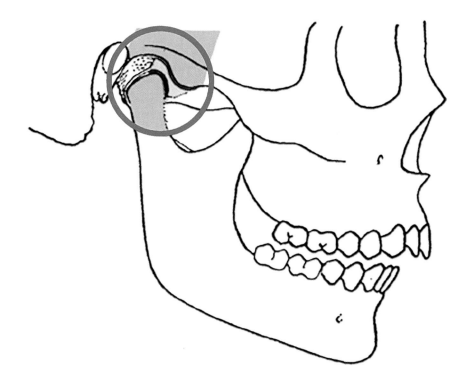

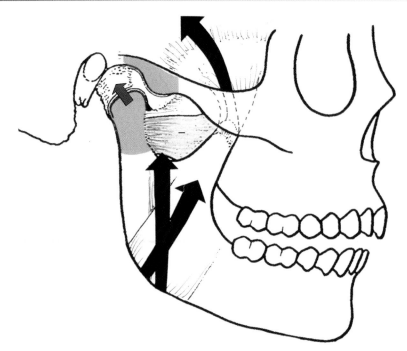

FIGURE 7-1 In coordinated muscle function, the triad of strong elevator muscles pulls the condyle-disk assemblies up the slippery posterior slopes of the eminentiae. The inferior lateral pterygoid muscles release and stay released through complete closure if there are no occlusal interferences to complete upward seating of the condyles into centric relation.

Because the position of the condyle-disk assemblies determines the maxillo-mandibular relationship during jaw closure, any variation in condylar position will change the closing arc of the mandible and thus affect the initial contact of the mandibular teeth against the maxillary teeth. If maximum intercuspal contact of the teeth is not coincident with the completely seated position of both condyles, the condyles must be displaced to achieve complete jaw closure into maximum intercuspation. Numerous electromyographic studies have confirmed that occlusal interferences to complete seating of the condyles (centric relation) disrupt the coordination of masticatory muscle function.[1-7]

The two most importat criteria for centric relation are:

1. The complete release of the inferior lateral pterygoid muscles, and
2. Proper alignment of the disk on the condyle. During jaw closure with intact temporomandibular joints (TMJs), the condyle-disk assemblies are pulled up the eminentiae by a triad of strong elevator muscles[8,9] (Figure 7-1).

UNDERSTANDING CENTRIC RELATION

Centric relation is the single most important factor of occlusion. Determination of centric relation is the most important skill required for predictable occlusal treatment. Verification of centric relation is an essential procedure in differential di-

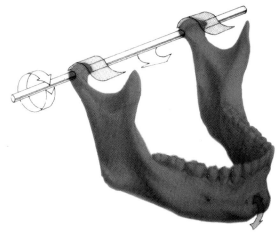

FIGURE 7-2 The condyles can rotate in a fixed axis in centric relation or they can rotate as they slide forward down the eminentiae.

agnosis of TMJ disorders. Recording of an accurate centric relation is critical for the most cost-effective, time-effective, trouble-free restorative or prosthetic dentistry.

Centric relation refers to both the position and condition of the condyle-disk assemblies. It is a specific position of the condylar axis. The condyles can freely rotate on a fixed axis in centric relation up to about 20 mm of jaw opening without moving out of the fully seated position in their respective fossa (Figure 7-2). Consequently, the mandible can be in centric relation even when the teeth are separated or even if there are no teeth in either jaw.

Definition: Centric Relation

Centric relation is the relationship of the mandible to the maxilla when the properly aligned condyle-disk assemblies are in the most superior position against the eminentiae irrespective of vertical dimension or tooth position.

At the most superior position, the condyle-disk assemblies are braced medially, thus centric relation is also the midmost position.

A properly aligned condyle-disk assembly in centric relation can resist maximum loading by the elevator muscles with no sign of discomfort.

Before we describe the reasons for each aspect of centric relation, let's clear up some common misconceptions.

1. *Centric relation* is a fixed axial position of the condyles. *This does not mean that the mandible is restricted* to centric relation during function. The rotating condyles are free to move down and up the eminence to and from centric relation, permitting the jaw to open or close at any position from centric relation to most protruded (see Figure 7-2).
2. Centric relation should not be confused with *centric occlusion,* an obsolete term that has been replaced with *maximum intercuspation.* Centric relation refers to the fully seated *condylar* position regardless of how the teeth fit.
3. Centric relation is not about teeth. It is about the position of the condyles. But remember that the position of the condyles determines the relationship of the mandible to the maxilla, even when no teeth are present (Figure 7-3). The edentulous mandible is in centric relation if the condyle-disk assemblies are completely seated.
4. Centric relation is not just a convenience position that is used because it is repeatable. It is the universally accepted jaw position because it is physiologically and biomechanically correct and is the only jaw position that permits an interference-free occlusion. The study that follows will demonstrate why this is so.
5. The fact that the definition of centric relation has changed from its original definition of "most retruded" does not make either the newer "uppermost" definition or the concept of centricity obsolete. The definition in this text should be absolutely clear in its meaning and is consistent with the glossary of prosthodontic terms. Furthermore, the current definition is consistent with the position described and advocated for more than 30 years. What has changed is a better understanding of the anatomy of the TMJ, and in particular the importance of disk alignment and the medial poles of the condyles. We learned that the temporomandibular ligament is not a factor in centric relation as was originally believed. However, the concept of "uppermost" instead of "rearmost" has not changed.

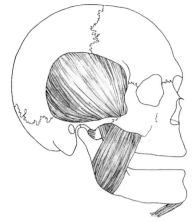

FIGURE 7-3   Edentulous mandible in centric relation.

6. In recent years, a barrage of misinformation about centric relation has been published in nonjuried publications. Dentists who have limited knowledge of the TMJs or occlusion can easily be misled.

To help you sort through the confusion, let's dissect the definition of centric relation and look at it bit by bit in light of what is known about the anatomy and biomechanics of mandibular function.

The Relationship of the Mandible to the Maxilla

If dentists understood the importance of determining a correct maxillo-mandibular relationship *before* analyzing and planning treatment, the value of properly mounted diagnostic casts (Figure 7-4) would be obvious and the importance of properly recording centric relation would be too apparent to disregard.

Remember that the purpose of the mounted casts is to see how the mandibular teeth relate to the maxillary teeth when the condyles are in centric relation. Mounted casts make it possible to determine the best treatment approach for bringing the teeth into harmony with the correct maxillo-mandibular relationship (Figures 7-5 and 7-6).

With casts mounted in this centric relation mandibular position, it is possible to accurately determine the best treatment option for making the teeth fit into the correct maxillo-mandibular relationship. Remember that the goal is to achieve maximum intercuspation without requiring displacement of the TMJs. With the condylar axis recorded, all treatment options can be explored including occlusal equilibration, orthodontics, restoration, or surgery.

Properly Aligned Condyle-Disk Assemblies

If the disk is not properly aligned, the condyle is not in centric relation. There are sound reasons for this description being part of the definition. Note that when the condyle and

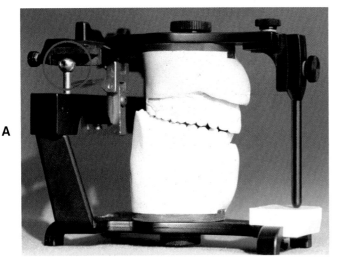

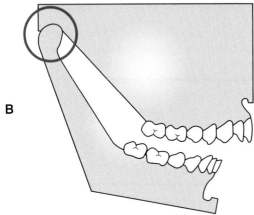

FIGURE 7-4 **A,** Casts mounted in centric relation enable the dentist to accurately determine what must be done to bring the teeth into harmony with the correct maxillo-mandibular relationship **(B).**

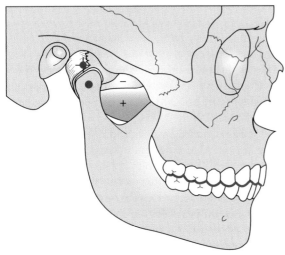

FIGURE 7-5 Ignoring the position of the TMJs when examining the occlusion is not acceptable. Just putting the casts together in maximum intercuspation does not provide the necessary information regarding how the mandibular teeth relate to the maxillary teeth when the condyles are in their completely seated centric relation position, nor does it show what must be done to achieve harmony between the occlusion and the TMJs. Unmounted casts are responsible for many mistakes of prosthodontic, restorative, and orthodontic treatment decisions.

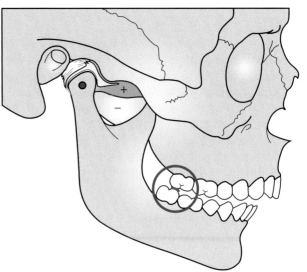

FIGURE 7-6 Analysis of the mandible-to-maxilla relationship when the condyles are in centric relation presents a completely different picture from maximum intercuspation. Now it becomes obvious why the molars are loose or are wearing excessively. Remember that this occlusal disharmony is incompatible with coordinated muscle function because the lateral pterygoid muscles must actively contract to pull the condyles down and forward in opposition to the elevator muscles every time the teeth are brought together.

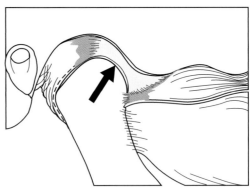

FIGURE 7-7 Note also that around the disk there are vascularized tissues with copious innervation. If the disk becomes misaligned, the loading forces are directed through highly vascularized and innervated tissues that respond with pain or discomfort. This is why load testing of the TMJs is an important step in determination of centric relation. This is one of the reasons the TMJs are not in centric relation if they cannot accept firm loading with complete comfort.

disk are properly aligned (Figure 7-7), all loading (compressive) forces are directed through avascular, noninnervated structures that were designed to accept loading. Sicher,[9] in his classic text on anatomy, *The Temporomandibular Joint,* ed. 2, cites this as proof that the TMJs are load-bearing joints.

Against the Eminentiae

One of the most prevalent misconceptions about the TMJs is that they are "hanging" joints that should not be subjected to loading forces because they overly compress the joint struc-

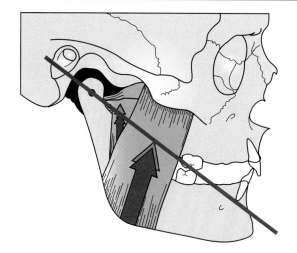

FIGURE 7-8 If the elevator muscles contract to pull the mandible toward the origination of each elevator muscle, the condyles will be pulled tightly against the eminentiae. Visualize the direction the condyles would move if the disk was removed.

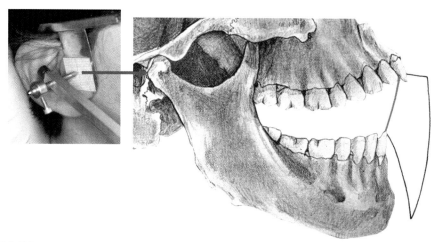

FIGURE 7-9 If the condyles are in centric relation, they can rotate on a fixed axis. Thus a bite record made at any point of opening on the correct centric relation arc *(shown in red)* is still in centric relation. If the casts are mounted on an articulator with the correct condylar axis, the vertical dimension can be increased or decreased without introducing any error.

tures. This mistaken idea fails in its understanding of basic biomechanics. The facts are clear. Contraction of the elevator muscles, which are all distal to the teeth and between the teeth and the TMJ, keep the condyle-disk assemblies loaded throughout the functional movements.

Muscles always work by shortening their length to pull the attached bone toward the bone site of muscle origin. Visualize what has to happen if you could remove the disk and position the condyles in space (Figure 7-8). What would happen to the condyles if the elevator muscles contract (to pull) the mandible toward the origination of each elevator muscle? It is obvious that the condyles would be pulled tightly against the eminentiae. This is exactly what happens. There are no muscles attached to the mandible in such a way as to pull the bones apart (distract the condyles). This basic observation is in accord with one of the inviolate laws of joint mechanics:

Strong contact between articulating bodies is found in all movable joints, because muscles are always arranged to pull across joints.[9]

—*Harry Sicher*

Irrespective of Tooth Position or Vertical Dimension

As previously stated, in centric relation, the condyles can rotate on a fixed axis to an opening of about 20 mm. This is an easily proven fact that can be demonstrated by a kinematic hinge axis recording (Figure 7-9) in which a needlepoint, attached by fixation to the lower arch, rotates on a fixed point when aligned with the rotational center of the condylar axis at the medial poles (see Figure 7-2).

The false conclusion that the condyles cannot rotate on a fixed axis has led some clinicians to discredit the use of face bow recordings and articulators, claiming that the vertical dimension cannot be accurately changed on an articulator . . . a provably false belief.

Most Superior Position

The most important condition to understand about centric relation is that in centric relation, the properly aligned condyle-disk assemblies are completely seated in the most superior position in their respective sockets. There are many

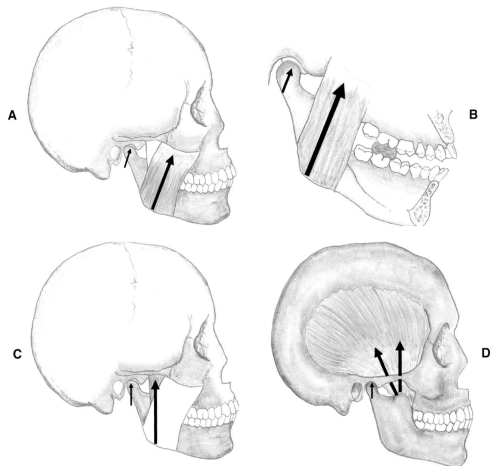

FIGURE 7-10 **A,** The superficial masseter pulls the condyles against the posterior slope and *up.* **B,** The internal ptery-goid muscles pull the condyles *up* from the lingual side of the mandible. **C,** The deep fibers of the masseter muscles pull the condyles *up.* **D,** The temporalis muscles attach to the coronoid process between the teeth and the TMJs and pull the condyle *up.*

important facets to this understanding, and every one has high clinical value.

Much of the confusion about the uppermost position of the TMJs comes from a mistaken but popular concept of "unloading" the joints. Failure to recognize that the TMJs are designed to accept loading has created a number of clinical approaches that attempt to "decompress" or "support" or "unload" the condyles. These concepts are the opposite of what is correct for a number of reasons.

COORDINATED MUSCLE ACTION SEATS AND LOADS THE TMJs

The elevator muscles are all distal to the teeth, between the teeth and the condyles. Action of the elevator muscles pulls the condyle-disk assemblies against the eminentiae and slides them upwardly. The posterior slopes of the eminentiae are convex and are made slippery by synovial fluid. All of the elevator muscles participate in pulling the condyles *up-ward* (Figure 7-10).

Now let's use some bio-*logic* by asking: If all of the elevator muscles are pulling the condyles upward, what determines the stopping point for the condyle-disk assemblies?

There are only two choices. The condyle-disk assemblies are either

1. Braced by muscle, or
2. Braced by bone

Anatomic dissections and EMG studies are consistent in their findings that the only muscle that can stop the condyles from moving up the eminence is passive during jaw closure unless activated by occlusal interferences to hold the jaw forward.

The inferior belly of the lateral pterygoid muscle is almost always completely inactive during clenching in the retrusive position (Figure 7-11).[6]

—*Mahan et al.*

Now add to your knowledge of coordinated muscle function and consider that the slope of the eminence that each

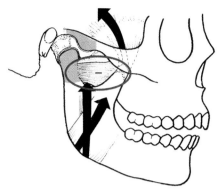

FIGURE 7-11 Inactivity of the inferior belly of the lateral pterygoid muscle releases the condyles to move up.

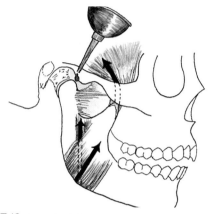

FIGURE 7-12 Synovial fluid provides lubrication for the condyle-disk assemblies.

condyle-disk assembly slides up and down against is lubricated by one of the slipperiest substances (synovial fluid) (Figure 7-12).

Now visualize the force that the lateral pterygoid muscle must resist if it must displace one or both the condyles down that slope and hold it there every time the jaw closes when there are deflective occlusal interferences.

THE POSITIONER MUSCLE: THE INFERIOR LATERAL PTERYGOID

All movement of the mandible, either forward, right, or left from centric relation, always involves the lateral pterygoid muscle because such movements are made by pulling one or both condyles forward and downward. Thus the inferior lateral pterygoid muscle[10–15] has the sole responsibility of forward positioning of the mandible to align with maximal interocclusal contact whenever centric relation is not coincident with maximal intercuspation. This puts the lateral pterygoid muscles in antagonistic isometric contraction in resistance to the upward force of the triad of strong elevator muscles every time the jaw closes. This becomes a more damaging problem if the patient has a tendency to clench or brux.

It is a mistake to think that there must be a major displacement of the TMJs to produce a problem. It has been my consistent experience that minute occlusal interferences are often the trigger for sore teeth and masticatory muscle pain. In fact, some of the most severe occluso-muscle pain can result from deflective occlusal contacts that slightly move a loose interfering tooth rather than cause a slide from centric relation to maximum intercuspation. I am convinced that many less than satisfactory occlusal equilibrations fail because minute interferences are allowed to remain. The key to perfecting any occlusion, however, is complete seating of the condyles up into centric relation. What might seem to be an insignificant displacement of the joints from centric relation is all that is needed to activate muscle incoordination and hyperactivity. Clinical experience has shown that to be true time after time.

Current elegant research into the role of the lateral pterygoid muscle has provided new insight on why minute occlusal interferences can provoke problematic muscle responses. Murray et al.[10] have provided evidence that suggests that a major function of the lateral pterygoid muscle is in the generation and fine control of the horizontal component of jaw movement. The isolation of subcompartments within the lateral pterygoid and EMG studies of single motor units (SMUs) indicate that a graded activation of internal segments of the muscle is involved in the generation of horizontal force vectors, as would be required in parafunctional activity and heavy mastication.

Measurements of displacement of as little as 0.1 mm were shown to recruit SMUs within the pterygoid muscle. This evidence for an association between SMUs and horizontal jaw displacements is consistent with predominantly aerobic fibers in the muscle that may correlate with fatigue resistance and low forces such as those used in speaking. However, Mao et al.[11] found that a significant proportion of fibers within the lateral pterygoid are predominantly anaerobic and are therefore fast-acting and fatigue-susceptible. These are the fibers that would most likely be involved in parafunctional motor activities involving protrusive and lateral grinding and clenching. The fatigue-susceptible characteristics of these fibers seem to correlate with our clinical findings of muscle discomfort from bruxing or clenching when only minute occlusal interferences were present. This observation is given further potential by findings that the inferior lateral pterygoid muscle was implicated in the development of isometric horizontal forces toward the end of the intercuspal phase of chewing.[12] Isometric muscle activity results from the lateral pterygoid muscle's resistance to elevator muscle contraction . . . exactly what we see in the presence of deflective occlusal interferences. Furthermore, it has been shown that both heads of the lateral pterygoid muscle are in active resistance[13] to prevent the condyle-disk assembly from complete seating during protrusive or contralateral clenching.

More studies are needed in which muscle activity is related to the relationship of maximum intercuspation to a precisely recorded and verified centric relation. In the meantime, our clinical observations are clear and consistent. In the absence of structural intracapsular disorders, precise occlusal correction to eliminate all premature or deflective interferences to centric relation is a highly predictable process for eliminating most problems of masticatory muscle pain. It routinely results in comfort for the patient and more stability of the dentition. The key to success seems to invariably be complete release of the inferior lateral pterygoid muscle during closure to maximum intercuspation. This can only be accomplished by eliminating all deflective interferences to centric relation.

THE EXTREMELY IMPORTANT SIGNIFICANCE OF TMJ SOCKET DESIGN

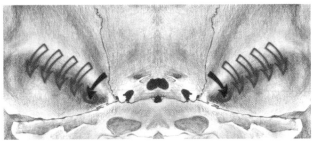

FIGURE 7-13 Direction of movement of the condyle-disk assembly.

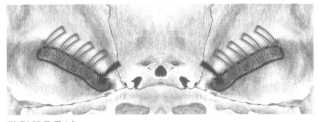

FIGURE 7-14 Note the outline of the condyle as it contacts the slope of the eminentia. It is not in contact with the thin roof of the fossa.

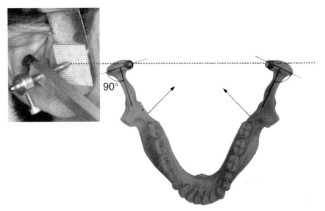

FIGURE 7-15 Hinge axis recordings are proof that the condyles can rotate on a fixed axis.

We've explained why muscle is not the ideal choice for stopping the upward movement of the condyle-disk assembly (Figure 7-13). Now let's look at what stops it very effectively: the bony socket that is referred to as the *glenoid fossa.*

Note the triangular shape of the fossae (Figure 7-14). The apex is toward the midline to accept the pure rotational axis of the medial poles of the condyles. The wide part of the fossa accommodates the movement of the lateral pole during rotation. The arrows represent the path of the condyles from protrusive to centric relation.

The term *centric* is an adjective that means "centered." The medial poles are centered in the middle of the medial third of the fossae (Figure 7-15).

When the condyles are fully seated, the front of the condyle (with disk interposed) contacts against the posterior slope of the eminence. The upward movement is stopped by contact of the medial pole with the heavily buttressed bone up in the medial third of the fossa (Figure 7-16). At this point, the condyle-disk assembly cannot move higher but it can rotate in that position, even under strong muscle loading.

IN CENTRIC RELATION, ONLY THE MEDIAL POLE ROTATES ON A FIXED AXIS

The lateral poles do not align with the fixed axis of rotation, so in all opening and closing movements of the mandible, the lateral pole must translate even when the condyles remain on a fixed centric relation axis (see Figure 7-16). This is why the glenoid fossae are triangular in shape with the apex at the medial poles.

The purpose of lateral pole translation during condylar rotation is to provide a sort of windshield wiper effect for spreading synovial fluid back and forth over the entire surface of the condyle and the bearing surfaces of the disk. The avascular bearing surfaces require this distribution of synovial fluid to provide nourishment and lubrication. If the convex condyle fits into a concave disk as a perfect ball and socket, the fit under compression would prevent synovial fluid from flowing through the entire interface of the condyle and disk. The irregularities in the surface of the condyle also aid the flow by providing indentations for the fluid to travel in.

Much confusion has resulted from misinterpretation of transcranial films of the TMJ because of failure to understand the mechanics of lateral pole travel. It appears on films that the condyle changes position as the jaw opens or closes. From such films, some have concluded that centric relation is not a *fixed axis. But the medial pole does not show on transcranial films and it can in fact stay on a fixed axis in centric relation. This can be clearly demonstrated by finding the fixed axis using a kinematic hinge axis locator.*

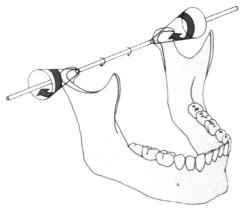

FIGURE 7-16 In centric relation only the medial pole rotates on a fixed axis.

Midmost Position

The braced position shown in Figure 7-17 is consistently simultaneous with the uppermost position. This medial pole stop also prevents the lower posterior teeth from moving horizontally toward the midline, an essential anatomic design that makes a normal curve of occlusion possible. It also explains why an immediate side shift is not possible from the fully seated position of the condyles in centric relation.

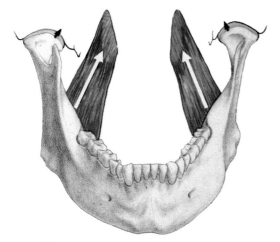

FIGURE 7-17 Medial pole bracing in line with internal pterygoid muscle contraction establishes the midmost position at centric relation.

Disk Alignment

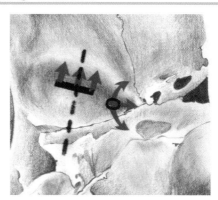

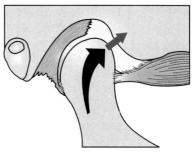

If the condyle-disk assembly is sliced through the center, it shows the disk on the front of the condyle. It is this perspective that misleads some to believe the condyle will slip off the back of the disk if it is not "supported" by teeth. This cannot happen if the disk and its ligaments are intact.

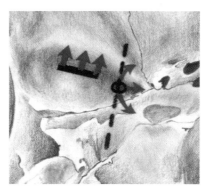

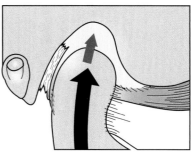

It is the medial third of the condyle that is well covered by the disk. A slice through this part of the condyle-disk assembly shows how the normal upward force of the elevator muscles is directed through the concavity of the disk and fossa.

Self-Centering Position

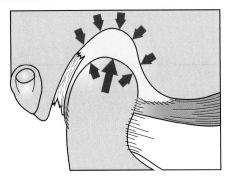

An intact condyle-disk assembly is self-centering on the condyle. The disk and ligaments must be damaged to permit displacement of the disk. The primary source of disk displacement is the tensive pull of incoordinated muscle activity that combines with damage to the ligaments.

The Apex of Force Position

There is an apex (point) of force at the uppermost bone stop at the medial part of the fossa. This is always a definite apex from which no forward or backward movement of the condyle-disk assemblies can occur unless they move *down* the bony slope of the fossae (Figure 7-18).

Because the medial pole of the condyle is braced at the uppermost part of its reciprocal fossa contour, it cannot move backward from that position without moving *downward*. The anterior surface of the condyle rests against the eminentia, so the condyle cannot move forward without being guided downward by the convex contour of the eminentia when it moves from its highest point.

Other factors can contribute to the downward movement when the mandible is pushed distally. The distal lip of the disk is quite thick and would force the condyle to move downward when it moves back. The position of the restraining ligaments could also be a factor according to some authorities. However, if the intact condyle-disk assembly is ob-

served carefully, it appears that the medial pole relationship is the dominant factor in guiding the condyle down from the apex position to a more distal relationship.

Numerous studies have verified the accuracy of the apex of force configuration as well as the repeatability of a precise centric relation position.[17-24] Our studies involving hundreds of recordings always show the uppermost position to be a *point*. There is no flat area at that apex so only *downward* movement from the apex is possible. This is a very important point to understand.

Why the Uppermost Position Is Mechanically and Physiologically Correct

The crux of why centric relation is the only condylar position that permits an interference-free occlusion becomes apparent when the apex of force configuration of the fossae is analyzed. When both condyle-disk assemblies are completely seated in centric relation, their medial poles should be at the highest point of concavity of that part of each fossa. From where the medial poles are stopped by bone, the fossae walls curve downward on three sides so that from a correct centric relation, the condyles cannot travel forward, backward, or medially without moving downward. The understanding of this apex of force position is extremely important to the concept of centric relation. It means that failure to completely seat the condyles when harmonizing an occlusion invariably results in a muscle-braced condyle-disk assembly instead of a bone-braced relationship. It also means that whenever the condyles go to their more upward centric relation position during function, the closing forces are directed more on the most posterior teeth, subjecting them to potential damage from occlusal overload (Figure 7-19).

Contrary to some opinions that centric relation is not a functional position, that observation has not been supported by extensive research by Lundeen and Gibbs[13] or in studies that show that the centric relation position is used frequently in swallowing.[16]

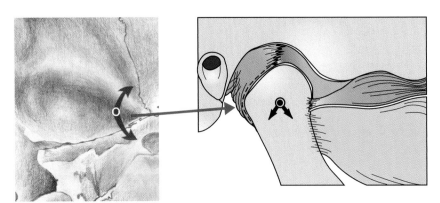

FIGURE 7-18 If the condyles are fully seated in centric relation, they cannot move horizontally forward, backward, or medially. They *must move downward*.

If the idea that the condyles do go repeatedly to centric relation is doubted, it would only be necessary to observe the facets of wear on the teeth of a number of patients. Casts mounted correctly in centric relation routinely show that if wear facets are present, the facets always extend to centric relation on tooth inclines that interfere with centric relation.

Centric Relation as Terminology

The term *centric relation* often comes under criticism as poor terminology for describing the condylar position. Actually, it is an accurate description. *Centric* is an adjective for describing a centered position. If the position of the condyle-disk assembly in its fossa is analyzed, it is apparent that the medial pole is centered in the medial third of the fossa (Figure 7-20). The medial pole is also centered at the

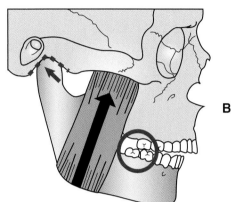

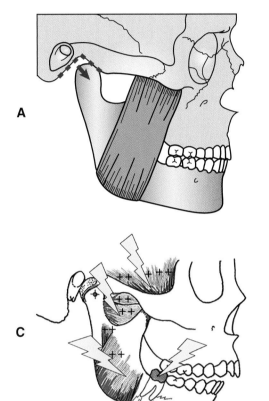

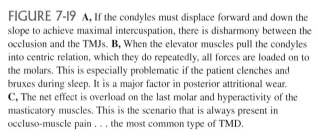

FIGURE 7-19 **A,** If the condyles must displace forward and down the slope to achieve maximal intercuspation, there is disharmony between the occlusion and the TMJs. **B,** When the elevator muscles pull the condyles into centric relation, which they do repeatedly, all forces are loaded on to the molars. This is especially problematic if the patient clenches and bruxes during sleep. It is a major factor in posterior attritional wear. **C,** The net effect is overload on the last molar and hyperactivity of the masticatory muscles. This is the scenario that is always present in occluso-muscle pain . . . the most common type of TMD.

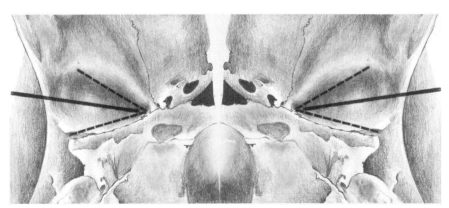

FIGURE 7-20   The medial pole is centered in the medial third of the fossa.

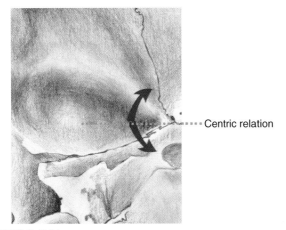

FIGURE 7-21 If maximal intercuspation requires the condyles to displace distally, the medial pole of the condyle must move downward from its apex of force position in the concave fossa. When it moves up and forward to centric relation, the posterior tooth becomes the pivot point.

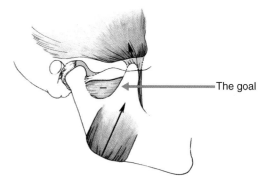

FIGURE 7-22 The goal of centric relation.

apex of force position as already described (Figure 7-21). There is no need to look for a different term to replace *centric relation.*

SUMMARY

The mandible is in centric relation if five criteria are fulfilled:

---

1. The disk is properly aligned on both condyles.
2. The condyle-disk assemblies are at the highest point possible against the posterior slopes of the eminentiae.
3. The medial pole of each condyle-disk assembly is braced by bone.
4. The inferior lateral pterygoid muscles have released contraction and are passive.
5. The TMJs can accept firm compressive loading with no sign of tenderness or tension.

TMJs that are not completely comfortable when loaded are not in centric relation.

The goal of centric relation (Figure 7-22) is a completely released inferior lateral pterygoid muscle on both sides. This is the essential requirement for a peaceful, coordinated musculature. It can only be achieved in the absence of deflective occlusal interferences to centric relation.

References

1. Ramfjord SP: Dysfunctional temporomandibular joint and muscle pain. *J Prosthet Dent* 11:353-374, 1961.
2. Bakke M, Moller E: Distortion of maximum elevator activity by unilateral tooth contact. *Scand J Res* 88(1):67-75, 1980.
3. Riise C, Sheikholeslam A: The influence of experimental interfering occlusal contacts on postural activity of the anterior temporal and masseter muscles in young adults. *J Oral Rehabil* 9:419-425, 1982.
4. Williamson EH, Lundquist DO: Anterior guidance: Its effect on electromyographic activity of the temporal and masseter muscles. *J Prosthet Dent* 49:816-823, 1983.
5. Hannam AG, DeCow RE, Scott JD, et al: The relationship between dental occlusion, muscle activity, and associated jaw movement in man. *Arch Oral Biol* 22:25-32, 1977.
6. Mahan PE, Wilkinson TM, Gibbs CH, et al: Superior and inferior bellies of the lateral pterygoid EMG activity at basic jaw positions. *J Prosthet Dent* 50:710, 1983.
7. Schaerer P, Stallard RE, Zander HA: Occlusal interferences and mastication: An electromyographic study. *J Prosthet Dent* 17:438-449, 1967.
8. Ramfjord SP, Ash MM: *Occlusion,* ed 4, Philadelphia, 1983, WB Saunders.
9. Sicher H: The temporomandibular joint. In Sarnat BG, ed: *The temporomandibular joint,* ed 2, Springfield, Ill, 1964, Charles C Thomas, Publisher.
10. Murray GM, Uchida S, Whittle T: The role of the human lateral pterygoid muscle in the control of horizontal jaw movements. *J Orofacial Pain* 15:279-291, 2001.
11. Mao J, Stein RB, Osborn JW: The size and distribution of fiber types in jaw muscles: A review. *J Craniomandib Disord Facial Oral Pain* 6:192-201, 1992.
12. Wood WW, Takada K, Hannam AG: The electromyographic activity of the inferior part of the human lateral pterygoid muscle during clenching and chewing. *Arch Oral Biol* 31:245-253, 1986.
13. Lundeen H, Gibbs C: *Advances in occlusion,* Boston, 1982, John Wright.
14. Uchida S: Electromyographic studies on the exhibition of isometric protrusive and lateral protrusive mandibular forces. *J Jpn Prosthodont Soc* 34:480-491, 1990.
15. Herring SW. The role of the human lateral pterygoid muscle in the control of horizontal jaw movements. *J Orofac Pain* 15(4):292-295, 2001.
16. Graf H, Zander HA: Tooth contact patterns in mastication. *J Prosthet Dent* 13:1055-1066, 1963.
17. Williamson EH: Laminographic study of mandibular condyle position when recording centric relation. *J Prosthet Dent* 39:561-564, 1978.
18. Gilboe D: Centric relation as the treatment position. *J Prosthet Dent* 50:685-689, 1983.
19. Long JH Jr: Locating centric relation with a leaf gauge. *J Prosthet Dent* 29:608-610, 1973.
20. Lucia VO: A technique for recording centric relation. *J Prosthet Dent* 14:492-505, 1964.
21. Woelfel JB: A new device for accurately recording centric relation. *J Prosthet Dent* 56:716-727, 1986.
22. Celenza FV, Nasedkin JN: *Occlusion: The state of the art.* Chicago, 1978, Quintessence.
23. McKee JR: Comparing condylar position repeatability for standardized verses nonstandardized methods of achieving centric relation. *J Prosthet Dent* 77:280-284, 1997.
24. Dawson PE: Optimum TMJ condyle position in clinical practice. *Int J Periodontics Restorative Dent* 3:11-31, 1985.

Chapter 8

Adapted Centric Posture

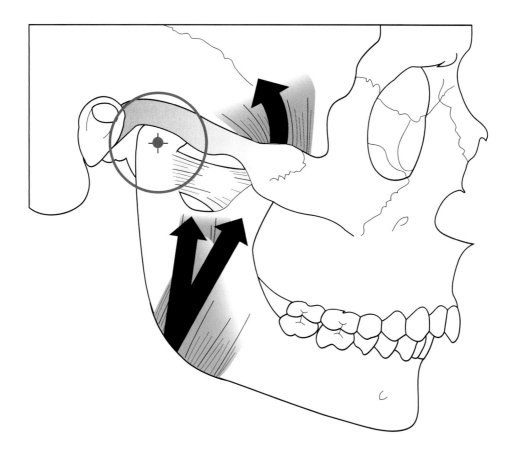

PRINCIPLE

In a deformed temporomandibular joint (TMJ), the type and degree of adaptation must be determined before addressing the relationship between the occlusion and the TMJs.

Centric relation is the accepted term for defining the condylar axis position of intact, completely seated, properly aligned condyle-disk assemblies. *A TMJ that is structurally deformed with a misaligned or displaced disk cannot be described as in centric relation because it does not fulfill the critical requirement of a properly aligned disk.* However, some structurally deformed temporomandibular joints (TMJs) may function comfortably even though they do not fulfill the requirements for centric relation. A wide range of intracapsular structural disorders from partial to complete disk derangements with or without reduction may adapt to a conformation that permits the joints to comfortably accept maximal compressive loading by the elevator muscles. Until the term *adapted centric posture* was introduced[1] there was no accepted terminology to define the condition or position of such joints.

Verification of successful adaptation is an important step in diagnosis because it rules out structural intracapsular disorders as a source of orofacial pain and establishes responsible guidelines for initiation of occlusal treatment or prosthetic dentistry. It also establishes a much needed terminology for more specific description of TMJ position and condition for clinical research on the relationship between occlusion and the TMJs.

Many TMJs function with complete comfort and apparent normalcy, even though they have undergone deformation caused by disease, trauma, or remodeling. Some TMJs click, or exhibit other signs of intracapsular disorder, but they do not prevent patients from functioning in an acceptable and comfortable manner. Whether a TMJ is in *adapted centric posture* is based on whether it can comfortably accept firm loading and whether it is manageably stable. Thus:

> Adapted centric posture is the manageably stable relationship of the mandible to the maxilla that is achieved when deformed TMJs have adapted to a degree that they can comfortably accept firm loading when completely seated at the most superior position against the eminentiae.

Like centric relation, adapted centric posture is a horizontal axis position of the condyles. It occurs irrespective of vertical dimension or tooth contact. It is also a midmost position, because even if a disk is completely displaced, the medial pole of each condyle adapts to the concavity of the fossae and maintains contact against the medial incline of each fossa wall.

The mandible is in adapted centric posture if five criteria are fulfilled:

1. The condyles are comfortably seated at the highest point against the eminentiae.
2. The medial pole of each condyle is braced by bone. (The disk may be partially interposed.)
3. The inferior lateral pterygoid muscles have released contraction and are passive.

4. The condyle-to-fossa relationship is manageably stable.
5. Load testing produces no sign of tension or tenderness in either TMJ.

The consequences of adaptive changes in the temporomandibular articulation may be positive or negative with regard to signs or symptoms. The same adaptive changes that result in reduction of symptoms may produce signs of serious and progressive deformation of intracapsular structures[2] as well as collateral damage to the teeth.[3] Excessive occlusal wear or hypermobility of teeth is a common result of disharmony between the TMJs and the occlusion. Damage to the teeth is progressive if deformation of the TMJs continues. Our clinical observation is consistent: Unstable TMJs result in unstable occlusions. That is why it is important to ascertain the condition of the TMJs before initiating any irreversible occlusal changes, and it is especially important to determine if any deformation has reached a point of manageable stability.

Adapted centric posture may be achieved in a variety of intracapsular deformations. The progression from a healthy, intact TMJ to one that is deformed and then adapted may include stages that produce pain and dysfunction in the early stages of deformation. An example is the painful compression of vascular, highly innervated retrodiskal tissue following a complete disk displacement. In time, the retrodiskal tissue may convert to a fibrous pseudo-disk at which point the discomfort dissipates and the TMJ can become comfortable. The more common scenario is for the retrodiskal tissue to break down and perforate from the compressive loading of the condyle. As the perforation enlarges, the condyle eventually develops a bone-to-bone articulation. When that occurs, the discomfort typically subsides but the bone-to-bone articulation is not as stable as an intact condyle-disk assembly. Nevertheless, a bone-to-bone articulation can often be classified as adapted centric posture because with a perfected occlusion, continuous deformation of the articulating surfaces can typically be slowed to a manageable level of stability.

Proper diagnosis requires an orderly evaluation of intracapsular structures, not just to see if deformation is present but to determine the specific stage of deformation. In most patients with so called "temporomandibular disorders (TMDs)," any discomfort is far more likely to be myogenous rather than intracapsular, even when some deformation has occurred within the intracapsular structures. This must be determined by specific testing. A combination of history, load testing, Doppler auscultation, and palpation can usually lead to a diagnosis, but some type of imaging may be needed for specificity.

Some of the most common intracapsular disorders that can evolve into an adapted centric posture include:

1. Lateral pole disk derangements
2. Complete disk derangement with formation of a pseudo-disk
3. Complete disk displacement with perforation
4. Other partial disk derangements and clicking TMJs

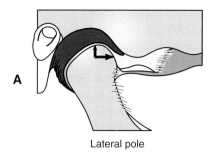

Lateral pole

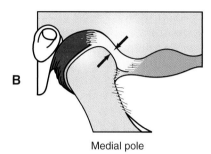

Medial pole

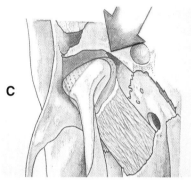

C

FIGURE 8-1 Complete comfort with an excellent chance for long-term stability is also possible, and this is true even if the lateral half of the disk has displaced and the deformation has progressed to a closed lock (A). If an intracapsular disorder is intercepted before the medial half of the disk becomes displaced (B), it is my consistent clinical experience that comfort and stability of the TMJ can be achieved with about the same success as a healthy, intact TMJ if harmony is established between the occlusion and the completely seated (but deformed) condyle disk assembly. C, The relationship from below. The pterygoid attachment to the neck of the condyle has been removed for this illustration.

LATERAL POLE DISK DERANGEMENTS

One of the most important diagnostic determinations to be made regarding any intracapsular disorder is whether a deranged disk is displaced off the lateral pole only. This is critical information because if the disk is not displaced off the medial third of the condyle, it is possible to achieve complete seating of the condyle with no discomfort (Figure 8-1).

The key to success is in establishing and maintaining a peaceful, coordinated masticatory musculature. This can be accomplished by complete elimination of all occlusal interferences to a verified adapted centric posture.

COMPLETE DISK DERANGEMENT WITH FORMATION OF A PSEUDO-DISK

In the early stages of a complete disk displacement, there is typically a period during which pain is a symptom. Even gentle load testing elicits a response of discomfort because of compression of the richly innervated retrodiskal tissue (Figure 8-2). At this stage, adapted centric posture cannot be achieved because the TMJ cannot accept loading without some degree of discomfort. Although not predictable, the retrodiskal tissue is sometimes converted to a fibrous connective-tissue pseudo-disk.

Pseudo-disk formation can be observed on magnetic resonance images (Figure 8-3). We have also observed such pseudo-disk formations in cadaver specimens and in open joint microsurgery. When pseudo-disk formation occurs, blood vessels and sensory nerves tend to evacuate the bearing area and the fibrous extension of the original disk is eventually able to accept loading with no discomfort. It may then be possible to achieve an adapted centric posture that appears to be as stable and as comfortable as an intact condyle-disk alignment.

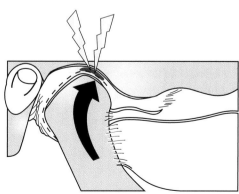

FIGURE 8-2 Painful compression of retrodiskal tissue when the disk is completely displaced.

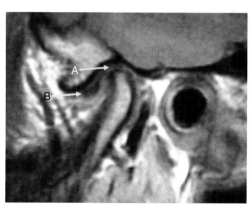

FIGURE 8-3 Magnetic resonance imaging showing pseudo-disk formation (A). Note how it extends from the original disk (B).

COMPLETE DISK DISPLACEMENT WITH PERFORATION

The most likely progression from a completely displaced disk with closed lock is to proceed through a painful stage of compression of the retrodiskal tissues, which become less painful as the condyle perforates the sensitive vascular tissues and begins to load against bone. As the soft-tissue perforation expands, a complete bone-to-bone contact may result (Figure 8-4) that permits loading with no impingement against innervated structures. At this stage, it is possible to verify an adapted centric posture by the absence of discomfort when the condyles are loaded (load testing.)

The typical sequence of events that occurs after the retrodiskal tissue is perforated is a progressive flattening of both the condyle and eminence. The osteoarthritic deformation starts at the articular cartilage, causing a loss of height of the condyle. Because of the perforation, the synovial fluid channel is damaged, disrupting the flow of synovial fluid. The loss or reduction of synovial fluid nourishment to the surfaces of the condyle and eminence results in breakdown of the bone surfaces.

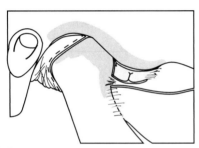

FIGURE 8-4 Typical pattern of flattened condyle against a flatter eminence after perforation of the retrodiskal tissue. The disk becomes deformed and is permanently locked in front of the condyle.

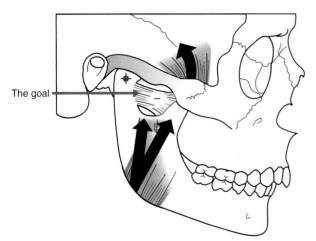

FIGURE 8-5 The goal for achieving adapted centric posture is the same as for centric relation. It is complete release of the inferior lateral pterygoid muscle. If the joints can comfortably accept loading at that position, a good result for occlusal treatment can be predicted.

Although the osteoarthritic joint is not completely stable, the joint is typically comfortable even under maximal load from the elevator muscles. The condyle will continue to lose height as its bearing surface breaks down. This shortened condylar height puts more load on the posterior teeth, which in turn activates an occluso-muscle disorder of hyperactivity and incoordination. As a result, any discomfort in this type of problem is almost always myogenous pain, frequently combined with soreness of the overloaded teeth. The intracapsular structure can be ruled out as a source of pain by load testing.

It is my consistent experience that patients with slowly progressing osteoarthritis can be made as comfortable as patients with intact TMJs if occlusal harmony is established with adapted centric posture. If both condyles can accept loading with no discomfort, relief of myofascial pain is highly predictable if all occlusal interferences to the bone-braced condylar position are completely eliminated so the lateral pterygoid muscles can release and stay released through complete closure to maximal intercuspation (Figure 8-5).

Typically it is necessary to periodically readjust the occlusion as condylar height is lost, but it does not create a management problem if patients are informed of this need in advance. Minimal corrections to the occlusion may be required every few months to maintain a harmonious occlusion that does not trigger occluso-muscle disturbances.

OTHER PARTIAL DISK DERANGEMENTS AND CLICKING TMJs

Reciprocal clicking is always a sign of damage to the ligaments that tether the disk in place. A disk cannot click if the posterior and collateral ligaments are intact. The variations in deformation of the ligaments and disk appear unlimited. However many clicking and deformed TMJs have adapted sufficiently so that they can comfortably accept loading. If a structural analysis shows that the condition is manageably stable, adapted centric posture may be achieved, even though the disk is deranged and a click is present. The key is whether the joint can be completely seated up into the bony stop in the fossa, so the inferior lateral pterygoid muscles can release contraction as the jaw closes to maximal intercuspation.

There is no difference in the procedure for determining either centric relation or adapted centric posture. Both should be confirmed by load testing to verify that the joint is completely seated and the lateral pterygoid muscle is released.

What is different is that a deformed joint that has adapted to a comfortable capacity to accept loading is not as stable as an intact TMJ. So patients should always be advised in advance of any occlusal treatment that there will be a need for periodic occlusal correction to maintain harmony with the changing joint position. Nevertheless, it is a manageable condition, and if the occlusion is meticulously corrected, follow-up corrections usually require only minimal changes.

For accuracy in research and for validity in communication, it is necessary to distinguish between centric relation and adapted centric posture. Long-term stability of the TMJs and thus the stability of any occlusal relationship is dependent on the condition of the intracapsular structures. Both the position and the condition of the TMJs must be classified and related to maximal intercuspation.

Many patients in adapted centric posture also display excessive attritional wear so they are often candidates for extensive restorative dentistry. If in doubt about the stability of the TMJs, it is wise to evaluate using a full occlusal splint long enough to ascertain that the TMJs are manageably stable. The occlusal splint should be meticulously adjusted with posterior disclusion via anterior guidance. If the occlusion stays acceptably stable for up to three months and there are no other concerns, proceed with the restorative phase.

SUMMARY

The condyles are in adapted centric posture (Figure 8-6) if five criteria are fulfilled.

1. The condyles are comfortable when fully seated at the highest point against the eminentiae.
2. The medial poles are braced against bone. (The disk may or may not be interposed at the medial pole.)

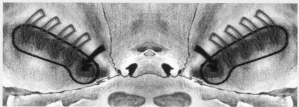

FIGURE 8-6 If the disk is completely displaced and the retrodiskal tissues have perforated, the bone-to-bone contact enlarges and flattens. While not as stable as an intact joint, it responds to occlusal harmony the same as does centric relation.

3. The inferior lateral pterygoid muscle has released its contraction and is passive.
4. The condyle-fossae relationships are at a manageable level of stability.
5. Just as in centric relation, the joints must be totally free of any tension or tenderness when load tested with firm compressive force up through the TMJs.

References

1. Dawson PE: New definition for relating occlusion to varying conditions of the temporomandibular joint. *J Prosthet Dent* 75(6):619-627, 1995.
2. Schellhas KP, Piper MA, Ornlie MR: Facial skeleton remodeling due to temporomandibular joint degeneration: An imaging study of 100 patients. *Am J Neuroradial* 11:541-551, 1990.
3. Lytle JD: The clinician's index of occlusal disease: Definition, recognition, and management. *Int J Periodont Rest Dent* 10:102-123, 1990.

Chapter 9

Determining Centric Relation

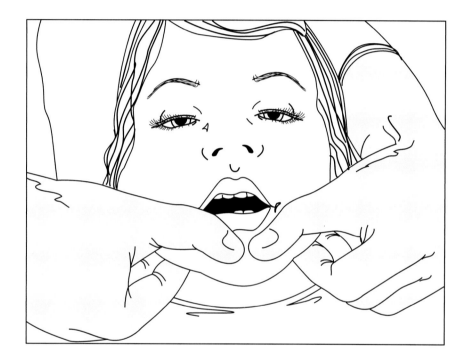

PRINCIPLE

Until the position and condition of the temporomandibular joints (TMJs) are precisely determined, an accurate maxillo-mandibular relationship cannot be verified and correct occlusal analysis is not possible.

DETERMINING CENTRIC RELATION OR ADAPTED CENTRIC POSTURE

Even though centric relation is a routinely used physiologic position, it is unreliable to use an unguided closure to determine the correct maxillo-mandibular relationship. This is because in an unguided closure, the condyles are not always completely seated in centric relation. An unguided closure has a tendency to close toward the maximal intercuspation position, which is why this type of closure is referred to as a "convenience position" or a "habitual closure." Unguided closures are also profoundly affected by muscle disharmonies that result from occlusal interference; so it is a key point that a hands-on technique is a requirement for a verifiable centric relation.

The purpose of manipulating the mandible is *not* to force the jaw into centric relation. Forcing the jaw almost invariably positions the condyles inaccurately. The most common method of chin point guidance has a strong tendency to shove the jaw back, forcing the condyles down and back.

Most important is the necessity of load testing to verify that the condyles can accept very firm pressure with no sign of tension or tenderness. This requires a hands-on method to direct the loading forces properly in an upward and forward direction. Once learned, bilateral manipulation can be repeated more precisely than any other technique tested. At least seven published studies have confirmed this.

Manipulation to find and verify *adapted centric posture* is done identically as for centric relation. Determination that the joints have been deformed but have adapted must come from the history, the use of Doppler imaging, and observation of signs and symptoms; but there should be *no* sign of discomfort when adapted joints are load tested.

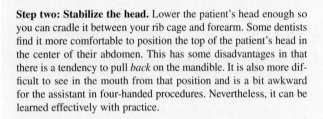

PROCEDURE   Using bilateral manipulation to find and verify centric relation or adapted centric posture

Step one: Recline the patient all the way back. Point the chin up. A supine patient is more relaxed and in a better position for the operator to work while seated. Pointing the chin up makes it easier to position the fingers on the mandible and prevents the tendency of some patients to protrude the jaw.

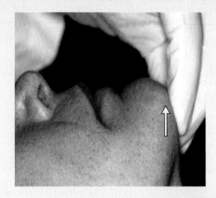

Step two: Stabilize the head. Lower the patient's head enough so you can cradle it between your rib cage and forearm. Some dentists find it more comfortable to position the top of the patient's head in the center of their abdomen. This has some disadvantages in that there is a tendency to pull *back* on the mandible. It is also more difficult to see in the mouth from that position and is a bit awkward for the assistant in four-handed procedures. Nevertheless, it can be learned effectively with practice.

Whatever method is used, it is essential that the head be stabilized in a firm grip so it will not move when the mandible is being manipulated. Failure to do this is a common mistake.

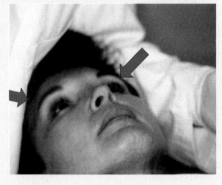

PROCEDURE   Using bilateral manipulation to find and verify centric relation or adapted centric posture—cont'd

Step three: After the head is stabilized, lift the patient's chin again to slightly stretch the neck. Be sure you are comfortably seated, with the patient low enough to allow you to work with your forearm approximately parallel to the floor.

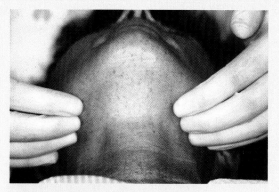

Step four: Gently position the four fingers of each hand on the lower border of the mandible. The little finger should be slightly behind the angle of the mandible. Position the pads of your fingers so they align with the bone, as if you were going to lift the head. Keep all four fingers tightly together.

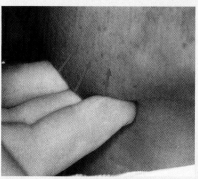

Step five: Bring the thumbs together to form a C with each hand. The thumbs should fit in the notch above the symphysis. *No pressure should be applied at this time. All movements should be made gently.*

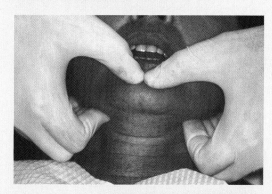

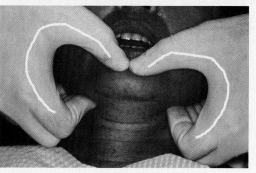

Continued

PROCEDURE   Using bilateral manipulation to find and verify centric relation or adapted centric posture—cont'd

Ensure that the fingers are properly positioned. The most common mistake in taking centric relation is positioning the fingers too far forward. Draw an imaginary line in the *center* of the inferior border of the mandible (dotted line). This separates the front half from the back half. *Do not let your fingers move forward off that line.* Keep the fingers tightly together and confined to the back half, where the elevator muscles are located.

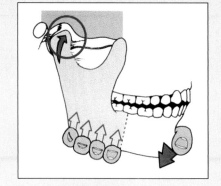

Step six: With a very gentle touch, manipulate the jaw so it slowly hinges open and closed. As it hinges, the mandible will usually slip up into centric relation automatically *if no pressure is applied.* Any pressure applied before the condyles are completely seated will be resisted by the lateral pterygoid muscles. The contracted muscles will be stretched by the pressure and will respond with greater muscle contraction (stretch reflex reaction). Once these positioner muscles have been stimulated to contraction, it is extremely difficult to seat the condyles into centric relation. The key at this point is *delicacy. There should be no pressure and no jiggling,* as this also activates muscle response. Use slow hingeing movements so the muscles are not triggered into contraction.

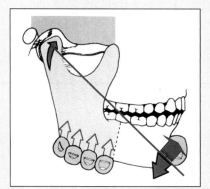

The whole purpose of this step is to deactivate the muscles. We often describe this procedure as *"romancing the mandible."* Remember that we are really just *letting* the condyles go where they physiologically want to be—properly seated in their respective fossa. When hingeing the jaw in this position, it is not necessary to open wide. An arc of one or two millimeters is acceptable. *When arcing, do not let the teeth touch.*

If the patient resists even gentle manipulation by holding the jaw in protrusion, position the hands *gently* and then *ask the patient* to hinge open and close. At the point that closing action starts to occur, the mandible will usually retrude automatically. If the hands simply ride along with the patient's own jaw movement, you will feel the jaw go back. *Then* hold it firmly on that hinge position in preparation for the next step.

Step seven: After the mandible feels like it is hingeing freely and the condyles seem to be fully seated up in their fossae, most experienced clinicians will assume that the mandible is in centric relation.

Key point
No matter how solidly the condyles seat and how freely the mandible hinges, you cannot tell by touch alone that the condyles are in centric relation. Centric relation must be verified by load testing.

We know of no other clinical test for verification of centric relation that is as reliable as load testing. We *never accept as accurate* any centric relation record that has not been verified by load testing.

The position and alignment of each condyle (Figure 9-1) must be tested by applying firm pressure **up** with the fingers on the back half of the mandible and **down** with thumb pressure in the notch above the symphysis. But it is very important that load testing be applied in increments starting with gentle upward pressure through the condyles while the thumbs keep the teeth apart. Sudden heavy loading could injure the retrodiskal tissue if the disk is displaced and could cause considerable pain. The same is true of intracapsular pathosis or edema from trauma. So always start with *gentle*

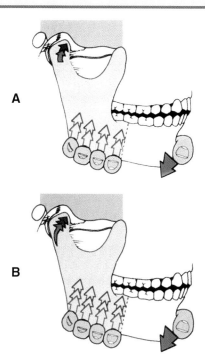

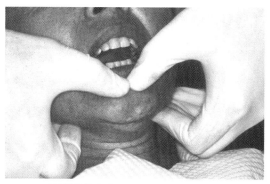

FIGURE 9-2 Proper hand positioning.

FIGURE 9-1 Testing position and alignment of each condyle. **A,** Always begin with gentle loading. **B,** Thumbs and fingers load the joints in an upward and forward direction.

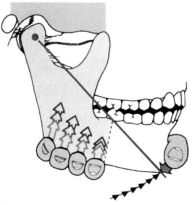

FIGURE 9-3 Condyles are kept firmly loaded while the mandible hinges to the first point of tooth contact.

loading. If there is no response of discomfort, proceed to moderate pressure and then firm pressure. With correct manipulation, there is a torque effect from the thumbs and fingers that loads the joints in an upward and forward direction.

With proper hand position, very firm upward pressure can be *maintained* through the condyles, while still allowing them to rotate freely.

Be certain that the direction of loading from the fingers is the same as the upward, forward pull of the masseter muscles to keep the condyle-disk assemblies loaded against the eminentiae. It is not possible to do this correctly if the four fingers are too far forward, which is one of the most common mistakes.

The instructions to the patient at this point must be very specific (Figure 9-2). Ask the patient, "Do you feel any sign of tenderness or tension in either joint when I apply pressure?" It is a good idea to lightly rub your finger on the skin over the joint area so the patient knows exactly where the joints are before pressure is applied.

Key point

If there is any sign of tenderness or tension in either joint when it is loaded, we cannot accept that position as centric relation. You must ask.

If the intracapsular structures are healthy and in proper alignment at the uppermost bone-braced position with no muscle bracing, there will be no tenderness or tension of any kind, even with very firm pressure.

If centric relation cannot be verified, it is essential to proceed with a differential diagnosis protocol to determine specifically what is wrong.

If centric relation can be verified, the condyles should be kept under loading pressure while the jaw hinges on its centric relation axis to the first point of tooth contact (Figure 9-3). At that point, the relationship between the TMJs and the occlusion can be studied.

After verification of centric relation or adapted centric posture, an interocclusal bite record should be made so casts can be mounted in a precisely correct relationship. The same manipulation procedure is used in order to hold the condyles up and maintain firm loading force while the bite record is being made.

IS CENTRIC RELATION REALLY REPEATABLE?

If any factor related to occlusion must be understood with complete clarity, it is that centric relation is *precisely* repeatable to within needlepoint accuracy. Dentists who do not understand TMJ anatomy are typically confused about such repeatability because they have a false idea of how the TMJs function. With a correct understanding of joint anatomy, it will be apparent why a precise centric relation is critical.

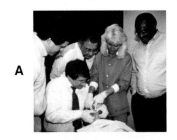

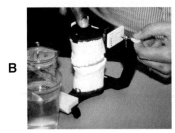

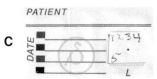

FIGURE 9-4 **A,** A group of dentists at the Dawson Center learn how to precisely determine, record, and verify centric relation. **B,** Multiple bites by the different attendees compared on the Centrichek. **C,** Identical needlepoint position of the condyles on five different centric relation bite records made by five different dentists on the same patient. This is a routine result achieved by almost every dentist with a day or two of hands-on instruction.

Centric relation can be precise because the condyle in its dense unyielding disk is *stopped by bone.* Only when it reaches that bony stop at centric relation will the inferior lateral pterygoid muscles release their contraction. This is the key to successful muscle coordination and peaceful function.

Dentists who clearly understand this concept can learn quickly how to manipulate the mandible to centric relation and *verify* that they have achieved it to needlepoint accuracy (Figure 9-4).

WHY USE BILATERAL MANIPULATION?

Bilateral manipulation is not the *only* way to position the mandible in centric relation.[1] But in our studies involving more than 3000 dentists attempting to record centric relation, we have found it to be the most consistently accurate method and the most repeatable. Several university studies agree with this finding.[2-5] Therefore, the first reason to use bilateral manipulation is its accuracy.

Bilateral manipulation achieves the most physiologic position and alignment of the condyle-disk assembly. Gilboe[3] studied condyle-disk alignment using arthrotomography, and he related the position and alignment of the condyle and disk to an optimum joint position. He then compared the optimum

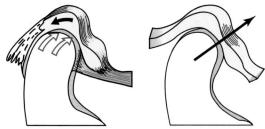

FIGURE 9-5 According to Gilboe,[3] "pressure exerted through the condylar articular surface on the slightly displaced posterior band tends to wedge the disk to its correct position."

position and alignment with results achieved by various methods of recording centric relation. He found that bilateral manipulation has a beneficial effect on slightly displaced disks while chin point guidance actually displaces the disk more anteriorly. Gilboe showed why manipulating the mandible in an appropriate way may seat a disk in the desired position if the malposition is not too great: "Dawson's bimanual manipulation technique positions the mandible posteriorly while simultaneously directing force superoanteriorly on the condyles" (Figure 9-5).

Bilateral manipulation is designed to achieve the most superior placement of the properly aligned condyle-disk assemblies. Williamson reported research findings from laminographic studies that support this concept.[8] "The need for achieving a superior position of the condyles becomes apparent and tends to support the hypothesis of Dawson who refers to centric relation as when the condyles are superior in the glenoid fossae."

Bilateral manipulation provides a quick verification of:

1. The correctness of the position.
2. The alignment of the condyle-disk assembly.
3. The integrity of the articular surfaces.

This is unquestionably the most important difference between bilateral manipulation and other jaw-positioning techniques. The ability to exert firm upward pressure through the condyles while the teeth are separated is the key to verifying the acceptability of the completely seated joint position. It is also an important step in the process of determining if an intracapsular structural disorder is present.

Bilateral manipulation is fast and uncomplicated. Once the correct method of manipulation has been learned, the centric relation position can usually be located *and verified* in a few seconds. Of course, the procedure must be learned and a level of skill developed before it can be totally reliable, but that is true of all techniques. Because a correct jaw-to-jaw relationship is so critical to all occlusal therapy, including the repetitious marking of centric relation interferences during equilibration or even simple bite adjustments after operative procedures, determining centric relation is the single most important procedure a dentist should learn. Once learned well, it gives the operator exceptional control over jaw movement. In most cases, it eliminates the need for extra procedures such as bite planes or repositioners and al-most completely eliminates the need for drugs to reduce muscle activity.

OTHER METHODS FOR DETERMINING CENTRIC RELATION OR ADAPTED CENTRIC POSTURE

Bilateral manipulation is not the only method for determining centric relation. Other methods can also be effective as long as the operator understands the goal of complete seating of both condyles and complete release of the inferior lateral pterygoid muscles.

Anterior Bite Stops

There are many different versions of anterior stops. They work well if they permit separation of all posterior teeth, and if the condyles are completely free to move horizontally and vertically to their uppermost seated positions. All of these appliances require a bite material for the posterior teeth after centric relation has been achieved. Some available methods follow.

Directly Fabricated Anterior Deprogramming Device

The earliest anterior deprogramming devices were fabricated directly, by molding autocuring acrylic resin to engage the incisal edges of the upper incisors (Figure 9-6). During the doughy stage, the mandible is manipulated to centric relation, or as close to it as can be achieved. The jaw is then closed so the lower incisors indent the soft acrylic, but closure is stopped short of posterior contact. After curing is completed, the tooth contact surface is ground to a smooth flat surface that permits full horizontal movement of the mandible. If the TMJs are intact and the lateral pterygoid muscles are completely released and passive, the patient can squeeze firmly to hold the condyles in centric relation as a fast-setting bite material is injected between the posterior teeth. All currently available anterior bite stop devices are patterned after these early appliances. They all work in exactly the same way by separating the posterior teeth so the condyles can completely seat up into centric relation. In spite of a variety of claims made for commercially available forms, none can claim superiority over the others.

The Pankey Jig

The Pankey jig (Figure 9-7) was designed many years ago by Dr. Keith Thornton. It is cost-effective and easy to use. It is fixated on the upper central incisors with autocure acrylic or any hard-setting material. The lower incisors slide freely against a flat surface to give unimpeded freedom for condylar movement to centric relation.

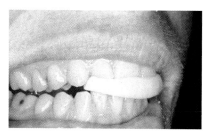

FIGURE 9-6   A directly fabricated anterior deprogramming device.

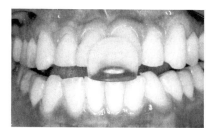

FIGURE 9-7   The Pankey jig.

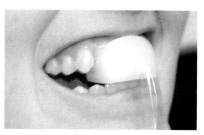

FIGURE 9-8   The Best-bite appliance.

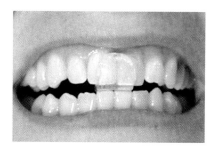

FIGURE 9-9   The Lucia jig.

The Best-bite Appliance

The Best-bite appliance (Figure 9-8) works exactly the same way as the Pankey jig. A kit is available with an injection material for stabilizing the appliance. A book by Dr. Jerry Simons can be used for patient education to explain the relationship of occlusal interferences to TMJ pain and headaches.

The Lucia Jig

The Lucia jig also works the same as other anterior stops (Figure 9-9). Lucia was one of the first to employ an anterior stop.[6] His original design was slanted to direct the condyles distally based on early misconceptions about cen-

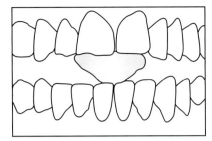

FIGURE 9-10 The NTI device.

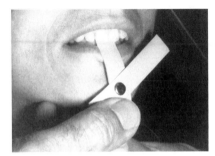

FIGURE 9-11 The leaf gauge.

tric relation being "most retruded." The jig was first modified by Dr. Peter Neff to permit upward condylar movement without the distalizing effect.

NTI (Nociceptive Trigeminal Inhibition)

The NTI device (Figure 9-10) has been heavily advertised as an appliance for treating migraine headaches and other facial pain problems. In reality, it is nothing more and nothing less than any of the other anterior bite stop devices. It works exactly like the other methods described above. If the cause of the masticatory system pain and the headache is an occluso-muscle disorder, as it often is, separation of the posterior teeth, complete seating of the TMJs, and release of the inferior lateral pterygoid muscles will result in centric relation and will relieve the pain, including related headache pain. If an intracapsular disorder is a primary cause of the pain, none of the above devices will completely relieve the pain, nor will they result in a correct centric relation. In fact, there can be a danger in the use of such appliances if an intracapsular disorder is present, as it can create an overload on painful misaligned tissues.

Leaf Gauge

The leaf gauge, one of the most popular aids for determining centric relation (Figure 9-11), was introduced by Dr. Hart Long many years ago.[7] This device consists of layers of flexible mylar that can be adjusted to varying thicknesses. The principle is to separate the posterior teeth by placing the gauge between the anterior teeth. The material is smooth and slick, so it allows the mandible to move horizontally as the

condyles seat up. It can be used as a deprogramming device for release of lateral pterygoid bracing. After centric relation has been confirmed (by load testing), layers of the gauge can be removed until the first tooth interference contacts.

Note: All of the above methods have value if used with an understanding of the goal of complete upward seating of the condyles. All methods require use of an accurate material for recording the bite relationship at the posterior teeth, as the anterior stop prevents posterior occlusal contact. *The ideal way* to use any anterior stop is to combine its use as a muscle deprogrammer with bilateral load testing after you think centric relation has been achieved. After centric relation has been verified, have the patient clench to hold the condyles in the fully seated position while the bite recording material is placed and set. My preference is to maintain joint position bimanually to ensure that there is no joint movement from centric relation until the recording material is set.

Load the Joints

Clinical experience with thousands of patients has proven its value. Firm loading of the TMJs during recording centric relation does make a difference. This became apparent in patient after patient as we evaluated our results from equilibrations. Finishing every equilibration by marking premature contacts that could only be observed with very firm loading of the joints has proven to be the answer to achieving what we refer to as the "wow" factor. What resulted from changing a "pretty good" result into an uncompromised success was the added factor of *very firm* loading of the joints to find and eliminate all premature contacts. For many years, we have observed the same practice for every centric relation recording, including those in which an anterior bite stop or a leaf gauge was used. The difference in joint position may be difficult to discern clinically, but the results of treatment will definitely be obvious.

Disadvantages of Anterior Bite Stops

The value of anterior bite stops is primarily in their usefulness as muscle deprogrammers. They do this by separating the posterior teeth so deflective posterior interferences cannot influence the musculature to displace the condyles. Thus they are an excellent aid in finding and verifying an accurate centric relation. Many dentists prefer the use of anterior bite stops as a routine step in locating centric relation. This is acceptable, but use of anterior bite stops does not eliminate the value or need for learning proper bilateral manipulation (Figure 9-12).

- During equilibration procedures, you cannot mark occlusal interferences with an anterior bite stop in place. Bilateral manipulation ensures correct condylar position during closure *all the way to tooth contact*.
- Even with an anterior bite stop in place, load testing to verify centric relation is the only sure way to ensure accuracy.

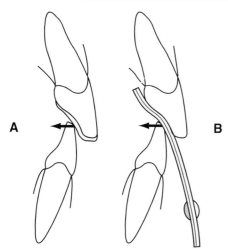

FIGURE 9-12 *Warning:* An improperly made anterior stop (**A**) can displace the condyles distally. Likewise, a leaf gauge (**B**) can force the condyles distally if used with strong elevator muscle contraction in combination with a steep, deep overbite.

- Load testing can be done in increments starting with gentle loading first to rule out intracapsular disorders before firm loading by elevator muscles when an anterior bite stop is in place.
- Bilateral manipulation with load testing has been proven to be accurate without the need for added appliances or extra steps. However, if combining bilateral manipulation with an anterior deprogrammer appliance is helpful to the operator, it should be used.
- Use whatever it takes to achieve accuracy in recording centric relation—but for accuracy with the highest level of efficiency, you will find that it is worth the time and effort to become proficient in bilateral manipulation. It is a skill that will be used on every patient.

References

1. Kantor ME, Silverman SI, Garfinkel L: Centric relation recording techniques: A comparative investigation. *J Prosthet Dent* 28:593, 1975.
2. Hobo S, Iwata T: Reproducibility of mandibular centricity in three dimensions. *J Prosthet Dent* 53:649, 1985.
3. Gilboe D: Centric relation as the treatment position. *J Prosthet Dent* 50:685-689, 1983.
4. McKee JR: Comparing condylar position repeatability for standardized versus nonstandardized methods of achieving centric relation. *J Prosthet Dent* 77:280-284, 1997.
5. Roblee R: A comparison of recording methods for centric relation. Thesis at Baylor University, 1989.
6. Lucia VO: A technique for recording centric relation. *J Prosthet Dent* 14:492, 1964.
7. Long JH Jr: Location of the terminal hinge axis by intraoral means. *J Prosthet Dent* 23:11, 1970.
8. Williamson EH: Laminographic study of mandibular condyle position when recording centric relation. *J Prosthet Dent* 39:561-564, 1978.

Chapter 10

Load Testing for Verification of Centric Relation

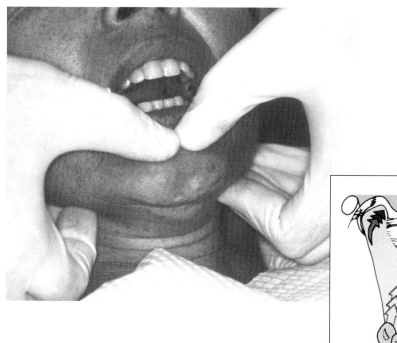

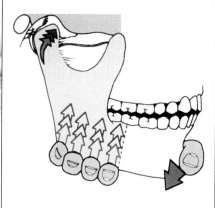

PRINCIPLE

If the temporomandibular joints (TMJs) are not completely comfortable when firmly loaded, they are not in centric relation.

One of the most significant procedures in the diagnostic process is also one of the most disparaged. Once understood, however, it will be obvious why *load testing* of the TMJs is an essential step in the determination and verification of centric relation or adapted centric posture. It is also an absolutely safe procedure to use on any patient if some simple rules are followed.

Load testing is not only an essential step in the verification of centric relation, it is a critical step in the differential diagnosis of intracapsular TMJ disorders. I have no doubt that if more dentists would learn and understand the proper method and rationale for load testing, there would be much less confusion about diagnosis and treatment selection for temporomandibular disorders (TMDs). In the specific classification of intracapsular TMDs, load testing is one of the explicit requirements in the classification process. Load testing is a simple process to understand and has application in every dental specialty or in general practice.

One of the most practical uses for load testing is that it is a fast, simple, and safe procedure for determining whether an intracapsular structural disorder is or is not a source of orofacial pain.

RATIONALE FOR LOAD TESTING OF TMJS

If the TMJs are in centric relation, all forces go through avascular noninnervated structures, and the inferior lateral pterygoid muscles have completely released their contraction (Figure 10-1).

There is no discomfort in the TMJs when loaded in this relationship, and there is no discomfort in the masticatory musculature from loading.

If the condyle-disk assemblies are completely seated up to the most superior position in the fossae, all upward movement is stopped by bone.[1-7] At this point, the inferior lateral pterygoid muscles release all contraction[8,9] (Figure 10-2). Even firm upward loading cannot stretch the muscles to

cause a response because the condyles cannot move higher. This is centric relation.

PROPER LOAD TESTING MUST BE DONE IN INCREMENTS

The first increment of load testing is always done with gentle compression. The loading process is not done to force the condyles into centric relation. Load testing is done to *verify* that the condyles are completely seated *after the operator has gently manipulated the mandible* to a freely hingeing position that is suspected of being in centric relation. There are many instances in which the condyles hinge freely and appear to be at a solid stopping point that feels like centric relation, but load testing produces tension or tenderness. *Any* sign of tension or tenderness on loading is an absolute indication that the condyle on the affected side is not fully seated, or that there is some form of intracapsular structural disorder.

Clinical experience has taught us much about the implications of load testing results. If the first increment of gentle loading produces discomfort, it is a fairly consistent indication that the discomfort is the result of compression on damaged tissue. The damage may be a displaced disk, or it may be pathology. Load testing does not readily distinguish the exact nature of the problem. What is does is warn us that a problem is present. A specific diagnosis must follow to determine the exact cause of the discomfort before proceeding with irreversible treatment. Remember that whenever there is a structural intracapsular disorder that cannot comfortably accept loading, muscle will also be involved as a source of discomfort when the joints are loaded. Muscle always attempts to protect a sore joint so the inferior lateral pterygoid muscle will be in contraction and will resist complete seating of the TMJs.

A response to *gentle loading* can also occur in the absence of an intracapsular disorder. The lateral pterygoid muscles can respond to occlusal interferences with intense hyperactivity that leads to painful spasm. Resistance to re-

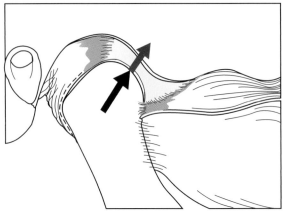

FIGURE 10-1 In centric relation, all forces are directed through vascular, noninnervated structures.

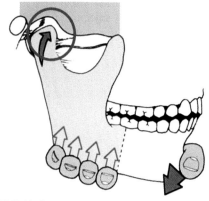

FIGURE 10-2 Proper load testing starts with gentle loading.

lease of that hypercontraction may produce pain on load testing even with a healthy, intact TMJ. It is important to recognize that load testing is but one of the tests used in evaluating the TMJs. Any response to load testing must be further evaluated by history, range and path of motion, auscultation, muscle palpation, and, if needed, imaging. If there does not appear to be an intracapsular disorder, the best diagnostic choice for separating a joint disorder from an occluso-muscle disorder is use of an anterior deprogramming device. The separation of the posterior teeth for even a few minutes is often all that is needed to verify that the TMJs are not the source of pain on loading. Once this decision has been made and the joints can be further loaded with moderate then firm compression, centric relation can be confirmed and an accurate bite record can be made. Properly mounted casts are always the logical choice for analysis of the occlusal relationship to determine the best way to bring the teeth into harmony with the correct maxillo-mandibular relationship.

A response to *moderate loading* is in most instances a response in muscle. TMJs that have deformed and have not completely adapted can sometimes require the second increment of loading before eliciting a response of discomfort. If the response is described as "tension" or "tightness," it is most likely a problem of muscle bracing rather than an intracapsular structural disorder.

If no response is elicited until the third increment of *firm loading,* it is my experience that it is most likely a response to muscle bracing. It is essential to the process of load testing that loading force start with gentle compression through the TMJs and only intensifies if there is no response. Intensification from gentle to firm should be a continuous process. Do not release compressive force before advancing to the next level of firmness unless the patient responds to a lower level with discomfort.

COMMON MISTAKES

The two most common mistakes we see in the load testing process are:

1. Applying too much pressure too soon
2. Not applying enough upward loading force at the final increment

Applying Too Much Pressure Too Soon

In spite of all admonitions against it, there is a tendency of some dentists to feel that they must overpower any resistant muscles and force the condyles into centric relation. This is the opposite of what is necessary. Too much force suddenly applied elicits a stretch reflex response in the lateral pterygoid muscle, which then attempts to protect the joint by tightly contracting to hold the condyle forward. The entire process of locating a precise centric relation axis is a gentle process. Load testing should not start until the operator assumes that the joints are fully seated. Then loading force should start with gentleness and become gradually firmer if there is no response to each increment of loading.

Not Applying Enough Upward Loading Force

If the patient has no response to lighter compressive force, the upward force through the TMJs must be increased until the loading force is very firm. After each increment of force is increased, the patient must be asked, "Do you feel *any sign* of tenderness or tension in either joint?" There will be many patients whose jaw hinges freely and seems to be at a definite centric relation stopping point. Their response to load testing is negative until very firm loading force is applied, at which point they report tension or tightness (only if asked). After deprogramming with a cotton roll between the teeth, one or both condyles may be able to move further up, sometimes a considerable distance before the joints are in a correct centric relation (Figures 10-3 and 10-4).

Hand position is very important for effective load testing. Note the position of the fingers on the back half of the mandible so firm upward pressure can be applied through the condyles. Thumbs should be positioned in the notch above the symphysis so downward pressure at the front of the mandible keeps the teeth apart while the condyles are being elevated.

MISLEADING CONCERNS ABOUT LOAD TESTING

When I first presented the concept of load testing before a national academy many years ago, a renowned clinician ran up on the stage after my presentation, shook his finger at me, and advised me, "If you keep shoving that jaw up in that socket, one day you're going to shove that condyle right into the brain." His advice was based on a misconception about the anatomy of the fossa, but nevertheless this misconcep-

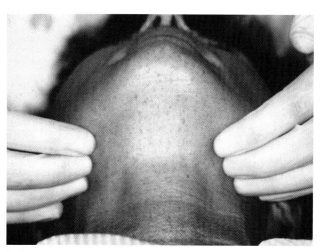

FIGURE 10-3 Fingers should be together on back half of mandible.

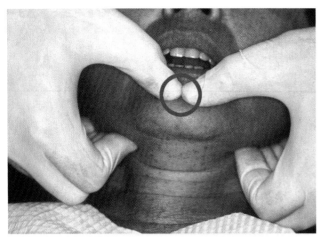

FIGURE 10-4 Thumbs should touch and should fit into the notch above the symphysis.

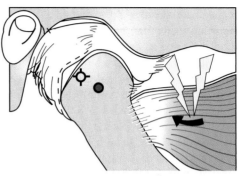

FIGURE 10-5 If the condyle is not completely seated to centric relation, it will be held down and forward by muscle. Load testing will then produce tension and tenderness.

tion has prevailed among some clinicians and is a major reason for much confusion about centric relation and occlusion in general.

This misconception arises from the fact that the roof of the fossa is paper-thin, and it is true that brain tissue lies just above that thin bone. However, the roof of the fossa never comes in compressive contact with the condyle-disk assembly, even if maximal force is directed upward through the condyles. The heavily buttressed medial third of the fossa is the very adequate stopping point for the condyle disk assembly. A meta-analysis of the world literature indicates that perforation of the roof of the fossa by a condyle is extremely rare and occurs only from severe traumatic injury.

Another misconception also arises from a mistaken picture of intracapsular anatomy. It is the warning that load testing compresses the retrodiskal tissues behind the condyle. It is not possible to compress retrodiskal tissue by load testing an intact TMJ unless the retrodiskal tissue has expanded by edema. It is precisely for this reason that load testing is such a valuable diagnostic procedure. It is also one of the reasons why load testing is always initiated by *gentle* loading first. If the retrodiskal tissue is swollen to a volume that prevents complete seating of the condyle, it will be apparent. Reduction of the edema then becomes a first order of treatment.

In a healthy intact TMJ, it is not even possible to compress retrodiskal tissue by forcing the mandible inappropriately toward the most retruded position. Forcing the mandible distal to centric relation requires the condyles to move down as they move back, directed by the posterior wall of the fossa at the medial pole.

If there is any clinical understanding that can be counted on with confidence, it is that a healthy intact TMJ can accept all loading forces that the maximal power of the elevator muscles can apply. If any TMJ cannot accept very firm load testing with total comfort, there is an absolute rule: Find out why before proceeding with specific treatment. That means that until centric relation or adapted centric posture can be verified, the patient is not ready for a final treatment plan.

RESPONSE TO LOAD TESTING IF THE CONDYLES ARE NOT COMPLETELY SEATED (MUSCLE BRACED)

If the condyle-disk assembly is down and forward from centric relation, it was pulled there by the contraction of the lateral pterygoid muscle. If the muscle does not release its contraction (Figure 10-5), upward pressure on the TMJ will have to be resisted by the muscle rather than bone. Upward pressure should be firm enough to stretch the shortened muscle so it will respond with a feeling of tenderness or tension. A *spastic* muscle will generally respond more painfully to forced stretching. If the condyle-disk assembly is completely seated, its upward movement is stopped by bone in centric relation. Then it is not possible to stretch the lateral pterygoid muscle because the condyle is already stopped from going higher and the muscle has released its contraction.

If upward pressure causes tenderness in either TMJ area, it has been our consistent experience that in most patients, the tenderness is in muscle. If the condyle is allowed to go further up the eminentia to its bone-braced stop for the medial pole, the need for muscle contraction is eliminated and upward pressure will then produce no tenderness or tension. The relief should be an immediate response when the condyle reaches centric relation. (Remember that all load testing must be done with the teeth apart.)

If gentle manipulation does not work to "romance" the condyle up, release of lateral pterygoid muscle contraction can be aided by any procedure that disengages the occlusal deflection. This takes away the sensory trigger that activates positioner muscle contraction. A cotton roll between the teeth generally works quite well in 5 to 20 minutes to release muscle contraction or spasm and permits easier manipulation to centric relation.

Bite planes permit a release of muscle spasm by providing a smooth surface to cover the deflective inclines. This gives the condyles the freedom to go to their physiologic po-

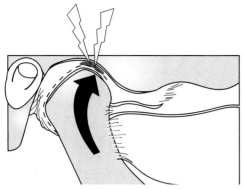

FIGURE 10-6 If the disk is displaced, compression of vascular retrodiskal tissue can produce discomfort.

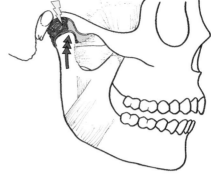

FIGURE 10-7 Trauma to the joint can result in edema and inflammation to the retrodiskal tissue. Compression of the swollen tissue can be painful.

sition rather than forcing the muscles to relate them to the malrelated occlusion.

The most effective bite plane is a flat, smooth surface that is contacted by the anterior teeth only. Separation of the posterior teeth permits one or both condyles to move upward without posterior tooth contact. This has the additional effect of shutting off about two thirds of the elevator muscles in addition to the inferior lateral pterygoid muscle.

RESPONSE TO LOAD TESTING IF THE DISK IS MISALIGNED

The stress-bearing area of the disk is fibrocartilage. It is avascular and has no sensory nerve endings, so when the condyle is properly aligned with the disk, it can resist great pressure with no discomfort.

The tissues around the periphery of the support area of the disk, however, are vascular and are innervated with sensory nerve endings. Pressure on these tissues stimulates a response of discomfort or pain (Figure 10-6). Therefore, upward pressure exerted on the condyle will produce discomfort if the disk is not properly aligned, especially if it is completely displaced off both poles.

If it is not possible to manipulate the condyles into a position that can resist pressure comfortably, and if separation of the teeth with a cotton roll gives no relief, we *suspect* a condyle-disk derangement or pathologic intracapsular problem.

It will be necessary to determine the specific classification of any intracapsular disorder *before* proceeding with treatment.

RESPONSE TO LOAD TESTING IF THERE IS INTRACAPSULAR PATHOLOGY OR INJURY

The third possibility to evaluate when upward pressure causes discomfort is the possibility of pathosis or injury to the intracapsular structures (Figure 10-7).

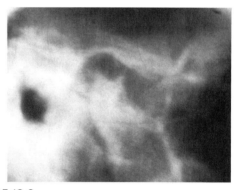

FIGURE 10-8 Degenerative bone disease can produce discomfort when load testing compresses the disordered tissues.

Trauma may result in a variety of problems, including inflammation and swelling of the retrodiskal tissues that make them painful to compression if the condyles are loaded. Fractures should always be a consideration when history of trauma is reported.

A variety of bone diseases including degenerative disorders, tumors, cysts, and growth disorders can cause deformation of intracapsular structures that causes discomfort when the joints are loaded (Figure 10-8).

The use of magnetic resonance imaging (MRI) has opened up new ways of evaluating the joints far more completely than previous methods allowed. Every general dentist should know and use basic diagnostic procedures for classification of TMJ disorders.

> Two inviolate rules for diagnosis:
> 1. Never accept a centric relation that has not been verified by load testing.
> 2. If load testing of the TMJs causes discomfort, always find out why.

References

1. Zola A: Morphologic limiting factors in the temporomandibular joint. *J Prosthet Dent* 13:732-740, 1963.

2. Kinderknecht KE, et al: The effect of a deprogrammer on the position of the terminal transverse horizontal axis of the mandible. *J Prosthet Dent* 68:123-131, 1992.
3. Hylander W: The human mandible: Lever or link. *Am J Phys Anthropol* 43:227, 1975.
4. Mansour RM, Reynik RJ: In vivo occlusal forces and moments: Forces measured in terminal hinge position and associated moments. *J Dent Res* 54:114-120, 1975.
5. Radu M, Mirandice M, Hottel TL: The effect of clenching on condylar position: A vector analysis model. *J Prosthet Dent* 91:171-179, 2004.
6. Hatcher DC, Blom RJ, Baker CG: Temporomandibular joint spatial relationships: osseous and soft tissues. *J Prosthet Dent* 56:344-353, 1986.
7. Ide Y, Nakazawa K: *Anatomical Atlas of the Temporomandibular Joint*, Chicago, 1991, Quintessence Publishing.
8. Uchida S, Whittle T, Wanigaratne K, et al: The role of the inferior head of the human lateral pterygoid muscle in the generation and control of horizontal mandibular force. *Arch Oral Biol* 46:1127-1140, 2001.
9. Mahan PE, Wilkinson TM, Gibbs CH, et al: Superior and inferior bellies of the lateral pterygoid muscle EMG activity at basic jaw positions. *J Prosthet Dent* 50:710-718, 1983.

Chapter 11

Recording Centric Relation

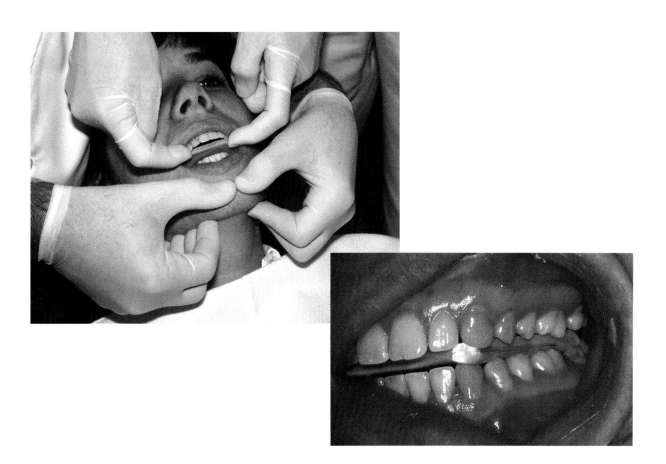

PRINCIPLE

The price for inaccurate bite records is wasted time, compromised results, and a lack of predictability.

ACCURATE RECORDING OF CENTRIC RELATION

One of the most common flaws in the literature regarding the relationship of occlusion to temporomandibular disorders (TMDs) is failure to verify that the intended joint position was actually achieved *and recorded accurately*. This same flaw is responsible for frustration, wasted time, and errors in treatment planning, and a cause for unacceptable grinding on new restorations. The price we must pay for a missed centric relation recording is always far more than the price in time to prevent it. Yet, a visit to almost any commercial dental laboratory will illustrate that accurate bite records for mounting casts are a rarity.

As shown in Chapters 9 and 10, practical methods exist for verifying the accuracy of joint positioning to within needlepoint repeatability. The preciseness of the determination of centric relation, however, can easily be lost if not matched by preciseness of the interocclusal bite record combined with an acceptable facebow record.

Some of the most published authors disagree that centric relation is a repeatable position. McNamara et al.[1] state that "a precise and reproducible method for determining the presence of occlusal supracontacts does not exist." Such a statement is provably wrong; centric relation can be reproduced on mounted casts to needlepoint accuracy. Furthermore, the process is learnable with a few hours of instruction. By using a Centrichek instrument (Teledyne, Fort Collins, Colorado), McKee[2,3] and 10 other clinicians with one morning of instruction were able to reproduce centric relation recordings to within a needlepoint hole in 10 of 10 recordings by 11 different dentists. Only 4 recordings of 110 were not perfectly centered. However, on 132 other recordings made on the same patients by 132 practicing dentists' "best method" (12 recordings on each of 11 patients), no consistent position was recorded (Figure 11-1). This study indicates why it is essential to verify condylar position in any research study purporting to analyze the effects of temporomandibular joint (TMJ)/occlusion relationships. Failure to do so explains why so many clinical studies in the literature fail to duplicate the results being claimed by careful, well-trained clinicians. Analysis of the 132 bite records representing the "best method" (see Figure 11-1) also shows why so many dentists have so much trouble with "high" crowns and deflective interferences built into new restorations.

Reasons for error in almost all of these recordings included the following:

1. Improper manipulation (chin point guidance or forcing)
2. No guidance or verification of centric relation
3. Flimsy bite-recording materials. Rubbery materials are consistently inaccurate because there is no stable position for seating the casts in the record.
4. Too-deep indentations into the bite material. This causes the compression of soft tissue in the mouth. On the casts, the soft tissue does not compress and prevents the casts from seating completely into the record.

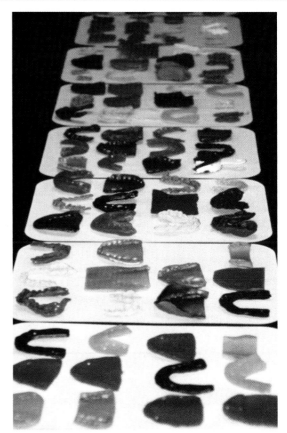

FIGURE 11-1 Sample of "best-method" centric relation bite records from 132 practicing dentists with no postgraduate training in recording centric relation.

5. Use of soft waxes that are easily distorted when casts are seated into the record.
6. Too shallow or nonexistent indentations into part of a bite record so there is no verifiable position for the casts to seat into the record.
7. Unstable bite-recording materials that warp or distort after the recording is made.

It is interesting to note that in spite of the almost universal inaccuracy of recorded bite records, none of the 132 dentists involved in the control group from diverse areas of the United States were aware that his or her bite record was flawed. Since this much unrecognized error is indicative of usual and customary dentistry, it indicates a serious shortcoming in dental education. The good news is that this is a very correctable problem as evidenced by the fact that the 11 dentists in the experimental group were able to learn a precise technique for recording centric relation in only one morning of instruction.

CRITERIA FOR ACCURACY

There are five criteria for accuracy in making an interocclusal bite record:

1. The bite record must not cause any movement of teeth or displacement of soft tissue.

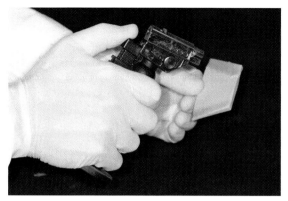

FIGURE 11-2 Using a torch to soften the wax.

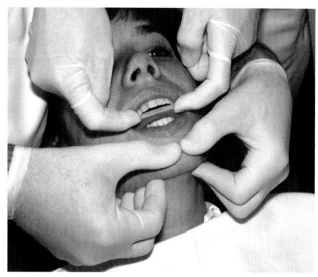

FIGURE 11-4 Closing into the wax.

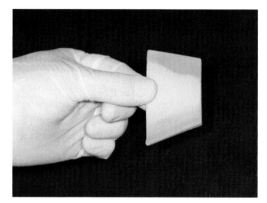

FIGURE 11-3 Shine produced by even heating on the edges.

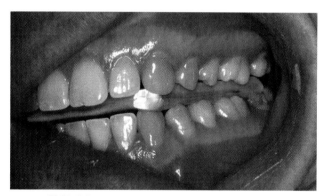

FIGURE 11-5 Wax trimmed back to buccal cusp tips.

2. It must be possible to verify the accuracy of the interocclusal record in the mouth.
3. The bite record must fit the casts as accurately as it fits the mouth.
4. It must be possible to verify the accuracy of the bite record on the casts.
5. The bite record must not distort during storage or transportation to the laboratory.

It should be possible to fulfill all five requirements for accuracy by proper selection of one of the techniques described below.

Wax Bite Record

The use of wax as a bite record is by far the most popular method. It is also easily abused. It is critical that the type of wax used is soft enough not to cause tooth movement when the wax is warmed; it must be brittle-hard when cooled. A wax that can bend without breaking when cool is not acceptable because it is too easily distorted during the mounting process. When cool, an acceptable wax should break with a snap when it is bent.

The bite record of choice for many years in our practice has been Delar wax. This brittle-hard wax is supplied in wafers that are thicker at the front for more even penetration by the teeth from back to front. The wax is softened at the edges by use of a small torch (Figure 11-2). Do not soften the middle section of the wafer. Don't overheat. Flame both sides several times to produce a shine (Figure 11-3). Let the heat soak in to soften the wax.

Place the wax against the upper arch, and compress it to lightly indent it. While the assistant holds the wax wafer in place against the upper arch, the mandible is manipulated to centric relation and verified by load testing before having the patient close into the wax. Keep upward loading compression on the condyles as the patient closes (Figure 11-4). Otherwise there is a tendency for patients to slightly protrude at the start of closing into anything between the teeth.

Be sure that the first premolars make a definite indentation. This ensures that all of the posterior teeth will be recorded with indentations that will hold the casts in a stable relationship with the bite record. While the wax is still warm, remove it and trim it back to the indentations of the buccal cusp tips so the fit of the bite record can be verified in the mouth (Figure 11-5). Note that there are no voids or cracks between the teeth and the bite record for a perfect tooth-wax-tooth fit.

Now is the time to verify the perfection of the bite record. Remove it and chill it in cold water to make it brittle-hard.

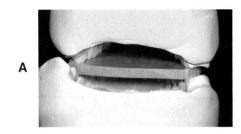

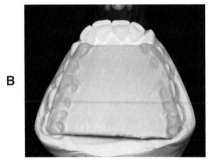

FIGURE 11-6 **A,** Wax should not touch palatal tissue. **B,** Extending across the arch.

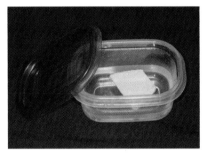

FIGURE 11-7 Storing wax in water in a sealed plastic container.

Replace it back in the mouth. Now seat the condyles and load test for verification of centric relation. Hold the condyles firmly in centric relation while the mandible hinges to bring the teeth into maximal contact with the bite record. Verify that both sides of the arch contact simultaneously with no premature contact or deflection into the hard wax. Verify that at complete closure there are no voids between the teeth and the wax.

Carefully examine the bite record to make certain there is no impingement into soft tissue. Any soft tissue contact at gingival margins should be trimmed back. If it is necessary to resoften the wax to correct for slight distortion, it is best to soften only the edge of the wafer where the teeth indent it. The wax is then placed back against the upper teeth and the mandible closed into it to readapt it.

The wax wafer should extend directly across the arch without touching palatal tissue (Figure 11-6). Wax should be thick enough so it does not bend. A one-piece wafer has a big advantage over individual quadrant bites that dislodge easily and are more difficult to adapt to casts. One-piece records are easy to control, and casts seat securely into across-the-arch indentations.

Store wax bites until needed by floating in water in a sealed plastic container (Figure 11-7). Careless handling of bite records is responsible for many mounting errors.

Once learned, the wax bite technique is the simplest and fastest way to record centric relation. It is also unsurpassed in accuracy for mounting casts because the casts fit so solidly in the record with no rocking. It is not the ideal method for every patient, and it is important to match the method used to the operator's skill and the particular needs of different patients. A second method that is particularly valuable and has many applications is the anterior stop technique.

Anterior Stop Techniques

Of all of the techniques for recording centric relation, methods using some form of anterior stop are the easiest to learn and have many applications. Anterior stop techniques can be modified to adapt to almost any clinical situation in which anterior teeth are present. Accuracy can be achieved with very loose posterior teeth, posterior edentulous ridges, and patients who are difficult to manipulate.

The term *anterior stop* as used here refers to contact in the incisor area only. When the mandible is closed, the lower incisors strike against a "stop" that is precisely fitted against the upper incisors. The stop should be thin enough so that the first point of tooth contact barely misses, but under no circumstances should any posterior tooth be allowed to contact when the anterior stop is in place (Figure 11-8).

The great advantage of the anterior stop is that it deprograms the lateral pterygoid muscles so they release contraction, allowing the condyle-disk assemblies to seat *up* without any deflection or restriction from posterior teeth. When complete seating of the TMJs is suspected, load testing should be used to verify that centric relation has been achieved. This can be done while the anterior teeth are in contact with the stop. When centric relation has been verified, a firm-setting bite paste can be injected between the posterior teeth and allowed to set (Figure 11-8, *B* and *C*).

Any of the anterior deprogramming devices shown in Chapter 9 (see also Figure 11-9) are acceptable for an anterior stop.

Power Bite

The power bite is a good idea that is often used improperly. Its misuse has fueled many controversial misinterpretations about occlusion and TMJ relationships. Proper use of the power bite method requires precise location of centric relation before closing power from the elevator muscles is applied. The power bite method starts with a bite record made between the upper and lower anterior teeth. The bite material is typically a softened compound that hardens after the indentations have been made between the upper and lower anterior teeth. The bite material is typically a softened compound that hardens after the indentations have been made by the anterior teeth. Closure of the jaw must stop short of any posterior tooth contact. The patient is then instructed to

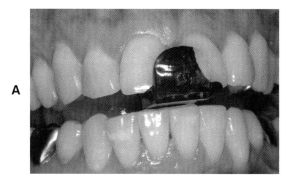

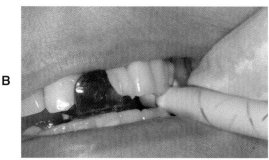

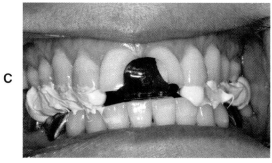

FIGURE 11-8 **A,** With an anterior deprogramming device in place, centric relation is verified by load testing, and the patient is instructed to clench to maintain the loaded joint position. No posterior teeth should be allowed to contact during bite registration. **B,** A firm-setting bite paste is injected between the posterior teeth while the patient maintains firm compression against the anterior stop. **C,** The bite material is allowed to set. The anterior stop is not used in the mounting procedure with the casts.

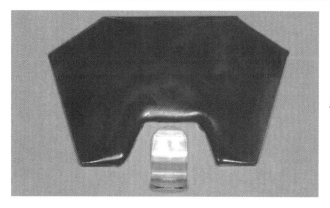

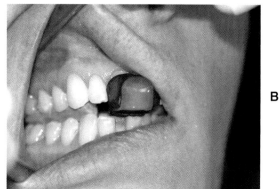

FIGURE 11-9 The wax bite record can be taken in combination with an anterior deprogramming device **(A).** The wax bite record can be cut out at the front. Bilateral manipulation should be used to seat the joints and verify centric relation as if the anterior jig **(B)** were not in place.

clench tightly to seat the condyles up into centric relation. The problem is that if the anterior segment of the bite is made with the mandible displaced from centric relation, the hardened material locks the jaw into that relationship and prevents the condyles from moving back and up (Figure 11-10).

Power bite methods only work if the bite indentations at the anterior teeth are in harmony with centric relation, or if a smooth flat surface is used at the anterior segment to permit free movement of the condyles as elevator muscles contract.

Anterior Index for Centric Relation

If centric relation can be achieved with bilateral manipulation, deprogramming the muscles is not necessary. In such cases, a different kind of anterior stop can be used that indexes the lower incisors into centric relation.

1. A little ball of red compound is softened and adapted to the upper central incisors so that their lingual surfaces are completely covered. It is extended over the incisal edges for stability.
2. With the patient in a supine position, the mandible is manipulated into centric relation and closed until the lower incisors indent the softened compound. The patient closes into the compound until the posterior teeth just barely miss contacting. The mandible is arced on its terminal axis to see whether there is any deviation off the axis as the lower incisors fit into the depressions in the compound. If there is any deviation off the arc of centric closure, the compound is resoftened and the procedure begun again.

The anterior stop should always be checked meticulously for accuracy before one proceeds with the bite record on the posterior teeth. This is done by checking against the hardened anterior stop. The centric relation axis of closure should be verified by load testing. If pressure produces tenderness in either joint area, the axis of closure is not correct.

When it is certain that the axis of closure is correct, the patient should close into the indentations in the compound. The lower incisors should go directly into the indentations with no movement of the teeth or deviation from the axis.

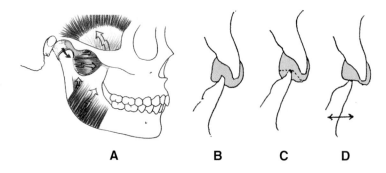

FIGURE 11-10 If the mandible is protruded (A) when anterior teeth indent an anterior stop (B) the condyles will not be permitted to go to centric relation even with a power clench. Indentations must be removed (C) and the surface must be flattened (D).

A   B   C   D

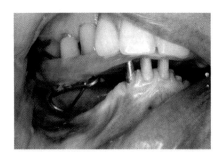

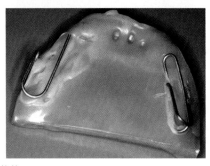

FIGURE 11-11 Premade wax base in the mouth (top) and with retention for future attachment of silicone putty (bottom).

3. When the accuracy of the anterior stop has been verified, the material for the bite record is mixed and placed on the lower teeth. The patient closes into the stop position and holds the jaws together with firm pressure. The firm pressure will hold the condyles up. The anterior stop will keep the patient from deviating from that position.

4. When the bite material has set, it is removed and trimmed back to the tips of the lower buccal cusps and the central grooves of the upper teeth. (This can vary with malposed or prepared teeth as long as the fit of the teeth against the bite material can be checked.) Now the bite record is trimmed back wherever it touched soft tissue.

5. The bite record is placed back on the upper teeth. It will usually fit snugly enough so that it will stay in place. The jaw is manipulated very carefully into a terminal axis closure, and any discrepancies between the teeth and the bite material are noted. If the record checks out as correct in the mouth, it can then be accepted for

mounting. It should be rechecked on the models to make sure it fits them as well as it fits in the mouth.

Edentulous Ridges

When large edentulous areas are present, a premade wax base can be adapted on a cast of the opposing arch. Retention can be added for future attachment of silicone putty. The wax base can then be fitted to the arch (Figure 11-11) and a manipulated centric relation closure can bring the lower anterior teeth into contact with the wax. While holding the TMJs firmly on their centric relation axis, ask the patient to lightly bite into the wax to form shallow indentations. Then chill the wax to harden it and add the putty silicone to the preformed wax base. Manipulate a verified centric relation and close into the indentations. The soft putty silicone will adapt to the opposing ridge (Figure 11-12).

The silicone should then be trimmed back so there is just a shallow groove for the ridge to fit into (Figure 11-13). Many different modifications can be made to this technique. The rule is that the casts must always fit solidly into the bite record with no rocking.

WHY CASTS MUST BE RELATED TO THE CONDYLAR AXIS

It serves no purpose to make an interocclusal bite record unless the relationship of the mandible to the maxilla is recorded when the condyles are in their uppermost physiologic position. There is very little, if any, value in studying unmounted casts, because the primary purpose of analyzing diagnostic casts is to observe tooth-to-tooth relationships in centric relation *at the correct vertical dimension*. This cannot be done on unmounted casts.

Remember that the centric relation bite record is taken with the teeth apart, so the articulator must be closed from that point to whatever vertical dimension allows maximal intercuspation. A correct axis allows changes in vertical dimension of occlusion (VDO) up or down without displacement from centric relation.

If the goal of treatment is to make centric relation (the condyle position) coincide with maximum intercuspation (the tooth-to-tooth position), how could an occlusion be analyzed

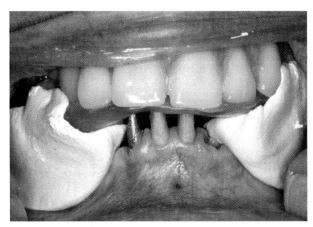

FIGURE 11-12 Silicone putty adapts to opposing ridge.

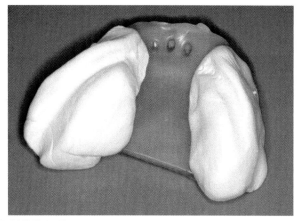

FIGURE 11-13 Shallow grooves in the silicone attached to the wax base where the edentulous ridge can fit.

without having the arc of opening-closing related around the correct condylar axis of rotation? Since it would create a considerable error to open the jaw on one hinge axis (for a bite record) and then close the casts on another hinge axis (on the articulator), the condylar axis must be located on the patient and transferred to the articulator. The *facebow* is used for this purpose. An open centric bite record without a facebow transfer has little if any value because it only records where the occlusal relationship is when the jaw is opened. *It does not show correct tooth-to-tooth relationships when the articulator is closed* to the most closed vertical dimension of occlusion, because without a facebow transfer, the arc of closure will be different on the articulator than it is on the patient.

Note the severe error in the path of a lower molar cusp when casts are mounted on a Galetti articulator and compared with the correct arc of closure related to the condylar axis (Figure 11-14). This is approximately the same type of error that results from unmounted casts.

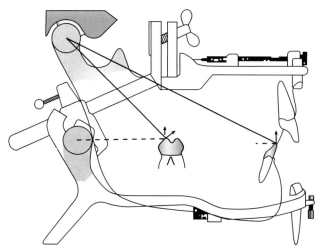

FIGURE 11-14 Direction of correct arc of closure *(solid lines)* compared to Galetti articulator *(dotted lines)*.

Effect of Arc of Closure on Bucco-Lingual Alignment

An extremely important value of correctly mounted casts (casts mounted in centric relation with a facebow to record the correct condylar axis) is that it facilitates accurate analysis of bucco-lingual relationships. To illustrate, look at the following arch alignment in centric relation as seen at the first point of contact from a front view only (Figure 11-15).

> **Key point**
>
> As the mandible closes in centric relation, the lower teeth follow an arc that moves the wider part of the lower arch forward into the narrower part of the upper arch. This has the effect of improving the bucco-lingual relationship if the lower cusp tips are lingual to the upper central groove at centric relation (Figure 11-16).
>
> If lower cusp tips are buccal to the upper central groove at centric relation, the bucco-lingual relationship will worsen.

Look again at the direction of the arc of closure on the Galetti articulator (see Figure 11-14), and relate that to unmounted casts.

Relating the Casts to the Correct Axis

A facebow relates the upper arch to the condylar axis (Figure 11-17). Transferal to the articulator maintains that relationship of the upper cast to the axis on the articulator. The lower cast is then mounted with a centric relation bite record so it is also related to the correct axis.

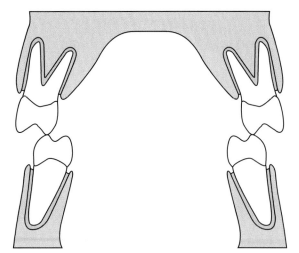

FIGURE 11-15 First point of contact in centric relation does not define where bucco-lingual relationship of arches will be when closed to correct VDO.

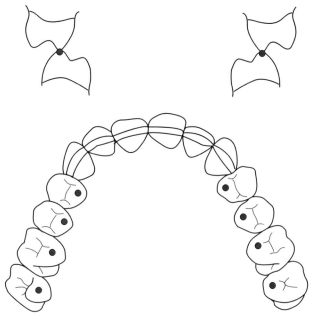

FIGURE 11-16 Red dots on the upper arch representing the lower cusp tips at centric relation contact. Plot where lower cusp tips will end up at complete closure if incline interferences are eliminated and the mandible can close without deflection from centric relation.

PROCEDURE   Facebow transfer

We use the Dénar Slidematic facebow. It is simple to use and is acceptable for all mountings. The discrepancy between the position of the earholes versus the correct condylar axis location is corrected automatically by the mounting procedure.

A facebow fork is fitted to the upper arch. Be sure the wax on the fork adapts to the upper teeth with no rocking.

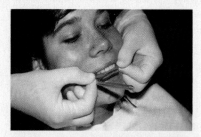

A special ruler is used to measure a spot on the face that will relate the casts to the center of the articulator. This is a convenience position. Preciseness is not required.

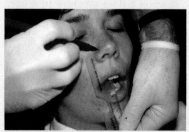

The bow is fitted onto the shaft of the bite fork. The earpieces are entered in the earholes and held in position by the assistant. The bow is leveled to the height where the pointer aligns with the mark on the face. Then the bow is secured in place by tightening the finger knobs in front.

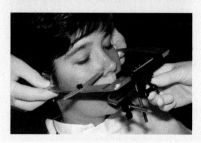

PROCEDURE   Facebow transfer—cont'd

The bite fork can then be removed (on its jig) from the facebow.

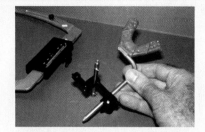

The jig and bite fork are then inserted into a positioner to be secured in place on the lower bow of the Combi articulator. This will relate the upper cast to the condylar axis. The difference between the ear-hole and the condyle position is automatically compensated for.

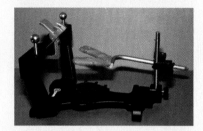

The upper cast is joined to the upper bow of the articulator. The upper bow must be locked in centric relation for this step.

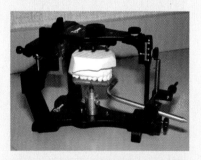

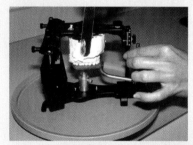

The centric relation bite record is then used to relate the lower cast to the upper cast.

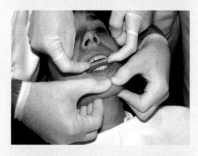

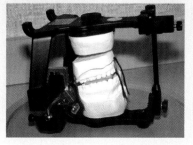

Continued

Casts are mounted on a Combi articulator in centric relation. With this mounting, the articulator can be opened or closed without changing the relationship of the casts to the centric relation axis. This is critically important when analyzing whether occlusal equilibration is an acceptable treatment option or if a different treatment choice would be better.

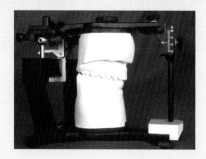

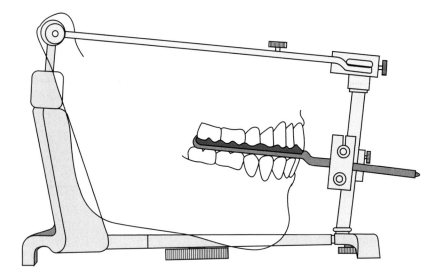

FIGURE 11-17 A facebow is an essential part of an acceptable mounting.

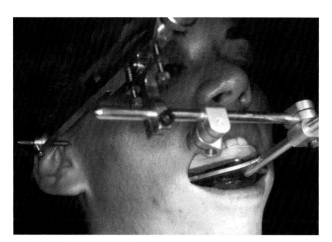

FIGURE 11-18 Kinematic hinge axis recording.

Facebow options

There are many different options regarding the use of a facebow. A facebow relates the upper cast to the horizontal condylar axis, an absolute necessity for accurate mounting of casts. In my early years of practice when gnathologic concepts were in vogue, I used a kinematic hinge axis recording to find the exact axis position (Figure 11-18).

I then learned that if I palpated the condylar fossa with the mouth wide open, the center of the indentation was rarely more than 1.5 mm from the true axis and many times it was identical. By marking the center point of the indentation with a felt pen (Figure 11-19), I eliminated the need for the hinge axis recording. Any facebow can be aligned to that axis with absolutely no loss of clinically acceptable accuracy (Figures 11-20 and 11-21).

There is no need to complicate the use of a facebow. One is as good as any other, including the most complex, as long as it relates the upper arch to the condylar axis. The simplest Hanau facebow is acceptable (Figure 11-22).

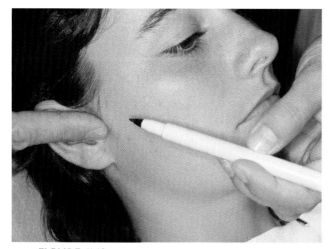

FIGURE 11-19 Marking the center point of the indentation.

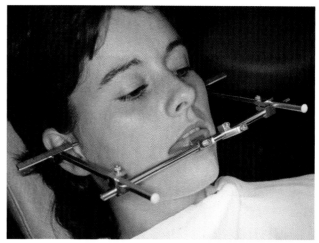

FIGURE 11-21 A facebow in alignment.

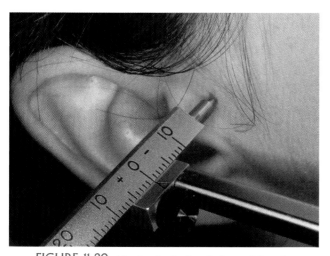

FIGURE 11-20 Aligning the facebow to the condylar axis.

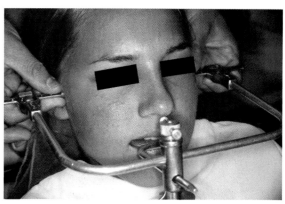

FIGURE 11-22 The Hanau facebow.

Why use an earbow?

The earbow is not as precise in locating the condylar axis. Instead of the locator rods lining up with the condyles, they are positioned into the earholes. The earbow is always used with a special jig that attaches to the front of the articulator. The jig compensates for the position of the condylar axis in relation to the earholes, so it self-corrects for the error of the earhole position. Is this correction acceptable? Some clinicians claim it is not, but I disagree. I have used earbow transfers for many years and thousands of mountings, including extremely complex diagnostic and treatment problems of occlusion. There have been no adverse effects on any restorative result from the use of an earbow. The earbow is the fastest and easiest bow to use, and you can use it with no concern whatsoever about accuracy. You'll be hard-pressed to find even the most purist gnathologist today who does not use the earbow for mounting casts. The most important thing to understand about a facebow or earbow is:

Even the most perfect centric relation bite record is inaccurate if used without relating it to the condylar axis. A facebow is a necessity for accuracy.

References

1. McNamara JA Jr, Seligman DA, Okeson JP: Occlusion, orthodontic treatment, and temporomandibular disorders: a review. *J Orofac Pain* 9:73-90, 1995.
2. McKee JR: Comparing condylar position repeatablilty for standardized versus non-standardized methods of achieving centric relation. *J Prosthet Dent* 77:280-284, 1997.
3. McKee JR: Comparing condylar positions achieved through bimanual manipulation to condylar positions achieved through masticatory muscle contraction against an anterior deprogrammer: a pilot study. *J Prosthet Dent* 94:389-393, 2005.

Chapter 12

Classification of Occlusions

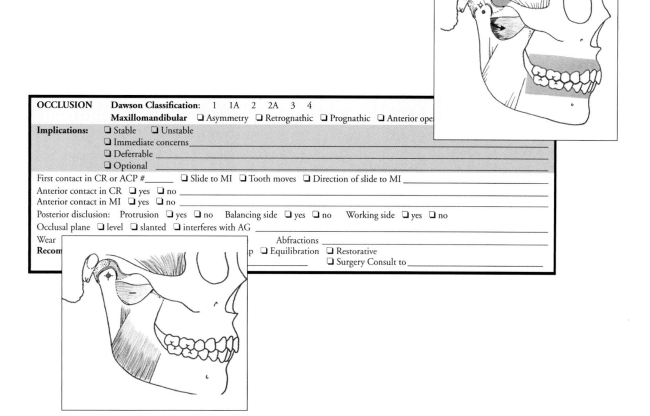

OCCLUSION	Dawson Classification:	1	1A	2	2A	3	4
	Maxillomandibular	❏ Asymmetry	❏ Retrognathic	❏ Prognathic	❏ Anterior ope		

Implications: ❏ Stable ❏ Unstable
❏ Immediate concerns_____
❏ Deferrable _____
❏ Optional _____

First contact in CR or ACP #_____ ❏ Slide to MI ❏ Tooth moves ❏ Direction of slide to MI _____

Anterior contact in CR ❏ yes ❏ no _____

Anterior contact in MI ❏ yes ❏ no _____

Posterior disclusion: Protrusion ❏ yes ❏ no Balancing side ❏ yes ❏ no Working side ❏ yes ❏ no

Occlusal plane ❏ level ❏ slanted ❏ interferes with AG _____

Wear _____ Abfractions _____

Recom_____p ❏ Equilibration ❏ Restorative
❏ Surgery Consult to _____

PRINCIPLE

To be valid, classification of occlusions must specify the relationship of maximal inter-cuspation to both the position and condition of the temporomandibular joints (TMJs).

EFFECTIVE CLASSIFICATION

It is axiomatic that maxillo-mandibular relationships cannot be right if condyle-to-fossa relationships are wrong. Regardless of how perfect an interocclusal arch-to-arch relationship may appear, if displacement of one or both condyles is required to achieve maximal intercuspation, the overall result will be occlusal disharmony and an obstacle to a coordinated peaceful neuromusculature (Figure 12-1).

For many years, the standard classification for occlusions has been *Angle's classification of malocclusion.*[1] The problem with Angle's classification is that it does not consider TMJ position or condition when relating the mandibular arch to the maxillary arch. The prevalent use of unmounted casts to document a "finished" Angle's class I occlusion is illustrative of the shortcomings in meaningful communication. The use of Angle's classification in research[2] purporting to evaluate the relationship between occlusion and temporomandibular disorders (TMDs) is too seriously flawed to be acceptable. This is because Angle's classification does not consider either the position or condition of the TMJs in relation to maximal intercuspation. In light of current knowledge regarding the exquisite sensitivity of the neuromusculature to minute deflective occlusal interferences,[3,4] it is all the more apparent that accurate diagnosis is dependent on accuracy in classification of the occlusion/TMJ relationship.

Angle's classification of malocclusion[1] has been used routinely to denote the relationship of the mandibular arch to the maxillary arch. Typically, Angle's class I occlusion is to depict a normal relationship of maxillary and mandibular arches of teeth. Class II or III occlusion indicates abnormal relationship of the arches. In class II, the mandibular arch is too distal, and in class III the mandibular arch is forward of the so called "ideal" relationship with the maxillary arch.

Analysis of any occlusion requires careful inspection of maximal intercuspation position in relation to both the position and condition of the TMJs. What might appear to be an ideal class I occlusion if joint position is not considered may be a severe class II maxillary overjet relationship when the condyles are completely seated in centric relation (Figure 12-2).

Class I arch relationship allows excellent esthetics and function with manageable stability if the class I occlusion is in harmony with the completely seated position of both TMJs. But if displacement of one or both TMJs is required to achieve a class I occlusion the result is not ideal because the deflective inclines have the potential for hyperactivating incoordinated muscle activity if occlusal contact is prolonged. The potential for muscle hyperactivity and pain is greatest if the premature deflective contact is unilateral. Tolerance to premature deflective occlusal contacts appears to improve when bilateral premature contact is simultaneous and the displacement is straightforward. However, clinical experience has shown that relief of incoordinated masticatory muscle hyperactivity is most predictable when the TMJs are permitted to seat completely up into centric relation during maximal intercuspation.

From the standpoint of stability or comfort of masticatory musculature, it is more important to have equilibrium of the total masticatory system (namely teeth, jaw joints, and

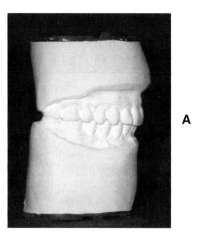

A

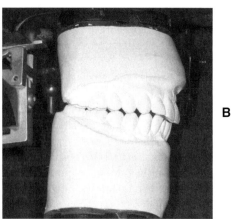

B

FIGURE 12-2 **A,** Casts articulated in maximal intercuspation without regard for the position of the correct condylar axis position. The casts appear to indicate an Angle's class I occlusion. **B,** The same casts mounted in centric relation. When the condyles are seated in their respective fossae, the entire character of the occlusal relationship is changed.

FIGURE 12-1 Any occlusal analysis that ignores the TMJs (**A**) is as incomplete as a mandible without TMJs (**B**).

musculature) than it is to develop an "ideal" class I stereotype that requires displacement of the TMJs to achieve maximal intercuspation. On the other hand, class II or III occlusion may achieve optimum stability and equilibrium with the joints and musculature and thus be the best occlusion for some patients if maximal intercuspation is not in conflict with complete seating of the jaw joints.

In Figure 12-3, note the perfect midline alignment and class I occlusal relationship that is achieved by displacement of the left TMJ. This type of displacement is often accompanied by masticatory muscle pain on the side of the displaced condyle. Treating the occlusion to conform to this jaw relationship is a mistake.

In order to achieve masticatory muscle harmony and relief of muscle pain, both condyles must be free to seat up into centric relation during maximal intercuspation. Note that when the condyles are both completely seated in centric relation, only the left side can contact, and that contact is on an incline (Figure 12-4). At this jaw position with the teeth apart, the TMJs are completely comfortable even when loaded. Elimination of the deflective posterior interference to allow complete closure to maximum intercuspation will predictably result in a comfortable occlusion, comfortable TMJs, and comfortable muscles. But the midline will no longer be centered.

Angle's classification is not an acceptable system for evaluating the relationship of occlusion to TMDs. Deflective occlusal interferences can occur in all of Angle's classifications including class I occlusions. Deflective occlusal interferences that require displacement of the TMJs to achieve maximal intercuspation are a primary cause of occluso-muscle pain, the most common type of TMD. Yet joint displacement is not a consideration in Angle's classifications, which are determined at maximal intercuspation regardless of whether the joints must displace to achieve it.

If there is significant condylar displacement, reliance on Angle's classification can result in severe misjudgments in treatment planning. Significant joint displacements are routinely missed if condylar position is not accurately determined before analyzing jaw-to-jaw relationships (Figure 12-5).

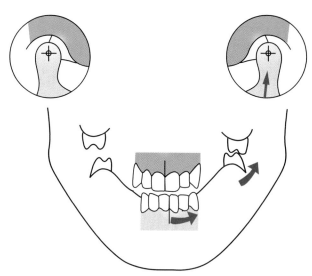

FIGURE 12-4 When condyles are seated in centric relation, occlusal interference occurs.

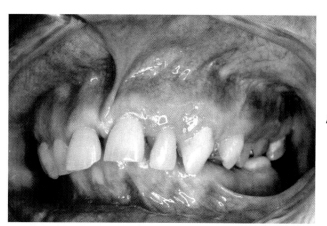

A

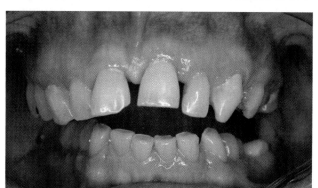

B

FIGURE 12-5 Compare the difference in how this dentition would be treatment planned if condylar position is ignored. In maximal intercuspation (**A**), it appears as a deep overbite problem. In centric relation at the first point of contact (**B**), the requirements for treatment are completely changed. Such major jaw malrelationships are commonly missed in both restorative and orthodontic treatment planning because decisions regarding jaw-to-jaw relationships are made from observation of maximal intercuspation.

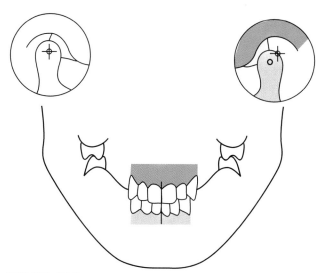

FIGURE 12-3 Masticatory muscle pain usually accompanies a displaced condyle.

Perhaps the problems inherent in Angle's classification would be more readily recognized if misconceptions about centric relation were not so prevalent in the literature.[10-13] A depiction of centric relation in the *Journal of Clinical Orthodontics*[14] expresses a common misrepresentation that "The term *centric relation* has become obsolcte . . . and does not exist in physical reality." The editorial continues, "It (centric relation) simply cannot be described in fixed positional terms." It is not fair to generalize but it appears that this bias against centric relation can be observed in much of the orthodontic literature and it would explain why joint position is so routinely ignored as a factor in maxillo-mandibular relationships. It can be easily demonstrated that centric relation can be accurately defined in precise positional terms, and the position can be verified and repeated with needlepoint accuracy[15-19] (see Chapters 9, 10, and 11).

Pullinger and colleagues[13] observed that occlusal factors do contribute to TMD and cannot be ignored, but they proposed that a new definition of "normal" should include deflective slides of up to 2 mm, unilateral tooth contacts in a retruded condylar position, and *all Angle classifications of occlusion*. Deflective interferences to complete seating of the TMJs may be a "normal"characteristic in most patients, but it can also be quite problematic. It is certainly not consistent with predictable treatment results of long-term stability and comfort. It appears from my clinical perspective that some of the most critical factors in occluso-muscle disorders, such as excessive tooth wear, hypermobility, sore or sensitive teeth, and other signs of instability, will go undiagnosed if centric relation is not determined precisely and all deflective occlusal interferences are considered as potential problems. Angle's classification does not address these issues because it ignores the position or condition of the TMJs when classifying arch-to-arch relationships.

The concept that a deflective slide from centric relation must be greater than 2 mm to cause signs or symptoms is clearly not consistent with what we observe in clinical practice. It is common for deflections of minute proportions to cause sore or sensitive teeth and/or masticatory muscle pain. Correction of the minute occlusal interference routinely eliminates the symptoms. It is clear from the literature that many "experts" do not accept the role of occlusal interferences as an important factor in TMD.[11] But it is also clear that the research literature cited to document the expert viewpoint is too flawed to be taken seriously.

Until research studies define and classify the specific type of TMD being studied, the position and condition of the TMJs are precisely defined and verified in relation to maximal intercuspation, and signs and symptoms of occlusal disease are evaluated accurately, the "experts" who have ignored what successful clinicians are doing to achieve predictable results will continue to confuse.

Cordray, in one of the exceptional orthodontic studies that verified condylar position,[20] demonstrated the importance of accurately mounted casts in relation to Angle's classification at maximal intercuspation. His study illustrates the importance of muscle deprogramming and mounting casts in a verified centric relation for analysis of a correct maxillo-mandibular relationship. This study revealed clinically significant deviations from Angle's classifications at the level of the occlusion as evidenced by posterior premature occlusal contacts, increased overjet, decreased overbite, and midline deviations. Analysis of the casts in centric relation showed deviations from Angle's classifications as dental arch discrepancy in centric relation were proven to be significantly different from arch relationships observed at maximal intercuspation. Cordray determined that one cannot assume that the condyles are positioned correctly before treatment just because the patient is asymptomatic. He found that the Angle's classification changed at either the canine or first molar in 40.9 percent of 596 asymptomatic patients as the mandibular relationship went from maximal intercuspation to centric relation. His conclusion agrees with our clinical experience that, just as in restorative dentistry, mounted diagnostic casts in centric relation are essential for accurate orthodontic diagnosis and treatment. Visual analysis of the mouth or handheld casts in maximal intercuspation are not accurate enough to be reliable for treatment planning. The requirement for accuracy in arch-to-arch analysis has been advocated by Williamson,[22-24] Roth,[25] and other respected clinicians.[26-29] A more accurate classification system that relates maximal intercuspation to a specifically defined condylar position is sorely needed and should be a step forward in improved communication and research.

DAWSON'S CLASSIFICATION[21]

In the analysis of any occlusion in relation to the TMJs, the condition and position of the TMJs must be determined *before* the occlusion can be analyzed.

Type I: Maximal intercuspation is in harmony with centric relation.

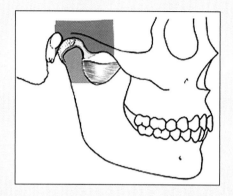

Implications for Type I

- Centric relation is verifiable with the teeth separated.
- There is no discomfort in the TMJ region even when firmly loaded.
- Treatment for TMD is not needed.
- The jaw can close to maximal intercuspation without premature tooth contacts or deflections.
- Occlusal equilibration is not needed except for possible excursive interferences.
- The patient can clench with no sign of discomfort.
- Use of an occlusal splint is not indicated.
- Type I occlusion can occur with any Angle's classification.

Type IA: Maximal intercuspation occurs in harmony with adapted centric posture.

The *A* signifies *adapted condition*.

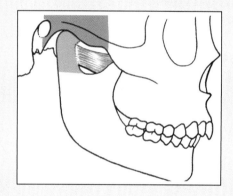

Implications for Type IA

- Intracapsular structures have deformation but have adapted.
- TMJs can accept loading with no discomfort.
- Treatment for TMD is not needed.
- Occlusal correction is not needed because there is no TMJ/occlusion disharmony.

A range of different types of intracapsular disorders may have previously occurred, followed by adaptive changes at the articular surfaces. The disk may be partially or completely displaced, or arthrogenous changes may have occurred. resulting in flattened bone-to-bone contact. If the joints can accept firm loading with no discomfort and are manageably stable, harmony between the occlusion and the TMJs can almost always be established.

If the TMJs have undergone deformative changes, the type and stage of the deformation should be ascertained and recorded. Piper's classification of intracapsular disorders (see Chapter 27) serves this purpose because it is specific for all types of intracapsular disorders.

It is important to recognize that deformed TMJs may not be as stable as normal, intact condyle-disk assemblies. It is also important to recognize that any changes in intracapsular structures may affect the TMJ/occlusion relationship. Clinical experience demonstrates that if adapted centric posture can be verified, the masticatory musculature can with few exceptions be kept comfortable. Occlusal harmony can be maintained with minimal occlusal corrections performed on an as-needed basis. Patients should be forewarned that periodic corrections may be required after initial treatment is completed.

Type II: Condyles must displace from a verifiable centric relation for maximum intercuspation to occur.

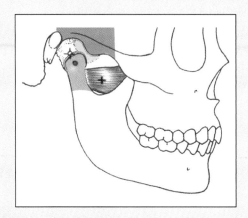

Type IIA: Condyles must displace from an adapted centric posture for maximum intercuspation to occur.

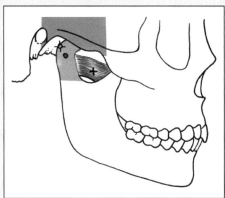

Implications for Type II or IIA

Centric relation or adapted centric posture has been verified, so discomfort from an intracapsular disorder has been ruled out. The source of pain will be in muscle or in interfering teeth. Prognosis is excellent if all occlusal interferences are eliminated. TMJ surgery, arthroscopy, joint injections, or lavage are contraindicated. The occlusal therapy goal is to achieve type I or IA.

Treatment may be reversible with use of an occlusal splint, or it may be direct using equilibration, orthodontics, or restoration to correct the TMJ/occlusion disharmony.

Type III: Centric relation cannot be verified.

TMJs cannot accept loading without tenderness or tension, so the relationship of maximal intercuspation cannot be determined until the TMJ problem is resolved.

Implications for Type III

Indicates the need for Piper classification of TMJs. Focus should be on correcting the TMD before occlusal treatment can be finalized. Selection of therapy depends on the specific type of TMD. Treatment will vary from a simple permissive occlusal device to relieve muscle spasm, to surgical correction for certain types of intracapsular disorders. Retrodiskal edema from trauma often prevents complete seating of the condyle until the inflammation and swelling are reduced. Thus it fits this category. The treatment goal is Type I or IA.

Type III classification applies to conditions that are deemed to be correctable with a potential for return to functional normalcy, but at the time of the examination, the TMJs cannot accept load testing without some degree of discomfort.

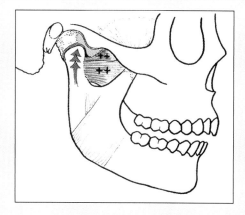

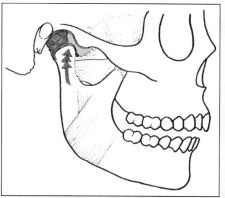

Type IV: The occlusal relationship is in an active stage of progressive disorder because of pathologically unstable TMJs.

Implications for Type IV

This indicates an actively progressive disorder of the TMJs that makes it impossible to establish a stable TMJ/occlusion relationship. Typical signs of type IV are:

* Progressive anterior open bite
* Progressive asymmetry
* Progressive mandibular retrusion

The goal is to stop the progression of the TMJ deformation until manageable stability of the TMJs can be confirmed.

Irreversible occlusal treatment is contraindicated at this stage.

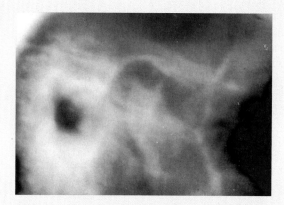

Discussion

Two essential skills must be learned to accurately classify occlusions: the skill of proper load testing and the ability to classify TMD into specific structural disorders.

The skill of proper load testing. Load testing is a standard procedure used routinely by orthopedic physicians when evaluating other joints in the body. Any response of tenderness or tension in the region of either TMJ during load testing is indicative that centric relation or adapted centric posture has not been achieved.

No reliable substitute exists for load testing. However, load testing may be used in combination with anterior deprogramming devices to relax the lateral pterygoid muscles and to separate all posterior tooth contacts.

Centric relation cannot be verified by unguided closure. Unguided closure can be seriously influenced by muscle incoordination patterns that result from deflective occlusal contacts. Muscle memory patterns guide the mandible around deflective tooth interferences and into a habitual closure into maximal intercuspation that requires displacement of one or both TMJs. Load testing is critical to verify that the joints are completely seated in centric relation.

The ability to classify TMD into specific structural disorders. The literature is rarely specific about the type of TMD being discussed, researched, or treated. Typically only symptoms such as joint sounds, limitation of motion, and discomfort in the region of the TMJ are listed. Any or all of these symptoms can be caused by a variety of structural disorders with different causes and thus require different treatment with vastly different expectations regarding treatment outcome. Piper's classification is the gold standard for specific diagnosis (see Chapter 27).

CLINICAL APPLICATION

In type I or IA occlusions, no discomfort should exist in the TMJ region or in the masticatory musculature even on maximal strength clenching. This is the first goal of proper occlusal therapy. Any discomfort in either joint or in any tooth from empty-mouth firm clenching, excluding some advanced periodontal conditions, is indicative of some occlusal interference to complete condyle seating. Thus the patient is not in a type I or IA classification.

In type II or IIA occlusions, centric relation or adapted centric posture has been verified, so any discomfort from intracapsular disorders has been ruled out. Prognosis is excellent for predictably successful elimination of masticatory muscle pain if all occlusal interferences are eliminated. With a corrected occlusion, type II is always reversible to type I, and type IIA is reversible to type IA.

In type I or II occlusions and their adapted subtypes, TMJ surgery, arthroscopy, joint injections, or lavage are contraindicated and unnecessary. The need for psychopharmacologic agents (as treatment of TMD) would be extremely rare, and long-term splint therapy would not be needed unless stabilization of the occlusion is a problem. Generalized muscle disorders, fibromyalgia, and neurologic factors may require additional therapy if muscle pain is not relieved by elimination of occlusal interferences for patients in whom an intracapsular disorder has been ruled out.

Type II or IIA occlusions focus on correcting the occlusion to an acceptably stable TMJ. Type III occlusions focus on correcting the TMD before occlusal treatment is finalized. The type of therapy selected should depend on the specific type of TMD, because it will vary from a simple permissive splint for relieving muscle hyperactivity to surgical correction of certain types of intracapsular disorders. When the TMJs reach the point at which they can accept loading with no discomfort, the goal is to establish a type I or IA occlusion so that a comfortable physiologic neuromuscular condition can be re-established.

Type IV occlusions are the most complex to treat, because they have no stable condyle positioning to relate to. The progressive deformation that causes a continuing change of condylar position makes it impossible to establish and maintain a harmonious TMJ/occlusion relationship.

This classification system includes the information that is critical to evaluation of the relationship between the occlusion and the TMJs. Any classification that does not include this information would automatically invalidate research data that presuppose to evaluate the relationship of occlusion to TMDs.

As a physician of the masticatory system, the dentist is the only health professional who has (or should have) the necessary education and training to properly evaluate the role of occlusal factors in relation to masticatory system disorders including, but not limited to, TMDs. This is an obligation that must not be treated with anything less than the thoroughness and professionalism that correct diagnosis requires.

References

1. Angle EH: *Classification of malocclusion of the teeth,* ed 7, Philadelphia, 1907, S.S. White Dental Manufacturing Company, pp. 35-59.
2. Dworkin SF, Huggins KH, LeRische L, et al: Epidemiology of signs and symptoms in temporomandibular disorders: Clinical signs in cases and controls. *J Am Dent Assoc* 120:273-281, 1990.
3. Robertson LT, Levy JH, Petrisor D, et al: Vibration perception thresholds of human maxillary and mandibular central incisors. *Arch Oral Biol* 48(4):309-316, 2003.
4. Jacobs R, van Steenberghe D: Role of periodontal ligament receptors in tactile function of teeth. *J Periodont Res* 29(3):153-167, 1994.
5. Ramfjord SP, Ash MM: *Occlusion,* ed 3, Philadelphia, 1983, WB Saunders.
6. Riise C, Sheikholeslam A: The influence of experimental interfering occlusal contacts on the postural activity of the anterior temporal and masseter muscles in young adults. *J Oral Rehabil* 9:419-425, 1982.
7. Dawson PE: Centric relation: Its effect on occluso-muscle harmony. *Dent Clin North Am* 23(2):169-180, 1979.
8. Kerstein R, Farrell S: Treatment of myofascial pain-dysfunction syndrome with occlusal equilibration. *J Prosthet Dent* Jun; 63(6): 695-700, 1990.

9. Ramfjord S: Dysfunctional temporomandibular joint and muscle pain. *J Prosthet Dent* 11:353, 1961.
10. McNamara JA Jr, Seligman D, Okeson JP: Occlusion, orthodontic treatment and temporomandibular disorders: A review. *J Orofac Pain* 9:73-86, 1995.
11. Glaros AG, Glass EG, McLauglin L: Knowledge and beliefs of dentists regarding temporomandibular disorders and chronic pain. *J Orofac Pain* 8(2):216-222, 1994.
12. Seligman DA, Pullinger AG: The role of functional occlusal relationships in temporomandibular disorders: A review. *J Craniomandib Disord* 5(4):265-279, 1991.
13. Pullinger AG, Seligman DA, Gornbein JA: A multiple regression analysis of the risk and relative odds of temporomandibular disorders as a function of common occlusal features. *J Dent Res* 72:968-979, 1993.
14. Keim RG: The editor's corner. *J Clinical Ortho* July 2003.
15. McKee JR: Comparing condylar position repeatability for standardized versus nonstandardized methods of achieving centric relation. *J Prosthet Dent* 77(3):280-284, 1997.
16. Wood DP, Elliott RW: Reproducibility of the centric relation bite registration technique. *Angle Orthod* 64(3):211-220, 1994.
17. Woelfel JB: New device for accurately recording centric relation. *J Prosthet Dent* 56:716-727, 1986.
18. Long JH: Locating centric relation with a leaf gauge. *J Prosthet Dent* 29:608-610, 1973.
19. Globe D: Centric relation as the treatment position. *J Prosthet Dent* 50:685-689, 1983.
20. Cordray FE: A three dimensional analysis of models articulated in the seated condylar position from a deprogrammed asymptomatic population—a prospective study. Submitted for publication 2004; Dr. Frank Cordray, 96 Northwoods Boulevard., Columbus, Ohio, 43235.
21. Dawson PE: A classification system for occlusions that relates maximal intercuspation to the position and condition of the temporomandibular joints. *J Prosthet Dent* 75:60-66, 1996.
22. Williamson EH: Laminographic study of mandibular condyle position when recording centric relation. *J Prosthet Dent* 39:561-564, 1978.
23. Williamson EH, Lundquist DO: Anterior guidance: Its effect on electromyographic activity of the temporal and masseter muscles. *J Prosthet Dent* 49:816-823, 1983.
24. Williamson EH, Evans DL, Barton WA, et al: The effect of bite plane use on terminal binge axis location. *Angle Orthod* 47:25-33, 1977.
25. Roth RH: Functional occlusion for the orthodontist Part 1. *J Clin Orthod* 5:32-51, 1981.
26. Kinderknecht KE, Wong GK, Billy EJ, et al: The effect of a deprogrammer on the position of the terminal transverse horizontal axis of the mandible. *J Prosthet Dent* 28:123-131, 1992.
27. Slavicek RO: On clinical and instrumental functional analyses for diagnosis and treatment planning Part 1. *J Clin Orthod* 22:358-370, 1988.
28. Karl PJ, Foley TF: The use of a deprogramming appliance to obtain centric relation records. *Angle Orthod* 69:117-123, 1999.
29. Cordray FE: Centric relation treatment and articulator mountings in orthodontics. *Angle Orthod* 66:53-58, 1996.

Chapter 13

Vertical Dimension

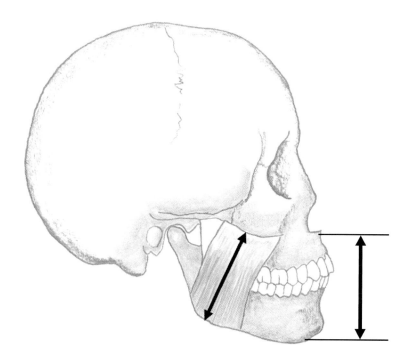

PRINCIPLE

The repetitive contracted length of the elevator muscles determines the vertical dimension of occlusion.

UNDERSTANDING VERTICAL DIMENSION

There are four serious misconceptions about vertical dimension to get out of the way. You need to know:

1. *You cannot determine vertical dimension based on whether the patient is comfortable.*

    We can make patients completely comfortable at an increased vertical dimension. We can make them just as comfortable at a decreased vertical dimension, or at the same vertical dimension they had. We can place an occlusal splint at an increased vertical dimension and make patients comfortable. We can remove the splint and correct the occlusion, and they will be just as comfortable. Patients can even lose all of their teeth and still be comfortable (as far as the temporomandibular joints (TMJs) and the muscles are concerned). In other words, using provisional splints or occlusal appliances to determine if a patient can "tolerate" an increased vertical dimension is a seriously flawed clinical approach. Patients can tolerate or even be comfortable at a wide range of vertical changes. Comfort is not a determinant of correct vertical dimension.

2. *Measuring the freeway space is not an accurate way to determine the correct vertical dimension of occlusion (VDO).*

    Patients readily adapt to changes in vertical dimension and quickly develop a new freeway space.[1-2] Freeway space is highly variable from patient to patient and at various times within the same patient.

3. *Determining the rest position of the mandible is not a key to determining vertical dimension.*

    One of the most serious flaws in the current promotion of so-called "neuromuscular dentistry" (NMD) is the use of an artificially stimulated rest position as a guide to occlusal relationships. That too often results in overtreatment by unnecessarily increasing the VDO. As a determining factor in measurement of the freeway space, the rest position is too variable to establish a consistent pattern regardless of how it is determined.

4. *Lost vertical dimension is not a cause of temporomandibular disorders (TMDs).*

    One of the most prevalent (and erroneous) concepts believed by many dentists is that TMDs are caused by a loss of vertical dimension. To understand why this is incorrect thinking, you must have an accurate perspective of the anatomy and biomechanics of the TMJs. The VDO is altered by *rotation* at the condylar horizontal axis. The misconception that the condyles move vertically up or down with changes in the VDO has led to misdirected attempts to "unload" the TMJs by increasing the VDO.

> The big question: If altering the VDO does not cause discomfort and does not cause TMDs, why should we even be concerned about the VDO?
>
> Answer: We should be concerned because failure to understand the physiology and biomechanics of vertical dimension has led to inappropriate overtreatment and has resulted in iatrogenic damage to dentitions and missed diagnosis of TMD, and because failure to understand the true nature of vertical dimension affects a major amount of the decisions every dentist must make in practice.

Let's start our understanding with a key point that throughout life there is an eruptive force that causes teeth to move vertically *with their alveolar bone* until they meet resistance that is equal to their eruptive force (Figures 13-1 and 13-2).

Usually the stopping point for eruption is contact with the teeth in the opposing arch (Figure 13-3, *A*). However, the eruption may be stopped by equal resistance from the tongue, the lips, or any object that is held between the teeth, including a thumb, a pipe, or appliances that cover the occlusal surfaces.

The critical point to understand is that the only intrinsic force that can supply resistance to the eruptive force is the elevator musculature (Figure 13-3, *B*).

> Thus the mandible-to-maxilla relationship, established by the repetitive contracted length of the elevator muscles, determines the VDO.

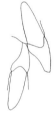

FIGURE 13-2 The eruptive process continues until the lower incisors contact the palatal tissue (unless the tongue is positioned to stop the eruption.)

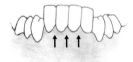

FIGURE 13-1 Note the typical elongation of the entire dento-alveolar process that occurs when there is no contact of the anterior teeth.

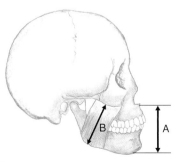

FIGURE 13-3 The teeth continue to erupt until they meet an opposite force of equal intensity to the eruptive force.

The Fallacy of Bite Raising for TMDs

Attempts at "unloading" the TMJs by increasing the VDO was popularized by advocates of posterior bite-raising appliances. The practice was based on a misconception that the TMJs could be vertically distracted. Such vertical unloading cannot occur as illustrated because all elevator muscles are posterior to the teeth.

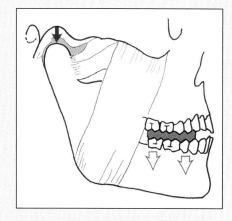

What "unloading" advocates believe happens but vertical unloading of the TMJs would be physiologically unacceptable within the closed intracapsular environment that requires any void to be filled because a vacuum cannot exist in a closed system. If such distraction of the joint were possible, loose areolar tissue that is rich with nerves and blood vessels would be sucked into the space.

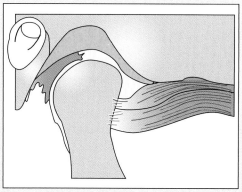

What really happens is that the upward pull keeps the condyles loaded because all of the elevator muscles are between the last molar teeth and the TMJs. The increased vertical dimension is achieved by *rotation* of the loaded condyles, placing the first occlusal contact on the last molar. The condyles must move forward down the eminentiae to pivot the anterior teeth up to gain more occlusal contact.

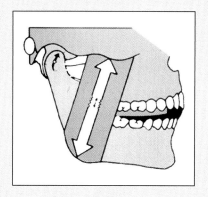

Then what happens is this results in increased bite force because the increased VDO interferes with repetitive contracted muscle length,[3–5] and results in increased bite force. The covered teeth are intruded while the uncovered teeth erupt with the alveolar process. A stepped occlusion is the typical end result.

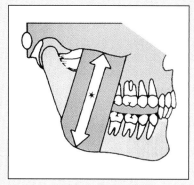

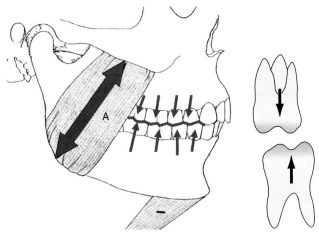

FIGURE 13-4 The teeth have an ever-present eruptive force that causes them to erupt toward their opposing teeth until they meet. The vertical point of contact is directly related to the repetitious *contracted* length of muscle *(A)*. Thus the jaw-to-jaw position determines how far the teeth erupt.

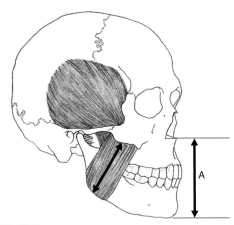

FIGURE 13-5 The VDO occurs when the eruptive force is stopped by the repetitious positioning of the mandible in relation to the maxilla. This dimension *(A)* results from the consistent length of the elevator muscles during repetitive contraction through their power cycle.

The VDO refers to the vertical position of the mandible in relation to the maxilla when the upper and lower teeth are intercuspated at the most closed position.

Even though the VDO occurs when the teeth are fully articulated, the teeth are not the determinants of vertical dimension. Rather, their position is determined by the vertical dimension of the space available between the fixed maxilla and the muscle-positioned mandible.

The most important thing to understand about vertical dimension is that the mandible goes repetitiously to the position dictated by the contracted elevator muscles (Figure 13-4). The upper and lower teeth erupt into the space until they meet at that jaw-to-jaw relationship (Figure 13-5). Thus the repetitive-contracted length during the power cycle of the elevator muscles sets the jaw-to-jaw relationship to which the teeth erupt.

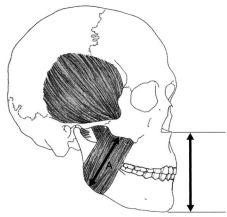

FIGURE 13-6 The jaw-to-jaw dimension is maintained with such consistent muscle contraction length that even rapid abrasive wear does not cause a loss of vertical dimension *(A)*. The alveolar process lengthens in an amount equal to the wear.

If muscle contraction length can be changed and maintained, the teeth will automatically adapt to the new dimension. However, the evidence supporting such change is not convincing. More study is needed.

The second important aspect of vertical dimension that must be understood is that the vertical position of each tooth is adaptable to the space provided, not vice versa, and that the capacity of the teeth to erupt or intrude is present throughout life. There is an ever-present eruptive force that causes teeth to erupt until they meet an equal, opposite force. If the opposing force is greater than the eruptive force, the teeth are intruded until the eruptive force equals the resistive force against them. If the resistive force is less than the eruptive force, the teeth will continue to erupt.

All resistive forces are solely the result of pressure exerted by the musculature-controlled elevation of the mandible toward the maxilla. The neutral point to which the teeth erupt is the optimum point at which the muscle contraction is completed in its repetitive power cycle. If there are no opposing teeth, it is possible to contract the muscles further by conscious demand, but the habitual pattern of closure is amazingly constant and is the controlling factor of vertical dimension. In fact, the dimension of this jaw-to-jaw relationship is consistent enough that even severe bruxing, clenching, and abrading parafunction do not alter the jaw-to-jaw dimension between bony landmarks in each jaw (Figure 13-6). This is evidenced by the consistent observation that eruption keeps pace with wear. Because of elongation of the alveolar process, even severe abrasion of teeth does not cause a loss of vertical dimension. The only explanation for this phenomenon is the constancy of the mandible-to-maxilla dimension at the completion of the elevator-muscle contraction cycle.

In some patients, it appears that severe wear can result in loss of face height. In analyzing such patients, it is important to ascertain if the obvious loss of facial height is at the anterior teeth accompanied by downward displacement of the condyles at maximal intercuspation. When this combination

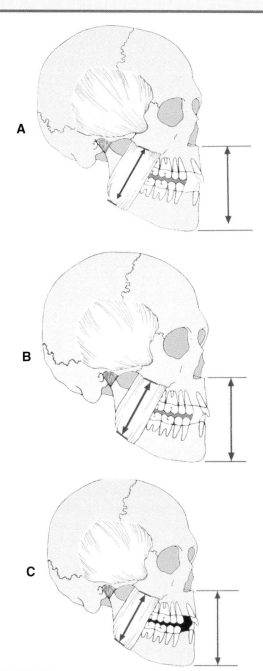

FIGURE 13-7 **A,** Bite-raising appliances increase the jaw-to-jaw dimension and interfere with the repetitive contracted length of the elevator muscle. The muscles can be expected to regain a vertical jaw relationship that is consistent with their contracted length. **B,** This occurs by intrusion of the covered teeth by an amount approximately equal to the thickness of the bite plane. **C,** When the posterior bite-raising appliance is removed, the teeth it covered will be out of contact. Intrusion of the teeth occurs within 6 to 12 months.

occurs, anterior facial dimension can be successfully increased by correction of posterior occlusal interferences. This allows upward seating of the condyles to centric relation and permits an increase of VDO at the anterior face without increasing the elevator muscle lengths. Studies that fail to consider condylar position as a factor in vertical dimension miss this important observation.

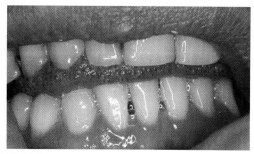

FIGURE 13-8 Eruption of teeth can be stopped by habitual tongue biting. The VDO at complete closure includes the thickness of the tongue, set by the repetitious contraction length of the elevator muscles. Such dentitions can be just as stable as if the teeth were in contact at complete closure.

Effect of Interocclusal Segmental Appliance on VDO

Examine Figures 13-7 and 13-8 for the various effects of these bite-raising appliances on the VDO.

Evidence for the Stability of Vertical Dimension

You will hear some clinicians claim that they routinely increase the VDO without any sign of relapse. A recent article (in a nonjuried journal) reported that the author had "increased the vertical dimension of over a thousand patients and every one of them had maintained the increased VDO." Such claims are never validated by any form of scientific verification, and they should not be believed. True scientific studies regarding vertical dimension are consistent in refuting such unsubstantiated claims.

Scientific research verifies that:

1. Decreases in tooth height are compensated for by a commensurate increase in alveolar bone height. This is true even in severe abrasive wear by habitual bruxers.[6–9]
2. Increases in tooth height are compensated for either by regressive remodeling of the alveolar bone to commensurately shorten the dento-alveolar process, or by intrusion into the alveolus of the teeth that had been lengthened.[10–12]

Several studies have shown that vertical facial dimension is essentially unaffected by even severe abrasion of the dentition because elongation of the dento-alveolar process matches the lost vertical dimension of the abraded teeth (Figure 13-9).

VERTICAL DIMENSION AT REST

When a muscle is neither hypotonic nor hypertonic, it is said to be "at rest." Even resting muscle is in a mild state of contraction. This mild contraction of antagonistic muscles is necessary to maintain the posture and alignment of the skeletal parts. Contraction of one muscle beyond its resting

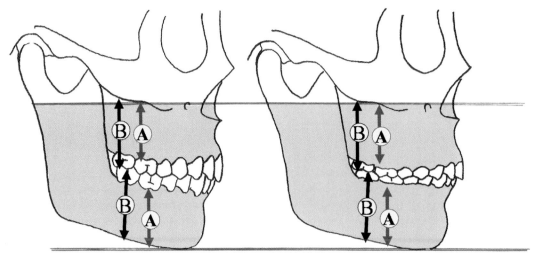

FIGURE 13-9   Measurements from fixed bony landmarks show that the dimension to the cementoenamel junction *(A)* increases with tooth wear. The dimension from bone landmark to occlusal surface *(B)* remains even with severe wear.[9]

length affects its antagonistic muscle to some degree. The antagonist must release and give the contracting muscle its way, or it must respond by isometrically contracting more forcefully itself to counterbalance the effect of the antagonist. Either way, the harmony of resting muscle is disturbed by any factor that interferes with its resting length.

From Niswonger's[13] early postulations that the rest position was constant and inviolate, numerous proponents of this concept have generated a variety of methods using the rest position for determining the VDO. Despite the popularity of using rest position as a starting point for determining VDO, it is an unreliable approach because the dimension between the teeth at the rest position is not consistent for different patients. The rest position is not consistent even in the same patient. Atwood[14] found variations as great as 4 mm at the same sitting and even greater variations at different sittings. Finding the vertical dimension of rest position and then arbitrarily closing a specific amount is an unsatisfactory approach.

The rest position is anything but constant. The jaw position at rest not only is highly variable, but it also changes noticeably in the same patient in response to a variety of factors including how much stress the patient is subjected to. The rest position is also altered by the presence of any noxious stimuli from occlusal interferences that can cause varying degrees of muscle incoordination. The effects of masticatory muscle incoordination can range from slight hypercontraction to severe trismus, all of which can have a profound effect on the postural position of the mandible at rest.

Although the length of the elevator muscles varies through a wide range in the so-called resting position, the *contracted* length in the power cycle appears constant.[3] This consistency results from the "all-or-none" contraction of a sufficiently constant number of muscle fibers to establish a repeatable dimension during the repetitious swallowing pattern.

To simplify the concept, the contracted length of the elevator muscles during the repetitive power cycle used in

swallowing is constant (at least within the range of clinical importance). The length of muscle at rest position is not constant, nor is the rest position consistently related to the VDO. Some muscles may contract to half of their resting length, whereas others shorten very little. The variations of muscle contraction are as great as the differences in people themselves.

Gibbs and Mahan[16] have pointed out that the maximum force with which muscle resists elongation is applied when it is completely committed to contraction. Since teeth erupt until they reach a resistance that equals their eruptive force, it is logical that the muscular placement of the mandible in relationship to the maxilla would determine the point at which that resistance is met. It is also apparent that an increase in the vertical dimension of the teeth would interfere with the length of muscle in its power-stroke contraction cycle.

If the vertical dimension can be established in harmony with the optimum repetitive length of the contracted elevator muscles, the muscles will be free to rest at whatever length is comfortable. The practical approach therefore is to concentrate on accurately recording the VDO and allowing the dimensions of the freeway space to be the natural result of the difference between the optimum length of contracted muscles and the length of the muscles at rest.

Attempts to determine a consistent rest position have been pursued using transcutaneous electrical nerve stimulation (TENS). The use of the Myomonitor to accomplish a TENS-induced relaxation of the masticatory muscles has become a popular procedure that allegedly leads to determination of the correct VDO. Williamson,[15] however, showed that the TENS-induced rest position differs significantly from the clinical rest position, and other researchers[17] have reported similar discrepancies, along with a frequent inability to duplicate the dimensions recorded. Williamson also showed that even after one hour of muscle pulsation to ensure adequate muscle relaxation, the vertical dimension at rest changed significantly on the same patient even while the Myomonitor was being used continuously. When the patient was subjected to varying levels of stress from playing a competitive electronic game, with electrical stimulation via surface electrodes from the Myomonitor continuing, the vertical dimension at rest decreased significantly.

Even if a transcutaneous electrical nerve type of stimulation could be used with consistent results to determine the vertical dimension at rest, it would still not be an acceptable method for determining the VDO. The muscle-contracted position is unrelated to any consistent comparison with the resting musculature, regardless of how resting length is determined. The finding that stress affects the resting posture of the mandible, even while the Myomonitor is being used, just adds another variable to an already questionable modality.

Rules for Determining the VDO on Patients with Teeth

1. The VDO that requires the least amount of dentistry to satisfy esthetic and functional goals is always the VDO of choice. Extensive treatment done solely for the purpose of increasing the vertical dimension to a perceived stereotypical dimension is contraindicated.

2. Maximal intercuspation of the posterior teeth determines the existing VDO. This dimension will be in harmony with the jaw-to-jaw relationship established by the repetitive contracted length of the elevator muscles.

3. The muscle-determined VDO must be measured from origin to insertion of the elevator muscles. This is best measured clinically from the zygoma to the angle of the mandible, the origin to insertion dimension of the masseter muscle.

4. The position of the condyles during maximal intercuspation must be considered when evaluating VDO. This is so because any change up or down of the condyles affects muscle length during maximal intercuspation.

5. If the VDO must be changed, it should be determined at the point of anterior teeth contact. If posterior interferences prevent anterior contact in centric relation and occlusal equilibration is determined to be the best choice of treatment, the posterior teeth may be adjusted until anterior contact is achieved in centric relation (see Chapter 38, "Solving Anterior Open Bite Problems" for exceptions to this rule).

6. Changing the VDO by either increasing or decreasing it is tolerated well by patients and within reason causes no harm to teeth or supporting structures if tooth contact includes the complete arches and the condyles are completely seated in centric relation during maximal intercuspation.

7. Changes in the true VDO are not permanent. The VDO will return to its original dimension measurable at the masseter muscle. Unnecessary increases in the VDO are contraindicated as they are not maintained.

Bite Raising

There was a time when bite raising was almost synonymous with oral rehabilitation. Even the finest dentists used bite-raising techniques with little or no concern for the consequences. The detrimental effects of bite raising are insidious, however, so it took years of practicing the procedure to learn that it was not a wise approach.

There are definite exceptions to the rules against bite raising, and it is sometimes necessary. With a better understanding we now have regarding the potential for vertical change within the alveolar process, we can often take advantage of alterations of vertical dimension during the treatment stage, knowing that the muscular control over jaw relationships will, in time, return the vertical dimension to its pretreatment measurement.

Although there are valid reasons for increasing the vertical dimension, most bite raising has been traditionally done for one of the following invalid reasons:

1. To relieve a TMD.
2. To "unload" the TMJs.
3. To restore "lost" vertical dimension in a severely worn occlusion.
4. To get rid of facial wrinkles.

None of these reasons is valid. Increasing the vertical dimension in each of these situations is based on erroneous concepts and may in fact be harmful.

It is almost always contraindicated. A better perception of each of these problems should be gained before any treatment is considered.

Bite raising for temporomandibular joint disorders
The VDO has in itself nothing to do with causing TMDs. If pain is from a true pathosis, vertical changes could actually increase the muscular loading of compromised tissues. The pain and dysfunction associated with occluso-muscle imbalances can be resolved at any vertical dimension up to the point of condylar translation or closed down to the point of coronoid impingement. As long as the correctly aligned condyle-disk assemblies are free to go to the most superior position against the eminentiae, the pain of muscle incoordination can be relieved. Condylar access to centric relation is not dependent on any given vertical dimension because the condyles are free to rotate on a fixed axis.

Dentists who have accomplished relief of occluso-muscle pain with the use of bite-raising appliances may erroneously give the credit to the increased vertical dimension. Actually, the same symptoms could have been relieved at a closed vertical dimension as long as the articulation is noninterfering with the centric relation axis of the joints.

Correcting the occlusion at an increased vertical dimension may indeed eliminate the patient's discomfort, but it appears that the increased vertical dimension almost always reverts to its original dimension by intrusion of the teeth that have been increased in height. If vertical stability is one of the goals of occlusal treatment, it seems more logical to work to the correct vertical dimension to start with, rather than to increase it and then wait for it to change back to where it was.

"Unloading" the temporomandibular joints

Increasing the vertical dimension does not "unload" the joints. This is a common misconception based on another erroneous concept that the condyles should be supported by the occlusion. The condyles are not supported by the teeth, and the condyles are not positioned by the teeth in a centered relationship with "space" around the condyle. That "space" is merely radiolucent tissue that is loaded by the elevator muscles, all of which are between the posterior teeth and the condyles.

Bite raising increases the vertical dimension by rotating the condyles (which remain loaded during the opening rotation), not by vertically distracting the condyles away from the eminence. If the bite-raising appliance attempts to distract the condyles away from their seated position, the elevator muscles will simply elevate the condyles against the eminentiae at whatever position may be dictated by the erroneous occlusal inclines. The most posterior tooth contact becomes the pivotal point in the dentition, and the elevator muscles behind that point elevate the condyles toward the eminentiae until they are loaded. If the bite-raising appliance is made at centric relation, the condyles can simply rotate the jaw more open, without joint displacement. The joints will still be loaded.

Even if no discomfort results, increasing the vertical dimension can have detrimental effects, especially if the condyles are not in centric relation during maximal intercuspation. Depression of the teeth can create excessive stresses on the periodontium and result in instability of the occlusion. Instability can lead to occlusal interferences that activate muscle incoordination and its detrimental consequences. Whenever possible, occlusal treatment should be performed as close to the original vertical dimension as possible. The vertical dimension the patient presents with has already stabilized in relation to contracted muscle length. Any changes will require adaptation that would be better to avoid whenever possible.

TMDs, such as disk derangements and other intracapsular problems, rarely benefit directly by changes in vertical dimension. The effects of various types of bite planes are the result of either permitting condylar access to centric relation or directing the condyles to a treatment position. The ability of the condyles to rotate from any position along their border paths enables them to assume any of those positions irrespective of vertical dimension.

Restoring "lost" vertical dimension

Much clinical evidence indicates that even severely worn occlusions do not lose vertical dimension.[6–9] Restoring "lost" vertical dimension in a worn occlusion really amounts to opening the bite because wear does not normally produce a loss of vertical dimension. Patients can wear their teeth down to the gum line and still not lose vertical dimension because the eruptive process matches the wear to maintain the original vertical dimension.

This process of eruption and alveolar development may continue throughout life as teeth are worn because of the continual addition of layers of cementum on the root and concurrent elongation of the alveolar process. So even with wear, the jaw-to-jaw relationship remains the same when the teeth are together.

The idea that eruption keeps up with wear comes as a surprise to some dentists, but it can be observed in many different ways. We notice what happens to the lower anterior teeth when they are not met by the upper teeth in some deep overbite situations. If the tongue does not substitute for the missing contact, the teeth erupt up into the palate. However, they do not erupt out of the alveolar bone. The bone develops vertically up with the teeth. Often the level of the anterior bone expands above the occlusal plane of the posterior teeth (see Figure 13-1). As another example, we notice how the tuberosity enlarges and grows down with an unopposed upper molar.

We have noticed what happens to natural teeth when they are opposed by plastic teeth on a bridge or partial restoration. As the plastic teeth wear, the natural teeth erupt. I have observed teeth that have worn all the way through a plastic partial restoration so that the erupted teeth were contacting the opposing ridge. Such problems are sometimes difficult to solve because the properly opposed teeth maintain their position as the others erupt, and the occlusal plane ends up with a stepped occlusion.

It might be asked whether or not there are exceptions to the rule. What about the tobacco chewer who wears his teeth down rapidly? Surely the eruptive process cannot keep up with that kind of wear. There is much clinical evidence to the contrary. Note the much-enlarged alveolar processes that are always evident when severe attrition or abrasion has shortened the posterior teeth. Several studies also show evidence that attrition of the teeth is compensated for by elongation of the alveolar processes except when condylar height is also lost due to bone disease.

Anyone who has observed what happens when a patient loses the temporary restoration on a crown preparation has seen firsthand how quickly teeth can erupt. In some cases, the prepared tooth may erupt all the way to contact within a couple of weeks. It is almost a certainty that the new restoration will be quite "high" any time a prepared tooth is not stabilized with a properly occluding temporary restoration.

We must not be fooled by worn teeth into believing that the bite has closed. Restoring "lost" vertical dimension is most often really bite raising when it is done on natural teeth. It is true that some occlusions are worn so badly that we have no logical alternative but to increase the vertical dimension slightly. When we do it, we must remember that the patient who wears the teeth badly is the one who can least afford to have disharmony with the musculature.

Opening the bite to eliminate facial wrinkles

On patients with natural opposing teeth, this procedure may have very detrimental effects. When the masticatory and facial muscles are at rest, the teeth should not be in contact. Increasing the vertical dimension to the extent of stretching the wrinkles out puts such an unnatural demand on muscles that it may actually accelerate further wrinkling. The increased length of the teeth positions them in continuous interference to normal contracting lengths of the muscles. Such continuous stimulation may cause reflex contraction of the muscles with damaging results to the teeth and supporting structures. The stresses exerted on the teeth are amplified by unfavorable crown-root ratios that result from increasing the length of the clinical crowns. Furthermore, the effect on the muscle may be to "age" it faster and produce worse wrinkles.

Patients who have previously had bite-raising procedures to eliminate wrinkles are often very insistent about further increases. As the teeth depress or the wrinkles return, they express the need for more and more increase in vertical dimension: Some patients tell us that they were more comfortable when the bite was first raised and that they would like to regain that comfort. It is difficult not to give in to such a request because it sounds so reasonable. If we understand that their early comfort was the result of an improved occlusal relationship rather than the increased vertical dimension, we can almost always regain the comfort by equilibration without further increase of vertical dimension.

The patient must be made to understand that the muscles should be allowed to position the jaw without interference from the teeth. "Support" from the teeth at an increased vertical dimension constitutes an interference to the contracted muscle in a normal power stroke.

Rather than trying to solve the wrinkle problem with a potentially destructive "solution," it would be far better to refer the patient to a plastic surgeon for cosmetic surgery. Cosmetic surgery techniques are quite successful when they are done by competent surgeons, and since such techniques do not involve the masticatory muscles, they have little if any effect on the VDO.

Several studies have shown that there is a significant relationship between the "power point" of muscular contraction and repeatable phonetic and comfort measurements. Using electronic means on dentures, Tueller[18] found an average variation of less than 0.5 mm from the vertical dimension established at the muscular power point when compared with either pre-extraction records or phonetic methods.

Silverman[19] has reported consistent results in measuring the VDO by phonetic methods. When a patient has lost natural occlusal stops for recording the vertical dimension, we have found that Silverman's closest speaking technique has provided consistently reliable results. The vertical dimension established in this manner is repeatable with extreme accuracy, even over a period of months.

WHEN THE VERTICAL DIMENSION MUST BE CHANGED

There are some problems of occlusion that would be very difficult to solve without increasing the vertical dimension. It is not always possible to restore an extremely worn occlusion without some increase, and sometimes the choice may be to either increase the vertical dimension or perform multiple pulp extirpations and endodontics to provide enough room for restorations. In some cases, the esthetic needs of the patient cannot be satisfied without the crown length being increased, and the choices may be either surgical crown-lengthening procedures versus increasing the vertical dimension. Some orthodontic results may be difficult to achieve without temporarily increasing the vertical dimension. The same may be true when one is restoring some severe arch malrelationships or extreme occlusal plane problems.

There are other types of occlusal problems such as anterior open bite that require a reduction of the vertical dimension in order to get an acceptable result. When the only alternative would be anterior teeth that are too long or smiles that would be too gummy, closure of the vertical dimension seems to be a far better choice.

Do all changes in vertical dimension lead to eventual problems in the dentition or its supporting structures? We know a bit more today about the adaptive capacity of the alveolar process to changes in vertical dimension, and we now know that in many patients, changes in vertical dimension can be managed. We also feel quite certain that changes in vertical dimension are only temporary. There is growing evidence to indicate that whether the vertical dimension is increased or decreased in adults, it will in time return to its pretreatment vertical dimension. This is not surprising if one considers how effectively muscle dominates skeletal form and function.

Ricketts[20] has described lower facial height in adults as staying constant with age. Using the same bony landmarks to measure the distance between the point on the mandible and the ANS point (at the anterior nasal spine), McAndrews[21] showed that adult orthodontic patients whose vertical dimension had been increased up to 8 mm had reverted to their pretreatment vertical dimension within one year. He also observed that decreases in vertical dimension of up to 7 mm regained the lost vertical dimension within one year!

An even more important finding in the McAndrews study, however, was that the change back to the original vertical dimension did not adversely affect the corrected arch alignments or the intercuspal relationships. This would indicate that changes back to the pretreatment vertical dimension occurred almost entirely within the alveolar bone by either progressive or regressive remodeling.[22] A further indication that changes in vertical dimension were the result of alveolar bone remodeling was the observation that the cementoenamel junction of the teeth retained the same relationship to the crest of bone.

Of great significance in the McAndrews study is the attention paid to achieving holding contacts for all teeth in centric relation. It appears that the response to increased vertical dimension is not the same if contacts are established only on posterior teeth. Where only segments of the occlusion are increased in height, there seems to be a tendency to intrude those teeth into the alveolar bone, whereas if the entire arch contacts simultaneously in centric relation, the changes take place by regressive remodeling of the alveolar process.

What this study and our own clinical observations seem to indicate is that it is permissible to alter the vertical dimension when necessary for achieving an improved occlusal relationship as long as all teeth are properly intercuspated at a correct centric relation. It is also a consistent finding that whenever the vertical dimension is increased, the number of postoperative occlusal adjustments required is increased and may be required repeatedly for up to one year before the occlusion stabilizes.

Before increasing any vertical dimension, one should evaluate the alveolar bone. Dense sclerotic bone with numerous exostoses does not have the same capacity to remodel as alveolar bone with normal trabeculae. Increasing vertical dimension in such unchangeable bone is contraindicated. (See Chapter 35.)

If the constancy of vertical dimension is perceived in detail, it will be obvious that promiscuous alteration of the vertical dimension should be avoided. There is no reason to change any vertical dimension unless it is the only way to achieve an acceptable result. If the vertical dimension must be changed, it should be changed as little as necessary because the increased dimension between the jaws will not be maintained in all probability.

Finding a "Comfortable" Vertical Dimension

Many clinicians advocate working with provisional restorations and varying the vertical dimension until a comfortable occlusovertical dimension is located. Despite the fact that this is the most popular way to determine vertical dimension for bite-raising procedures and other restorative vertical changes, it is absolutely without merit. There is no recognizable difference in the comfort level through a wide variation of changes in vertical dimension if the condyles are in centric relation when occlusal contact is made bilaterally on nondeviating surfaces.

Regardless of how comfortable a patient may be at an increased vertical dimension, it is not an indication that the vertical dimension is correct.

If opposing, reasonably stable posterior teeth occlude, the jaw relationship at maximum intercuspation is the correct vertical dimension. If that relationship is uncomfortable, it is because the intercuspation does not occur at centric relation, an intra-articular problem exists, or a continuous clenching pattern exists. Correction of any of these problems will permit an optimum level of comfort without increasing the vertical dimension. The same level of comfort can also be achieved at an increased or decreased vertical dimension, so the use of "comfort" as an indication of correct vertical dimension is not valid.

Intrusions into the Interocclusal Space

If the vertical dimension is perceived to be a jaw-to-jaw relationship, it will be apparent that there is only so much space between the jaws to accommodate the teeth. If any object is placed between the teeth for an extended period, the teeth will be intruded by the thickness of the object so that the dimension between the jaws can remain the same.[12]

Whether the intruding object is a bite plane, a high crown, or a tongue, the result is the same. The muscles will eventually bring the mandible back or very close to its original vertical relationship to the maxilla, and the teeth will be intruded by whatever amount is necessary to allow that to happen. The length of the contracted muscle will prevail. The teeth, being the most movable part of the masticatory system, will adapt.

This concept is illustrated dramatically by the thumb-sucking child. Placing the thumb between the anterior teeth may temporarily open the bite, but eventually the mandible regains its normal relationship to the maxilla as the teeth around the thumb are intruded to conform to the shape of the thumb. Notice also that the alveolar process conforms to the position of the teeth. The basal bone of the mandible and maxilla retains a fairly constant relationship to the contracted elevator muscles, whereas the teeth and their alveolar bone adapt to conform, sharing the limited space with whatever intrudes into that set dimension.

WHY NOT INCREASE VERTICAL DIMENSION?

A major goal of all occlusal treatment is to develop harmony in the masticatory system. Any disharmony in the system provokes adaptive responses designed to return the system to equilibrium. There is always some price to pay for adaptation, and even though the adaptive process may be beneficial, it is not always predictable. Adaptive responses to increased vertical dimension may simply cause the lengthened teeth to intrude into the alveolar bone to regain the original jaw-to-jaw relationship, or there may be an attempt to wear away the increased dimension by bruxing. There is increased loading on the lengthened teeth from muscle that is attempting to regain its normal length of contraction, and if the added compression of the supporting tissues exceeds their capacity to remodel acceptably, we will see hypermobility of the teeth and a lowered resistance in the periodontal structures.

With adequate care and attention to the details of a perfected centric relation occlusion, the adaptive responses can be managed and controlled. However, if it is not necessary to disturb the equilibrium in the first place, it makes sense to plan treatments that do not require adaptive changes to correct for an increased vertical dimension that was of no benefit to the patient and could not be maintained at the treatment level.

Most increases in vertical dimension have no benefit over time to the patient whatsoever. If there is no benefit to be derived from the treatment, it is difficult to rationalize doing it. The goal of occlusal therapy is to minimize the requirements for adaptation. Unnecessary increases in vertical dimension do the opposite. They increase the requirements for adaptation, and once the adaptive process is in accelerated activity, it is not always completely predictable.

If the increased vertical dimension is achieved by restorations that have no other purpose, the procedure is clearly contraindicated. In dentitions that have no need for extensive restorative dentistry, using restorations to increase the vertical dimension is an unnecessary expense and inconvenience to the patient and has no ultimate benefit, since the increase in vertical dimension cannot be maintained anyway.

Increasing the vertical dimension on only part of the dentition is clearly contraindicated because it leads to an instability of the entire occlusal harmony. Segmental bite raising causes intrusion of the covered teeth and supraeruption of the uncovered teeth. The damage to occlusal harmony is the same whether the segmental coverage is removable or fixed, but the use of fixed restorations to segmentally increase vertical dimension is also an irreversible insult to the teeth themselves that is more difficult and more costly to repair.

If the constancy of vertical dimension is perceived in detail, it will be obvious that promiscuous alteration of the vertical dimension should be avoided. There is no reason to change any vertical dimension unless an acceptable result cannot be achieved at the patient's given vertical dimension. If the vertical dimension must be changed, it should be changed as little as necessary to reduce the requirements for adaptation to the minimum. In all probability, the increased vertical dimension will gradually revert to the original jaw-to-jaw measurement.

WHY SOME PATIENTS REQUEST BITE RAISING

Some patients request an increase in vertical dimension based on a feeling of greatly improved comfort if they can have added height to their occlusions. They routinely justify such requests by explaining how uncomfortable they are when their teeth are together. Often there are esthetic implications of a "collapsed" bite or an "old-woman look" with fear that their nose-to-chin distance will continue to close together until they meet, unless the teeth can be built up to stop the closure.

Such observations may be valid if one or both arches are edentulous because the loss of alveolar bone often occurs when the teeth are extracted. Denture wearers do in fact lose vertical height if ridge resorption occurs.

The problem with the dentulous patient, however, is rarely the result of lost vertical height, and increasing the vertical dimension will usually be the first of a continuing series of bite raisings that eventually close back down to the original dimension. Notice that many of the patients who request such treatment have had it done previously. I have had patients request bite-raising treatment who have had as many as seven previous attempts at increasing the VDO.

Patients need to understand the consequences of such treatment before it is rendered. They also need to understand the reason for their discomfort at the occluded position as well as their apparent lost facial height.

The primary thing patients (and dentists) must understand is that the teeth should not be in contact except fleetingly during chewing and during swallowing.

The teeth do not and should not support the facial height. At the resting jaw position, the teeth should be separated. It is the posture of the lower jaw as dictated by the musculature that determines the lower facial profile. Tooth contact is not necessary or desirable at the jaw position of best profile appearance.

The feeling of overclosure, or the strained feeling that occurs when the teeth are held together, is a normal response to prolonged elevator muscle contraction. The masticatory muscles are designed for intermittent tooth contact. They are not designed for the extended contraction required to hold the teeth together. Patients who feel uncomfortable when they hold their teeth together should be educated to correct jaw posture without tooth contact. The old adage "lips together–teeth apart" is physiologically correct, and patients must often be taught its importance. Some patients are under the mistaken impression that they are supposed to keep the teeth together. Such a position is extremely tiresome.

Building the occlusion up to provide comfortable "support" may make the clenching patient more comfortable during prolonged tooth contact, but the increased vertical dimension will interfere with the normal contracting length of the elevator muscles, and so it will not be maintainable. Furthermore, it is unnecessary because the muscles will actually be more comfortable if the patient allows the mandible to be suspended by the resting musculature without tooth contact.

There is such a wide variation between resting and contracted muscle length in different patients that there also may be some patient-to-patient variation in the response to increasing the vertical dimension. More research is needed to analyze these differences more critically, but it is doubtful that such increases will be maintained, even in patients with large freeway space.

Patients should always be examined carefully to notice the type of musculature. Any evidence of hypertrophy or the effects of strong muscle pull on the bony parts should alert the examiner to avoid any increases in vertical dimension if there is any way to plan the treatment at the given VDO.

Patients with minimal freeway space often have shorter and thicker muscles with a smaller range of difference between the contracted length and the resting length. On palpation, the muscles appear firmer and more unyielding than normal, and the gonial angle may be more acute. Evidence of strong masseter and internal pterygoid complex may be related to formation of an antegonial notch. The concavity at the base of the mandible is evidence of the limiting power of the contracted elevator muscles. When it is present, the vertical dimension should not be increased regardless of how much freeway space is present.

Patients with greater freeway space may or may not accept an increased vertical dimension, depending on the character of their muscle contraction. We have seen patients with the appearance of a long, lean musculature who had masseteric hypertrophy and a severe antegonial notch, but an obvious freeway space of over 10 mm. Regardless of the high interocclusal dimension at rest, the contracting force of the muscle would overpower even the slightest extension of teeth into the vertical dimension at full contraction.

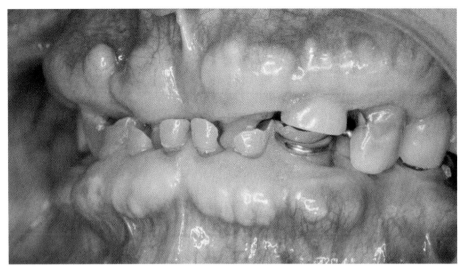

FIGURE 13-10 When increasing VDO is a problem: Some delta-stage bruxers have severe attritional wear that requires restoration. There are two important concerns about any increase in VDO on these patients. First, the response in the alveolar process is often a buildup of dense, almost sclerotic bone that does not regressively remodel as normal alveolar bone does when the VDO is increased. Nor does it permit the intrusion of teeth into the alveolar bone if the VDO is increased. Second, because of the extreme muscle hypertrophy that is characteristic for delta-stage bruxers, any increase in vertical dimension puts a severe overload on the teeth, often resulting in destruction of the restorations or the teeth themselves. Therefore, be cautious in treating patients with extreme muscle hypertrophy and multiple exostoses on enlarged alveolar processes. See Chapter 35 for details on diagnosis and treatment.

The amount of freeway space at rest is not an automatic indication of whether the vertical dimension can be increased. But if the musculature is fairly weak and not too resistive to palpation, there may be a better chance of maintaining an increase in vertical dimension if there is ample freeway space to permit. Patients with weak muscles and large freeway space rarely need an increase in vertical dimension (Figure 13-10).

CLOSING THE VERTICAL DIMENSION

Unless it results in labially directed stress on the upper anterior teeth, there do not appear to be any problems associated with closing the vertical dimension on natural teeth. It does not produce stress because a closed vertical dimension does not interfere with muscle lengths.

It appears that even when a natural occlusion is closed down all at once, it eventually regains its original vertical dimension, probably in less than one year. We know that slight reductions in vertical dimension often permit us to harmonize an occlusion with reduced need for restorations. When all teeth are in harmonious contact, any readjustment of the vertical dimension seems to take place with minimal disturbance to that harmony. At least it does not normally present any clinical problems.

Closing the vertical dimension to an extreme degree could cause coronoid impingement against the zygoma, but it is highly unlikely that there would ever be a need for that much closure. Tenderness to palpation in the zygoma area would alert us to this.

Relationship of the Anterior Teeth to Vertical Dimension

One of the most important considerations in any change of vertical dimension is the direction of the arc of closure. As the mandible is elevated, the lower incisors travel forward on the closing arc. Any time the VDO is reduced, the lower incisal edges are automatically moved forward at the more closed vertical dimension.

If the lingual surfaces of the upper anterior teeth are in the way of this forward movement of the lower teeth, it results in horizontal stress directed labially against the upper anterior teeth and lingually against the lower anterior teeth. As obvious as this stressful relationship may seem, it is easily missed by many dentists because of carelessness in recording the correct vertical dimension and failure to record the correct horizontal axis with a facebow.

The axis of closure on most simple articulators is much closer to the occlusal plane level than the true condylar axis (which is higher). The arc of closure on the erroneous "simple" articulators is nearly vertical, rather than forward. If the bite is closed during restorative procedures, the interference to the front teeth is not noticed on the improperly mounted models.

If such restorations are placed in the mouth, the resultant stress against the anterior teeth is not easily picked up without digital examination. The incline contacts are so steep and the vector of force is so horizontal that the upper anterior teeth are forced out of the way and the lower anterior teeth are forced inward. The result is continuous complaints by the patient that the front teeth "hit too hard." If the upper lingual surfaces have been restored, it is often necessary to grind completely through the metal to adjust the anterior oc-clusion on such closed vertical cases. If the vertical dimension has been closed enough, it may be impossible to reduce the horizontal stress on the anterior teeth without restoring the posterior teeth back to a correct vertical dimension or inducing their eruption by using an anterior bite plane.

The vertical dimension can sometimes be closed to improve anterior relationships in anterior overjet problems. Closing the vertical dimension may arc the lower incisors forward into contact that they did not have at their original VDO.

Regardless of whether teeth are being restored or equilibrated, care must be taken to assure that the harmonious relationship of the anterior teeth is never disturbed by imprudent or careless changes in vertical dimension.

HOW THE CONDYLE POSITION AFFECTS VERTICAL DIMENSION

The dimension that determines vertical dimension is located at the elevator muscles *(B)* because it is the repetitive contracted length of the elevator muscles that determines the repetitive end point of closure of the mandible. That, in turn, determines the point at which the erupting teeth contact and the point at which the eruptive forces are neutralized (Figures 13-11 to 13-13).

If optimal muscle length occurs with a downward displacement of the condyles, the zygoma-to-angle dimension may be shortened as the condyle seats upwardly to centric relation. As the condyle moves up, the most posterior tooth becomes the pivot point producing an anterior open bite in centric relation. Thus, the dimension at the anterior teeth may increase without increasing the muscle length. In some instances of condylar displacement, the vertical dimension at the anterior teeth may be increased at the same time the zygoma-to-angle dimension is decreased. This makes it possible to increase the anterior dimension further without interfering with the repetitive contracted length of the elevator muscles. This is why it is often possible to increase the length of the lower face or to show more length of anterior teeth for improved esthetics and achieve a stable result in which the teeth are in harmony with the musculature.

How to Measure Vertical Displacement of the Condyles

Determinant index
The *determinant* index on the Dénar® Combi articulator (Figure 13-14) can be used to determine vertical displacement of each condyle during maximal intercuspation. Casts are mounted in centric relation with the condylar path insert in place. Remove the condylar path insert and replace it with the *determinant index*. The condyle ball should be against the back wall and roof of the index. Then position the casts into maximum intercuspation, and measure the space between the top of the condyle and the roof of the index (Figures 13-15 and 13-16).

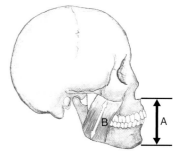

FIGURE 13-11 If there are no deflective occlusal interferences that require downward displacement of the TMJs from centric relation to achieve maximum intercuspation, the vertical dimension at *(A)* will stay constant. If you increase the vertical dimension, it will always revert back to this dimension at the anterior teeth as the muscles close the bite back to where it was.

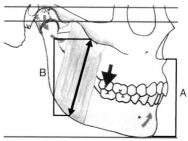

FIGURE 13-12 If the vertical dimension of the anterior face at *(A)* is achieved by downward, forward displacement of the condyles from centric relation, it is at this jaw relationship that muscle length *(B)* establishes the VDO. Note the upward movement at the front of the mandible as the condyles move down. The pivot point is usually at the most distal tooth.

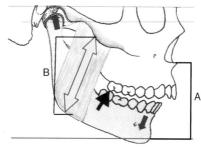

FIGURE 13-13 Note that as the condyles are seated up into centric relation, the vertical dimension at the front is increased. Because the condyles move upward, the muscle length at *(B)* is shortened. This permits an increase in vertical dimension *(A)* that can occur without lengthening the muscles at *B*. Such an increase at the front could be stable because it does not interfere with repetitive muscle contraction length.

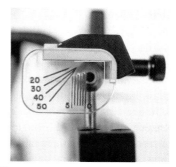

FIGURE 13-14 The determinant index on the Dénar® Combi articulator.

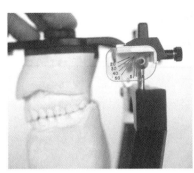

FIGURE 13-15 Casts are positioned from centric relation into maximum intercuspation. Condyle displacement can be observed through clear plastic.

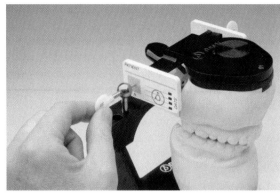

FIGURE 13-17 Using a Centrichek recording to determine vertical displacement (Dénar® Combi articulator). *(Courtesy Water Pik, Inc., Fort Collins, CO.)*

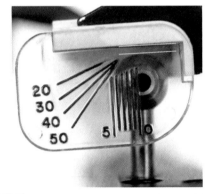

FIGURE 13-16 The distance between the top of the condyle and the roof of the fossa can easily be seen and measured.

This measurement tells you how far the condyle must move up to get from the maximal intercuspation to centric relation. There is usually more vertical displacement than horizontal displacement in the maximum intercuspation position. This determination can simplify determinations regarding changes in vertical dimension at the anterior teeth.

> A safe rule: For each millimeter of vertical displacement at the condyle (from centric relation to maximal intercuspation), the vertical dimension at the anterior teeth can be increased by 2 mm without affecting the repetitive contraction length of the elevator muscles.

Using a Centrichek Recording to Determine Vertical Displacement (Teledyne Dénar® Combi articulator)

1. Record the needlepoint indentation with the casts seated in a centric relation bite record (Figure 13-17).
2. Remove the bite record and seat the casts into maximal intercuspation (MIP).
3. Record another needlepoint indentation at the MIP.
4. Measure the vertical displacement from the centric relation indentation to the MIP indentation.

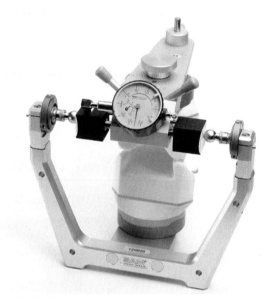

FIGURE 13-18 SAM® articulator with CPI (Condylar Position Indicator). *(Manufactured by SAM Präzisionstechnik GmbH, distributed exclusively by Great Lakes Orthodontics, Ltd. Image provided courtesy Great Lakes Orthodontics, Ltd., Tonawanda, NY.)*

Other methods

Condylar position indicators are available for several semiadjustable articulators (Figure 13-18). The process is the same. Record the position of the condyles at centric relation. Remove the centric relation bite record, and record the condylar position at maximal intercuspation. Then simply measure the vertical displacement from the centric relation position to the MIP position.

Note: The process of determining vertical displacement of the condyles is primarily useful when an increase in the VDO is desired *for the anterior teeth*. If there is no need to increase anterior facial height or to display and *maintain* more anterior tooth length, it is not essential to measure condylar displacement.

Work toward the VDO that can be achieved with the least amount of invasive treatment. As long as maximal intercuspation can be effectively achieved in centric relation, even if by equilibration at a more closed vertical dimension, the VDO will be re-established by the musculature.

The question of whether increased anterior length can be maintained becomes important when one of the objectives of treatment is to display more tooth surface or to increase nose-to-chin dimension. If a permanent increase is not essential for esthetics, it is okay to temporarily increase the VDO to make room for restorations. The rule is to add only as much VDO as needed because it will close back to the original vertical dimension established by the musculature. Also remember that if you increase the VDO, you must increase it for the complete arch. Segmental bite raising creates a stepped occlusion and potential problems of intrusion of teeth into the alveolar bone.

ESTABLISHING VDO WHEN THERE ARE NO OPPOSING TEETH

The Closest Speaking Position

Patients with opposing natural teeth should be maintained at the vertical of their maximum intercuspation position whenever practical. The phonetic technique is used when there are no opposing teeth in contact. It is an ideal method for use in full denture construction but has equal value for the restorative dentist when a restored arch is opposed by a denture, when the vertical has been altered by improper restorations, or in any relationship without adequate opposing tooth contacts.

As a way to understand the principle, one may perform the following steps on a patient with opposing teeth, as outlined by Silverman and Pound[23,24] (Figure 13-19).

1. The patient is seated in an upright position with the occlusal plane parallel to the floor. The patient is asked to close firmly (centric occlusion), and a line is drawn on a lower anterior tooth at the exact level of the upper incisal edge (see Figure 13-19, A). This line is called the *centric occlusion line.*

2. Now the patient says "yes" and continues the *s* sound like *yesssssss.* While the patient is pronouncing the *s* sound, a line is again drawn on the same lower anterior tooth at the level of the upper incisal edge. This line is called the *closest speaking line* (see Figure 13-19, B). The space between the lower centric occlusion line and the upper closest speaking line is called the *closest speaking space.*

3. To analyze how repeatable this record is, the patient should be asked to count from 60 to 66. One should notice how the upper incisal edge comes right back to the closest speaking line with the pronunciation of each *s* sound. If it does not, the line should be altered slightly to match the *s* position when the patient reads or talks fairly rapidly.

4. If such a measurement is to serve as a pre-extraction record, the difference between the closest speaking line and the centric occlusion line is recorded. The

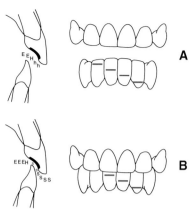

FIGURE 13-19 **A,** A centric occlusion line. With the patient's teeth in maximum occlusal contact, a line is drawn on a lower anterior tooth at the exact level of the upper incisal edge. This is the *maximal closure line.* **B,** The position of the line when the patient says *yessssss.* Notice that the distance from the line to the incisal edge on the *s* sound is about 1 mm. A new line is drawn at the incisal edge position that is repeated during the *s* sound. This is called the *closest speaking line.* Observe how precisely the closest speaking line is repeatedly aligned with the upper incisal edge on *s* sounds.

closest speaking space must be maintained in the finished denture.

5. If the determinations are being made on a patient who has already lost the natural VDO, the missing teeth can be substituted for on temporary restorations or on fabricated bases. After proper lip support, esthetics, and incisal-edge position have been determined, the phonetic method can be used to establish the vertical dimension (Figures 13-20 to 13-22). Since the VDO is unknown, we determine the closest speaking position first and then close the vertical dimension 1 mm from that point. A wax esthetic control rim can be used in place of upper teeth. It can be attached to the upper denture base and adjusted for lip support, smile-line esthetics, and the like. If it interferes during the phonetic exercises, it can be easily corrected. By placing several marks on the lower anterior teeth or lower esthetic rim, we can observe which mark aligns with the incisal edge of the esthetic control rim or the artificial upper anterior teeth when the *s* sounds are made.

There should be no bumping of the teeth during speaking. Such contacts would indicate either interference with the correct vertical dimension or insufficient overjet. When normal phonetic function can take place comfortably, the closest speaking level should be noted and the centric bite record should be made by closing 1 mm further to the VDO.

The vertical dimension has long been regarded as one of the variables of occlusion, but with time more and more evidence has been found that points to an inability to permanently defy the effect of muscle on the vertical relation of the mandible to the maxilla.

Perhaps some of the confusion comes from the loss of vertical dimension that occurs in denture patients as the ridges resorb. However, natural teeth do not react the same

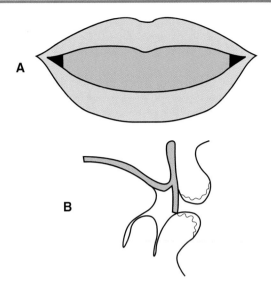

FIGURE 13-20 **A,** A wax esthetic control rim is adapted to the denture base and contoured to relate to the smile line. **B,** The wax is then adjusted to contact the inner vermillion border of the lower lip when an *f* sound is made at a soft-speaking level. This will be used later to establish the incisal edge positions for the teeth on the denture.

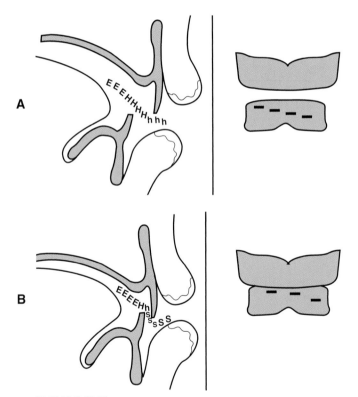

FIGURE 13-21 **A,** Another wax esthetic rim is attached to the lower denture base to conform to where the lower incisors will be placed. The wax can be contoured or bent until an *s* sound can be made comfortably (**B**). By noting which line on the lower rim aligns with the upper incisal edge, the closest speaking position can be determined. A centric relation bite record is then made at a closure of 1 mm past the speaking alignment. This is the VDO.

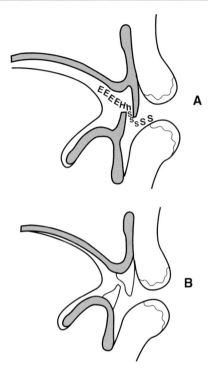

FIGURE 13-22 The denture teeth (**B**) are then set up so their incisal edges and labial surfaces are exactly in line with the esthetic control wax rims (**A**).

as edentulous ridges. More scientific study is needed, but on the basis of clinical evidence and studies of muscle physiology, the safest approach for restorative patients with natural teeth is to work as close to the existing VDO as possible.

When bone and muscle war, muscle never loses.

—*Harry Sicher MD*

When teeth and muscle war, muscle never loses.

—*Peter E. Dawson DDS*

SUMMARY

If the VDO must be altered, do the most conservative dental treatment possible to achieve an optimal esthetic and functional result.

References

1. Hellsing G: Functional adaptation to changes in vertical dimension. *J Prosthet Dent* 52:867-870, 1984.
2. Gross MD, Ormianer Z: A preliminary study on the effect of occlusal vertical dimension increase on mandibular postural rest position. *Int J Prosthodont* 7(3):216-226, 1994.
3. Prombonas A, Vlessides D, Molyvdas P: The effect of altering the vertical dimension on biting force. *J Prosthet Dent* 71:139-143, 1994.

4. Manns A, Miralles R, Palazzi C: EMG, bite force, and elongation of the masseter muscle under isometric voluntary contraction and variation of vertical dimension. *J Prosthet Dent* 42:674-682, 1979.

5. Marimote T, Bekura H, Tokuyama H, et al: Alteration in the bite force and EMG activity with changes in the vertical dimension of edentulous subjects. *J Oral Rehabil* 23:336-341, 1996.

6. Hylander WL: Morphological changes in human teeth and jaws in a high attrition environment. USBHS Grant DE173 & Department of Anatomy, Duke University.

7. Varrela TM, Paurio K, Wouters FR, et al: The relation between tooth eruption and alveolar crest height in a human skeletal sample. *Arch Oral Biol* 40:175-180, 1995.

8. Berry DC, Poole DF: Attrition: Possible mechanisms of compensation. *J Oral Rehabil* 3:201-206, 1976.

9. Crothers A, Sandham A: Vertical height differences in subjects with severe dental wear. *Euro J Orthod* 15:519-525, 1993.

10. Dahl BL, Krogstad O: The effect of a partial bite raising splint on the inclination of upper and lower front teeth. *Acta Odontol Scand* 41:311-314, 1983.

11. Ramfjord SP, Blankenship JR: Increased occlusovertical dimension in adult monkeys. *J Prosthet Dent* 45:74-83, 1981.

12. Ramfjord SP, Ash MM: *Occlusion,* ed 4, Philadelphia, 1995, WB Saunders.

13. Niswonger ME: Rest position of the mandible and centric relation. *J Am Dent Assoc* 21:1572, 1934.

14. Atwood DA: A critique of research of rest position of the mandible. *J Prosthet Dent* 16:848, 1966.

15. Williamson EH: Myomonitor rest position in the presence and absence of stress. *Facial Orthop Temporomandibular Arthrol* 3(2):14-17, 1986.

16. Gibbs CH, Mahan PE, et al: Occlusal forces during chewing: Influences of biting strength and food consistency. *J Prosthet Dent* 46(5):561-567, 1981.

17. Reigh JD: Vertical dimension: A study of clinical rest position and jaw muscle activity. *J Prosthet Dent* 45:670, 1981.

18. Tueller VM: The relationship between the vertical dimension of occlusion and forces generated by closing muscles of mastication. *J Prosthet Dent* 22:284, 1969.

19. Silverman MM: Determination of vertical dimension by phonetics. *J Prosthet Dent* 6:463, 1956.

20. Ricketts RM: *Orthodontic diagnosis and planning: Their roles in preventative and rehabilitative dentistry,* Denver, 1982, Rocky Mountain Orthodontic.

21. McAndrews I: Presentation to Florida Prosthodontic Seminar, Miami, Florida 1984. Also personal communication, 2001.

22. Seega S: Bone remodeling in oral region. *J Dent Res* 64:736, 1985.

23. Silverman MM: The speaking method in measuring vertical dimension. *J Prosthet Dent* 85:427-431, 2001.

24. Pound E: The vertical dimension of speech: The pilot of occlusion. *J Calif Dent Assoc* 6(2):42-47, 1978.

Chapter 14

The Neutral Zone

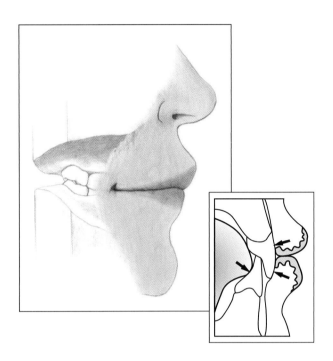

PRINCIPLE

Teeth will not stay stable where muscle does not want them to be.

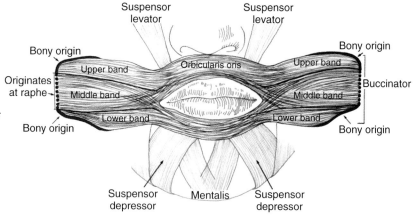

FIGURE 14-1 The three bands of the buccinator muscle. *(From Frederick S: The buccinator–orbicularis oris complex, Manual prepared for Florida Prosthodontic Seminar, 1987.)*

UNDERSTANDING THE NEUTRAL ZONE

Factors That Determine the Horizontal Positioning of Teeth

Teeth are the most movable part of the masticatory system. If outward horizontal forces from the tongue are greater than inward forces exerted by the buccinator muscle bands and the lips, the teeth will move horizontally until the opposing forces are equal. This is the *neutral zone.* As teeth erupt into the mouth, they are guided into a specific zone of neutrality that determines the horizontal position of each tooth in the arch.

The three bands of the buccinator muscle become the *orbicularis oris* (Figure 14-1). We refer to this as the *perioral musculature,* and in combination with the tongue, it plays a profound role in determining a precise horizontal relationship for the anterior and posterior teeth.

The Corridor Between the Tongue and the Buccinator–Orbicularis Oris Muscle Bands

The neutral zone determines the position of each tooth and establishes the dimensions of the entire arch, including the shape and position of the alveolar processes. In effect, the boundaries of the neutral zone form a matrix for the dental arches (Figures 14-2 and 14-3). Any attempt to move any part of the dental arch, including the alveolar structures outside the neutral zone, will result in increased pressure against the part that intrudes.

> There is no occlusal scheme that can stabilize teeth if they are in an unbalanced relationship with muscular forces against them.

The neutral zone has not been given enough importance in the literature, but as a determinant of occlusion it cannot be ignored. Understanding of the neutral zone makes it readily apparent why so many orthodontic results do not remain stable. It also explains why many postrestorative problems occur and even why some periodontal procedures are unsuccessful. Relapses with orthognathic surgery can almost

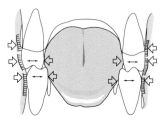

FIGURE 14-2 As the teeth erupt, they are directed horizontally into position by opposing forces from the tongue pressing outward versus the perioral musculature pressing inward. Any factor that affects size, strength, or position of either the tongue or the perioral musculature will affect the position of the neutral zone.

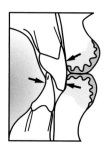

FIGURE 14-3 The combined effect of the position and strength of the buccinator–orbicularis oris muscle and the size, strength, and posture of the tongue determines the precise horizontal position and inclination of the anterior teeth.

always be explained by neutral zone imbalance. And complete or partial denture failures are often related to noncompliance with neutral zone factors.

Regardless of the method of treatment, any part of the dentition out of harmony with the neutral zone will result in instability, interference with function, or some degree of discomfort. Thus the neutral zone must be evaluated as an important factor before making any changes in arch form or alignment of teeth.

The landmark work regarding the limiting effect on arch size was done by Sidney Frederick.[1] He showed that the perioral musculature was erroneously described in the majority of anatomy texts. He also observed the effects of muscle pressure against the dento-alveolar structures in hun-

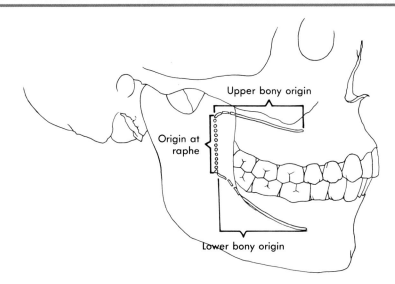

FIGURE 14-4 Origin of the three bands of the buccinator muscle. See text for description. *(Redrawn from Frederick S: The buccinator–orbicularis oris complex, Manual prepared for Florida Prosthodontic Seminar, 1987.)*

dreds of patients. His findings are important to every phase of dental treatment that deals with arch contour or tooth alignment. Understanding of the neutral zone is incomplete without knowledge of Frederick's contributions regarding the perioral musculature.

The outer limits of the neutral zone are determined by the perioral musculature. The main determinant of length, strength, and position of the perioral musculature is the buccinator muscle (see Figure 14-1). The buccinator muscle is a flat, thin muscle composed of three bands.

The upper band has a wide bony origin that starts at the base of the alveolar process above the first molar and extends distally on the skeletal base above the alveolar process to the suture between the maxilla and palatine bone. From that bone, the line extends down to the lower surface of the pyramidal process of the palatine bone and continues on a short ligament to the tip of the pterygoid hamulus (Figure 14-4).

The lower band also has a wide bony origin that starts at the skeletal base below the alveolar process at the first molar. It extends back and up along the external oblique line where it then crosses over behind the last molar at the lower end of the retromolar fossa and proceeds onto the internal oblique line. Its bony origin stops where the middle band starts at the end of the internal oblique line.

The middle band fibers originate from the pterygomandibular raphe, a ligament that extends from the tip of the pterygoid hamulus down to the posterior extremity of the internal oblique line on the mandible. This middle band does not have a bony origin like the upper and lower bands, and because of its soft origin, it cannot exert the strength of contraction that the upper and lower bands can apply to their underlying structures (Figure 14-5).

The upper and lower bands are continuous from side to side without decussation (Figures 14-6 to 14-8). The middle band fibers decussate and join into the fibers of the orbicularis oris. Because the muscle fibers form a continuous band from origin to origin, the size of the arch is limited by the length of the muscles when they are contracted repetitiously.

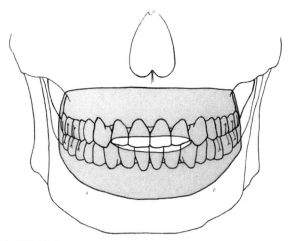

FIGURE 14-5 The combined width of the three bands of the buccinator muscle covers both the teeth and the alveolar processes. This has a limiting effect on the overall size and shape of the dental arches. Crowding occurs in the dentition when the teeth are too large to fit within this dimension.

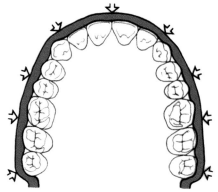

FIGURE 14-6 The upper band of the buccinator muscle extends around the arch from origin to origin, and even though it becomes part of the orbicularis oris muscle, it is effectively one band of muscle. Thus it influences the dimensions of the arch to the limits of its repetitive contracted length.

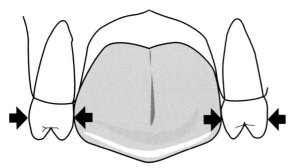

FIGURE 14-7 The tongue is postured up in the vault and in direct opposition to the inward force of the perioral musculature.

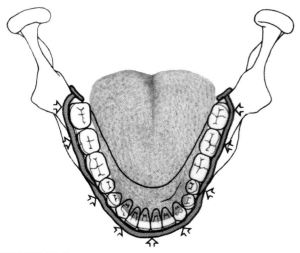

FIGURE 14-8 The lower band of the buccinator muscle is usually the strongest band that, like the upper band, extends from origin to origin. If tongue posture is normal, it resists the inward force to form a corridor of neutrality between opposing forces. Notice how the buccinator muscle originates on the internal oblique line and extends around the last molar following the external oblique line. At this molar position, the widest, strongest part of the tongue opposes the strongest, most unyielding part of the buccinator muscle.

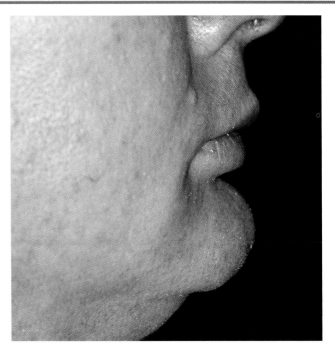

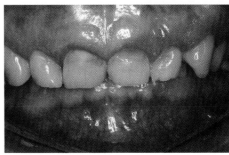

FIGURE 14-9 The combination of a strong lower band of buccinator muscle versus growth of the skeletal base of the mandible results in a deep cleft with a protruded chin. The dental arches are actually held back as the mandible grows forward. The restrictions from the perioral musculature also dictate vertical or even lingual inclination of the upper anterior teeth.

The tonus of the buccinator–orbicularis oris muscle band may very well be controlled by the central nervous system. However, regardless of the reason for variations in muscle tonus in different patients, the strength of that contractile force at the length of the muscle band during contraction forms an inviolate outer limit for arch size.

Problems of alignment occur when the size of the teeth is too large to fit into the arch-size dimension dictated by a constrictive perioral musculature.

The effects of neutral zone confinement on the dento-alveolar structures can also play a critical role as a determinant of facial profile. A restrictive perioral musculature may prevent the dento-alveolar arches from expanding to a normal alignment with the skeletal base. Thus mandibular skeletal growth may extend the chin point forward while the dental arches are restricted by the band of muscles that prevent them from growing commensurately with their skeletal base (Figure 14-9).

Variations in length and strength of the three bands of the buccinator muscle can further affect the profile by controlling the axial inclinations of the anterior teeth, especially when combined with the myriad variations of tongue size and pressure.

Other factors, such as the size of the mouth, must also be evaluated when a change in arch size is being contemplated. A very small orifice is far more restrictive than a large broad opening that exposes the dentition all the way around to the molars.

A series of statements may give perspective to an evaluation of neutral zone considerations:

1. The teeth and their alveolar process are the most adaptive part of the masticatory system. They can be moved horizontally or vertically by light forces.
2. There is a neutral zone within which muscular pressure against the dentition is equalized from opposite

directions. The entire arch form falls within that zone of neutral pressure.

3. If irregularities of tooth position, alignment, or contour can be corrected within the neutral zone, the prognosis for long-term stability is good.

4. A problem occurs when the neutral zone is not where we want the teeth to be.

5. A treatment decision then must allow determination of if and how we can change the neutral zone to orient it where we want the teeth to be.

Because the neutral zone can assume so many variations of form from different types of confinement by the same musculature, any irregular dental alignment or arch form should be evaluated in relation to the directional pressures exerted by the tongue, lips, and cheeks. It should be determined why the dental arches are where they are before it can be determined if they can be altered. Several different arch configurations may be possible without any changes in muscle lengths.

RELATING MALOCCLUSION TO THE NEUTRAL ZONE

The high-vaulted, constricted maxillary arch is a good illustration of how aberrant pressures relate to the configuration of the dento-alveolar arches (Figure 14-10). It also serves as an example of the cause-and-effect influence by muscle pressures, explaining why the problem occurs and how it can be treated. In the case of a patient with a high, narrow vault, the maxillary arch is squeezed inward by buccinator pressure that is unopposed by outward tongue pressure.

The reason for the lack of outward tongue pressure against the posterior arch segments is a forward tongue posture that possibly develops as the effect of an inadequate airway space. With enlarged tonsils or adenoids, there is no room for the posterior width of the tongue in its normal position, so it must be postured forward to provide an airway.

The forward tongue posture causes two effects. It pushes the anterior teeth forward, and it evacuates its normal space up in the vault, thus eliminating the outward tongue pressure as resistance to buccinator pressure against the posterior teeth (see Figure 14-10). The narrowing of the arch form in back also permits a lengthening of the arch forward, without altering the length of the perioral musculature.

As the upper anterior teeth are forced forward, the lower lip drops back behind them (Figure 14-11). This lip relationship can actually be a stabilizing effect on the anterior teeth as the aberrant lip positions establish a neutral zone, albeit a very unesthetic relationship.

The arch configuration is determined by the pressures exerted against the dento-alveolar structures during tooth eruption, and even though the airway space may be enlarged during growth, permitting a more posterior tongue posture, the narrowed space between the posterior segments will not permit a normal tongue position up in the vault. Thus the arch

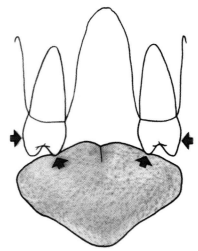

FIGURE 14-10 See text for description.

malformation will persist along with an aberrant neutral zone.

One can correct both the narrow arch and the anterior disharmony by changing the neutral zone orthodontically. Expansion of the dento-alveolar arch width at the posterior segments creates room for the tongue to fit up into the vault where it can then direct outward pressure against the posterior teeth to resist the inward buccinator pressure (see Figure 14-11, *B*).

As the posterior arch width is expanded, the perioral band of muscle pulls back on the anterior teeth thus allowing for correction of the pointed protrusion in the anterior segment (see Figure 14-11, *B*). The corrected arch form can then be quite stable because the widened vault not only permits normalized outward tongue pressure against the posterior teeth, but it also reduces the forward pressure against the anterior teeth as the tongue is allowed to posture back into the widened vault space. The combination of firmer perioral muscle pressure against the anterior teeth versus lessened forward tongue pressure results in a changed neutral zone position that is consistent with the corrected arch form.

The above correction also alters the direction of lip pressures against the upper anterior teeth. When the upper anterior segment is protruded, the lower lip tucks in against their lingual and incisal edges with forward-directed pressure (Figure 14-12). Correction of the overjet alters the neutral zone by allowing the lower lip to pass in front of the labial surfaces and thus reverse the lip pressure to hold the teeth in the improved alignment (Figure 14-13).

How Combined Vertical and Horizontal Factors Influence the Neutral Zone

By understanding that teeth move both vertically and horizontally to a position of neutrality with opposing muscle forces, you can understand how these forces can be misdirected by inappropriate treatment. A classic and all too common example of this is a segmental interocclusal appliance (posterior bite-raising appliance).

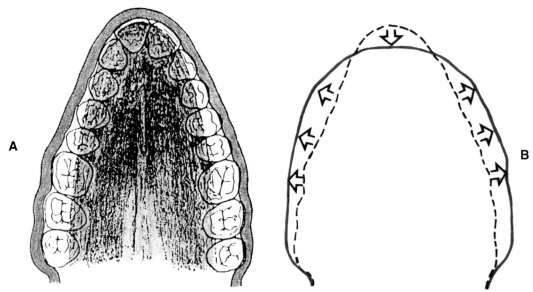

FIGURE 14-11 The arch form that can result from an airway problem due to a forward tongue thrust. The linear dimension of the perioral musculature is limited, but it can be altered in shape. The arch form in **A** resulted from a malposed neutral zone. As the tongue pushes the anterior segment forward, the unopposed posterior segments are pulled inwardly. By expanding the arch at the posterior segments **(B),** the anterior segment is brought back. The contour of the arch is corrected without changing the linear dimension of the perioral musculature. The wider arch form also accommodates the tongue in the vault to stabilize the arch form.

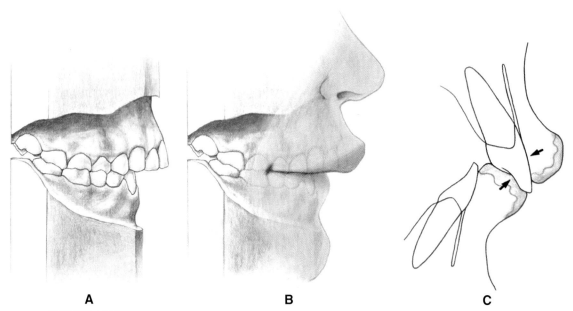

A   **B**   **C**

FIGURE 14-12 Analysis of any malocclusion should include analysis of the neutral zone that contributed to the malrelationships to see if the neutral zone can be changed. **A,** Diagnostic casts tell only part of the story. **B,** Observation of lip position in relation to the anterior teeth is essential. **C,** When the lower lip has insufficient linear dimension to posture in front of the upper incisors, it takes a position behind them and contributes further to the malposition. Diagnosis is critical in this type of malocclusion. It can result from a skeletal retrognathic mandible, which might require a surgical solution. If it is an airway problem, an orthodontic solution may be correct.

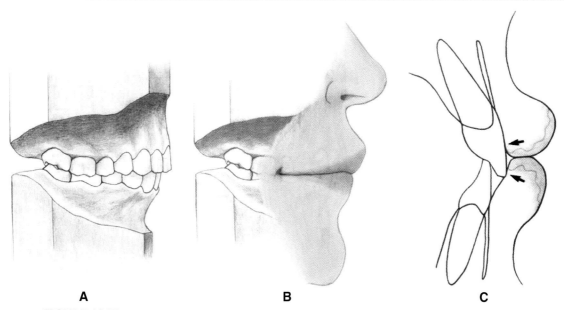

A   B   C

FIGURE 14-13 **A,** Repositioning the anterior teeth back makes it possible for the lower lip to bypass the upper in-cisors to form a proper lip seal **(B).** This in turn postures the lips to resist the forward tongue pressure **(C),** which is also reduced by the expansion of the arch width at the posterior segments. This is an example of changing a neutral zone po-sition to achieve a better esthetic profile. Such a result, however, will not be stable unless the airway problem is also cor-rected, regardless of the type of treatment selected.

Combined effect of neutral zone problem and interference with the VDO.

A posterior segmental bite appliance increases the vertical dimension and interferes with the repetitive contracted length of the elevator muscles. The muscles start to intrude the posterior teeth.

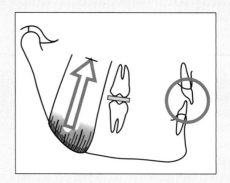

The bite opening also prevents the anterior teeth from contacting. Therefore, the lip pressure back is not resisted by the tongue, which is blocked by the lower anterior teeth, and the upper teeth start to move lingually.

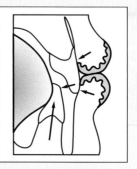

Because the lower anterior teeth are taken out of contact, they start to erupt.

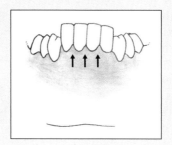

This is the typical result of a posterior bite-raising appliance after one year. Posterior teeth are intruded because the added dimension of the appliance has interfered with the repetitive contraction length of the elevator muscles. The anterior teeth have supraerupted with their alveolar bone to form a stepped occlusion. Lingualization of the upper anterior teeth has steepened the anterior guidance and interfered with the envelope of function in addition to interfering with the arc of closure to centric relation.

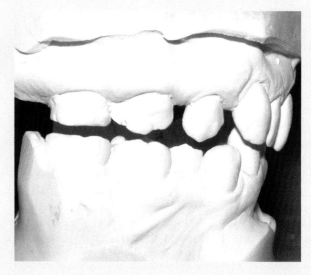

Determining the Neutral Zone for Posterior Teeth

Unless posterior teeth have been recently moved or restored, they will be in their current neutral-zone relationship. Teeth will never spontaneously move vertically or horizontally out of neutral-zone harmony. If muscle pressures change in intensity or direction, the teeth will change position to accommodate. Thus any tooth that has remained in a stable position is in neutral-zone harmony. This position should be carefully evaluated in relation to muscle forces before one makes a decision to alter shape or position.

Inclination and alignment of second and third molars are particularly subjected to the strongest pressures from the widest part of the tongue versus the most unyielding part of the buccinator muscle near its origin. Attempts at uprighting or perfecting alignment in this segment are often unsuccessful because the neutral zone does not conform to the textbook norm. Pretreatment observation can be very enlightening regarding the location of the neutral zone, and if realignment can take place within that established zone, the prognosis for stability will be excellent.

In replacement of teeth on posterior edentulous ridges, there are no teeth to indicate the neutral-zone location, but one can precisely determine it by allowing the musculature to form a moldable material during swallowing. The procedure is described in Figure 14-14.

Observation of several neutral-zone recordings is a convincing exercise that is highly recommended. One will notice the consistency in the width of the recorded neutral zones, and it will be apparent that it relates to the normal width of natural teeth. It will also be apparent that even in mouths that have been without posterior teeth for extended time periods, the outward tongue pressure is still resisted by inward buccinator pressure that is sufficiently strong to position the neutral zone in a reasonably normal alignment over the ridge. This repeated finding raises doubt about the popular belief that the tongue expands when teeth are lost.

The effectiveness of some functional appliances is based on blocking the pressure from one side of the neutral zone. By placing a shield on the cheek side to prevent inward pressure, one can see that the unopposed tongue forces will then move the teeth toward the cheek. Regardless of the method of creating uneven pressure, teeth will move toward the neg-

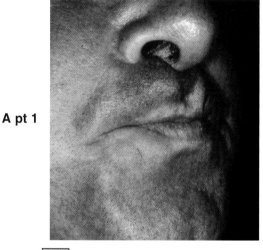

A pt 1

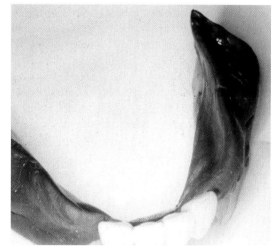

A pt 2

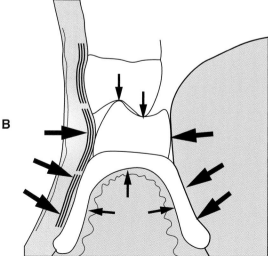

B

FIGURE 14-14 The neutral zone for an edentulous ridge can be formed in moldable compound during swallowing. **A,** Notice how the tongue pressure has formed the lingual contour. Pressure from the buccinator muscle forms the buccal contour and defines the neutral zone where the posterior teeth should be placed. **B,** A lower denture in harmony with the neutral zone is stabilized as much by the tongue and cheek musculature as it is by the adaptation on the ridge. When both vertical and horizontal harmonies are achieved, there are no dislodging forces.

ative side of imbalanced forces and away from the side with stronger pressure. The long-term effectiveness of functional appliances is ultimately related to the *balance* of pressures at the completion of treatment.

Determining the Neutral Zone for Anterior Teeth

Because the neutral zone is determined by the functional relationship of the tongue versus the perioral musculature, locating an unknown neutral zone starts by observation of the positional relationships of these structures during specific functions. Several different functions require rather precise mechanical interrelationships between the teeth, the tongue, and the lips in order to perform the function correctly. The value of understanding how these interrelationships work mechanically is that it provides known reference points for determining how the teeth must interrelate in order for correct function to occur. Functional harmony and anatomic harmony are almost always coincidental.

Phonetic methods can be used with a high degree of accuracy because the shaping of sounds results from precise approximation of upper and lower teeth with each other, with the lips, and with the tongue. The near contact of structures that constrict the airflow into particular sound forms can also be used as a guideline for incisal edge position and the entire incisal plane. The lip closure path can be used to determine labial contours, and methods for determining the anterior guidance can direct the contouring of the upper lingual surfaces. When all of these functional relationships are correct, the teeth will be in harmony with the neutral zone.

The methods for determining all the necessary anterior relationships are described in detail in Chapter 16.

Methods for Altering the Neutral Zone

The neutral zone may be altered in several ways, as follows:

Orthodontics
By realigning the teeth for improved balance between the tongue and the perioral musculature, one can most often improve it without the need for lengthening muscle.

Elimination of noxious habits
Thumb sucking, lip biting, or forward tongue posturing all tend to increase outward pressure against the perioral musculature, thus moving the neutral zone accordingly. Elimination of such habit patterns allows the perioral muscles to move the teeth back into harmony with normal tongue position. It should be noted, however, that success in changing habit patterns is often difficult or impossible if they involve long-standing tongue-thrust patterns.

Myofunctional therapy
If lip pressure can be increased by strengthening the perioral musculature, the neutral zone will move accordingly. Any change in muscle pressure will affect the neutral zone, but results are often disappointing for long-term effectiveness in mature adults.

Reduction of tongue size
Surgical reduction of tongue size will reduce outward pressure and allow the perioral muscles to move the teeth lingually into a new neutral zone. For some reason, this procedure has not had popular acceptance.

Surgical lengthening of the buccinator muscle band
Surgical lengthening of the buccinator muscle band can be used to reduce restrictive pressure that limits arch size. Frederick[1] has reported increased thickness of labial tissues over the roots of teeth, along with increased stability of the teeth after arch expansion when restrictive muscle pressure is released. It is usually done to lengthen the lower band of the buccinator muscle.

The procedure involves four steps:

1. Surgically cut through the mucosa with a vertical incision.
2. Vertically cut through the lower band of the buccinator muscle on each side.
3. Suture the mucosa only. Leave the muscle segments unattached.
4. Add lip pressure to increase the length of muscle with a Frankel-type appliance.

Scar tissue will fill in between the two cut ends, effectively lengthening the perioral band around the arch.

Vestibuloplasty
Vestibuloplasty, either alone or in combination with muscle-lengthening procedures, appears to cause a reduction of perioral pressure. It should extend around the anterior arch to the bicuspid area.

More study is needed to evaluate the full effect of the surgical approach. However, clinical results appear to be beneficial in reducing the thinning out and clefting of labial tissues when arches are expanded beyond the normal boundaries of a tight neutral zone.

Neutral-zone considerations in orthognathic surgery
Surgical advancements tend to relapse if the advanced section causes extension of any connected muscle or interferes with the length of the perioral musculature. Modern surgical techniques all consider muscle relationships and move either the muscle origin or insertion to compensate for the change in position of the skeletal part.

Reference

1. Frederick S: The buccinator–orbicularis oris complex, Manual prepared for Florida Prosthodontic Seminar, 1987.

Chapter 15

The Envelope of Function

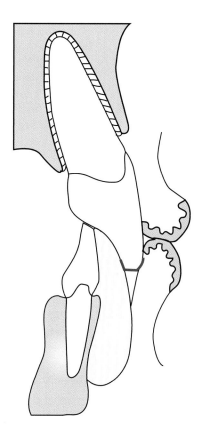

PRINCIPLE

The envelope of function dictates incisal edge position and consequentially determines the anterior guidance.

FUNCTION

The functional movements of the mandible constitute the most fundamental basis for ideal occlusal design. A discussion about the *envelope of function* may appear to be a merely academic exercise, but that would be a mistaken viewpoint. The entire context of occlusal harmony is based on a precise relationship of the teeth to how the mandible moves in function versus pathofunction.

The starting point for understanding the envelope of function is to first understand the *envelope of motion*.

THE ENVELOPE OF MOTION

Every tooth in the mandible (the only moving jaw) has an *envelope of motion* that outlines the outer limits to which each lower tooth can be moved. These limits of movement are imposed on the mandible. To a larger degree, the limits of mandibular movement are directly related to limits imposed by ligaments, bone, and muscle on the temporomandibular joints (TMJs). The condyles can go back and up only so far, rotate to open the mouth only so far, move forward only so far, and rotate the mandible laterally only so far. Therefore, the TMJs have an envelope of motion that sets the border paths (the envelope) for all movement of the teeth that are attached to the mandible. The envelope of motion can be altered in a limiting way by teeth that interfere with physiologic masticatory muscle function.

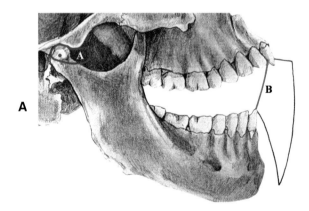

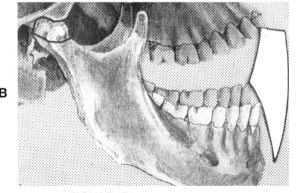

FIGURE 15-1 See text for description.

The Envelope of Motion of the Condyle

From centric relation *(red dot)* in Figure 15-1, *A* the condyles cannot move up or back any further (unless forced back by external pressure). The condyles can move forward and down the posterior slopes of their eminentiae. They can move anywhere within their envelope of motion and can rotate around both a horizontal and a vertical axis as they move forward and back and laterally. Pure rotation in centric relation can occur until stopped by the lateral temporomandibular ligament at which point the condyles *must* move forward to continue opening rotation.

The Envelope of Motion of the Lower Incisors

Figure 15-1, *B* reflects the limitation of condylar movement. The red line is the most posterior border path that can be made by the lower incisors and also represents the maximum length of the opening/closing arc in centric relation before the mandible must move forward in order to open wider. The lower incisors can move anywhere within the envelope of motion, but they cannot move outside of the border paths that define the envelope of motion.

Some early pioneers in occlusion and restorative dentistry surmised that if the border movements of the condyles controlled the envelope of motion of the mandible, recording the condylar path and copying it on a fully adjustable articulator would provide a precise method for occlusal analysis and treatment. Out of this concept, *gnathology* was born. The development of pantographic recording devices was perfected, and the recording of condylar pathways became the standard for quality occlusal treatment by a fast-growing cadre of "gnathologists." I must admit that for some time I was a proponent of gnathologic concepts. I studied them intensely with some of the "fathers of gnathology" (Stallard, Stuart, Thomas, Paine, Luccia, Granger, Guichet). All were great contributors to dentistry. There was much to learn from practicing gnathology, but in time, some of the flaws in the concept became apparent and some of the major tenets have since been discarded. For a more complete analysis of gnathologic instrumentation, see Chapter 22. For now, we'll concentrate on conceptual changes that relate to the *envelope of function*.

THE ENVELOPE OF FUNCTION

The first thing to understand about the *envelope of function* is that the functional movements of the mandible occur *within* the envelope of motion and cannot be determined by recording the border movements of the condyles. Pantographic tracings use a central bearing point to separate the teeth so the condyles are free to travel along all of their border paths without interference from deflective tooth inclines. These tracings do a good job of accurately recording the condylar border paths. But they record *only* the condylar border paths.

That is not enough information to determine an envelope of function that occurs *within* the envelope of motion.

The Influence of Teeth

Let's look again at the determinants of occlusion. You will see that the condylar path dictates how the back end of the mandible moves. That is the first determinant of occlusion. The second determinant is controlled by teeth. Ideally, that is the anterior guidance, which determines how the front end of the mandible moves. In a perfected occlusion, the combination of condylar guidance and anterior guidance determines the path that the mandible follows in function. In an ideal occlusal relationship, all contact by posterior teeth is determined by the combined border paths at both the front and back ends of the mandible. Thus, the anterior teeth play a dominant role in establishing the *functional* path that the mandible can travel (Figure 15-2).

This means that the position, inclination, and lingual contour of the upper anterior teeth combine to establish the anterior guidance. This also means that the position of the upper incisal edges is critically important in determining whether or not an anterior guidance is in harmony with an ideal envelope of function, or is interfering with it. Determination of precisely correct incisal edges is the second most important decision a dentist must make regarding occlusion (centric relation is first in importance). Incisal edge position is highly variable from patient to patient and cannot be determined from even the most sophisticated recording of the envelope of motion (Figure 15-3).

The early gnathologists did not understand that the anterior guidance is *not* determined by the envelope of *motion.* Rather the anterior guidance is determined by the envelope of *function,* and it varies from patient to patient regardless of the condylar path or the envelope of motion. There is no need or advantage of any kind for the anterior guidance to be the same as the condylar guidance. It is a completely separate entity and requires separate clinical procedures for determination (see Chapter 17).

The Concept of Harmony

When restoring upper anterior teeth, the lingual contours should be *in harmony with* the envelope of function from centric relation contact to incisal edge positions. It is not enough to be in noninterference to the envelope of function. If best appearance, best function, best phonetics, and best long-term stability are to be achieved, the upper incisal edges must be *in harmony with* the envelope of function.

Of all mistakes that can be made in restorative or orthodontic treatment, *restriction* of the envelope of function is one of the most problematic. Putting anterior teeth into a relationship that restricts a more horizontal envelope of function is an almost certain cause of excessive wear, mobility, or forced movement of the anterior teeth. Unfortunately, it is a common mistake. When you see excessive wear on the labio-incisal edges of lower anterior teeth or on the lingual surfaces of upper anterior teeth, always look for restriction of the envelope of function as a potential cause.

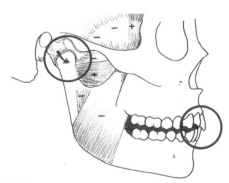

FIGURE 15-2 Both the condylar guidance at the back and the anterior guidance at the front should determine the functional pathways of the mandible. The posterior teeth should contact in centric relation but should be discluded when the mandible moves from centric relation. Posterior teeth must not interfere with either condylar guidance or anterior guidance during functional jaw movements.

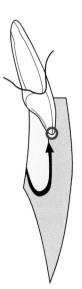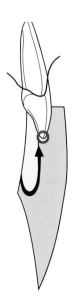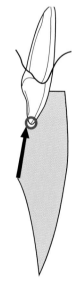

FIGURE 15-3 Variations in the envelope of function result naturally from how the anterior teeth were guided during eruption into their neutral-zone position by the tongue and the lips. Mechanoreceptors in and around the teeth program the muscles for functional jaw movements. The incisal edge position should be in harmony with the envelope of function. The outer limits of potential jaw pathways (the envelope of motion) are not a factor in location of the incisal edges or the envelope of function.

Restorations must be *in harmony with* the envelope of function

In harmony with the envelope of function

STABLE

Results in the best esthetics, comfort, and patient satisfaction.

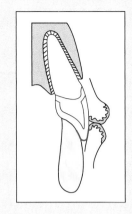

Incisal edges *too far back*

Interferes with the envelope of function.

UNSTABLE

May result in fremitus, excessive wear on the labio-incisal contours of lower incisors or the lingual contours of upper incisors, tooth movement, or fracture of anterior laminate restorations.

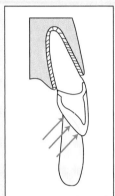

Incisal edges *too far forward*

Interferes with the lip closure path and neutral zone.

UNSTABLE

May result in phonetic problems or feeling that teeth are too long or too thick. Compromised esthetics is a common result as teeth appear too large and too far forward.

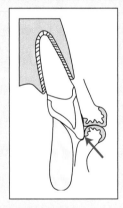

LATERAL ENVELOPE OF FUNCTION

After the stability of the TMJs has been ascertained, and after the anterior guidance has been determined to be in harmonious function in all excursions, the next goal is to establish stable holding contacts of equal intensity on all posterior teeth. In dentitions in which there are posterior interferences to centric relation, the centric relation interferences must be corrected before the anterior guidance can be finalized. Then all excursive interferences must be removed so the harmonized anterior guidance can maintain contact from centric relation through all excursions. The usual goal is for the posterior teeth to be separated in all eccentric jaw movements (Figure 15-4).

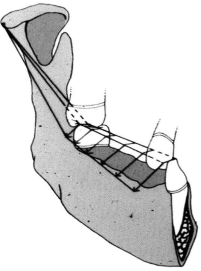

FIGURE 15-4   The lateral pathway of the mandible is controlled by the lateral anterior guidance, which will remain stable only if it is in harmony with the envelope of function. The long-term stability of the posterior teeth is dependent on the anterior teeth not wearing away or moving, so it is important to establish an anterior guidance that does not interfere with either the neutral zone or the natural envelope of function through all excursive pathways.

How the Envelope of Function Is Programmed

More than any other factor, the neutral zone programs the envelope of function. This is so because the neutral zone is the major determinant of how the anterior teeth erupt into the mouth, and it is the position of the anterior teeth that influences the neuromuscular programming of functional jaw movements (Figure 15-5).

> The envelope of function is directly related to the neutral-zone positioning of the anterior teeth.

The envelope of function depends on complex integrative neural processes that dictate the motor behavior of the neuromusculature. It involves the cerebral cortex, cerebellum, basal ganglia, and brain stem. Control of masticatory system motor responses is integrated with and is dependent on mechanoreceptive and proprioceptive information from the teeth, tongue, TMJs, and reflex responses in the musculature.[1-5]

The criteria for reflex responses in the musculature typically relate to stimuli that are fairly constant in their application, but modulation of motor responses, including jaw reflex movements, may be produced by periodontal pressoreceptors, receptors in the mucosa, pain fibers, and muscle spindle afferents.

One thing appears certain: The repetitious movements of the mandible that determine the envelope of function are far more complex, and far more influenced by exquisitely sensitive sensory systems than can be explained by simplistic explanations. But clinical observation is too consistent to be ignored: The mandible does have favored pathways of function, and if teeth interfere with these favored paths, there will be a price to pay in deformation or dysfunction. The weakest link will be the prime focus of the damage.

THE EXQUISITELY SENSITIVE MECHANORECEPTOR SYSTEM

It has generally been accepted that horizontal and vertical pressure sensation is generated entirely from pressure and tension sensors located in the periodontal ligament. Research studies have shown conclusively that such sensory nerve endings do exist, and that they play an important role in the way masticatory muscle activity is coordinated or stimulated into incoordinated hyperactivity (Figures 15-6 and 15-7).

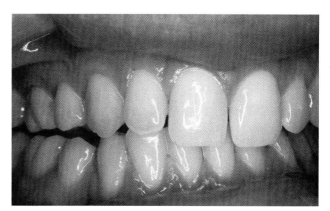

FIGURE 15-5   Vertical inclination of the anterior teeth is the natural result of a tight neutral zone. Inward force from strong perioral musculature dictated the eruption of the teeth into this relationship (shown in mandibular protrusion). Mechanoreceptors in and around the teeth program the neuromuscular system to function in a vertical pattern of jaw movement. This 42-year-old patient has stable TMJs and a stable dentition with no signs of wear or mobility. If the incisal edges of these upper anterior teeth were moved forward, they would interfere with the strong neutral zone, the lip closure path, and comfortable phonetics. Strong lower lip pressure would have a tendency to move the teeth back to a position that is more conformative to the neutral zone.

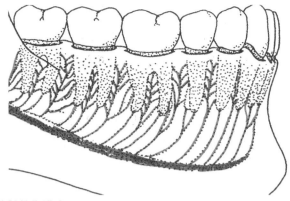

FIGURE 15-6 Major innervation supply to the periodontal ligaments indicates the importance of the sensory response to compressive and tensive forces on teeth.

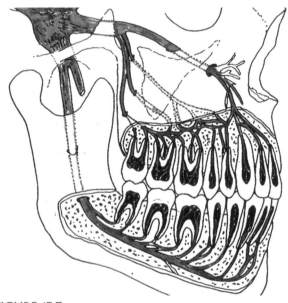

FIGURE 15-7 An even greater supply of sensory innervation goes to interdental structures. Several million nerve receptors associated with the odontoblastic sensory units within each tooth relate to motoneurons that control masticatory neuromuscular reflex responses to the most minute forces.

(*Note:* The term *proprioception* has been used almost universally in the dental literature to connote what should be more correctly termed *mechanoreception.* Proprioception refers to awareness of a body part in space. Mechanoreception refers to sensory recognition of mechanical tension, compression, or torque applied, in this discussion, to teeth.)

Williamson's[6] landmark work of 1983, showing the direct effect on reducing elevator muscle activity that results from anterior disclusion of posterior teeth, can only be explained by some form of mechanoreceptive input from the dentition. Conversely, the hyperactivity that occurs in the same muscles when posterior teeth interfere with the anterior guidance is further evidence of sensory input from the teeth to the musculature.

Any dentist who becomes even marginally aware of the role tooth mechanoreception plays in masticatory muscle activity will start to see daily evidence of a causal relationship with many symptoms that may otherwise be blamed on stress or psychologic factors. But new evidence and new understanding of mechanoreception from teeth are presenting strong reasons for believing that the sensitivity of teeth is far more exquisite and far more important as a stimulus for neuromuscular activity than previously understood. Levy[7] has opened up an expanded understanding of tooth mechanoreception by showing that the mechanoreceptive input generated by strains from within the teeth may have a greater influence on the neuromusculature than the sensory input from the periodontal ligament.

Levy has postulated that the component materials of teeth form a multilayered structural system with an elaborate *integrated* neural sensory network that responds to minute deformations of odontoblastic tubules and provides rapid feedback to enable the neuromusculature to control applied forces. Levy supports his hypothesis based on the coincident presence in the dentinal tubules of specialized ultra-structural and neurologic components.

Levy has also shown through beam analysis correlated to finite element analytical models that extreme elevations in stress levels are produced *within* dentin by lateral forces on teeth, and that these deformations also occur in the odontoblastic tubules. It is quite probable that the odontoblastic sensory units with their abundant tie-in to major sensory nerve pathways form a very important and exquisite relationship to the total neuromuscular reflex patterns of the masticatory system. Far from being inert stonelike forms, teeth have an internal system of sensors that can discern the slightest compression or torque—and teeth do bend and twist far more than we have realized. Many now suspect that the formation of abfractions, as an example, may be caused in part by microscopic chipping away of crystalline structures as the tooth is bent by occlusal forces.

The increased understanding of the exquisite nature of tooth mechanoreceptors is consistent with many of the clinical observations regarding reflex muscle responses to *minute* occlusal interferences, and it supports the concept of precise occlusal harmonization as a logical approach for achieving a peaceful neuromusculature.

The major portion of sensory innervation of one of the largest cranial nerves (the trigeminal nerve) is directly stimulated by variations in intensity and direction of contacts on the teeth. The fact that so much innervation should be assigned to the teeth, plus the relationship of that sensory input to reflex jaw movements activated by associated motoneurons, is an indication of how exquisitely sensitive the neuromuscular system can be even to minute occlusal prematurities or deflections.

A prime purpose of occlusal therapy is to achieve a peaceful neuromusculature. Occlusal therapy will lack predictability unless the preciseness of the system is understood and the skills for refining occlusions precisely enough are developed.

An understanding of the clinical implications of the *envelope of function* is a necessary preparation for understanding many of the most important essentials of occlusal diagnosis and treatment. Certainly a complete understanding of anterior guidance would not be possible without being aware of its relationship to each individual's envelope of function.

References

1. Robertson LT, Levy JH, Petrisor D, et al: Vibration perception thresholds of human maxillary and mandibular central incisors. *Arch Oral Biol* 1294:1-8, 2003.

2. Jacobs R, van Steenberghe D: Role of periodontal ligament receptors in the tactile function of teeth: a review. *J Periodont Res* 29:153-167, 1994.

3. Ash MM, Ramfjord SP: *Occlusion,* ed 4, Philadelphia, 1995, WB Saunders.

4. Hannam AG, et al: The relationship between dental occlusion, muscle activity, and associated jaw movement in man. *Arch Oral Biol* 22:25, 1977.

5. Taylor A: Proprioception in the strategy of jaw movement control. In Kawamura Y, Dubner R, eds: *Oral-facial sensory and motor function,* Tokyo, 1981, Quintessence.

6. Williamson EH, Lundquist DO: Anterior guidance: Its effect on anterior temporalis and masseter muscles. *J Prosthet Dent* 39:816-823, 1983.

7. Levy JH: University of Oregon research: personal communication.

Chapter 16

Functional Smile Design

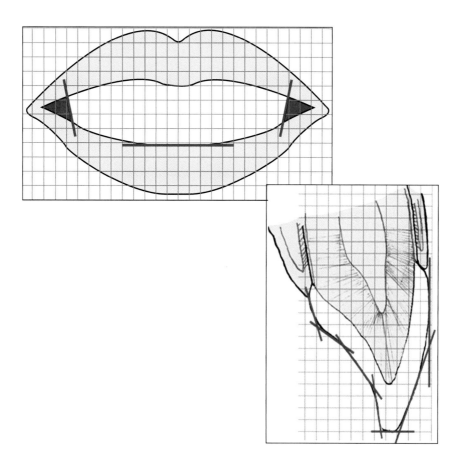

PRINCIPLE

The better the function, the better will be the smile design.

NATURAL ESTHETICS

As more patients are saving their teeth into their golden years, the desire for a more esthetic smile has become one of the most powerful incentives for a visit to the dentist. The esthetic revolution is a fact. The demand for beautiful smiles has become a phenomenal trend that shows no sign of diminishing. And with this increased demand comes unprecedented opportunities for any dentist who is willing to learn the principles of smile design that are compatible with predictable comfort, function, and long-term stability. It comes as a surprise to many dentists that none of these goals has to be achieved by trial-and-error guesswork. There is a learnable reason for every tooth contour, position, or inclination. There is a definite process for designing any and every smile. If that process is understood and followed, there will be no reason to ever end up with anterior teeth that look artificial, or are uncomfortable or unstable.

Let's just be openly honest about what we see far too often. Look at almost any magazine cover showing celebrities smiling with teeth that are obviously artificial. Watch TV celebrities, and there is no mistaking many smiles that are anything but natural. I cringe when I see friends, acquaintances, or even other dentists with their new "cosmetic" veneers or crowns that are obviously unrelated to any of the guidelines for either natural esthetics or normal function.

There seems to be a mass departure from naturalness in smile design and a trend toward bigger, longer teeth with little consideration for normal contours, including embrasure contours. Some clinicians explain unnatural design as "what patients want." I'm confident that if you follow the concepts and procedures outlined in the chapters that follow, you will see firsthand that it is a rare patient who will not choose a naturally beautiful smile over artificially contoured anterior teeth. The principles and procedures of functional smile design will lead you through a step-by-step process. The process defines every tooth position and contour toward an end result that is specifically related to functional harmony. To achieve functional harmony requires harmony of form that patients will choose almost every time if given the opportunity.

With this said, it is nevertheless a fact that some patients do want smiles that are not natural in appearance. The process I am advocating will never produce a finished smile that is not in compliance with the esthetic wishes of the patient, even if those wishes depart from a natural appearance. It is my experience though that such a choice is rare if the process is followed.

DECISIONS IN SMILE DESIGN

Two critical decisions are required to produce any smile that is in harmony with function:

1. The position of each anterior tooth
2. The contour of each anterior tooth

There are many different factors that influence these two ultimate decisions. The decision-making process for restoring anterior teeth requires following a specific sequence. You must be faithful in completing each and every step in proper sequence. If you want the ultimate predictability, here is the rule: *There should be no shortcuts.*

The Importance of Mounted Casts

If there is any step in the process of smile design that dentists fail to complete, ignoring the importance of properly mounted diagnostic casts surely leads the list. Because the horizontal condylar axis is the determinant of the arc each lower tooth travels as the jaw opens or closes, mounted casts are the only certain way of knowing the correct relationship of the lower incisal edges to the upper anterior teeth. Since the anterior guidance must start at centric relation to achieve immediate posterior disclusion, functional smile design cannot even be achieved until a decision is made regarding how to ensure that the posterior teeth don't interfere with the condyles in centric relation or the anterior guidance. The easiest, fastest, and surest way to make that decision is with mounted casts. The price in lost time paid for not having that information is always greater than the time required to take a facebow and centric bite record.

There will be times when increasing the vertical dimension of occlusion (VDO) improves the anterior relationship. There will be times when closing the VDO creates the best alignment for centric relation contacts of the anterior teeth. There will be times when vertical displacement of the condyles is required to achieve maximal intercuspation, and such condylar displacement can have a profound effect on the choice of treatment for anterior teeth. Design of cosmetic restorations that does not consider the entire temporomandibular joint (TMJ)/occlusion condition is shortsighted and an invitation for problems. Until the displacement of the condyles is corrected, accurate analysis of the anterior relationship is not possible.

Restoring Anterior Teeth: Where Do You Start?

Before starting anterior restorations, it is absolutely critical that the planning stage includes analysis of the TMJs. You must determine if the TMJs can be completely seated into centric relation. Load testing should always be a part of this process to verify that centric relation has been achieved. If there is any sign of tenderness or tension in either joint, you are not ready to proceed with planning for anterior restorations. There are many reasons for verifying that the TMJs are stable and can comfortably seat into centric relation before proceeding.

After the condyles are completely seated, they should be held in centric relation while closing the jaw to evaluate the relationship of the anterior teeth. The goal is anterior contact in centric relation (or adapted centric posture) without interference or premature contact of the posterior teeth. It is not possible to accurately analyze an ideal relationship for anterior teeth if posterior teeth interfere with complete closure to anterior contact in centric relation, or at least to maximal intercuspation if anterior contact in centric relation is not possible.

If there are posterior interferences that require displacement of the TMJs to achieve anterior contact, the result will be the potential for any or all of the following:
1. Overload on posterior teeth
2. Hyperactive incoordinated muscles
3. Mandibular slide forward into anterior overload
4. Excessive wear, hypermobility, and tooth migration (unstable dentition)

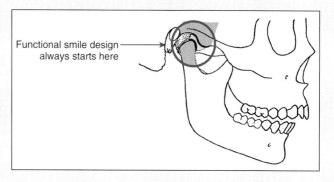

Functional smile design always starts here

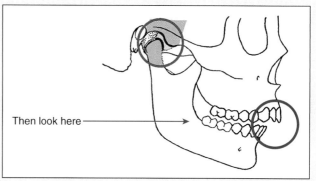

Then look here

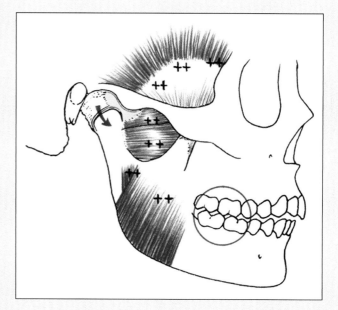

Posterior interferences to centric relation make it impossible to do this. Remember that a major function of the anterior guidance is immediate disclusion of the posterior teeth the moment the mandible moves from centric relation. This is the only occlusal scheme that permits peaceful coordination of the masticatory musculature. It also prevents excessive wear on posterior teeth, and actually reduces the forces on the anterior teeth.

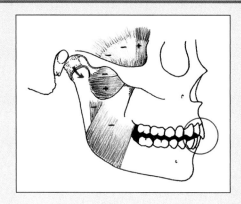

So before the anterior teeth can be designed or corrected to achieve immediate disclusion of the posterior teeth, the treatment planning must be directed at achieving noninterference of the posterior teeth with both anterior contact and the fully seated condyles. Immediate disclusion of posterior teeth is dependent on centric relation contact of the anterior teeth. Proper smile design requires this as a starting point.

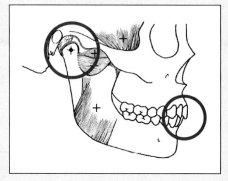

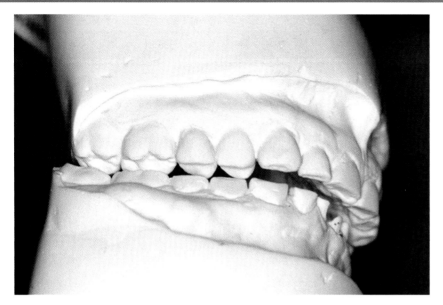

FIGURE 16-1 Facebow-mounted cast in centric relation.

So, your first key thought process in treatment design is . . .

> Get the back teeth out of the way so the front teeth can contact in centric relation.

You cannot be effective in making the best treatment decisions without facebow-mounted casts in centric relation. It is in analysis of your casts that you determine which treatment options you select for achieving anterior contact in centric relation. Until that decision is made, you are not ready to make other decisions about the front teeth. If anterior restorations were planned for this patient (Figure 16-1) at maximal intercuspation instead of in centric relation as shown, the result would be an invitation to many problems.

Options for Achieving Anterior Contact

1. **Reshape.** Consider reshaping the posterior teeth to close down the VDO in order to gain anterior contact.
2. **Reposition.** Consider repositioning either posterior or anterior teeth.
3. **Restore.** Consider restoring the anterior teeth to achieve contact, or posterior teeth to achieve more closure
4. **Surgery.** Consider surgical reposition of a segment of the dento-alveolar process.

The four primary options for treatment are discussed in detail in Chapter 30 on programmed treatment planning. It is a process of evaluating all options for treating all types of occlusal problems, and should be studied in detail. For now, we will apply some of those sequences to show the importance of proper treatment planning for smile design and to illustrate the folly of attempting anterior restorations without recording the correct jaw-to-jaw relationship on mounted casts. Also notice how problematic it would be to attempt anterior restorations without knowing the correct jaw-to-jaw relationship in centric relation. Because the casts are mounted with a facebow, the VDO can be changed, if necessary, without changing the relationship of the casts to the centric relation axis.

Reshaping the casts

Before smile design can be achieved with accuracy, the best option for getting the back teeth out of the way has to be determined. Analysis of the posterior occlusion can be done on the casts mounted in centric relation. Marking ribbon is used to mark interferences that prevent anterior contact in centric relation. The articulator should be locked in centric relation for this step.

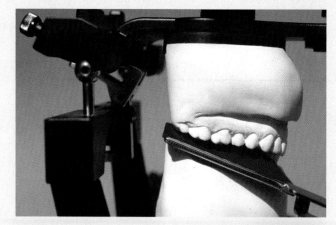

If reductive reshaping is selected as the best option, the posterior teeth can be equilibrated to close the VDO and bring the anterior teeth closer together for centric relation contact.

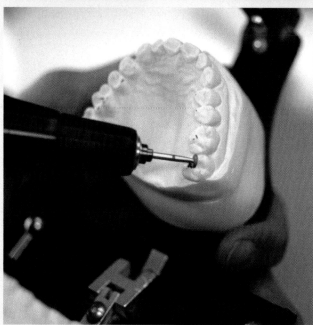

The diagnostic wax-up on the lower anterior teeth is an important planning step to get an idea of what can be accomplished by restorative reshaping to achieve anterior contact in centric relation.

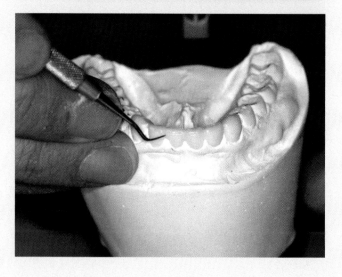

Analysis of the results of reductive reshaping of the posterior teeth and additive reshaping of the lower incisors. By improving the position of the lower incisal edges, it now can be seen that restorative reshaping of the upper anterior teeth can establish acceptable centric relation contacts.

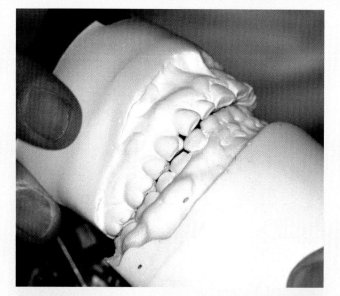

The completed diagnostic wax-up. It is very important to understand that the diagnostic wax-up is rarely the final contour of the anterior teeth. It is a very good guide for selecting the best option for treatment, and it will be used to fabricate a matrix for the provisional restorations when the teeth are prepared. But final determination of the incisal edges, labial contour, and anterior guidance must be worked out in the mouth. Whenever a restorative change is required for incisal edge position, it should always be worked out in provisional restorations.

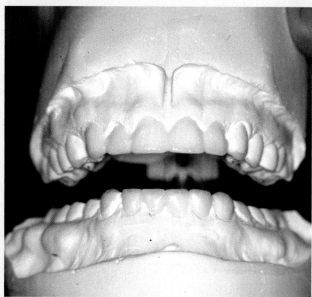

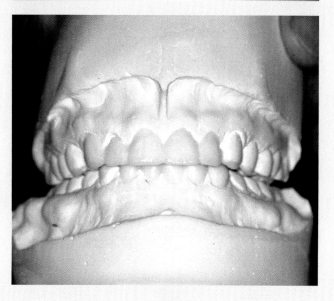

Compare the bucco-lingual relationship of the lower posterior teeth to the upper posterior teeth before and after equilibration was done on the casts. Observe the improvement in this relationship when the VDO was closed (see previous figure). With facebow-mounted casts, the correct arc of closure shows how the relationship improves as the wider part of the mandibular arch arcs forward to a better alignment with the narrower part of the maxillary arch. Closing the VDO also improves the relationship of the lower anterior teeth to the upper anterior teeth.

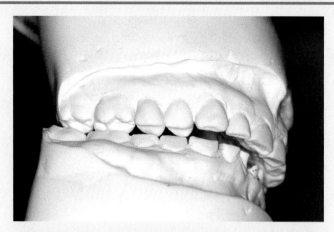

Treatment planning with a diagnostic wax-up has many advantages. One of the main advantages is that the wax-up provides an ideal starting place for refinement of all the anterior teeth contours, including the precise location of the incisal edges and the anterior guidance. A putty silicone matrix is made from the wax-up, to be used for fabricating the provisional restorations after the teeth are prepared.

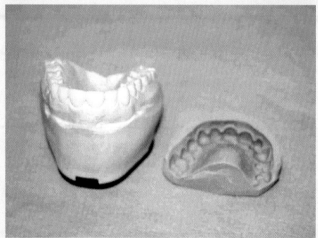

It is in the refinement and contouring of the provisional restorations that the details of smile design are brought into final form. If you want to have the most physiologic, most natural, stable anterior restorations, you will follow this rule:

> You cannot trust a diagnostic wax-up regardless of how beautifully it is done.

It is the rare diagnostic wax-up that cannot be improved in the mouth. The *matrix of functional anatomy* can only be determined in the mouth.

THE MATRIX OF FUNCTIONAL ANATOMY

For many years and thousands of anterior restorations, I studiously observed the functional relationships that matched up with the contours and positioning of anterior teeth. As a restorative dentist, I had many opportunities to alter incisal edge position and anterior guidance and then observe the effects. Working with provisional restorations, it is possible to make instant changes and then objectively analyze the effect on the lips, phonetics, comfort, and the appearance of the smile.

All patients were given these instructions on the day the provisional restorations were placed: "I want you to be extremely fussy about how these teeth feel. If they are not completely comfortable; if they bother your speech; if there is anything about the appearance that is not to your liking, I want to know about it. These teeth are made of a plastic resin, and if there is anything that doesn't feel like they are your own teeth we can change them . . . and we will change them until you tell me you are completely happy. We won't proceed with the final restorations until you are totally happy with these provisional ones."

By observing patient responses and the changes that make a positive difference, patterns emerge that can be used as guidelines for every aspect of anterior tooth position, inclination, and contour. There are six specific contour decisions that must be made for upper anterior teeth. These six decisions dictate the form of a matrix of functional anatomy.

> Understanding the matrix of functional anatomy is the key to smile design.

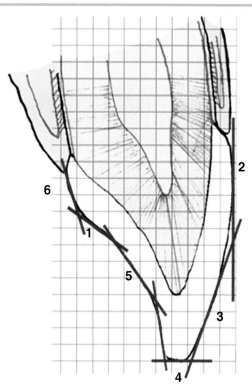

FIGURE 16-2   The *matrix of functional anatomy* describes six specific surfaces of upper anterior teeth that define their contour boundaries.

Each contour decision must be made in proper sequence (Figure 16-2).

The first decision determines the relationship of the lower incisal edges to the upper anterior teeth (Figure 16-3). It is the surface contour that establishes an ideal holding contact for the anterior teeth when the mandible is in centric relation. This is always the starting point for smile design because it is the beginning point of functional movements that establish the anterior guidance.

This decision is the only decision that can be determined almost solely from the articulated casts in centric relation. Selection of the best treatment choice for accomplishing this is made by evaluating all treatment options as just described in the previous example.

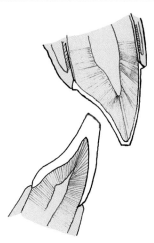

FIGURE 16-3 Determining the relationship of the lower incisal edges to the upper anterior teeth is always the starting point for smile design.

After centric relation stops have been determined, the second most important decision is to determine the exact position and contour of the incisal plane. That involves the determination of each upper incisal edge. Since the incisal plane of the upper teeth is located within the envelope of motion, it cannot be determined precisely on an articulator.

The incisal edges of the upper teeth must be in harmony with the envelope of function, so smile design at this point relates more to the lips than to the condylar path. But do not make the mistake of thinking that the front teeth are only about esthetics. Remember that the anterior guidance is the dominant factor in establishing the morphology of the posterior teeth. Remember also that the anterior guidance cannot be accurately determined until the incisal edges are in place. Because this cannot be done accurately on an articulator, the diagnostic wax-up is used as a "best-guess" starting point for fabricating provisional restorations that are then modified as needed in the mouth.

Modification of the provisional restorations continues the sequence for determining the other five contour boundaries that result in a perfected smile design. It also establishes a correct anterior guidance. Follow the process in the next chapter to understand why it is necessary to establish the labial contours *before* the incisal edges can be located, and why the incisal edges must be located before the anterior guidance can be determined in harmony with the envelope of function.

Because the anterior guidance has such a critical relationship with functional anterior esthetics, the study of smile design cannot proceed until anterior guidance is understood. Anterior guidance is a continuation of the functional matrix concept.

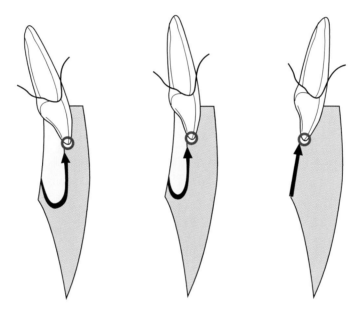# Chapter 17

Anterior Guidance and Its Relationship to Smile Design

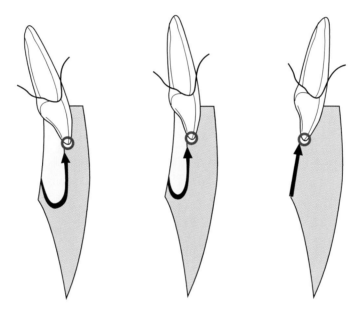

PRINCIPLE

The anterior guidance must be in harmony with the envelope of function.

THE IMPORTANCE OF ANTERIOR GUIDANCE

Next to centric relation, the anterior guidance is the most important determination that must be made when one is restoring an occlusion. The success or failure of many occlusal treatments hinges on the correctness of the anterior guidance. Yet the dentist who clearly determines specific guidelines and communicates precise information to the technician about the anterior guidance is a rarity. Dentists who are not utilizing methods for precisely establishing correct anterior guidance can make a quantum improvement in patient satisfaction with their restorative efforts by adhering to some very learnable concepts for determining, communicating, and verifying the accuracy of every anterior restoration.

The anterior guidance has similar importance in orthodontic treatment. Failure to properly establish the correct guidance is a major cause of posttreatment instability. Unfortunately, the occlusal problems that result from an inadequate anterior guidance are usually slow enough in causing damage that the orthodontist is not aware of the problems or the reason for the instability. Furthermore, a clear understanding of the functional rationale for a correct anterior guidance can simplify orthodontic treatment planning and often shorten the time required for treatment.

Besides being the most visible part of the smile, the relationship of the anterior teeth in function is the principal determinant of posterior occlusal form. How precisely the anterior guidance is harmonized to individual patterns of function determines each patient's comfort. We now know that it is also critically important to the coordinated muscle function of the entire masticatory system. Normal function includes the lips and tongue in a variety of functional relationships, and the anterior teeth must fit into all of those relationships with far greater preciseness than is possible without definitive methods of determination.

The contour and position of upper and lower anterior teeth are so critical that an error of less than a millimeter in incisal edge location can feel grotesque to some patients. It is a rare dentist who has not been stung by a patient's displeasure at what the dentist felt was a beautiful anterior restoration. We have all heard the adage, "It is harder to fit the patient's mind than it is to fit the mouth," and we tend to explain away most patient dissatisfaction as more psychological than real. There is no question that there are some patients with irrational expectations, but I have come to believe that they are rare. We have learned that anterior relationships must be determined with extreme preciseness if we are to be predictably successful in restorations involving anterior teeth. Fortunately we do have definitive guidelines for determining every aspect of anterior teeth relationships, so there is no reason to guess at a single determination of position, contour, or arch-to-arch correlation. Radical change in lip support, incisal edge position, and lingual contours may affect more than a patient's natural appearance. Along with the discomfort and the look of artificiality, improperly

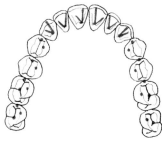

FIGURE 17-1 Keep this formula in mind as you analyze the anterior guidance: *Dots in back* signify centric relation contact only, on posterior teeth. *Lines in front* signify the role of the anterior teeth to disclude the posterior teeth in all excursions. A principal role of the anterior guidance is to protect the posterior occlusion.

restored anterior teeth may contribute to the destruction of the entire dentition.

One thing every dentist should know before attempting to restore anterior teeth is that besides being the key to esthetics, the anterior teeth are also the key factor in protecting the posterior teeth. So important is this job of anterior relationship that posterior teeth that are not protected from lateral or protrusive stresses by the discluding effect of the anterior teeth will, in time, almost certainly be stressed or worn detrimentally. Recall the formula for a perfected occlusion (Figure 17-1). Also, keep it in mind as your goal for anterior guidance. There are exceptions to this rule that require posterior group function on the working side when the anterior teeth are not in contact. These other considerations are explained for anterior open bites and anterior cross bites in Chapters 37, 38, and 41.

CUSTOMIZING THE ANTERIOR GUIDANCE

There is no way to standardize anterior guidance. There are no cephalometric norms that work for all patients, and there are no arbitrary guidelines for interincisal angulation that fit all patients. One of the most important concepts to understand about anterior guidance is that it is highly variable from patient to patient. Minute changes can make a major difference in patient comfort, but even if comfort is not a problem, slight mistakes in incisal edge position can profoundly affect the stability of the anterior teeth over time (Figure 17-2).

The Centric Relation Contact

The most critical tooth contour in the entire occlusal scheme is also the most universally mismanaged. The contours that establish stable, holding contacts for the anterior teeth are so important because any instability of the anterior guidance has the probability of allowing posterior occlusal interferences to be introduced. Correct contouring of anterior holding contacts requires attention on both upper and lower anterior teeth.

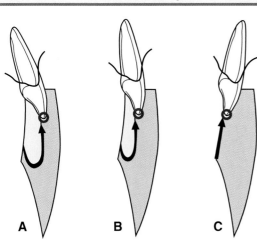

A   B   C

FIGURE 17-2   Three different anterior guidance patterns represent variations in the inclination of the upper anterior teeth. The differences in incisal edge position also reflect major differences in the envelopes of function. If the incisal edges on **A** or **B** were moved more lingually, there would be a conflict with jaw function and the result would be excessive wear or tooth mobility. If the incisal edges on (**C**) were moved toward the labial, there would be no interference to the envelope of function, but there would be interference with the neutral zone, phonetics, and lip-closure path. The process of customizing the anterior guidance is designed to *precisely* locate the correct incisal edge position.

Lower incisal edges

The leading edge of each lower anterior tooth should be formed by a definite labio-incisal line angle. Rounding off this contour is a common mistake that reduces the stability of the anterior contact. A definite line angle contour is also the most natural looking. If the casts are analyzed in centric relation, it may appear advantageous to move the incisal edges slightly forward or back to achieve a solid stop. That decision may be resolved orthodontically, restoratively, or surgically.

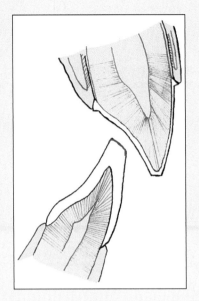

Note: Lower anterior teeth require several key determinations to ascertain the shape and the position of their incisal edges. The contour of the lower incisal plane also has great significance. To elaborate on the most important considerations without disrupting the discussion on anterior guidance, the details regarding lower anterior teeth are explained in a separate chapter that follows.

The contour of the centric relation contacts on the upper anterior teeth must be shaped to form a definite stop for the cingulum whenever that can be achieved. Any contacting contour that does not prevent further eruption of the lower teeth will be unstable. A high percentage of anterior wear and instability problems are the result of improper centric relation stops.

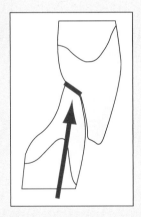

Unstable contact

This is a common mistake in many orthodontically treated occlusions. Failure to provide a definite stop allows the lower teeth to continue erupting. As the lower incisors erupt into a converging space, crowding is the ultimate result. Attempts to stabilize the lower incisors with a permanent lingual retainer will not be necessary if adequate holding contacts are provided.

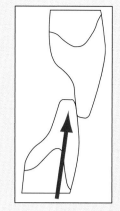

An all too common problem results from improperly contoured upper anterior restorations. The lack of a stable holding contact combined with contours that interfere with the envelope of function invariably leads to severe wear on the lower labio-incisal contact area.

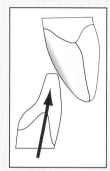

This is a typical wear pattern that results from improperly contoured lingual surfaces on upper anterior teeth. Loss of the labio-incisal line angle and the resulting tapered wear pattern always leads to progressive wear into the dentin on the lower anterior teeth.

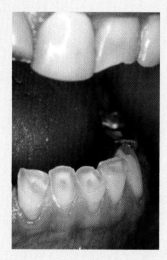

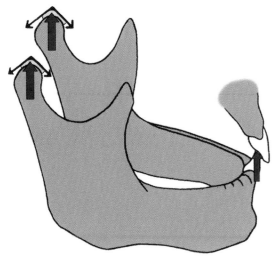

FIGURE 17-3 Visualize the mandible as an inverted tripod. The posterior determinants (the condyles) have a stable uppermost stop in centric relation at their apex of force position. At this position, the condyle-disk assemblies are stopped by bone, so they cannot move any higher, even under firm compression by the elevator muscles. The anterior determinants (the anterior teeth) also have a stable stopping point if the contacts at centric relation are properly contoured to a solidly stopped jaw closure.

The Inverted Tripod Concept

Visualizing the mandible as a stable inverted tripod at centric relation (Figure 17-3) gives a good picture of the goal of perfected anterior teeth contours at the centric relation contacts.

No posterior tooth should interfere with any one of the three legs of the tripod. The condyles should be free to move down and forward of the apex position. If all of the lower anterior teeth contact simultaneously against stable centric stops at the correct vertical dimension, the first requirement for a good anterior guidance has been fulfilled. No other decision about anterior guidance can be made with certainty until this first requirement has been satisfied.

DETERMINING INCISAL EDGE POSITION

Incisal edge position is second in importance to centric relation, but two other decisions must be made before it can be determined. Those decisions involve the inclination of the upper anterior teeth, and the labial contours. Incisal edge position cannot be determined solely from a photograph, although photographs of a person's smile can be very helpful. However the horizontal position of the incisal edges is extremely important to all aspects of anterior guidance as well as appearance. The vertical position of the incisal edges is dependent on the horizontal position, which is not discernible on two-dimensional photographs (Figure 17-4).

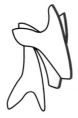

FIGURE 17-4 The vertical position of the upper incisal edges is affected by the inclination of the teeth. Thus determination of the horizontal position of the incisal edges must precede the determination of the length of the upper anterior teeth and the steepness of the anterior guidance.

Determining the Horizontal Position of the Incisal Edges

The controlling factor in determination of the horizontal position for the upper incisal edges is the contour and position of the labial surfaces. The labial surfaces of each tooth involve two planes (see figure below).

Decision #2

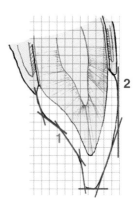

The second step in the process of defining the functional matrix is to determine the upper half of the labial surface. This can be done with reasonable accuracy from the study cast.

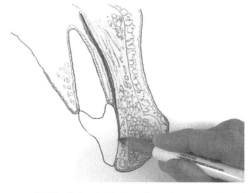

The upper half of the labial surface is a continuation of the contour of the labial surface of the alveolar process. There should be no change in direction or curvature from alveolar process to the tooth surface. To facilitate this decision, study casts should include the entire labial surface of the alveolar process. This process is particularly useful for doing the diagnostic wax-up when teeth are missing or when poorly contoured restorations are being replaced.

Decision #3

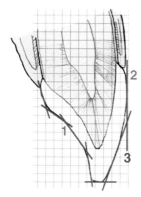

The next step is a very important step in determining horizontal position of the incisal edges. Failure to correctly determine the lower half of the labial contour is a far more common mistake than most dentists realize. Variations in this contour can be subtle and easily missed. Even minute changes can profoundly affect the comfort and long-term stability of the anterior teeth. At this stage of the process, it is not yet time to determine the vertical position of the incisal edges. In fact, it is an advantage to wax-up for provisional restorations that are slightly longer than needed. For now, the concentration should be on contouring the surface back until the lower lip can easily slide by the incisal third to seal contact with the upper lip. We refer to this as the *lip-closure path*.

To achieve an ideal contour for the lip-closure path, it is important to prepare the teeth in two planes. Restorations in which the incisal edges are too far forward are often the result of inadequate preparation for the lower half of the labial surface.

If incisal edge position is to be maintained unchanged
Preparing the incisal half of the labial surface first can ensure adequate room for restorative materials. By sinking the diamond to the full depth of a measured width (Figure 17-5, *A*), parallel to the lower plane of enamel surface, the resulting tooth reduction enables the technician to position the incisal edge where it should be (Figure 17-5, *B*). For many restorations, the goal is to copy the existing contour of the labial surface and duplicate the incisal edge position. Both the preparation of the teeth and the precise communication with the technician are necessary to achieve this goal.

If incisal edge position is to be changed
If restorative changes are contemplated for existing incisal edge positions, they should always be completed on provisional restorations first. The diagnostic wax-up determines the contours on the provisional restoration, but remember that the wax-up is, at best, a guess. Some modification of provisional restorations is almost always necessary to

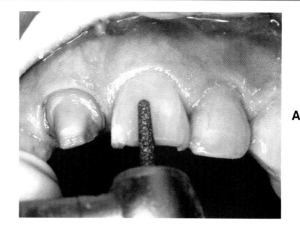

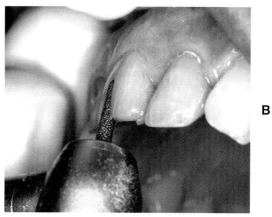

FIGURE 17-5 See text for description.

achieve an ideal contour (Figure 17-6). The starting point for modification is always the labial contour to make it conform to the lip-closure path. Until the two planes of the labial contour are determined, refinement of the incisal plane will be by trial and error without knowing its horizontal positioning. In such cases, the tendency will almost always be to position the incisal edges too far labially.

Decision #4

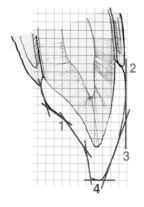

Decide on the exact position and contour of the incisal edges, and the contour of the incisal plane.

At this stage, the incisal plane is usually fairly close to where it should be. But this is the step where minute

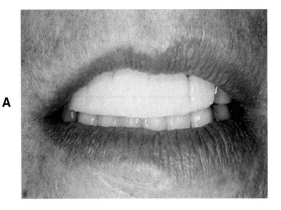

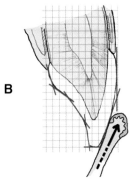

FIGURE 17-6 Modification of the provisional restorations can sometimes require major reduction of the labial contour. **A,** On this patient with a tight neutral zone from strong lower-lip pressure, the reduction obliterated the labial embrasure contours to achieve an unstrained lip-closure path. There is no way to know this contour from the articulator mounting. If the original diagnostic wax-up had been accepted, the incisal edges would have been too far forward. After the labial contours are determined to be satisfactory **(B),** the vertical position of the incisal plane can be established and the labio-incisal contours can be further refined within a correct matrix of functional anatomy.

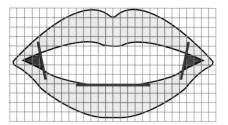

FIGURE 17-7 The incisal plane should follow the contour of the lower lip when the patient smiles.

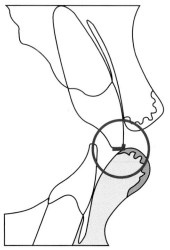

FIGURE 17-8 Contact *(in circle)* shows correct vertical and horizontal position for the incisal plane.

changes often make the difference between perfection versus "getting used to it." When doing the diagnostic wax-up, it is helpful to make the anterior teeth slightly longer because it is easier and faster to outline and then reduce the length of the provisional restorations than it is to add to the length. Remember that all you are trying to do at this stage is define the boundaries of the matrix of functional anatomy. Once you are certain of the matrix form, the labial view of each tooth can be outlined and the labial embrasure contours can be completed. So at this step in the process, the overall contour of the incisal plane must be established.

Determining the Contour of the Incisal Plane

If the labial contours have been positioned and shaped correctly, the incisal edges should fit the internal contour of the lip when the patient smiles gently (Figure 17-7). If the incisal edges compress into the outer lip surface during the smile, the incisal edges are too far forward. More labial reduction of the incisal half of the provisional restorations will be needed before the incisal plane can be accurately determined (see Figure 17-6).

The contacts of the incisal edges at the inner vermillion border of the lower lip during a gentle smile (Figure 17-8) determine the correct vertical and horizontal position for the incisal plane. It is also the correct relationship of the anterior teeth to the lower lip that is ideal for comfortable, unstrained phonetics.

There is a physiologic reason for making the incisal plane fit the smile line. The masticatory system is also the organ for speech. Phonetic sounds are actually shaped mechanically by various combinations of teeth, lips, and tongue. The *F* sound is one of the most useful guides for precisely positioning the upper incisal plane because to make an *F* sound, air is compressed into a broad, flat band between the lower lip and the upper incisal edges (Figure 17-9).

The secret to using the *F* sound as a guide to locating the exactly correct incisal plane position and contour is to speak *softly and very gently* to determine the unstrained lip contour and position that is compatible with *F* and *V* sound production.

The lip can accommodate to any incisal edge position to form *F* and *V* sounds. But the facial muscles become fatigued if the incisal plane requires abnormal lip activity to squeeze the sound into a flat band. If a patient complains about a tired face when talking a lot, or if facial fatigue occurs at the end of the day, it is probable that there is a mismatch between the lips and the teeth (Figure 17-10).

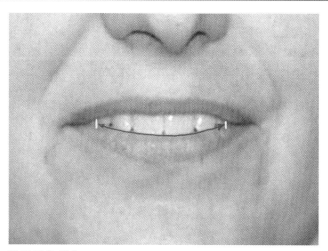

FIGURE 17-9 Contour of the lower lip and upper incisal edges when making an *F* sound.

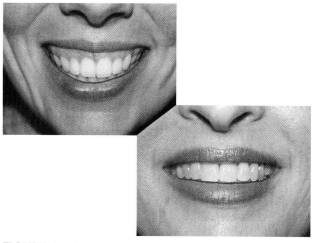

FIGURE 17-10 The display of tooth length and incisal plane contour varies greatly from patient to patient and must be evaluated in the mouth. Articulators do not have lips. Note how the curvature of the incisal planes on two different patients conforms to the natural curvatures of the smile lines. No unusual lip activity is required for either patient to shape the air for *F* or *V* sounds.

The process

Sit the patient in a relaxed position. Ask the patient to completely relax, look straight ahead, and very gently and softly count from 50 to 55. Carefully observe the relationship of the upper incisal edges to the *inner* vermillion border of the lower lip when the provisional restorations are in place. As you learn to observe and correct tooth contours to specifically relate to the lip, you will be able to observe the difference that small changes make. It will also be obvious that as you perfect the functional relationships, you will also be improving esthetics.

Decision #5

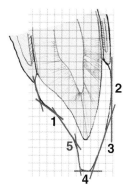

Now you are ready to determine the contour of the anterior guidance. Remember that the goal for the anterior guidance is that it be in harmony with the envelope of function. The process up to this point was to determine the starting point (centric relation) and the end point (incisal edge position) of the functional envelope. The anterior guidance cannot be precisely determined until both of these landmarks have been established.

STEPS IN HARMONIZING THE ANTERIOR GUIDANCE

The refinement and restoration of anterior guidance contours are greatly simplified once the centric relation contacts and incisal edge positions have been determined (see Figure 17-11).

While the sequence of steps is simplified at this point, it is still essential to understand the reason for any change made.

The effect on esthetics and phonetics should be considered in advance, and a clear insight should be developed regarding the variations of periodontal support, the mechanics of stress, and the role of the anterior teeth as protectors of the posterior teeth. Unless these factors are understood and tempered with clinical judgment, no technique will achieve dependable results. This is true for the procedures that follow. Nevertheless, it is a practical sequence to use when the anterior guidance needs modification. The same steps can be utilized to determine whether changes are needed. The procedures are practical whether the anterior teeth are to be restored or merely modified. If restoration is necessary, the correctness of any changes can be tested before they are accepted.

Preliminary steps

1. When indicated, the lower anterior teeth should be reshaped or restored first.
2. If restorations are not needed on the posterior teeth, they must be equilibrated before the anterior guidance can be worked out. All interferences to centric relation must be eliminated on both anterior and posterior teeth to establish stable contacts at the most closed position. Eccentric interferences should then be eliminated on the posterior teeth. The goal is to move all excursive contact on to the anterior teeth if they are in a position to function in that capacity. Thus any posterior incline that causes separation of the anterior teeth should be reduced until anterior contact can be maintained through the complete excursion.

> If posterior interferences prevent a full range of anterior guidance function, it will not be possible to determine or work out a correct anterior guidance.

Remember that full functional contact of the anterior teeth depends on their ability to contact in centric relation. If there is no anterior contact because of tongue postures, lip postures, or arch malrelationships, a normal anterior guidance may not be achievable. Various degrees of anterior open bite should be analyzed carefully before you make an attempt to achieve anterior contact (see Chapter 38).

If restoration of the posterior teeth is indicated, you can take advantage of the opportunity for precise harmonizing of anterior guidance. By preparing the posterior teeth in one arch before completing the correction of the anterior inclines, you can eliminate the influence of posterior contacts completely. This is helpful because taking the posterior teeth out of contact eliminates their mechanoreceptor influence and makes it easier to record centric relation stops on the anterior teeth. It also makes it easier to observe mobility patterns during function when the anterior teeth are the only teeth in contact.

Any reduction of posterior support is helpful because the fewer posterior teeth that contact, the easier occlusal adjustments can be made and the simpler it is to observe hypermobility patterns on the teeth that remain in contact.

The Five Steps to Harmony

Step 1. Establish coordinated centric relation stops on all anterior teeth (Figure 17-11).

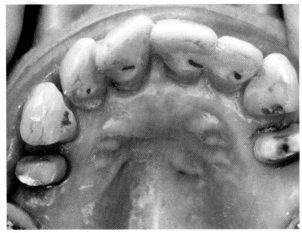

FIGURE 17-11   Centric relation stops marked in red.

The dentist must manipulate the mandible and guide it into a terminal axis closure, marking the contacts with thin marking ribbon and adjusting them until each lower incisor makes a definite mark. In most mouths, minimal adjustment is required to establish good centric stops. In others, major decisions may have to be made. Some of the common problems faced at this step are the following:

Deviation from first centric contact into a more closed position. All interferences should be eliminated so that the mandible may close all the way to maximum closure without any deviation. This is the most common problem and the easiest to solve.

No contact on some teeth after deviation is eliminated. This condition occurs in the patient who has solid centric stops, but not on all teeth. What do we do with the teeth that are not in contact? We have three choices:

1. We can close the vertical dimension by grinding down the centric stops until all teeth contact. This may sound harsh, but a slight closure of the vertical dimension does no harm. In teeth with severe bone loss, this may be an advantage because it improves the crown-root ratio. Even with firm teeth, slight closure to gain contact is usually better than having to restore teeth to contact.
2. We can build up teeth to contact. It is often necessary to make temporary restorations to build out the lingual contours into contact. All of the steps of working out the anterior guidance are then finalized on the temporary restorations before the contours are accepted as a guide for the permanent restorations.
3. We can "do nothing." Sometimes nothing is what we should do. Anterior teeth that are not in contact but are stable because of a substitute contact such as lip or tongue position are sometimes better left as they are. However, we must be certain that they are stable without tooth contact before electing to leave them that way. If noncontacting teeth need to be restored and if we can establish enough centric stops from other teeth to program the customized guide table, we do not have to be concerned about missing contacts. The restorations can be corrected on the articulator.

Missing Anterior Teeth. This problem is solved when a provisional anterior bridge is made from articulated casts and then all contours are finalized on the temporary bridge in the mouth. Correct esthetics can be established right along with correct lingual contours.

Arch-relationship problems that do not allow centric contact on all teeth. These problems are discussed in separate Chapters 37 and 38. However, as a general rule, we must determine which teeth should contact in centric relation before proceeding to the next step. If lower anterior teeth need to be moved or reshaped, their position and contours must be correct before we proceed with finalizing the anterior guidance.

If orthodontic movement or gross reshaping of either upper or lower anterior teeth can improve the finished result, such changes should always be worked out in advance on articulated casts. Temporary acrylic restorations that reflect the changes can be placed after orthodontic movement has been completed. Refinements can then be made in the mouth.

Habits that keep anterior teeth from contacting. Before any noncontacting tooth is brought into contact, we must make sure it is not being held out of contact by an unbreakable habit. Many habits of lip biting actually result from unconscious attempts to cushion the teeth from interfering contacts. Such habits usually disappear when the occlusion is corrected. Other habits such as chewing on a pipe stem can be broken if the patient wants to, but this should be determined before restoring the lost contact. If the habit remains, the restored teeth will simply be pushed further out of alignment. Equilibration procedures should be carried out to produce as much stability as possible before preparation. Any anterior teeth that could touch but do not touch should be evaluated carefully before they are brought into contact.

Contouring the centric stops. It is not necessary for the entire incisal edge of the lower incisors to contact in centric relation. This usually produces too much of a ledge in the upper teeth. If upper contours are correct, contact with only the labial half of the lower incisal edge is sufficient. The shape of the upper contacts should direct the forces as close as possible up the long axis, but contacts on slight inclines are not as stressful as they may seem because the labial vector of force is counteracted by inward pressure from the lips. Posterior support that is harmonized to the anterior stops will also minimize the potential stress.

When all centric stops have been refined, each tooth should be checked digitally to make sure it is not being moved by centric closure. Any teeth jarred by a manipulated closure should be re-marked while slight pressure is applied to keep the tooth from moving.

Step 2. Extend centric stops forward at the same vertical dimension to include light closure from the postural rest position.

Such extension occurs when we determine how much "long centric" the patient requires. It is also the step that enables us to have centric contact with the anterior teeth without fear of stressing them excessively toward the labial. "Long centric" is explained in detail in Chapter 19, so there is no need for repetition here regarding its rationale.

After centric stops have been established by manipulation of the mandible into terminal axis closure, the patient should sit up in a postural position. Remove the headrest, and instruct the patient to "tap lightly with the lips relaxed." Insert the red ribbon between the teeth, and have the patient repeat the tapping. The mouth should be held open while the patient is returned to the supine position, and a manipulated centric closure into a darker marking ribbon is made (green or blue works fine). If the red marks extend onto inclines forward of the centric marks, the centric stops should be extended at the same vertical so that the teeth can be closed either into centric relation or slightly forward of it without bumping into inclines. The amount of freedom from centric relation required rarely exceeds 0.5 mm. Regardless of the amount needed, we can determine it quite precisely by following this procedure.

Extension of the centric stops is accomplished nicely with a sharp inverted-cone Carborundum stone. Care should be taken not to touch the centric stops themselves. The re-

sults should be checked digitally to make sure that no teeth are jarred when the patient taps.

Step 3. Determine the incisal edge position.

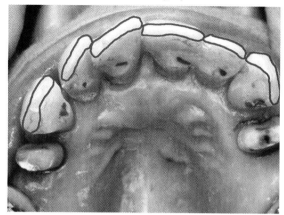

FIGURE 17-12 The incisal edges must be precisely determined before the anterior guidance can be worked out.

Location of the incisal edges is second in importance only to centric relation holding contacts (Figure 17-12). If the anterior teeth are stable and no contour changes are needed, the incisal edge position should be maintained. If incisal edges are to be altered restoratively, the changes should always be determined in provisional restoration first and then copied in final form only after the patient has approved the comfort and appearance.

Step 4. Establish group function in straight protrusion.

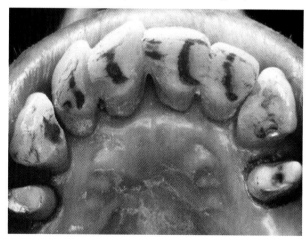

FIGURE 17-13 The protrusive path starts at centric relation and ends at the incisal edges.

Before protrusive paths can be established, the precise location of each incisal edge must be determined (Figure 17-13). Since there are so many factors that determine the incisal edge position, this is discussed in separate detail in Chapter 16. For simplicity's sake, we will assume that all the aspects of lip support, phonetics, and esthetics that dictate incisal edge position are correct. If so, we only need to selectively grind from the centric and "long centric" stops forward to the incisal edges. In most cases, the four incisors fall right into group function as individual tooth interferences are reduced. All reductions should be done on the upper teeth. Interferences are marked by sliding forward on marking ribbon from centric relation to end-to-end. If one tooth marks by itself, the marked area is hollow ground until the second tooth shares the load, and on until all four incisors have continuous contact forward.

For patients with a regular to deep overbite, the protrusive paths are almost always concave. However, as the amount of overbite lessens, the path becomes progressively straighter. Near end-to-end relationships produce nearly straight-line protrusion. By maintaining incisal edge positions and being careful not to destroy centric or "long centric" contacts, we can work out the protrusive paths with amazing simplicity for a variety of arch-relationship problems. Patients with very large central and small lateral teeth may have to be content with protrusive group function on the central incisors only. If the central incisors are not strong enough to carry the load, it would be better to splint them to other teeth than it would be to give the lateral incisors a bizarre shape to bring them into function. Protrusive paths should always be checked digitally. It is easy for an interfering, hypermobile tooth to move slightly and allow other teeth to mark evenly. If an individual tooth is displaced by protrusive movements, the tooth is simply held in place with the finger and re-marked. It is adjusted by selective grinding until it is no longer moved.

If all incisors are stressed to movement, even with good group function, the incisal edge position should be re-evaluated. It may be too far lingually. If it is necessary to shorten the upper incisors or move the incisal edges labially to flatten the protrusive guidance, the patient should test the changes under function before accepting them as final. If the hypermobility results from loss of bone support, splinting should be considered. At the completion of the protrusive movement, the incisal edges of the lower central incisors should meet the incisal edges of the upper central incisors. If the lateral incisors can also meet edge to edge, so much the better, but it is not always possible without ruining the esthetics.

Step 5. Establish ideal anterior stress distribution in lateral excursions.

It is incorrect to think that every mouth should have anterior group function in lateral excursions (Figure 17-14). It is just as big a fallacy as giving every mouth canine protection. Some dentitions function well and maintain excellent stability with only the canines carrying all lateral excursions, and there is no reason to change such an occlusion. However, if the canine is showing signs of hypermobility, accelerated wear, or loss of periodontal support, both stress and wear can be diminished when the canine is brought into group function with other anterior teeth. Although it is often advantageous to change a canine-protected occlusion to anterior group function, there appears to be no sound reason for changing anterior group function to canine protection.

Since we do not know for sure what the resistance level is in a deteriorating mouth, the safest approach is to minimize stresses as much as practical. Group function of the an-

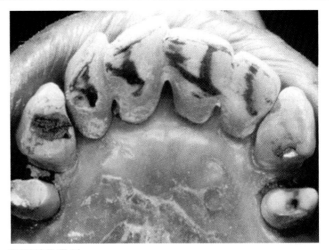

FIGURE 17-14   Lateral excursion with group function anterior guidance.

terior teeth accomplishes this, and if the teeth in group function are also in harmony with the envelope of function and if their inclines have been adjusted according to the quality of periodontal support, the lateral anterior guidance can be said to be customized to produce minimal stress.

The procedure for customizing the lateral anterior guidance starts with closing the mandible into centric contact. With firm help from the operator, the patient is asked to slide the jaw laterally and any movement of any teeth is noted. The excursion is repeated with marking ribbon interposed between the teeth and the marked lateral contacts selectively ground until there is continuous contact from centric to the incisal edge of the upper canine. In some mouths, this will bring the lateral and central teeth into contact. However, it may not be sufficient to stop individual teeth from being moved by the stresses.

To reduce the lateral stress on any tooth or teeth, the contacting surfaces must be flattened from centric contact laterally. However, it is not necessary to extend the flat surface all the way through the teeth. The canine is the key tooth in lateral excursions, and as the jaw moves laterally on a fairly flat plane, the teeth in front of the canine begin to share more of the load. This permits the lateral lingual inclines to be gradually steepened, forming a concave path. The downward excursion of the balancing condyle also contributes to a tendency for a natural opening movement as the jaw moves laterally to form a concave over-and-down path of the lower front teeth.

Just as in protrusive excursions, the tendency toward concave inclines lessens as the amount of overbite decreases. However, it is not uncommon to have fairly straight lateral inclines that are compatible with concave protrusive inclines. For best esthetics, protrusive inclines are almost always steeper than lateral inclines.

In working out lateral inclines, we reach a point when the lower anterior teeth seem to function smoothly against the upper inclines. The patient may volunteer that the teeth feel good. Stressful movement of the teeth has been minimized or eliminated when the jaw moves laterally. There are no hang-ups. Esthetics is good, and there is fairly even symmetry to the right and left inclines. Now the inescapable need for clinical judgment enters the picture. Do we accept what we have worked out or do we adjust further? If in doubt, the patient should try it for a few days and see whether or not he or she can find fault with any aspect of the anterior teeth. Any dentist who understands the importance of the anterior teeth to the success of the entire restorative case will be willing to make sure that all aspects of anterior guidance are correct before proceeding.

Decision #6

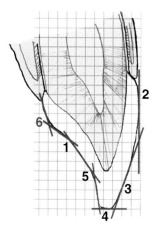

The final matrix decision is the contour from the centric relation stop to the gingival margin. This is a simple decision, but contour mistakes here can interfere with *T, D,* and *S* sounds as the tongue positions against this area. Avoid sharp ledges. Round off the cingulum contour to blend into the centric relation stop. Preserve the forward half of the stable stop for contact with the lower incisal edge.

ESTHETIC CONTOURING

Up to this point, the boundary lines for functional anatomy have been established. In most cases, the diagnostic wax-up is relatively close to the correct contour, so major changes are not required. Small contour changes in the provisional restorations are almost always needed to perfect the labial contours and the incisal edge position. Remember that the incisal edge position determines the general angulation of the anterior guidance, and is the key to harmony with the neutral zone. So minor alterations can affect the long-term stability of the anterior restorations as well as the phonetics, lip-closure path, and perfection of esthetics.

Requirements for major changes to the provisional restorations are more common than might be expected if attention to functional contours has not been a regular part of your process. When major contour changes are required to the labial surface, it may obliterate the labial embrasure form established in the diagnostic wax-up (Figure 17-15). In such cases, you will be working with surfaces devoid of tooth outline form. This is particularly common in complex restorative cases in which there are arch misalignments, occlusal plane problems, or severe damage to the remaining

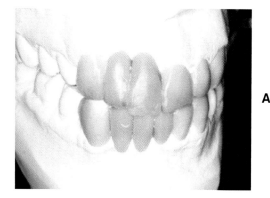

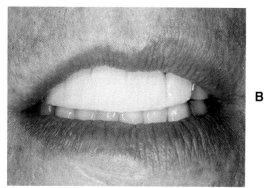

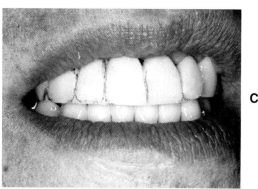

FIGURE 17-15 **A,** A diagnostic wax-up on mounted casts of severely damaged anterior teeth involves both upper and lower arches to ascertain tentative positioning of centric relation stops and incisal edge positions. **B,** When provisional restorations are placed, contour changes obliterate individual tooth contour because labial contour and incisal edges had to be moved back to accommodate very tight neutral zone and lip-closure path. **C,** The labial surface is then used as a matrix on which individual teeth are drawn. Understanding some basic guidelines for individual tooth contour is a learnable and important skill.

teeth. It is also common in many previously restored mouths that have poorly positioned or contoured anterior teeth. As we proceed into treatment planning for problems of occlusion, you will learn how provisional restorations can be used in many different circumstances for determining esthetic and functional guidelines, and also for communicating these guidelines to the technician for the final restorations.

It would take an entire volume to address all issues related to esthetic contouring of anterior teeth, but the following basic fundamentals can be used as a guide when contours must be changed.

Guidelines for Upper Anterior Tooth Contours

Midline should always be vertical regardless of incisal plane. A slanted midline is one of the most noticeable detriments to good esthetics.

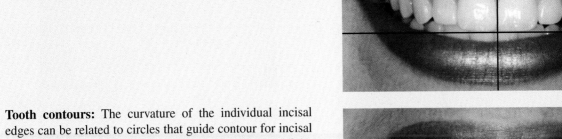

Tooth contours: The curvature of the individual incisal edges can be related to circles that guide contour for incisal embrasures. Starting at the mesial of central, the size of the circle progresses from $1/3$ width to $2/3$ width at the distal. The lateral is $2/3$ at mesial and $3/3$ of the width at distal. This is an easy guide to follow when shaping anterior teeth.

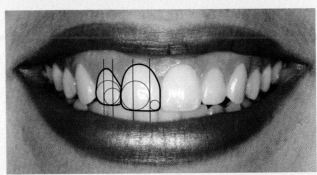

Gingival contour formed as trigonal shape with apex slightly toward distal. Height varies, with centrals slightly higher than laterals.

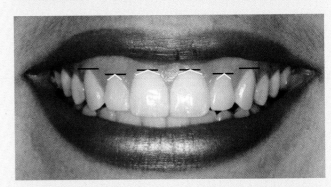

Canine inclination should converge inwardly from front view. From side view, canines should be straight vertical for best appearance.

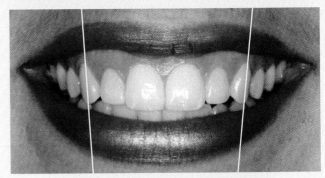

Canine contours: The ideal position for canines is facing to the side. Front view should display the mesial surface, and there is typically a line angle at the mesio-labial juncture. Try also to avoid roundness of the labial surface. Note that it is rather straight. Correct positioning creates a high contact with the lateral.

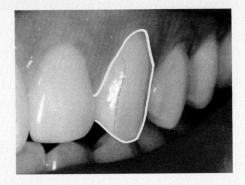

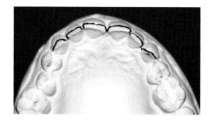

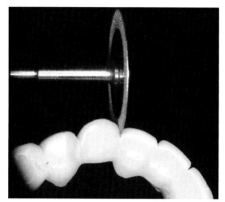

FIGURE 17-16 Recontouring labial embrasure form.

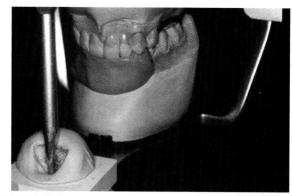

FIGURE 17-17 The cast of the corrected and approved provisional is the best of all possible ways to communicate exact details to the technician. Incisal edge position, contour, and plane can then be copied. The anterior guidance, as determined and tested, can be duplicated by use of the customized anterior guide table. This process also permits verification by the dentist that the technician has followed all details.

Contouring Labial Embrasure Form

To recontour labial embrasure form that has been obliterated, follow the outline drawn on the labial surface and shape a sharp-pointed *V* using a thin diamond disk (Figure 17-16). Note that labial embrasures are formed by abutting convex surfaces. The provisional restorations must be considered to be more than just a temporary bridge. They are the medium for working out, testing, and communicating every important guideline for the anterior teeth. The technician can improve on the final details, but must adhere to the specific guidelines established in the provisional restorations.

After testing the provisionals for all guidelines including phonetics, lip-closure path, smile line, esthetics, and comfortable anterior guidance, place the resin provisional restorations using temporary cement. Now invoke the rule that can save time, expense, and frustration.

> Never proceed with construction of final anterior restorations until the patient is happy with the provisional restorations.

When I first developed the concept of a true *matrix of functional contours* and worked out those contours before fi-

nalizing the individual tooth form, it was apparent that the process saved a significant amount of trial-and-error time expenditure. Most notable is how quickly patients not only accept the contour results, but enthusiastically accept all aspects of esthetics as well as comfort. As you use this approach to anterior esthetics, you will find that you quickly become proficient at going through the step-by-step process. As you develop that proficiency, you will also find that your patients will rarely ask you to alter what you work out at the first seating of the provisional restorations. However, there is no need to rush into final restorations until both you and the patient are completely satisfied at the provisional stage.

COMMUNICATING PRECISE DETAILS TO THE TECHNICIANS

After the patient has approved the provisional restorations, an impression of the provisionals in the mouth is made. A stone cast is poured and mounted with a facebow and a centric relation bite record (Figure 17-17). The cast must be precisely interchangeable with the exact position of the master die model on the articulator. If possible, it can be mounted with the same centric bite record used to mount the master die model. A putty index can communicate exact incisal edge position and contour. A customized anterior guide table communicates exact lingual contours. Both procedures make verification possible.

PROCEDURE   QUICK REVIEW: Determining anterior tooth position and contour

Step 1: Refine and verify lower incisal edge position, shape, and plane. If upper anterior position has not been determined, it must be done in combination with lower determinations.

Step 2: Establish centric holding stops. This is always the first step. The correct anterior guidance cannot be determined until all interferences to centric relation have been eliminated.

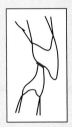

Step 3: Lip support in line with alveolar contour. The upper half of the labial contour can be determined fairly well on the cast. The upper impression must include the complete contour of the alveolar process.

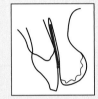

Step 4: Lip-closure path. This is a critical determinant for the incisal half of labial contour. It can only be determined in the mouth.

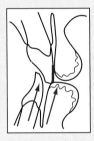

Step 5: Determine incisal edge length (using the smile line). This relationship is important for phonetics of the *F* and *V* positions as well as for the best esthetics.

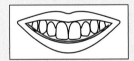

Step 6: Refine incisal edge position (using *F* and *V* sounds). Determination must be made with gentle, softly spoken sounds. Make sure incisal plane contacts inner vermillion border during gentle speech.

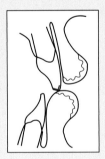

Step 7: Adjust for long centric (if needed). Follow the rules for anterior guidance after centric relation and incisal edges have been determined.

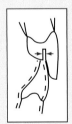

PROCEDURE   QUICK REVIEW: Determining anterior tooth position and contour—cont'd

Step 8: Establish lingual contours (anterior guidance) in harmony with the envelope of function:
a. in straight protrusive
b. in lateral excursions

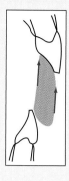

Step 9: Evaluate *S* sounds. The closest speaking position should produce no whistle or lisp.

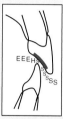

Step 10: Evaluate cingulum contours (using *T* and *D*). Round into centric stops.

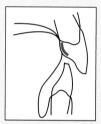

Key point

For optimum stability, comfort, and function, the anterior teeth must be:

In harmony with the neutral zone
In harmony with the lips
In harmony with phonetics
In harmony with centric relation
In harmony with the envelope of function

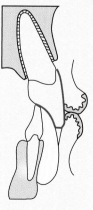

This results in tooth position and contours that are in harmony with a matrix of functional anatomy that also produces the most natural esthetics.

Chapter 18

Restoring Lower Anterior Teeth

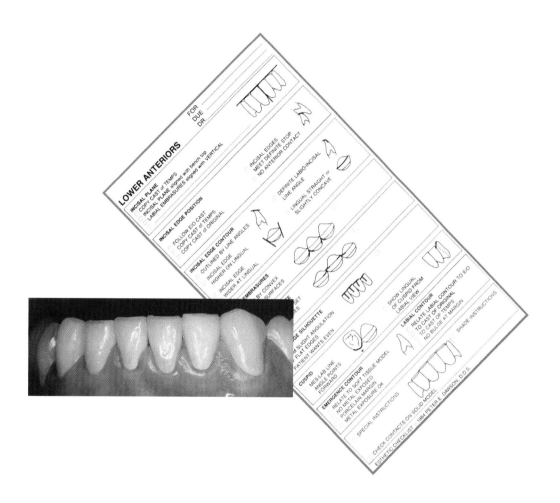

PRINCIPLE

Lower incisal edges are the starting point for anterior guidance and "the view" when speaking.

THE STARTING POINT FOR THE OCCLUSAL SCHEME

Lower Anterior Teeth

Do not downplay the importance of the lower anterior teeth. The arrangement of the entire occlusal scheme starts with the lower anterior teeth. Just as the erupting lower incisors are guided into position by the tongue and lips before the upper anterior teeth erupt, so too must lower incisal edge position be determined before the position and contour of the upper anterior teeth can be finalized.

Determining the correct position for lower anterior teeth is one of the most important decisions we must make in planning restorative treatment. The position of the lower incisors is also recognized as the first priority in orthodontic diagnosis and treatment planning. Occlusal stability, esthetics, and space available in the mandibular arch all depend on correct positioning of the lower anterior segment. Many of the failures we see in orthodontics and restorative dentistry could have been avoided with even slight modifications in position or contour of the incisal edges of the lower anterior teeth.

Five important goals in occlusal treatment depend on correct position and contour of the lower incisal edges, as follows:

1. *Esthetics:* During speaking, the most visible part of the dentition is the incisal half of the lower anterior teeth. Also, correct positioning of the upper anterior teeth depends on correct lower incisal edge placement.
2. *Phonetics:* The spatial relationships between the lower incisal edges and the opposing tooth surfaces are critical to the formation of various sound patterns. Their relationship to the tongue and lips also affects phonetic formations.
3. *The occlusal plane:* The lower incisal plane is the starting point in front for the occlusal plane. An incorrect incisal plane on the lower jaw may require compensations to be made in all other occlusal segments including the upper anterior teeth.
4. *The anterior guidance:* The lingual surfaces of the upper anterior teeth are determined by how the mandible, in function, moves the lower incisal edges. If the lower edges are incorrectly positioned or contoured, the position or contour of the upper anterior teeth must be compromised.
5. *Stability:* Long-term stability depends on harmony between the teeth and the structures that relate to them in function. If the teeth interfere with anatomic or functional harmony of those structures, the adaptive process will attempt to correct the imbalance. The result will be either loosening of teeth, excessive wear, or tooth migration.

Analysis of lower anterior teeth

The correctness of the lower anterior segment can be analyzed from several different perspectives. If the teeth are stable, function comfortably, and are esthetically acceptable to the patient, there would rarely be a need to change them. If there are signs of instability, evidenced by excessive wear, hypermobility, or tooth migration, or if functional or esthetic problems are present, changes in tooth position or contour may be required. Likewise, if teeth are missing or improperly restored, so that positional landmarks have been lost, the correct relationship can be determined if a sequential approach is used in analysis. Some determinations must be made in a certain order. As an example, it is difficult to finalize incisal edge *contours* until after incisal edge *position* is determined. Incisal edge position cannot be refined until an acceptable incisal plane determines the height of each incisal edge.

Analysis to determine the best esthetics may seem unrelated to occlusion, but every contour has a purpose that is related to function. Thus, it is almost always true that the better the esthetics, the better the function will be, and vice versa. It is also important to the patient that occlusal therapy does not destroy the appearance of a natural smile. For that reason, esthetically correct contour should always be a goal along with the determination of what is functionally correct since the incisal edges are the most visible part of the lower teeth when speaking.

LOWER ANTERIOR QUALITY CONTROL

The restoration of lower anterior teeth requires two key determinations:

1. Incisal edge position
2. Incisal edge contour

The contour of lower incisal edges cannot be precisely determined until their position as part of the incisal plane has been defined. Quality control for restoring lower anterior teeth is a three-step process that must be followed in proper sequence. The steps are:

1. *Determination:* Determining exact guidelines for every contour and position is always the starting point.
2. *Communication:* After each specific guideline has been determined, it must be communicated to the laboratory technician. Instructions must be so clear that nothing is left to chance.
3. *Verification:* Any method of communication that cannot be verified is not acceptable. Both the technician and the dentist must be able to verify that each communicated guideline has been correctly followed.

The Esthetic and Restorative Checklist

In my early years of practice, communication with my technician was by written prescription and word of mouth. Even though I had my own private laboratory in which I would sit with my technicians and explain in detail what I wanted, it was easy (and common) for some specific details to be missed. As I learned how important minute details were to the finished result, it became obvious that we needed more pre-

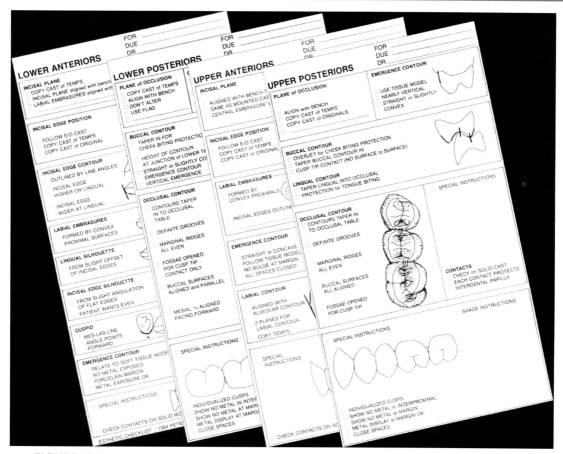

FIGURE 18-1 The esthetic and restorative checklist is a quality control outline that is used to communicate all of the key guidelines for anterior and posterior restorations. It is divided into four sections.

cise, verifiable methods of communicating every detail. It also meant that before I could communicate any precise detail, I had to determine *exactly* what I wanted. The result of our efforts to achieve a reliable system of verifiable communication is a combination of clinical steps to determine each guideline coupled with a specific method for precise communication utilizing a checklist for quality control (Figure 18-1). The system revolutionized my practice and gave me control over every restorative case. It eliminated major waste of time. This system has been in continuous use in my practice ever since its inception. It is the cornerstone for quality control for all restorative cases. We will demonstrate its use as we outline the requirements for perfecting lower anterior restorations.

If all guidelines on the *Esthetic Checklist* for lower anterior teeth are followed (Figure 18-2), the result will be a natural appearance that is functionally correct. Thus the checklist serves as a constant reminder of correct contour for both the technician and the dentist. Used properly, it requires the dentist to determine each guideline before the patient is dismissed from the operatory. It also requires the dentist to determine the method of communicating each guideline so the technician has clear instructions. It further serves as a verification checklist to insure that each guideline has been faithfully followed.

INCISAL EDGE POSITION

The determination of incisal edge position requires three decisions:

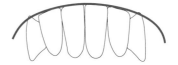

1. The curvature of the incisal plane

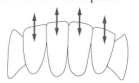

2. The height of the incisal plane

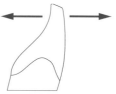

3. The horizontal position of the incisal edges

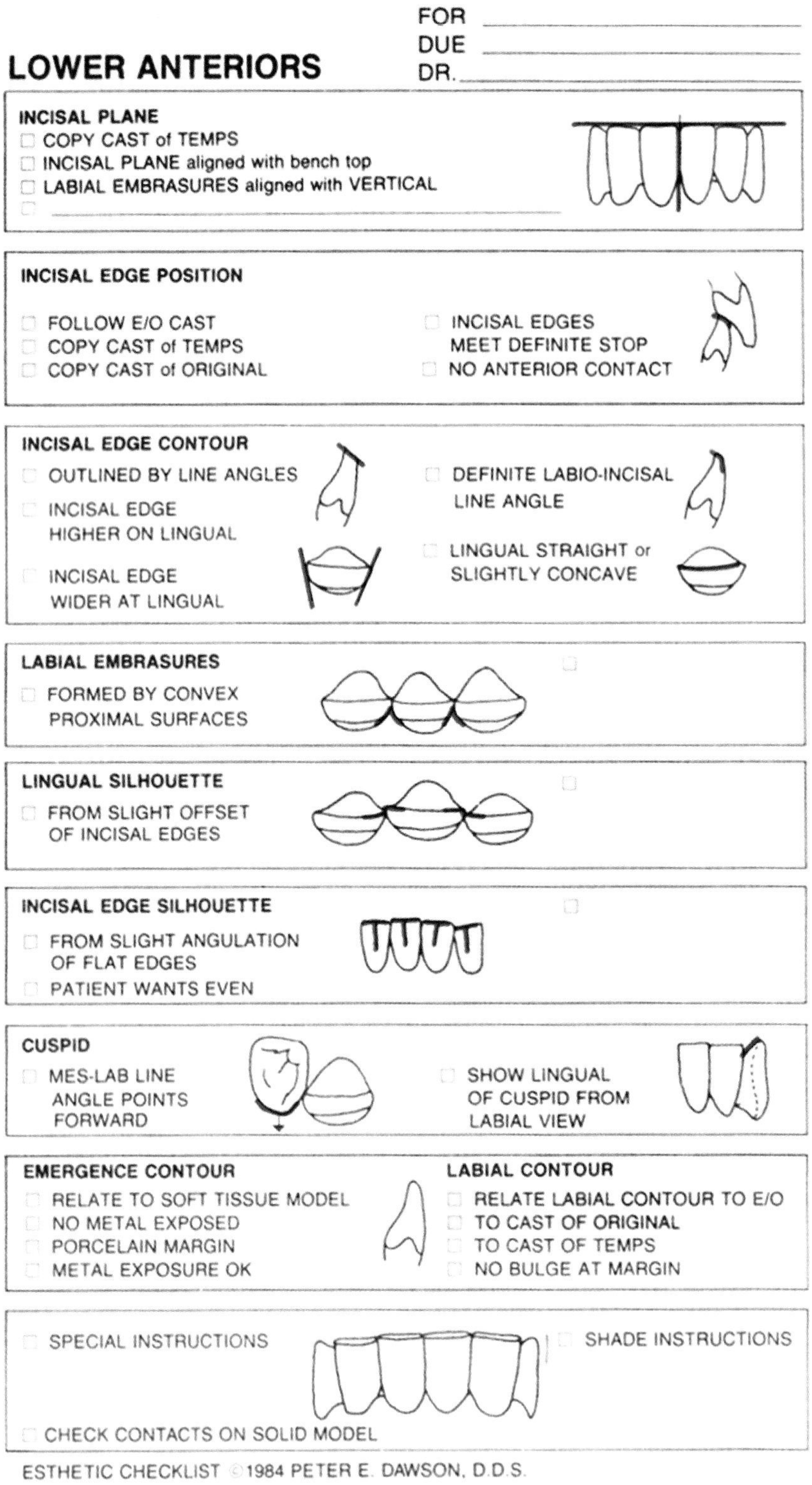

LOWER ANTERIORS

INCISAL PLANE
- ☐ COPY CAST of TEMPS
- ☐ INCISAL PLANE aligned with bench top
- ☐ LABIAL EMBRASURES aligned with VERTICAL
- ☐ _____

INCISAL EDGE POSITION
- ☐ FOLLOW E/O CAST
- ☐ COPY CAST of TEMPS
- ☐ COPY CAST of ORIGINAL
- ☐ INCISAL EDGES MEET DEFINITE STOP
- ☐ NO ANTERIOR CONTACT

INCISAL EDGE CONTOUR
- ☐ OUTLINED BY LINE ANGLES
- ☐ INCISAL EDGE HIGHER ON LINGUAL
- ☐ INCISAL EDGE WIDER AT LINGUAL
- ☐ DEFINITE LABIO-INCISAL LINE ANGLE
- ☐ LINGUAL STRAIGHT or SLIGHTLY CONCAVE

LABIAL EMBRASURES
- ☐ FORMED BY CONVEX PROXIMAL SURFACES
- ☐

LINGUAL SILHOUETTE
- ☐ FROM SLIGHT OFFSET OF INCISAL EDGES
- ☐

INCISAL EDGE SILHOUETTE
- ☐ FROM SLIGHT ANGULATION OF FLAT EDGES
- ☐ PATIENT WANTS EVEN
- ☐

CUSPID
- ☐ MES-LAB LINE ANGLE POINTS FORWARD
- ☐ SHOW LINGUAL OF CUSPID FROM LABIAL VIEW

EMERGENCE CONTOUR
- ☐ RELATE TO SOFT TISSUE MODEL
- ☐ NO METAL EXPOSED
- ☐ PORCELAIN MARGIN
- ☐ METAL EXPOSURE OK

LABIAL CONTOUR
- ☐ RELATE LABIAL CONTOUR TO E/O
- ☐ TO CAST OF ORIGINAL
- ☐ TO CAST OF TEMPS
- ☐ NO BULGE AT MARGIN

- ☐ SPECIAL INSTRUCTIONS
- ☐ SHADE INSTRUCTIONS

- ☐ CHECK CONTACTS ON SOLID MODEL

ESTHETIC CHECKLIST ©1984 PETER E. DAWSON, D.D.S.

FIGURE 18-2 Checklist for lower anterior teeth.

The Curvature of the Incisal Plane

The curvature of the incisal plane is as important to phonetics as it is to esthetics. This relationship to phonetics has a profound effect on function, and mistakes in the contour of the incisal plane are often responsible for problems of discomfort as a result of phonetic disharmony. If the jaw must be repeatedly moved to a strained position to shape certain sounds, the result can be muscle fatigue. Patients may complain of a tired face and difficulty in being understood when they have been talking a lot (Figures 18-3 and 18-4).

To ensure that the jaw-to-jaw relationship during *S* sounds is in harmony with the envelope of function, remember this rule:

> Always use relaxed, gentle, softly spoken *S* sounds for harmony with a comfortable, unstrained envelope of function.

As a general rule, *the more convex the incisal plane is on the upper teeth, the more convex it will be on the lower teeth.* The reason for this relationship is apparent if one understands the necessity of a wide, flat flow of air to make the sharp *S* sound. A convex upper incisal plane cannot fit end to end with a convex or flat plane on the lower teeth without leaking air out the sides (Figure 18-5). Thus the *S* sound is necessarily made with the upper teeth overlapping the lower teeth so that the lower edges can evenly approximate the concavity of the lingual arch form.

If a patient with convex incisal planes is accustomed to making *S* sounds with an overlapped anterior relationship, altering the lower incisal plane can create a significant problem with speech. If a naturally convex lower incisal plane is mistakenly flattened, it will no longer fit the concave lingual arch form and the air will be funneled into an open area in the center, rather than maintained as the flat band that is required for a crisp clear *S* sound (Figure 18-6).

If the lower incisal plane is made concave to fit the convex upper plane in protrusive relation, the patient will be able to make a clear *S* sound by protruding the mandible to the edge-to-edge position. But such mandibular movements are not normal for patients who are used to speaking with less horizontal motion of the jaw, and they will routinely complain of tiredness or strain when they talk a lot. In addition, the natural harmony of the lower incisal edges is lost, and the esthetic result is often severely compromised.

It is a common but very erroneous belief that all upper and lower incisors must be in contact throughout the entire protrusive range and that all four incisors should meet edge-to-edge at the end of the protrusive path. If the upper and lower anterior teeth are in harmony with the functional movements of the mandible, there is no tendency to overload them whether there be two teeth or four teeth in protrusive contact with the opposing arch. With very convex upper incisal planes, it would be unusual to have more teeth in edge-to-edge contact than the central incisors in the maxil-

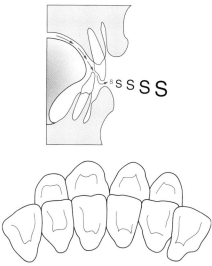

FIGURE 18-3 If *S* sounds are made at an overlap position, the lower incisal plane must be curved to fit the lingual contour of the upper lingual surfaces. This is necessary to constrict the air into a broad flat band between the hard surfaces of the lower and upper teeth. Because the air must be constricted rather uniformly for the width of the incisal plane, the lower incisal edges must relate to the upper teeth with near contact at the jaw relationship that is in harmony with the normal envelope of function.

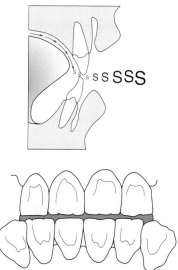

FIGURE 18-4 If *S* sounds are normally made at an end-to-end relationship, the incisal plane on the lower anterior teeth will be fairly flat, to match up with the incisal edges of the upper teeth. This is often what is found on near end-to-end occlusions. A flat smile line that dictates flatter incisal plane contours for the upper teeth does not necessarily result in an end-to-end phonetic relationship. The dictating factor that controls phonetics is the jaw-to-jaw relationship that is in harmony with the envelope of function during *S* sounds. A flat smile line may dictate a flat upper incisal plane because the upper incisal edges contact the lower lip in F sounds. The lower incisal edges relate to the upper tooth surfaces at the *S* sound, and that relationship can be anywhere between overlapped and end-to-end, as dictated by the envelope of function.

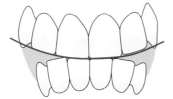

FIGURE 18-5 Convex upper and lower incisal planes cannot make a clear *S* sound at the end-to-end position because air leaks out at the sides. A broad band of air is necessary for a clear *S* sound.

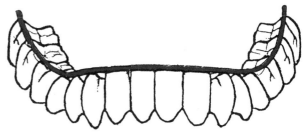

FIGURE 18-7 Ideal occlusal curve along lower incisal edges.

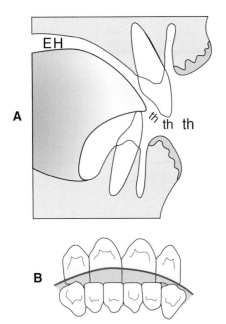

FIGURE 18-6 **A,** If a convex lower incisal plane is flattened, it will no longer relate correctly to the concave upper lingual contour. This creates an open area in the center and destroy the relationship required for a clear *S* sound. **B,** To compensate, the patient must fill the space with the tongue, but this results in a lisp and produces a typical *eth* sound. This is a common mistake that is made because of an erroneous belief that all incisal edges must contact edge-to-edge during the protrusive position. Some patients will compensate by protruding the jaw to an end-to-end tooth relationship in order to make a crisp *S* sound, but that is not in harmony with their envelope of function. It produces fatigue in the facial and masticatory muscles.

lary arch and the four incisors in the lower arch. It is not unusual for the lower lateral incisors to also be discluded.

If the lower incisal plane does not closely approximate the contour of the upper arch during the *S* sound, another common problem of speech may also be caused. Lisping is the result of using the tongue to fill in the void so that the air can be squeezed into the flattened band that is necessary for making a crisp *S* sound. There is a characteristic difference, however, between the *eth* sound made with the soft tongue surface versus the clear *S* sound that comes from approximation of hard tooth surfaces.

If the lower incisal plane relates to the upper arch form in a manner that produces a small roundish opening instead of the uniform space across the width of the incisors, the result is a whistle.

Remember that the organ of mastication is also a critical component of the organ of speech. The masticatory system was designed to be compatible with both functions. By using phonetics as a guide for functional relationships, we will rarely find that it is inconsistent with either masticatory function or esthetics.

The Height of the Incisal Plane

Relating lower incisal edges to the occlusal plane
In ideal instances, the lower incisal edges form a continuous gentle curve that is an extension of the posterior occlusal plane (Figure 18-7). There should be no sudden variation in height between the incisal edges and the posterior cusp tips. As wear occurs, there is a tendency for the plane to become flatter, but there should still be no sudden changes in height.

If the incisal plane is greatly higher than the posterior occlusal plane, that is an indication of elongation of the anterior segment, almost always the result of no stable holding contacts on the anterior teeth. When the lower incisors erupt, they do not erupt out of the alveolar bone. Rather the alveolar process itself elongates, moving the teeth vertically until a stable stop is met. That stop preferably is the opposing tooth, but it also may be the tongue or the lip. The absence of any stop allows the lower anteriors to erupt all the way to the palatal tissue, creating an incisal plane that is at a different level from the posterior plane of occlusion.

The critical element in determining the height of the lower incisal edges will in most instances be the relationship with the upper anterior teeth. It is often necessary to reshape or reposition the upper anterior teeth to get an acceptable position and contour of the lower incisors. This working out of both the upper and lower anterior teeth relationship is the first step in solving most of the complex problems of occlusal malrelationships. The goal is to establish stable holding contacts for the lower incisors at an esthetically acceptable height.

Relating lower incisal edges to the lips

Every patient does not look like the ideal norm in the textbook, so trying to adapt every patient's dentition to the average can result in some very unacceptable results. There is merit, however, in knowing what the norms are because they serve as basic guidelines toward which treatment can be directed.

We can relate the height of the incisal edges to the lips using three norms. If we analyze a large number of attractive dentitions, we find a consistency in the amount of lower anterior tooth surface that is exposed during certain lip relationships, as listed in the following section.

1. Lips sealed: The lower incisal edge is at the height of the juncture of the upper and lower lips when the teeth are together. On a lateral cephalometric radiograph, this usually positions the incisal edge slightly above the functional occlusal plane. If the lower incisal edges are much below that juncture, there is a tendency for the upper anterior teeth to be positioned too low, producing a gummy smile. A quick analysis of incisal edge height relates it to the height of the first molar and even with the juncture of the lips together.

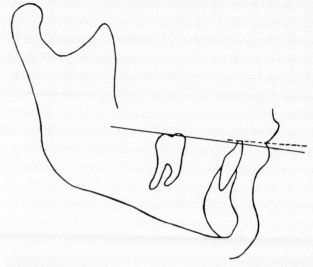

2. Speaking: "The view" when speaking is of the incisal edges of the lower anterior teeth. A varying amount of labial contour may also be on display. The upper teeth are usually hidden during speech.

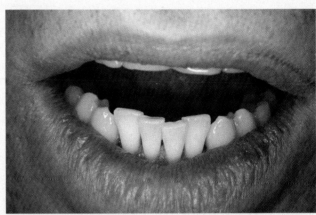

3. Smiling: Only the upper anterior teeth are typically on display during smiling. The lower incisors are usually hidden during a big smile.

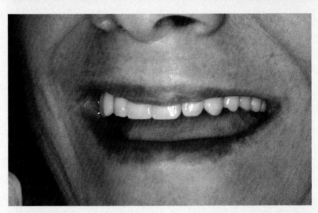

4. Lips slightly parted: When the jaw is at rest and the lips are slightly parted in a half smile, both upper and lower labial surfaces are about equally on display.

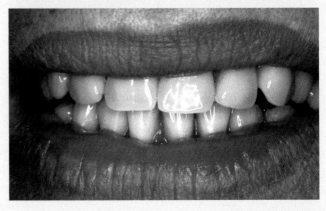

Exposure of the lower teeth varies with lip positions required for phonetics in different patients, and it must be remembered that every smile is an individual characteristic that cannot be stereotyped. If a patient is happy with his or her smile, and the anterior teeth are stable, there is rarely a reason to change it just because it does not fit an exact pattern of average "normalcy."

Some attractive smiles do not fit the norms described above, and in many situations the length of the lips or other configurations simply does not permit a "normal" relationship. Common sense and clinical judgment must prevail.

The Horizontal Position of the Lower Incisal Edges

The key to determining the horizontal position of lower incisal edges lies in establishing stable holding contacts with the upper anterior teeth. If there is doubt about where the upper anterior teeth should be, that question must be resolved before a final decision can be made for the lower teeth.

The question of horizontal position for lower anterior teeth is one of the most important decisions that must be made on every anterior restorative patient. It is a decision that cannot be made without knowing the jaw-to-jaw rela-

tionship in centric relation, which is the reason for using mounted diagnostic casts.

The diagnostic wax-up is the best possible way to determine lower incisal edge position (Figure 18-8). On many occasions, it is necessary to alter the upper anterior teeth to accommodate an acceptable lower incisal edge position (Figure 18-9). Remember that the diagnostic wax-up is used with a putty matrix to fabricate the provisional restorations, which then must be refined to a final contour in the mouth (Figure 18-10).

Upper and lower provisionals are placed and refined in the mouth until the patient approves. Following this process will show any clinician how important minute changes in contour can be to patient comfort. In this very tight neutral zone, the correct position of the upper incisal edges is close to the lower labial surfaces, indicating a very vertical envelope of function. As the upper labial contours had to be reduced back to accommodate the lip-closure path and phonetics, the lower incisal edges also had to be moved lingually before functional jaw movements could be made with total comfort. This degree of accuracy can only be achieved in the mouth, and it requires a sequential process for determining what is correct.

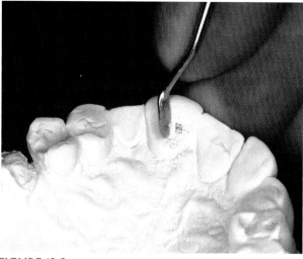
FIGURE 18-9   Adjusting upper anterior teeth to accommodate lower incisal edge position.

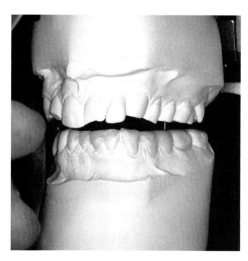
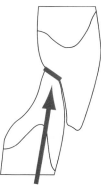
FIGURE 18-8   Diagnostic wax-up helps determine lower incisal edge position.

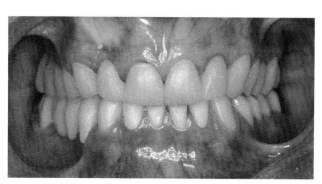
FIGURE 18-10   Provisional restorations in the mouth.

PROCEDURE   Communicating details to the technician

After the lower provisional restorations are approved, an impression is made, and a putty silicone index is adapted to the cast and trimmed to conform with the contour of the labial surfaces.

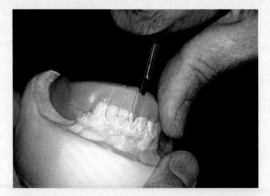

The index is used by the technicians to precisely locate the incisal edges and labial contours so the finished restorations copy the cast of the temporary restorations.

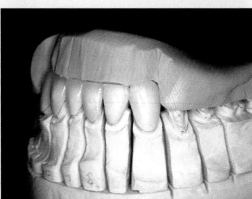

When the technician is sure that all details have been faithfully duplicated, the checklist is checked off. This process eliminates all guesswork and results in restorations that are precise and correct.

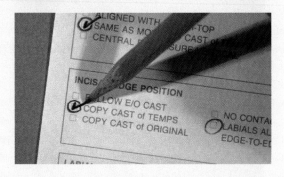

LOWER INCISAL EDGE CONTOUR

The most important contour on the lower incisal edges is the labio-incisal line angle (Figure 18-11). The "leading edge" is important for natural appearance but also to achieve a stable holding contact against the upper lingual stop. Use of the *Esthetic Checklist* reminds the technician to do this on every lower anterior restoration (Figure 18-12). Loss of this leading edge contour is usually the start of progressive wear and instability of the anterior guidance.

The lingual-incisal line angle is an important key to natural-looking incisal edges and a consideration before the teeth are prepared for restorations (Figure 18-13). As lower incisors wear into the thicker part of the tooth, the incisal edges get thicker and rounder (and unesthetic). If extensive wear also occurs on the upper anterior teeth, the lower teeth tend to move forward and the upper teeth may move lingually (the neutral zone is compressive). If the diagnostic wax-up indicates a need to move thick incisal edges lingually to permit better lingual contours on the upper anterior teeth, the preparation for lower anterior restorations will require more reduction on the labial to permit thin normal incisal edge contours on the restorations. If the incisal edges need to be moved labially, the bulk of the reduction will be on the lingual. What you don't want is convex contours on the lingual, so more tooth reduction may be needed on severely worn teeth to produce natural looking contours on the incisal edges.

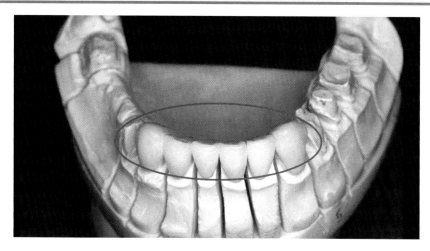

FIGURE 18-11 *Red circle* shows area of labio-incisal line angle.

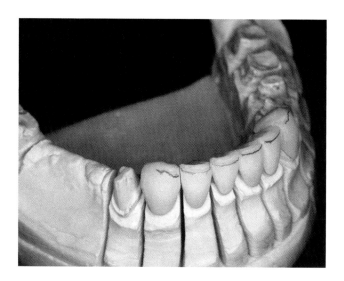

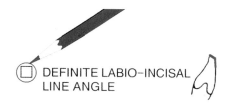

DEFINITE LABIO–INCISAL LINE ANGLE

FIGURE 18-12 Corresponding *Esthetic Checklist* area reminds technician to check labio-incisal line-angle on every restoration.

LINGUAL STRAIGHT or SLIGHTLY CONCAVE

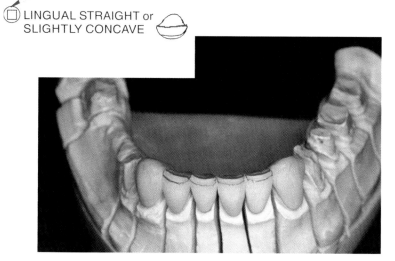

FIGURE 18-13 Corresponding *Esthetic Checklist* area reminds technician to check lingual-contour on every restoration. Convex contours on lingual is never desirable.

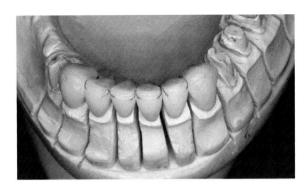

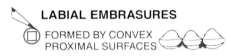

LABIAL EMBRASURES

FORMED BY CONVEX
PROXIMAL SURFACES

FIGURE 18-14 Checking proper contour of labial embrasures.

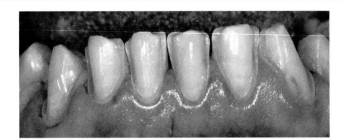

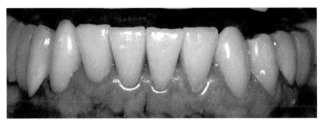

FIGURE 18-16 Preparation and placement of bonded veneers have been an excellent solution for restoring defective incisal edges. Note the definite labio-incisal line angles on the leading edges.

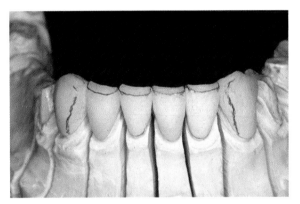

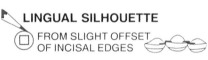

LINGUAL SILHOUETTE

FROM SLIGHT OFFSET
OF INCISAL EDGES

FIGURE 18-15 Checking lingual silhouette.

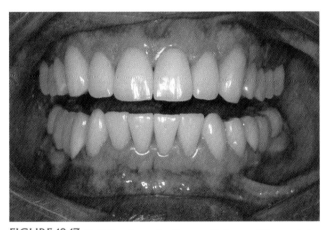

FIGURE 18-17 Both function and optimum esthetics result from anterior restorations in harmony with a precise and correct anterior guidance as restored by Dr. Michael Sesemann, DDS.

Proper contouring of the labial embrasures completes the outline of the incisal edge contour (Figure 18-14). A common mistake is to round the incisal edges. Incisal edges, except in prepuberty, have a flat surface outlined with definite line angles. The incisal edge is higher on the lingual, and there are no embrasures on the lingual (Figure 18-15).

The principles that relate to the incisal edge's position and contour apply regardless of the type of restoration. The use of laminates for restoring deformed incisal edge contour is an excellent way to restore the leading edge of lower anterior teeth when the labio-incisal line angle has been worn down to a steep angular contour.

The importance of correct position and contour of lower incisal edges cannot be overemphasized. The entire occlusion can be compromised by instability if lower incisal edges are not correct. It is a critical point for analysis and treatment of anterior teeth (Figures 18-16 and 18-17).

Chapter 19

Long Centric

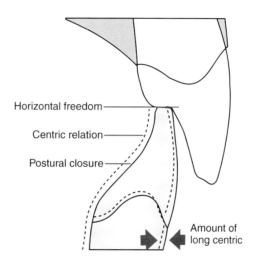

Horizontal freedom

Centric relation

Postural closure

Amount of
long centric

PRINCIPLE

Long centric is really just a "short protrusive."
—*Frank Celenza*

THE CONCEPT OF LONG CENTRIC

Centric relation refers to the exact point at which the loaded condyle-disk assemblies are braced by bone at the most superior position possible against the eminentiae. At this loaded position that occurs from firm contraction of the elevator muscles, the disk is compressed and the condylar axis reaches what we refer to as the *apex of force position.* It is this position that can be located repeatedly and recorded with needlepoint accuracy. Consequently, it is somewhat confusing to think of such a precise point as being "long."

The term *long centric* is misleading because there cannot be such a thing as a long precise point. It is even harder to accept the concept of a long centric with the current understanding that the medial pole of the condyle-disk assembly is stopped by bone, which is unyielding, at least within the range of normal function. The original concept of long centric probably garnered some advocates for the wrong reason, because of clearly erroneous beliefs that the condyle either rested in a yielding mass of soft tissue or was simply suspended in space. Because both of these beliefs portray the condyle as resting on rather spongy articulations, it was postulated that a precise occlusal relationship was incompatible with an imprecise centric relation. Thus an "area" of centric on the teeth must be created to accommodate an "area" of centric at the condyle.

Because of similar misconceptions about the firmness of the medial-pole stops, the "midmost" concept of centric relation was also considered to be a spongy articulation. Thus long centric was also quite often combined with a lateral area of freedom that was referred to as a "wide centric."

On the opposite side of the long centric argument were those who believed that centric relation was such a precise point that occlusal contacts should be contoured to provide no horizontal freedom forward of centric relation. Advocates of this belief often contoured the occlusal surfaces to lock the teeth into this restricted relationship by tripod contacts on three sides of each cusp, relying on the downward movement of the condyles to unlock the centric relation contact. Great pains were taken to relate cusp inclines to precise condylar border paths, and then the anterior guidance was arbitrarily steepened or flattened to conform to the condylar path angulation. This produced a very precise occlusal relationship with possible restrictions on horizontal freedom during functional jaw movements.

Since the downward movement of the condyles was in fact usually able to disclude the posterior tripod contacts, the effect of the restricted occlusion was more related to the arbitrary confinement by the lingual inclines of the upper anterior teeth. Patients often complained that the front teeth hit hard or bumped, even though no interference could be shown in centric relation. Explanations that "my bite is different when I'm sitting up" were frequently ignored.

To recapitulate, the most common attitudes about the concept of long centric can be boiled down to two beliefs:

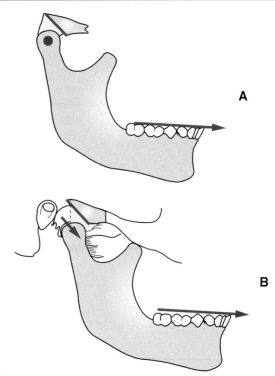

FIGURE 19-1 A flat long centric is not needed on the posterior teeth even if it is incorporated into the anterior guidance. **A,** The condyles cannot move horizontally forward because they are up against the eminentiae at centric relation. **B,** They must move downward from centric relation to protrude the mandible. The molars must move down with the condyles.

1. Horizontal freedom was needed in the entire occlusion to accommodate a resilient relationship at the articular surfaces.
2. Horizontal freedom was not needed in the occlusal relationship because there is no resilience of the articulation at the centric relation position.

We need to understand what the term *long centric* is intended to mean even if we disagree with the semantics. Perhaps then, some of the confusion can be eliminated. I will define the term *long centric* as: *freedom to close the mandible either into centric relation or slightly anterior to it without varying the vertical dimension at the anterior teeth.*

Two points about long centric should be clarified to facilitate further understanding:

1. *Long centric involves primarily the anterior teeth.* In a healthy articulation of the condyles, there can be no horizontal protrusive path of posterior teeth. Even with a zero-degree anterior guidance, the condyles must move downward as the jaw moves forward. The lower posterior teeth must move downward with them (Figure 19-1). Thus a flat protrusive area is usually not necessary on posterior teeth, especially in the molar region.
2. *Long centric refers to freedom from centric, not freedom in centric.* The principal concern regarding long centric is the restrictive effect that can result from the

lingual inclines of the upper anterior teeth. If the lower

lingual inclines of the upper anterior teeth. If the lower incisal edges are in contact with steep lingual inclines at the centric relation jaw position, those same inclines may interfere with postural closing patterns that do not conform to the centric relation axis. If no horizontal freedom is provided for a slightly protruded postural closure, the lower incisal edges will strike the lingual inclines of the upper anterior teeth. If those inclines are steep enough, they can provide a wedging effect at first contact, which, in varying degrees, may interfere with the normal pattern of postural jaw closure.

The provision for long centric simply moves the lingual incline forward so that the jaw is free to close without restriction either in centric relation or in the slightly protruded relationship that occurs at various postural positions of the head. A flat long centric is not needed on the posterior teeth even if it is incorporated into the anterior guidance. The condyles cannot move horizontally forward because they are up against the eminentiae at centric relation. They must move downward from centric relation to protrude the mandible. The molars must move down with the condyles.

A basic rule for optimizing the comfort and stability of any occlusal relationship is as follows:

> When the teeth come together in a postural closure, the lower incisors should not strike an incline before reaching full closure.

Contact in centric relation

Before long centric can be recorded, all posterior interferences to centric relation must be completely eliminated so anterior contact in centric relation can be verified.

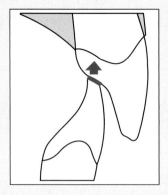

Postural closure

With the patient in an upright, relaxed, postural position, gentle tapping of the teeth together should not result in striking the upper lingual incline before complete closure to the most closed position.

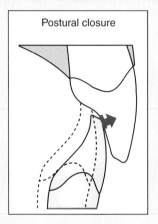

Clearance for long centric

The goal is for the patient to be able to close either into centric relation or slightly protruded during gentle postural closure without striking the lingual incline. This means a slight extension of the centric stop on the upper anterior teeth.

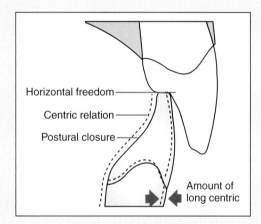

Interference to postural closure is marked with a red marking ribbon during unguided closure. The patient is instructed to tap lightly while the fresh marking ribbon is held as shown. The teeth should be dried before marking.

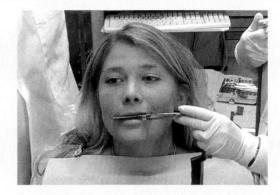

If the incline forward of centric relation marks, it is relieved so the incline does not touch during gentle unguided closure. The amount of relief required is never more than 0.5 mm, so it should not be necessary to mutilate teeth to accommodate long centric.

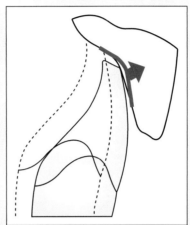

The cleared incline allows complete closure to centric relation when closing firmly, or gentle closure from a postural position without wedging into the lingual incline. About 50 percent of patients require no freedom for long centric because they close directly into centric relation even when in postural position.

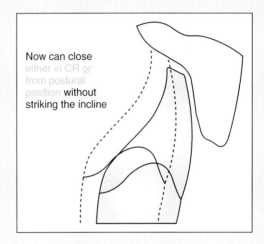

Now can close either in CR or from postural position without striking the incline

There are anatomic and physiologic reasons for accepting the concept of long centric. The fit of the condyle into its disk is not like the fit of a machined ball in a bearing. Rather, there is some front-back play permitted by the disk that allows the condyle to hinge freely anywhere within the limits of the anterior and posterior lips of the disk. When the mandible is closed firmly, the strong contraction of the muscles of closure pulls the condyle to the back of the disk against its posterior lip. Light closure from the rest position may be of insufficient intensity to completely pull the condyle into such a terminal position, and there will consequently be a slight difference between the firm terminal hinge closure of centric relation and a light closure from rest position.

A further difference between centric relation closure and a light closure from rest position could occur if the position of the mandible is influenced through a less intense closure by muscles of posture and facial expression. The postural position of the mandible during light closure can affect the position of the entire condyle-disk assembly as well as the position of the condyle in its disk.

Regardless of the cause, we do know from clinical studies that many patients exhibit a difference between centric closure and light closure from rest when they are in their postural position, and it is precisely this difference between the two positions that dictates the amount of long centric that any patient should have.

In establishing the need for long centric in any given patient, it is absolutely essential that all interferences to terminal hinge closure be eliminated. If centric relation interferences are present, the path of closure will be dictated by the mechanoreceptors of the teeth instead of by the normal physiologic function of the muscles.

In the absence of any centric relation interferences, it has been our experience that the difference between centric closure and light closure from rest rarely exceeds 0.5 mm. The usual long centric would be close to 0.2 mm, and many patients require no long centric because their light closure from rest is identical to their firm closure into centric relation.

It might be difficult to understand how such minute differences in the paths of closure can be significant, but it is just such minutiae that make the difference between just acceptability and complete predictable comfort. The dentist will only have to provide a needed long centric for one patient who has been "locked in" to centric relation (even a perfect centric relation) to get an idea of the usual reaction of patients to their new freedom.

If the vertical dimension is less when the teeth contact in centric relation than it is when they touch at the front end of the long centric area, light closure (which would be slightly protruded from centric closure) would direct the lower teeth against upper inclines instead of into stable contacts. If the patient requires a long centric and does not get its built-in freedom, the lower incisors may strike the lingual inclines of the upper incisors in a manner that has a tendency to wedge the upper teeth labially. It is probably this "wedging effect" that causes most of the instability of occlusions that have not been provided with a long centric.

It might be argued that the wedging contacts would occur with such light pressure that they could not possibly cause any harm. Such reasoning would continue to point out that when firm muscular pressure is exerted, the condyles would then be pulled into centric relation, and at this point the pressure would be properly directed by correct centric stops.

To understand how such light pressure on such minute interferences can cause problems of comfort and stability, it is necessary to have an acute appreciation for the exquisite sensitivity of the mechanoreceptor sensory system. When teeth are in the way of any functional border position, the muscles moving the mandible have two choices: they can move the mandible in a pattern of closure and function that avoids the interference, or they can move the mandible in a pattern of erasure to get rid of the interference.

Careful observation will convince one of the consistent pattern of grinding or clenching that occurs when an interference restricts functional jaw movements. Patterns of wear or movement of teeth are too routinely found in relation to such interferences to ignore their potential as targets for bruxism, if not the actual trigger that activates much of the parafunction. It appears that the erasure mechanism may actually be part of the adaptive process that is activated to regain lost equilibrium in the system by grinding away or moving the offending interference. What is not generally appreciated is how the bruxism pattern can be activated by such delicate contact on tooth surfaces that interfere so minimally with functional jaw patterns.

Clinical experience has been consistent, however, in the observation of accelerated wear of anterior teeth when inclines strike before full closure, or when an anterior guidance is restricted in any way from functional movements that occur during upright posture. The patterns of wear will be noticed on the labial surfaces of the lower incisors, or on the lingual surfaces of the upper incisors, or both.

Often the patient's subconscious attempt to regain the freedom of a muscularly coordinated closure ends up as forced protrusion, with the lower jaw trying to push the upper teeth forward to move them out of the way. Because of this forward thrust against the upper teeth, it is not uncommon for "locked-in occlusions" to develop slides. If the centric holding contacts on posterior teeth have been locked in with steep inclines that also interfere in the protrusive range of long centric, pressure against upper distal inclines can have a tendency to move them forward. This brings the upper mesial inclines into interference, and the slide results.

Not all patients require long centric. Their centric closure and their light closure when they are in a postural position are identical. If such patients are given a long centric, they will not use it, but it will not hurt them either. In fact, there are no contraindications to providing the freedom that goes with long centric. Problems occur when we fail to realize that long centric starts with a perfectly harmonized centric relation and that we are only providing patients with the freedom to close slightly anterior to that point at the same vertical. They are not forced to use either position, but they are free to use both positions or any point in between.

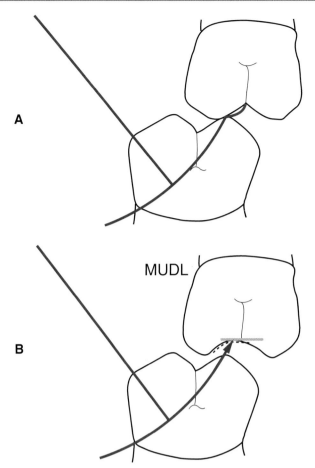

FIGURE 19-2 Equilibration usually results in an "automatic long centric." This results from elimination of the inclines that interfere with closure into centric relation (**A**) so that contact can be made at the most closed vertical either in centric relation or the original maximal intercuspation position (**B**). The patient is free to use either position, or both.

PROVIDING LONG CENTRIC BY EQUILIBRATION

When interferences to centric relation are eliminated by equilibration, long centric is usually provided automatically unless the vertical dimension is closed.

If the vertical dimension of the acquired occlusion is maintained, the first step in equilibration consists simply in eliminating all interferences from that point back to centric relation. The result is a long centric area that goes from centric relation all the way to the point of the original "acquired centric" (see Figure 19-2). The equilibrated patient is then free to close either into centric relation or into his or her original convenience position, or anywhere in between.

Our clinical experience has clearly and consistently shown that when interferences to centric relation are eliminated, the acquired position of occlusion is immediately forgotten. There is no need to maintain a long centric that includes the original acquired position because, given the freedom to do so, the mandible will close either directly into

centric relation or within a fraction of a millimeter forward of it, the amount depending on vagaries of anatomy and on how much pressure is exerted by the closing musculature.

There is no relationship between the length of a "slide" and the length of the long centric. The length of the slide is a result of interferences of the teeth. The length of the needed long centric is dependent on the anatomy of the condyle-disk relationship and the varying patterns of muscle activity in different patients. Many patients with long slides require no long centric when the interferences are eliminated (Figure 19-2). However, when the equilibrated mouth ends up with a longer long centric than the patient needs, it is not usually an indication for restoration of the entire occlusion. It will cause no discomfort or harm, since the patient will use only as much of the long centric as is needed.

In some patients, the interferences to centric relation are so severe that their elimination requires extensive flattening out of the occlusal areas between the convenience contacts and centric relation. Although such gross contouring will not cause any actual discomfort, some patients may complain that the flat surfaces make it difficult to chew meat or other fibrous foods. They may relate the feeling that their teeth are not "sharp enough." It is sometimes necessary to restore cuspal anatomy to such occlusions to give patients efficiency along with the comfort that goes with a harmonious gnathic system.

If there are no indications for restorative procedures other than a feeling of inefficiency, it would always be wise to give the patient a little time to see whether it is just a matter of adapting to the changed occlusion. The improvement in comfort is usually so great after proper equilibration that most patients will gladly accept the change in chewing efficiency that sometimes occurs when severe malocclusions are corrected. In many cases, it is the lesser of evils when compared with the otherwise unnecessary restoration of an entire occlusion.

It should be very clearly stated that reduced chewing efficiency should not result from normal equilibration procedures. The preceding discussion refers only to the unusual occlusal problems that cannot be corrected without extensive flattening out of the occlusal surfaces from the acquired position of maximum occlusal contact back to centric relation—in other words, the patient who ends up with the long centric that is much too long. In almost all other cases, judicious and correct equilibration should not "flatten out" an occlusion. The careful use of small stones on interfering inclines almost always improves efficiency without destroying the occlusal anatomy.

I should also point out that orthodontic procedures should be considered as an alternative to equilibration procedures that would mutilate. In many instances, minor tooth movement through use of simple appliances will minimize the need for occlusal reshaping.

Although the establishment of long centric is usually an automatic part of equilibration, it is not always so. There is never a concern about this if both condyles are deviated to some degree of protrusive movement. If occlusal interferences cause a definite lateral shift of the mandible with no protrusion whatsoever of the rotating condyle, elimination of the interferences could produce a "locked-in bite."

Reading the Marks

By using a red ribbon for postural closure and then using a black ribbon to manipulate for centric relation closure, you may compare the centric contacts with the contacts made by allowing the patient to close from the rest position. Variations in marking may occur if red is used for light closure from rest and black is used for a manipulated centric marking. The following is a list of the various marking combinations along with the interpretation and treatment suggestions for each combination.

1. When each red mark is covered by the black centric mark. Exact coverage would indicate that terminal hinge closure and light closure from rest are identical. A long centric is not essential in such cases.
2. When red marks extend forward from black centric marks. Forward extension would show a need for long centric. To provide the necessary amount, each centric stop should be extended forward at the same vertical for the length of the red mark. One should not grind the black centric marks. Equilibration for long centric is complete when there are no red marks on inclines. Allowing the patient to tap the teeth together should not cause movement of any tooth. This should be noted by careful digital examination of each tooth while the patient taps. Teeth that are jarred by the tapping should be re-marked while being held in place and then adjusted accordingly by selective grinding. The final result should produce no perceptible jarring of any tooth on closing, either when manipulated into centric relation or when the patient closes from the relaxed postural rest position.

   The red marks on the perfected occlusion will still extend forward from the black centric marks, but both red and black marks should be at the same vertical dimension of occlusion, as measured in the anterior part of the mouth. The vertical dimension of occlusion will open slightly in the posterior region as the protruding condyles move downward, but because of the minute distances involved, the difference in vertical between the front and the back of the average long centric is minimal.
3. When red marks extend backward from black centric marks. Backward extension can mean only one thing: the dentist has not manipulated correctly into centric closure. The black marks made by correct manipulation into centric closure will always be at the back border of any red mark. The red mark may be the same as the black mark, but it cannot be behind it.
4. When black centric marks are missing from red marks. If posterior teeth are marked by the red ribbon when the patient taps but some of them do not mark with the black ribbon when the mandible is manipu-

lated into a centric closure, the equilibration for centric relation is incomplete. The equilibration must be perfected to permit free, unobstructed access into centric relation before the correct long centric can be determined. If red marks are not accompanied by black marks, it may be because teeth with some degree of mobility are being moved when the teeth are tapped together. Compression of mobile teeth permits more teeth to mark when they are squeezed together into the red ribbon than are permitted to touch with controlled manipulation for centric relation.

To check for such mobility, the dentist should manipulate into centric relation with different degrees of firmness, varying from a feather touch to a very firm contact. A different-color ribbon should be used for comparing the light contacts with the firm contacts. There should be no difference in the position of marks made by varying degrees of firmness when the mandible is manipulated into centric relation. This is accomplished by grinding interferences that are detected by marking with the lightest pressure so that the interfering tooth is not moved out of the way.

When the centric stops have been perfected to this degree, you are then ready to determine the long centric. An occlusion that has been properly equilibrated in this manner will always show the black centric marks contiguously with the red marks made by allowing the patient to close from the postural rest position.

PROVIDING LONG CENTRIC WHEN THE OCCLUSION IS TO BE RESTORED

If all posterior teeth of either arch are to be restored, an excellent opportunity is presented to see the difference, if there is one, between a firm closure into centric relation and a light closure from the postural rest position.

By preparing all of the upper or lower posterior teeth, you eliminate the possibility of any mechanoreceptor influence from them. Since the prepared teeth have been reduced occlusally and cannot contact the teeth in the opposing arch, they certainly cannot interfere with any pattern of closure. With all such chance of any posterior interference eliminated, it is then rather simple, when needed, to correct any inclines on the anterior teeth that cause a deviation from terminal hinge closure. By manipulating the mandible to make sure it does not deviate from its terminal axis, mark and reshape the interferences by selective grinding to provide centric relation stops on as many anterior teeth as possible. Properly adjusted centric stops on anterior teeth should be stable enough that not one of the teeth is jarred when the teeth are firmly tapped together in a terminal hinge closure.

When this is accomplished, the muscles that move the mandible are free to close it in any manner that best suits them. Since there are no interferences to terminal axis closure, the mandible is free to go there if the physiologic action of the muscles dictates. If the muscles close the mandible into any

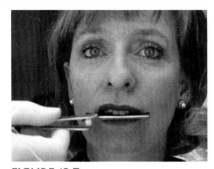

FIGURE 19-3 Gentle tapping (unguided) on a red marking ribbon shows interferences to postural closure.

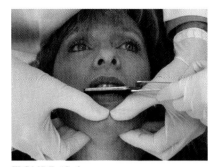

FIGURE 19-4 Manipulation to centric relation with guided closure overlays black centric relation contacts on red postural contacts

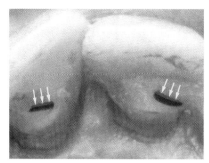

FIGURE 19-5 If red marks appear on inclines forward of centric relation contacts *(arrows)*, it indicates a need to extend the centric relation contact forward.

position other than centric relation, it is easily observed by checking with thin marking ribbon on the anterior teeth. Consequently, this is the ideal time to determine whether the restorative patient requires a long centric and, if so, how much.

After the anterior centric relation stops have been perfected, the patient should sit up in a normal postural position. The headrest should be removed, and then the patient should lightly tap the teeth together from a relaxed jaw position. Thin red ribbon should be interposed between the teeth, and the patient should repeat the light tapping (Figure 19-3). The red marks made from this procedure will indicate on the lingual surfaces of the upper anterior teeth the first points that the lower teeth contact when the mandible is closed lightly by the unrestricted, unaided, physiologic action of the muscles when the patient is in a postural position.

For comparison of such a closure with the terminal axis closure of centric relation, the mouth should be held open to preserve the red marks while the patient is placed back into a supine position for marking of centric relation with a darker-colored ribbon (Figure 19-4). If black ribbon is used to mark centric relation contacts over the red marks, it is simple to see whether there is a difference between a manipulated terminal hinge closure and the unmanipulated light closure from a postural rest position.

If the patient requires the freedom of a long centric, the red marks will extend forward from the black centric marks. If the red marks are on wedging inclines, the centric stops should be extended forward at the same vertical dimension for the length of the red marks (Figure 19-5).

When extending the centric stops to include closure from postural rest position, the dentist should be sure never to grind on the black centric marks. A knife-edged inverted-cone Carborundum stone is practical to use for accurate grinding.

Interference to Long Centric

An example of a restricted envelope of function is shown in Figure 19-6. If this patient closes in centric relation (red marks), there are no incline contacts and tapping the teeth together is comfortable and produces no fremitus. In this patient, the lingual surfaces of the upper anterior teeth will interfere with postural closure of the jaw and will certainly be

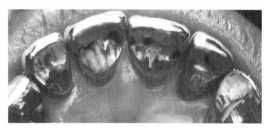

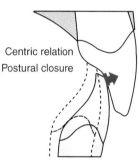

Centric relation
Postural closure

FIGURE 19-6 Do not be confused by the use of a different color sequence for the marking ribbons *(green* was used for postural closure; *red* was used for centric relation). Note the wedging effect of striking the steep lingual inclines during postural closure (shown in *green*).

a factor in accelerated wear of the lower incisors and/or mobility of the upper anterior teeth. This is a common finding in anterior restorative cases in which provision for a needed long centric is neglected.

> It is very important to check each tooth digitally for any jarring from the light rest closure.

It is easy for mobile teeth to be moved rather than marked by the ribbon. Checking each tooth for such movement while the patient taps is sometimes the only way such interferences are picked up. It is often necessary to hold mobile teeth in place with one finger while the patient taps in order to correctly mark them.

For those who are skeptical about the value of long centric, the preceding procedures can be very enlightening. It is quite convincing to see teeth jarred when the patient sits up and taps that were not jarred by tapping when the patient was lying back. It is also quite enlightening to see other patients who tap directly and precisely into a terminal hinge axis closure, despite the fact that before the interferences to centric relation were removed their habitual closure was far from their centric closure.

When patients tell us that their teeth feel fine when they are lying down but that the teeth are in the way when they are sitting up, they are really giving us important information. They are telling us, in effect, that their centric relation is all right but they need the freedom of a long centric. To provide them with less than both is to fall short of potential comfort and stability. We like to provide our patients with occlusions that are comfortable when they are either sitting up or lying down, whether biting hard or lightly closing. This is not always possible to do with an occlusion that is restricted by tooth inclines to terminal hinge closure only.

If patients complain that their teeth fit fine when the dentist "pushes the jaw back" but hit only on the front teeth if they close it themselves, they are referring to the same type of restricted occlusion that often occurs when the dentist fails to provide a needed long centric.

If restricting an occlusion only to centric relation is sometimes bad, restricting it only to an acquired habitual closure is worse. We have never seen a temporomandibular disorder that was directly caused by failure to provide a long centric if centric relation was correct. Failure to provide a needed long centric may lead to clenching and bruxism and

a locked-in feeling of mild discomfort, but in itself it cannot cause true joint pain-dysfunction.

On the other hand, failure to provide access to centric relation not only can cause severe problems of discomfort, clenching, and bruxism, but, as already pointed out, it can also cause pain and dysfunction of the muscles that move the mandible.

Occlusal inclines restricting mandibular movement are potential stress producers. Long centric is permissive. It frees the mandible to close either into centric relation or slightly anterior to it. When the mandible is free to go where the muscles wish to move it, the result is predictable comfort with minimal stress to the entire gnathic system.

Because of the permissiveness of long centric, there are really no disadvantages to providing it. Since we are talking about a freedom of rarely more than 0.5 mm, it does not create any problems for restoring the posterior occlusal form with good morphology. If the patient has it and does not need it, he or she does not have to use it.

Suggested Readings

Ash MM, Nelson SJ: *Wheeler's dental anatomy, physiology, and occlusion,* ed 8, Philadelphia, 2003, WB Saunders.

Ramfjord SP, Ash MM: *Occlusion,* ed 3, Philadelphia, 1983, WB Saunders.

Schuyler CH: Factors in occlusion related to restorative dentistry. *J Prosthet Dent* 3:772-782, 1953.

Chapter 20

The Plane of Occlusion

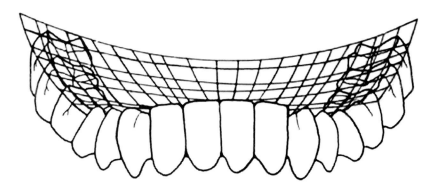

PRINCIPLE

The plane of occlusion is acceptable if it permits the anterior guidance to do its job without interference.

OCCLUSAL PLANE DESIGN

The configuration of the occlusal plane is one of the most beautiful examples of design that can be found in nature. The conformity to that design by the other parts of the masticatory system is so subtle it is often missed. However, the logic of these interrelationships is important to understand because even slight variations from this intended configuration can lead to unexplained occlusal instability. The irritating reductions in comfort or function that bother the patient and frustrate the dentist are often related to unnoticed occlusal plane problems.

The term *plane of occlusion* refers to an imaginary surface that theoretically touches the incisal edges of the incisors and the tips of the occluding surfaces of the posterior teeth. Because the term *plane* refers geometrically to a flat surface, it is not entirely correct to describe the occlusal surface as following a true plane. Instead of a flat surface, the plane of occlusion represents the average curvature of the occlusal surface. Despite the problem of semantics, it is probably the most practical way of relating the occlusal surfaces of the teeth to one another and to other structures of the head. Each curvature of the plane is related to specific effects it should produce. Its acceptability should be analyzed on that functional basis rather than on its conformity to a set ideal.

The curvatures of the anterior teeth are determined by the establishment of an esthetically correct smile line on the upper and the relationship of the lower incisal edges to the anterior guidance and the requirements for phonetics. These factors are covered in Chapter 17.

The curvatures of the posterior plane of occlusion are divided into (1) an anteroposterior curve called the curve of Spee (Figure 20-1) and (2) a mediolateral curve, referred to as the curve of Wilson (Figure 20-2).

Together, the composite of the curve of Spee, the curve of Wilson, and the curve of the incisal edges is properly referred to as the *curve of occlusion*. Popular usage combines both the curve of occlusion and its relationship to the cranium into the plane of occlusion (Figure 20-3). This chapter will discuss each aspect of it individually.

THE CURVE OF SPEE

The curve of Spee refers to the anteroposterior curvature of the occlusal surfaces, beginning at the tip of the lower canine and following the buccal cusp tips of the bicuspids and molars and continuing to the anterior border of the ramus. If the curved line continued further back, it would ideally follow an arc through the condyle (Figure 20-4). The curvature of the arc would relate, on average, to part of a circle with a 4-inch radius.

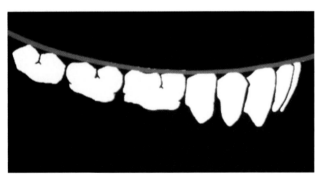

FIGURE 20-1   The curve of Spee is the anteroposterior curve. It begins at the tip of the canine, and touches the cusp tips of all the posterior teeth.

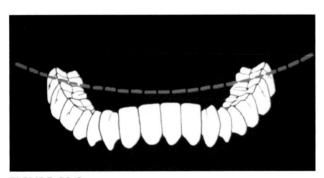

FIGURE 20-2   The curve of Wilson is the mediolateral curve that contacts the buccal and lingual cusp tips on each side of the arch.

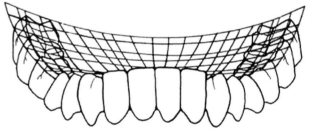

FIGURE 20-3   The plane of occlusion represents the average curvature of the occlusal surface.

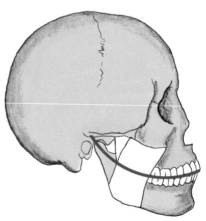

FIGURE 20-4   An ideal curve of Spee is aligned so that a continuation of its arc extends through the condyles. The curvature of this arc relates on average with a 4-inch radius.

There is a purpose behind the curve of Spee design as well as its location in relation to the condyle. The curve results from variations in axial alignment of the lower teeth. To align each tooth for maximum resistance to functional loading, the long axis of each lower tooth is aligned nearly parallel to its individual arc of closure around the condylar axis (Figure 20-5). This requires the last molar to be tilted forward at the greatest angle and the forward tooth to be at the least angle. This progression positions the cusp tips on a curve that is directly related to the condylar axis by a progressive series of tangents.

The relationship of the curve of occlusion to the condylar axis also relates to the condylar path in protrusion. If the occlusal plane is on an arc that passes through the condyle, the posterior part of the occlusal plane will always be flat enough and low enough to be discluded by the normal condylar path on its steeper eminentia (Figure 20-6). Thus even with a flat zero-degree anterior guidance in protrusion, the occlusal plane on the lower will be discluded by the forward movement of the condyle that is directed downward at an angle that is steeper than the posterior part of the occlusal plane.

It is because of this geometric design that the 4-inch radius of the Monson curve works so effectively if the condyle is used for a survey point, as it is in the SOPA technique described below.

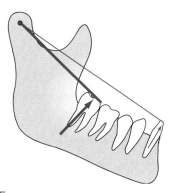

FIGURE 20-5 The curve of Spee results, in part, from aligning each lower tooth parallel with its arc of closure. This requires the last molar to be inclined at the greatest angle.

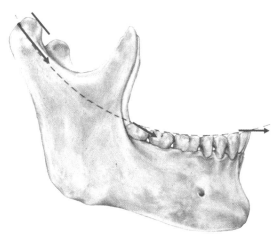

FIGURE 20-6 If the curve of Spee arc extends through the condyle, the occlusal plane will always be flat enough in the posterior segment to be separated by the downward path of the condyle against a normally steeper condylar path. This is so even with a flat anterior guidance.

Determining an Acceptable Occlusal Plane for Restorative Cases

PROCEDURE   Using a simplified occlusal plane analyzer (SOPA)

This simplified method reduces the time required for occlusal plane analysis because the analysis point for surveying the occlusal plane is already related to the condylar axis. The pencil point is simply positioned at the desired height for the lower canine, and the point of the compass is placed on the center line of the SOPA. The compass pencil is then arced back to show the occlusal plane that would correctly relate to the condyles. If this plane would require mutilation of either upper or lower posterior teeth, the compass point can be repositioned on the front or back line on the SOPA to compensate. If an acceptable occlusal plane cannot be surveyed, it is probable that the facebow mounting is incorrect.

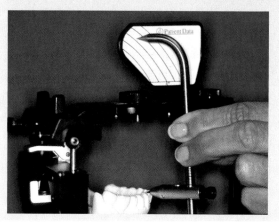

Continued

PROCEDURE   Using a simplified occlusal plane analyzer (SOPA)—cont'd

An ideal occlusal plane starts at the canine tip and goes through the condylar axis. If all positive cusp tips relate to this plane, disclusion of posterior teeth is never a problem. However, remember that this is an arbitrary plane based on an arc around a survey point that is 4 inches from the tip of the canine. It is an excellent aid for establishing an ideal occlusal plane if all posterior teeth are to be restored. It should not be used to determine whether or not restorations are necessary.

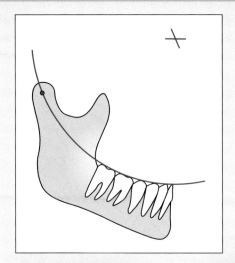

A SOPA is preset at 4 inches from the condylar axis. The SOPA works with Dénar® (Teledyne Waterpik™) articulators. The Broadrick flag accomplishes the same occlusal analysis on almost all types of semiadjustable articulators.

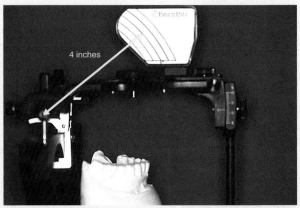

By setting the caliper scribe at 4 inches and aligning the marking point at the tip of the canine, an occlusal plane can be scribed on the lower cast that will go through the condylar axis in one simple step.

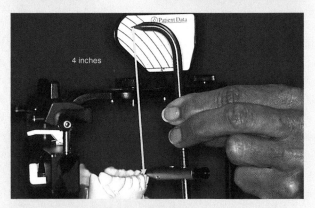

A line drawn on the cast represents an acceptable occlusal plane. The caliper scribe can be lengthened to a preparation height. This process is only used if the posterior teeth are to be restored. It is never used to determine whether or not teeth must be prepared.

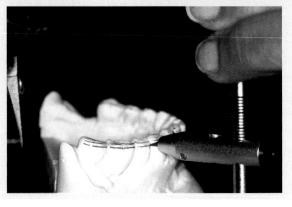

PROCEDURE   Using a simplified occlusal plane analyzer (SOPA)—cont'd

A simple wax index can be adapted to the cast and the desired occlusal plane can be scribed on the wax, which is then trimmed to the line.

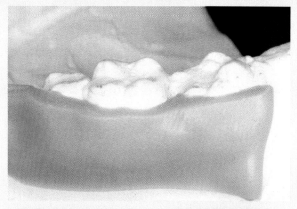

With the wax index in place, the teeth can be marked to the indicated preparation height and occlusal plane.

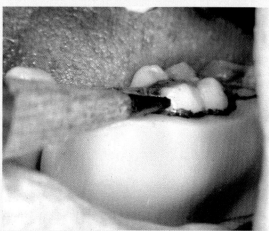

Tooth reduction that follows the predetermined preparation height and contour ensures that there will be sufficient room for restorative materials when the restorations are fabricated. Preparations are completed after the occlusal reduction is verified.

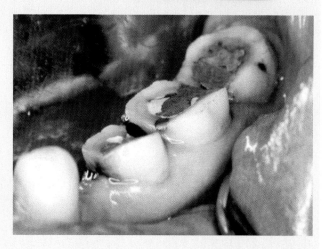

The anteroposterior curvature of the occlusal plane is designed to permit protrusive disclusion of the posterior teeth by the combination of anterior guidance and condylar guidance. The separation of posterior teeth during excursive contact of the anterior teeth results in more efficient incisive function as the anterior teeth slide past each other to the overlapped relationship that makes the shearing action possible.

To separate the posterior teeth for better incisive function during protrusive excursions, all forces of the elevator muscles must be loaded entirely onto the condyle and the anterior teeth. This results in a strong horizontal vector against the upper anterior teeth, since all the contacts are against their lingual surfaces. To protect the anterior teeth from being overloaded, an ingeniously designed sensor system shuts off most of the elevator muscle activity at the precise moment of complete posterior disclusion. This reduction of pressure against the anterior teeth depends on a correct occlusal plane because if there is any interfering tooth contact posterior to the canines during excursions, the elevator muscles are triggered into hypercontraction.

This prevention of increased muscle loading on the teeth and the joints is the dominant reason for making certain that the occlusal plane is correctly evaluated as a part of every complete examination. If it does not permit the anterior guidance to separate the posterior teeth in excursive movements, there is a real possibility of eventual damage to the teeth, the joints, and the periodontal structure.

THE CURVE OF WILSON

The curve of Wilson is the mediolateral curve that contacts the buccal and lingual cusp tips on each side of the arch. It results from inward inclination of the lower posterior teeth, making the lingual cusps lower than the buccal cusps on the mandibular arch; the buccal cusps are higher than the lingual cusps on the maxillary arch because of the outward inclination of the upper posterior teeth.

There are two reasons for this inclination of posterior teeth. One has to do with resistance to loading, and the second has to do with masticatory function.

If the buccolingual inclination of the posterior teeth is analyzed in relation to the dominant direction of muscle force against them, it will be apparent that the axial alignment of all posterior teeth is nearly parallel with the strong inward pull of the internal pterygoid muscles (Figure 20-7). The strongest component of lateral function occurs from the outside in, nearly parallel with the direction of the internal pterygoid muscles, which bilaterally pull the condyles medially to the midmost position of centric relation. Aligning both upper and lower posterior teeth with the principal di-

rection of muscle contraction produces the greatest resistance to masticatory forces and creates the inclinations that form the curve of Wilson (Figure 20-8).

There is another reason for the curve of Wilson that relates it definitively to masticatory function. Because the tongue and the buccinator complex must repetitively place each bite of food onto the occlusal surfaces for mastication, there must be easy access for the food to get to the occlusal table. The inward inclination of the lower occlusal table is designed for direct access from the lingual, with no blockage by lower lingual cusps (Figure 20-9).

The outward inclination of the upper occlusal table provides access from the buccal for the food to be tossed directly onto the occlusal table by the action of the bands of the buccinator muscle (Figure 20-10). The longer lingual cusps of the upper posterior teeth serve as a baffle for food tossed on from the buccal; and the lower buccal cusp serves the same purpose for food tossed on by the tongue.

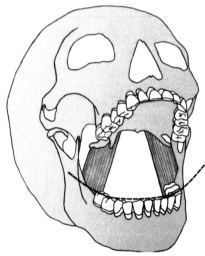

FIGURE 20-8 Alignment of the posterior teeth to parallel the direction of loading from the internal pterygoid muscles results in the curve of Wilson.

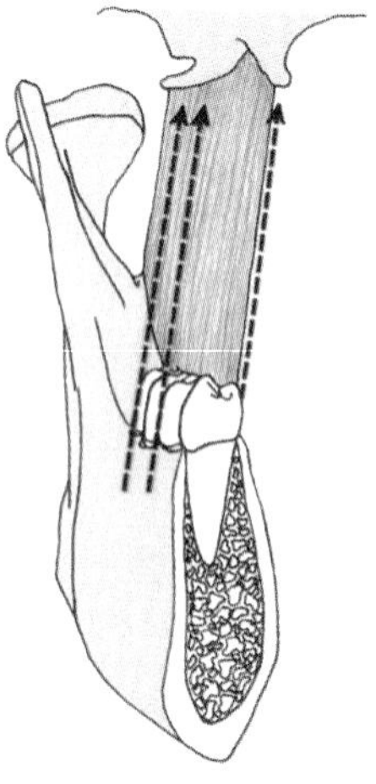

FIGURE 20-7 The principal loading force against the posterior teeth occurs during the outside-inward chewing stroke. The posterior teeth are thus aligned parallel to the internal pterygoid muscles for optimum resistance to this functional stress.

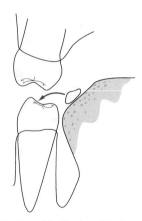

FIGURE 20-9 The lingual inclination of the lower posterior teeth positions the lingual cusps lower than the buccal cusps. This design permits easy access to the occlusal table. As the tongue lays the food on the occlusal surfaces, it is stopped from going past the chewing position by the taller buccal cusps.

When the curve of Wilson is made too flat, ease of masticatory function may be impaired because of increased activity required to get the food onto the occlusal table. The greater the relative height of the lower lingual cusps, the greater the problem of chewing efficiency may become. Unless the problem is understood, it is easily missed because patient complaints do not pinpoint the problem.

Condylar Path Protection for Posterior Teeth

The inclination of the posterior teeth coordinates their masticatory function with the necessary function of the tongue and cheeks to put the food where it can be chewed. This coordination of functional design creates a need for further design coordination in the articulation of the jaw joints. The

upper lingual cusps would be in jeopardy of great horizontal stress from the lower buccal cusps if the lower teeth were permitted to move horizontally toward the midline (Figure 20-11). The articulation of the medial pole of the condyle is designed to prevent that from happening. The same configuration of the fossae that braces the condyle-disk assemblies in the midmost position also prevents them from traveling medially without first moving downward (Figure 20-12). In short, the lower posterior teeth must travel down before they can shift medially. This important aspect of design makes it possible to have a curve of Wilson without creating balancing incline interferences.

The concept of an immediate side shift, which allows the condyles to translate horizontally before any rotation oc-

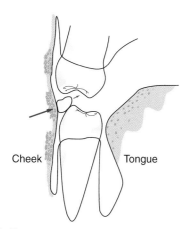

FIGURE 20-10 The outer inclination of the upper teeth positions the buccal cusps higher for easier access from the buccal corridor. The buccinator muscle squeezes the bolus onto the occlusal table where it is stopped by the longer lingual cusp.

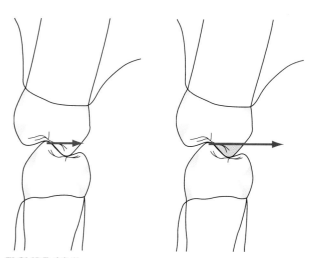

FIGURE 20-11 The concept of an immediate side shift is a very popular misconception that somehow persists. The purpose of the curve of Wilson to aid in positioning food on the occlusal table would not be possible if the posterior teeth could travel horizontally toward the midline. Fortunately, the condylar path prevents such a movement.

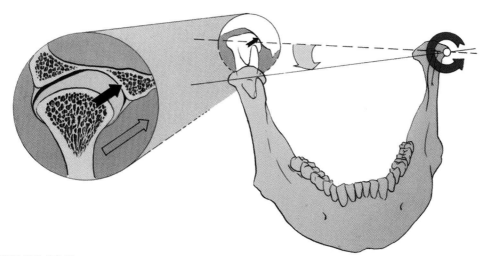

FIGURE 20-12 The design of the functional curve of Wilson would not work if the lower posterior teeth could travel horizontally toward the midline, because the longer lower buccal cusps would clash with the longer upper lingual cusps. The medial pole bony stop prevents any side shift until after the condyle has moved down the eminentia and permits the curve of Wilson design to function without interference. This necessary functional relationship of the joints is also responsible for the solid "midmost" position in centric relation. It also explains why the concept of an immediate side shift is incorrect.

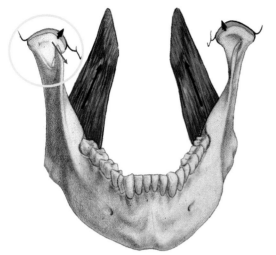

FIGURE 20-13 The condyles are braced medially in centric relation. They must move down to permit any lateral jaw movement.

curs, was a popular notion. However, it cannot occur in a healthy joint if the condyles are in centric relation at the start of motion (Figure 20-13). If it could occur, the curve of Wilson would result in balancing incline interferences. The only way this can occur is if there is severe alteration of the shape of the articulating surfaces.

It would be very unlikely to have flattening of the condyle and eminence without similar adaptation of the curve of Wilson. The effect of such changes in the joints is seen in the flattening of the curve of Wilson by wearing away of the upper lingual cusps. This type of wear cannot occur in a correct occlusal plane with normal, healthy temporomandibular joints. The presence of severe wear on upper lingual cusps should alert the diagnostician to adaptive changes in the articular surfaces of the joint.

The occlusal plane is a marvelous example of the interplay between form and function. Analysis of the occlusal plane should be important to any dental examination because of its importance to coordinated function of the entire masticatory system. Adaptive changes in the occlusal plane are signals of possible dysfunction somewhere in the system.

SUMMARY

The form of the occlusal plane is directly related to specific functional requirements. In addition to alignment of teeth in relationship to the arc of closure for best resistance to loading, it should permit ease of access for positioning of the food on the occlusal surfaces. If these two functional requirements are met, an occlusal plane is acceptable if it permits the anterior guidance to do its job.

The occlusal plane is a critical consideration in solving many different problems of occlusion. But if basic requirements for acceptability of an occlusal plane are understood, resolution of problem occlusions can be achieved more readily.

Suggested Readings

Boucher DO: Current status of prosthodontics. *J Prosthet Dent* 10:418, 1960.

Craddock HL, Lynch CD, Fraulslin P, et al: A study of the proximity of the Broodrick ideal occlusal curve to the existing occlusal curve in dental patients. *J Oral Rehabil* 32(12):895-900, 2005.

Mann AW, Pankey LD: Use of the Pankey-Mann instrument in treatment planning and in restoring the lower posterior teeth. *J Prosthet Dent* 10:135, 1980.

Monson GS: Applied mechanics to the theory of mandibular movements. *Dent Cosmos* 74:1039, 1932.

Spee FG: *Prosthetic dentistry,* ed 4, Chicago, 1928, Medico-dental Publishing.

Wilson GH: *Dental prosthetics,* Philadelphia, 1917, Lea & Febiger.

Chapter 21

Posterior Occlusion

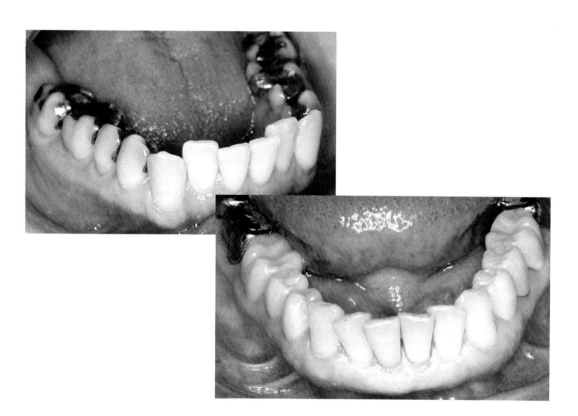

PRINCIPLE

Posterior teeth should have equal intensity contacts that do not interfere with either the temporomandibular joints (TMJs) in the back or the anterior guidance in the front.

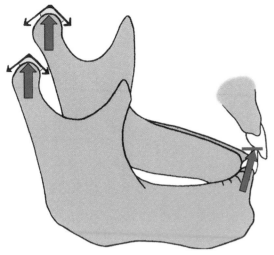

FIGURE 21-1 The mandible as an inverted tripod.

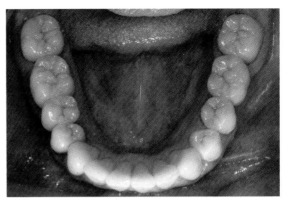

FIGURE 21-2 Note the beautiful occlusal contours restored in full-coverage restorations by Dr. Michael Sesemann, DDS, and Lee Culp, CDT.

NONINTERFERING POSTERIOR TEETH

The third requirement for successful occlusal treatment is noninterfering posterior teeth. This means that posterior teeth should not interfere with complete seating of the jaw joints (the first requirement) and should not interfere with the anterior guidance (the second requirement). The ideal occlusal scheme is complete separation of all posterior teeth by the anterior guidance the moment the condyles leave centric relation. When the condyles are completely seated up into centric relation, the goal is to have simultaneous, equal-intensity contact of all posterior teeth at the same instant that the anterior teeth contact.

Let's review the visualization of the mandible as an inverted tripod (Figure 21-1) with two TMJs in back that are solidly seated against bony stops so they cannot move upward. If centric stops are properly contoured on the anterior teeth, jaw closure is stopped against solid contacts at the front of the mandible. The ideal starting point for posterior teeth is to align and contour the teeth so they fit into the space between these front and back stops without interfering with either of them.

In occlusions in which anterior contact in centric relation can be achieved, the only contact on posterior teeth should be in centric relation. As soon as the mandible moves in any direction, all posterior teeth should be discluded. In dentitions that cannot achieve anterior contact in centric relation (see discussion of anterior open bite in Chapter 38), it is often necessary to achieve group function contact on the working side. Teeth on the nonworking side should never contact during excursions.

LOWER POSTERIOR TEETH

With advancements in materials and methods, posterior teeth can be restored to natural beauty without sacrificing strength or stability (Figure 21-2). Even the best materials,

however, will not hold up if the occlusion is not correct. The requirements for perfected posterior occlusions start with the lower posterior teeth.

Three Key Determinations

Three important determinations must be made for successful posterior occlusions. Each of these determinations involves the lower posterior teeth. These determinations are in order of priority as follows:

1. Plane of occlusion (see Chapter 20)
2. Location of each lower buccal cusp tip
3. Position and contour of each lower fossa

These three determinations are important because once these decisions are made, all other aspects of posterior occlusion are relative to them.

Restoration of posterior teeth should not be considered until the condyles can be positioned with acceptable comfort in centric relation. Restoration of posterior teeth should not be attempted for the purpose of determining if uncomfortable condyles can be made comfortable. Condyles should be comfortable before restorations are completed.

Restoration of posterior teeth should not be completed until the anterior guidance is correct. The fossa contours are directly related to the anterior guidance and cannot be determined accurately until after the anterior guidance paths have been finalized.

It is not necessary to restore upper and lower posterior teeth together to ensure correct occlusal contours. Even when upper occlusal surfaces are to be changed, every aspect of lower occlusal form can be correctly determined and accurately restored before the upper posterior teeth are prepared.

There are advantages to completing the lower posterior segment before the upper teeth are prepared. It is easier for both the dentist and the patient. The lower posterior preparations can be made, and impressions, bite records, and temporization can be accomplished in a reasonably comfortable time period. There is no need for extremely long, tiring appointments, repeated removal of temporary restorations, and extra anesthetics. The cumulative errors of cementation are reduced to the effect of cement thickness on

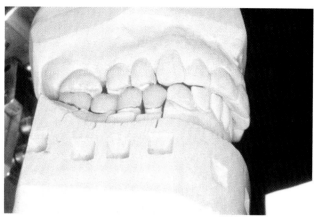

FIGURE 21-3 **A,** Determining the alignment of lower cusp tips is uncomplicated when analyzed on mounted casts in centric relation. It is not necessary to place cusp tips in a stereotyped position. What is important is that the contact is favorable to the axial alignment of both upper and lower teeth. Contact is preferable in a fossa but may be on a marginal ridge if a second contact can be achieved on the same tooth. **B,** A simple dot on the opposing teeth is all that is needed to communicate lower cusp tip alignment to the technician.

a single arch. Laboratory procedures are more easily carried out, and the coronal reference points left intact on the upper segment can be used to indicate the degree of buccolingual tilting of each tooth.

Every aspect of occlusal form has a purpose, and every contour can be determined by measurable and recordable factors. For example, the lower cusp–fossae inclines are determined by the anterior guidance and the condylar guidance. If the lower lingual cusp is to have functional contact in working excursions, its buccal incline must be the same as the lateral anterior guidance, with some modifications to maintain simultaneous conformity to condylar paths. If the lower lingual cusp is to be discluded in working excursions, its buccal incline must be flatter than the lateral anterior guidance. These facts of occlusal morphology will hold true whether the upper and lower teeth are waxed up together or separately. The inclines will not change simply because the technique changes. If the controlling determinants can be recorded, the results of the determinants can be captured.

Lower lingual cusp excursive contact unnecessarily complicates the fabrication of occlusal surfaces without any improvement in function or stability. So from a practical standpoint, lower cusp–fossae angles should be flatter than the lateral anterior guidance. This is one simplification that can be utilized without any concern that quality is being compromised.

Posterior teeth in the lower arch can be accurately restored with cusp-tip–to–fossa contact if the following determinations can be made (Figure 21-3):

1. Correct height and placement of buccal cusps
2. Correct height and placement of lingual cusps
3. Correct placement of fossae
4. Correct inclines for fossae walls

None of the above ascertainments is complicated if the objectives and determinants of each occlusal segment are understood. Following a logical sequence simplifies each de-

termination and provides a reference point from which the next decision can be made regarding occlusal configurations.

The starting point for determining lower occlusal contours should be the buccal cusps.

Placement of Lower Buccal Cusps

Placement of lower buccal cusps is determined on the basis of providing the optimum effect for buccolingual stability, mesiodistal stability, and noninterfering excursions.

Buccal cusp placement for buccolingual stability

The correct location of each lower buccal cusp should be one of the first determinations made when the original treatment plan is outlined. Preparation for restorations should not be made until the lower teeth are in their most acceptable relationship to the upper teeth. When necessary, arch expansion is usually a simple orthodontic procedure that can be accomplished in a matter of weeks. Lower teeth that are not in acceptable buccolingual relationship with their related upper teeth should have their alignment corrected before restorative procedures are initiated, rather than be restored with "warped" contours that misdirect stresses off the long axis. The need for orthodontic correction can be determined from correctly mounted study casts. It is frequently necessary to equilibrate the casts to make a final determination regarding the acceptability of interarch relationships. To make such a determination, casts must be mounted with a facebow recording and an interocclusal bite record at the correct centric relation.

The buccolingual position of lower buccal cusps is determined in the following manner on mounted casts.

1. Upper central groove position is analyzed. On each upper occlusal surface, a line is drawn from mesial to distal in the central groove. The ideal contact point for each lower buccal cusp tip is usually located somewhere on this line. However, the correctness of the

central groove should be analyzed on each tooth. In some tilted teeth, it is advantageous to move the central groove to gain better direction of forces through the long axis. As an example, an upper second molar, which is tilted toward the buccal, can have the stresses directed to better advantage if the central groove is moved toward the lingual. When the upper teeth have not been prepared, the tilt of each tooth can be more easily determined and points of contact can be more accurately selected. If moving the central groove will enable the stresses to be directed more nearly through the long axis of any upper tooth, the improved central groove position should be so noted on the upper cast by drawing a new line.

2. Optimum contact for stress direction on lower posterior teeth is determined. While we disregard the upper central groove position, the buccal cusp position that would most nearly direct stresses down through the long axis of each lower posterior tooth is determined. This may be done at the study model stage, or in cases with acceptable arch alignment, it may be done after the lower posterior teeth have been prepared. At this point, we are concerned only with buccolingual relationships.

   A mark is made on each lower tooth to indicate the position of the buccal cusp that would be optimum for buccolingual stability and direction of force. In selecting this point, we disregard the upper teeth and determine only what is best for the lower teeth. Next, we evaluate the relationship of the selected lower cusp position against the ideal upper central groove position.

3. Alignment of the optimum lower buccal cusp position against optimum upper central groove position is evaluated. This is easily done if we close the articulator and observe how the lower marks line up with the upper marks. If the marks do not line up precisely, the positions of both the upper central groove and the lower buccal cusp tip are equally changed. The new cusp-tip positions are re-evaluated to make certain that they are compatible with acceptable stress direction through the long axis of each lower tooth (Figure 21-4). The upper groove position is similarly evaluated.

If the altered buccal cusp-tip position does not provide acceptable stress directioning for both upper and lower posterior teeth, the arch relationship is unacceptable and the treatment plan should be designed to correct the problem. Orthodontic movement is usually the best way to correct malrelated arches, but it is not always possible or practical. There are many subtle factors to be considered before arch expansion or contraction is initiated, and a competent orthodontist should be consulted. When it is practical, arch expansion or contraction can usually be done rather easily and seldom takes very long to accomplish.

There are some arch relationship problems that are better off being left as they are. The chapters on treating end-to-end occlusions and solving crossbite problems (Chapters 39 and 41) should be studied carefully. "Warping" posterior oc-

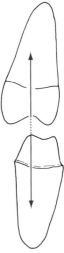

FIGURE 21-4 When determining the buccolingual placement of the lower buccal cusp, the resulting direction of force should be favorable to both upper and lower teeth. The main force vector should be as parallel as possible to the long axis of both.

clusal contours to "correct" such conditions is very often more damaging than corrective.

> The basic rule to follow regarding the buccolingual position of the lower buccal cusp is: The lower buccal cusp must be positioned so that its contact directs the stresses through the long axis of both upper and lower teeth.

When the buccolingual line of the lower buccal cusp tips has been determined, the next determination to make is the mesiodistal position of each cusp tip on that line.

Mesiodistal placement of lower buccal cusps

Two considerations should determine the mesiodistal position of lower buccal cusps: mesiodistal stability and noninterfering excursions.

Attaining mesiodistal stability

The best mesiodistal stability is attained by placement of the lower buccal cusps in upper fossae. Placement in the fossae directs the stresses properly through the long axis, eliminates any possibility of plunger cusp food impaction at contact, and is stable. There is no tendency for cusp tips to migrate out of properly contoured fossae (Figure 21-5).

There will be times when it is not practical to place the lower buccal cusp in an upper fossa, and it will be necessary for it to contact on the marginal ridges of two upper teeth. Plunger cusp food impaction can be avoided by proper design. The upper marginal ridges should be contoured with sluiceways from the adjacent fossae that permit the crushed bolus to slide away from the contact. The contact itself should be wide enough to protect the interdental papilla. Whenever possible, another lower buccal cusp of the same tooth should be brought into centric contact, or the upper lingual cusp should be used as an additional centric stop to

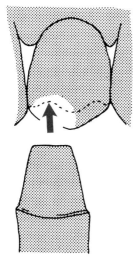

FIGURE 21-5 For mesiodistal stability, the cusp tip has a tendency to stay centered in a correctly designed fossa far better than against an incline or even a flat surface contact.

MES

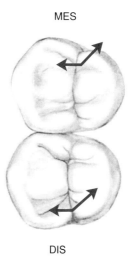

DIS

FIGURE 21-6 When the lower buccal cusp tip placement is being located, the path of egress from the upper fossa should be evaluated. If the cusp tip is placed in the mesial fossa, above, it moves into space on its excursion toward the lingual. If it is placed in a distal fossa, below, it may meet interference with a lingual cusp.

eliminate plunger activity. Of course, the main cause of plunger cusp impaction is the wedging open effect of incline contacts. Incline contacts in centric relation should be avoided.

Although acceptable tooth to two-teeth contact can be accomplished, it is usually rather simple to warp the lower buccal cusp mesially or distally the 1 or 2 mm required to place the cusp tip into an upper fossa. Whenever it can be done with practicality, this is what I try to do.

Locating the lower buccal cusps for noninterfering excursions

Determining which fossa the lower buccal cusp should contact depends on where the cusp travels when it leaves centric relation. The mesiodistal placement of each lower buccal cusp is determined when one locates it in the fossa that permits excursions from centric relation without interference (Figure 21-6). This may sound complicated, but learning the border paths of each lower tooth can be a rather simple exercise.

By first selecting appropriate fossae on the upper mounted model, one can quickly determine the paths of the lower cusps from each fossa, since they will travel at right angles to the rotating condyle. By visualization of a straight line from the rotating condyle to the selected contact point in the fossa, it is a simple matter to determine the general path of the lower cusp as it travels in either a working or balancing excursion. Protrusive paths are easy to determine since all cusps move straight forward in that excursion.

When each upper fossa position is selected, the articulator should be closed to see whether the upper fossa location would also be acceptable as a buccal cusp position for the lower tooth. The selected contact points should direct the forces through the long axes of both upper and lower teeth.

If stress direction is acceptable to both teeth, the paths of movement from the selected fossa should be evaluated. If

the lower buccal cusp can move out of the fossa in protrusive working and balancing excursions without colliding with another cusp, its position is acceptable. By evaluating each lower buccal cusp placement in this manner, we are taking an essential step to assure in advance the correct contouring of the upper posterior teeth after the lower teeth are completed.

Placement of the lower cusp tip directly between the upper buccal and lingual cusps not only is unstable, but it also necessitates the destruction of upper occlusal anatomy to permit excursions. Placement of a lower premolar cusp tip in the distal fossa of the upper may provide a free path from centric relation out to a working excursion toward the buccal, but the upper lingual cusp can be in the way of balancing excursions toward the lingual.

It is usually best to place the lower buccal cusps of premolars in a mesial fossa when possible. This allows egress from centric relation through all excursions with the least chance of destroying tooth anatomy in the process.

Molar cusp tips should be placed so that they will not collide with upper cusps. They may be placed in the mesial fossa, the same as premolars, or in the distal fossa with nonfunctional egress through the transverse groove. Molar cusp-tip placement is also permissible in the upper central fossa, since it can pass to the mesial of the upper mesiolingual cusp in its nonfunctioning excursion and it can pass between the buccal cusps in working excursion.

Because the nonfunctioning-side condyle must move down the eminentia for a lateral excursion to take place to the opposite side, the buccal inclines of upper lingual cusps on the nonfunctioning side can usually be steeper than the anterior guidance. However, since we never want these inclines to contact in any jaw position, it provides a safety factor to have the buccal inclines of upper lingual cusps slightly more concave than the anterior guidance. If the anterior

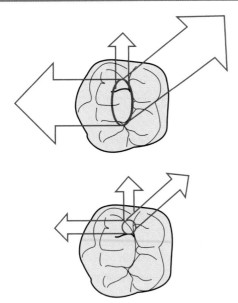

FIGURE 21-7 Wide cusp tips produce neither better function nor better stability. A properly contoured small cusp tip fits into the base of a saucer-shaped fossa that helps to stabilize it because the cusp does not have a tendency to migrate down the inclines of the fossa. The smaller cusp can pass through opened-out grooves and does not destroy the occlusal anatomy. A cutter blade extends distally from the small lower cusp tip, but it does not touch in centric relation. It barely misses lateral contact with the grooved fossa walls of the upper tooth.

guidance is very steep, there is rarely a problem, since jaw movements are restricted to near-vertical function.

Contouring cusp tips

For cusp-tip–to–fossa contact, the tip of each lower buccal cusp should be small enough to fit into a normally contoured fossa. If the anterior guidance permits a lateral side shift, the cusp tip should be able to contact the base of the fossa without touching the fossa walls in centric relation. If the anterior guidance is steeper than the fossa walls and no lateral side shift is permitted, the side of the cusp may contact the fossa walls.

When the tip of the cusp serves as the centric contact, it should be wide enough to provide optimum wear resistance. A sharp, pointed cusp tip would have too little surface contact to resist accelerated wear. A broad, flat cusp tip could require the upper fossa to be opened out too much to permit good occlusal contour. It is difficult to be specific about the size of a cusp tip that would be suitable for all fossae because contours vary as border paths vary, but in general the tip of the cusp should have a fairly flat area about 1 mm or so wide. This is wide enough to withstand wear when the tip contacts in centric relation and small enough to permit good fossa contours in the upper. In lateral excursions, if group function is desired, the side of the cusp contacts the wall of the fossa rather than the tip. The centric contact on the tip itself is subject to very little wear if the occlusal contours are correct.

If a cusp tip is to be placed in a fossa, the tip must not be wide mesiodistally. This is a common fault, and it should be

remembered that each cusp must follow border paths from its point of centric contact. If a cusp is too wide, the path that must be cleared for its excursive movements will destroy the anatomy of the opposing tooth.

Wide cusp tips require more force for bolus penetration, and therefore they put more stress on the supporting structures. Narrow cusps require less force, so they produce less stress (Figure 21-7).

Placement of Lower Lingual Cusps

In normal tooth-to-tooth relationships, the tip of the lower lingual cusp never comes in contact with the upper tooth. Even though the buccal incline of the lower lingual cusp can be made to contact in working excursions, there is no apparent advantage in doing so. For reasons of practicality, we treat the lower lingual cusp as a nonfunctioning cusp as far as contact is concerned. This does not mean, however, that it should be ignored. It should still act as a gripper and a grinder by passing close enough to the upper lingual cusps to aid in tearing, crushing, and shearing the food that is caught between the opposing surfaces.

The lower lingual cusp has another job to do, since it is primarily responsible for keeping the tongue from getting pinched between the posterior teeth. The position and contour of the cusp tip should reflect this responsibility without causing irritation to the tongue. The cusp tip should be rounded and smooth on its lingual aspect. The position of the tip should have enough lingual overjet to hold the tongue out of the way, but it should always be located over the root, within the long axis.

The distance between the lower buccal and lingual cusp tips is the same as the distance between upper cusp tips; so once the lower buccal cusp tip has been located, this measurement can be applied to position the lingual cusp. The measurement between buccal cusp tip and lingual cusp tip should not be much greater than half of the total buccolingual width of the tooth at its widest part.

The lingual cusp height can vary in relation to buccal cusp height because of variations in the lateral anterior guidance, but such variations are not necessary from a practical standpoint. Generally the lower lingual cusp height should be about a millimeter shorter than the buccal cusp. Cusp height can be lowered further in the first premolar. If upper and lower posterior teeth are to be restored, simply following the occlusal plane dictated by the simplified occlusal plane analyzer (SOPA) or the Broadrick flag will be acceptable for both the curve of Spee and the curve of Wilson. Any one of the accepted types of occlusal form can be fabricated on such an occlusal plane.

Contouring the lower fossae

As the mandible moves right or left from centric relation, its front end should be guided down the lingual incline of the upper canine. When it serves as the lateral anterior guidance, the lingual incline of each upper canine dictates the fossa contour of each lower incline that faces it (Figure 21-8).

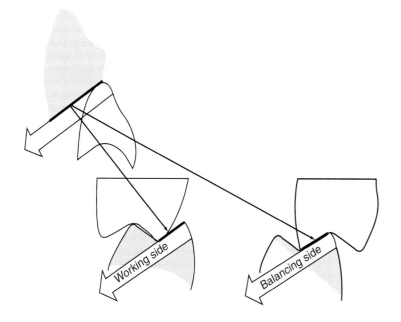

FIGURE 21-8 The inner incline of the upper canine dictates the incline limitations of the lower posterior inclines facing it. The lower working side incline cannot be steeper than the lateral anterior guidance incline of the canine. From a practical standpoint, it should be made flatter, since it is not necessary for the lower incline to contact in function. The balancing incline should never be allowed to contact, so it too should be flatter than the lateral guidance of the canine. This incline also usually gets some downward movement from the orbiting condyle, but for simplicity this can just be considered as insurance. If the canine is steeper than the lower balancing incline that faces it, the balancing incline will be discluded (if the occlusal plane is correct).

The lateral guidance incline of each upper canine dictates the fossa contours of the buccal inclines of each lower lingual cusp on the same side and the lingual inclines of each lower buccal cusp on the opposite side. When the canine is not in position to function individually or in group function as the lateral anterior guidance, the lingual incline of the most anterior upper tooth that can assume the role becomes the dictator of the lower fossa inclines facing it. As the lower posterior teeth follow the mandible down its lateral path, any fixed upper lingual cusp seated into the lower fossa becomes an interference if the lower incline is steeper than the upper guiding incline it faces.

Since this is such an important aspect of occlusal form, we will look at lower fossa contours in still another way. When the mandible moves right or left, the tooth with the steepest fossa incline carries all the stress. This is modified slightly on the balancing side by the downward movement of the orbiting condyle, but for now we do not need to consider that as anything but a safety factor to help disclude the balancing side. With that in mind, the following is a good rule to follow: from the contact point of each upper lingual cusp, the lower fossa inclines should be no steeper than the lateral anterior guidance inclines they face. Any posterior incline that is steeper discludes the anterior guidance and adds to its own lateral stress. If the lower cusp-fossa angle is steeper than the lateral anterior guidance, the upper lingual cusps will be locked into the lower fossae and the back teeth will clash stressfully when lateral excursions are made.

To accommodate upper lingual cusps as centric holding contacts without interference to excursions and to achieve the desired posterior disclusion, the cusp-fossa angle of the lower posteriors must be flatter than the lateral anterior guidance angle. If the anterior guidance has been freed laterally to permit a concave path of the mandible, the lower fossae must be opened up accordingly or interference will result. A concave anterior guidance requires concave fossa contours.

The simplest and most practical approach is to open up the lower fossae by providing more than enough freedom for lateral paths and making the cusp-fossa angle flatter than the lateral anterior guidance angle. This takes away nothing that is needed while facilitating an extremely stable centric holding pattern.

If Only Lower Posterior Teeth Are to Be Restored

If the upper posterior teeth do not need to be restored, cusp tip position and fossa contours for lower posterior restorations are aligned and contoured in relation to the existing upper teeth on the opposing cast. Lower fossa contours will be established to conform to the upper lingual cusps. Fossa walls can be carved to be discluded by the anterior guidance without complication. To ensure complete disclusion, the condylar path on the articulator can be set flatter than the patient's condylar path. This will guarantee posterior disclusion when the restorations are placed in the mouth if the master casts are mounted correctly in a verified centric relation.

If Both Upper and Lower Posterior Teeth Are to Be Restored

When all posterior teeth are to be restored, it is not always evident where the upper lingual cusps will be when they are restored. In my early gnathologic training, it was considered essential to wax upper and lower arches together starting with wax cones to represent all the cusps. This was done on fully adjustable articulators programmed with pantographic recordings to copy the condylar paths.

Fossa contours were waxed in only after it was ascertained that the lower cusps would not collide with the upper cusps during border movements of the mandible. The process produced beautiful occlusal anatomy but it was time-consuming and tedious. Most importantly, however, was that it was also unnecessary. What we learned that completely changed and dramatically simplified the restorative process were four important discernments:

1. Immediate posterior disclusion by the anterior guidance was desirable over posterior contact in excursions. It had the effect of reducing muscle forces on the entire occlusion.
2. The anterior guidance is the dominant determinant of excursive paths.
3. The anterior guidance is independent of condylar guidance and is not determined by condylar paths.
4. There is no immediate side shift of the condyles toward the midline.

As the above discernments became accepted, more attention to precise determination of the anterior guidance has taken the place of focus on condylar border movements. If posterior disclusion is the goal, it is easily achieved by making fossa walls flatter than the lateral anterior guidance, and establishing an acceptable occlusal plane that permits the anterior guidance to disclude the posterior teeth in all excursions. After the anterior guidance has been finalized, the simplest method for ensuring that fossa walls will be discluded in lateral excursions is through the use of a fabricated *fossa contour guide.*

Determining and Carving Lower Fossa Contours

The following technique was designed to simplify the carving of occlusal fossae of lower posterior teeth. It has one purpose: to ensure a noninterfering accommodation for the upper lingual cusps. It will provide a fossa contour that is compatible with the lateral anterior guidance regardless of the contour of the anterior guidance. It can be easily modified to provide extra freedom.

The procedure involves making a fossa contour guide that can be used in any stage of wax-up or even porcelain application. It can be fabricated by auxiliaries in the office in just a few minutes. The guide should accompany the articulated die model to the technician and should be returned with the finished restorations for use by the dentist in his or her evaluation of the finalized occlusal contours.

Making the Fossa Contour Guide

The fossa guide is used only if both upper and lower posterior teeth are to be restored. The anterior guidance must be correct before the guide is fabricated or before occlusal contours can be determined for lower posterior restorations. The anterior guidance may be corrected in provisional restorations, and a centrically mounted cast of the provisional restorations in place may be used to determine the allowable fossa-wall angulation for the posterior restorations. The guide is usually made when the casts are mounted, but it is not used until the posterior wax-up is done or the porcelain is being applied and contoured.

PROCEDURE   Making the fossa contour guide

Step 1: The regular incisal guide pin is removed and replaced with the special fossa-contour pin. The blade of the pin is indented into a mound of wax on a flat plastic guide table.

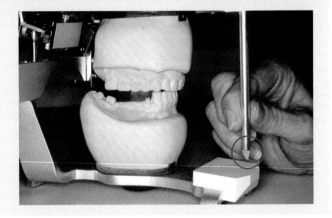

PROCEDURE   Making the fossa contour guide—cont'd

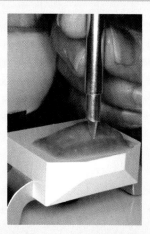

Steps 2 and 3: The upper bow is moved into left and right excursions, allowing the contours of the lateral anterior guidance to determine the path that the guide pin cuts into the wax.

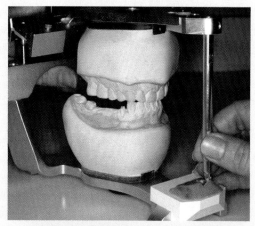

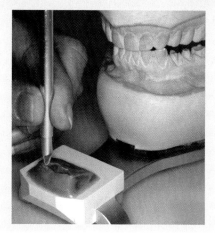

Continued

PROCEDURE   Making the fossa contour guide—cont'd

Steps 4 and 5: When the lateral guidance paths have been cut sharply into the wax, the special pin is raised. It is then used to hold a handle for the fossa guide. Make the handle by cutting off the tip of a plastic protector for a disposable needle. The large end fits snugly onto the raised special pin.

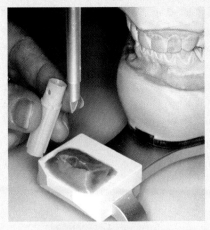

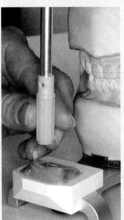

Step 6: A creamy mix of self-curing acrylic resin is flowed into the indentation in the wax.

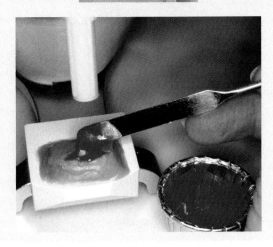

PROCEDURE   Making the fossa contour guide—cont'd

Steps 7 and 8: Resin is wiped into the hollow end of the handle, and the pin is lowered so that the two portions flow together. The resin is allowed to set hard. The guide can then be removed. The wax on the guide table is then no longer needed, and so it can be cleaned off after the guide is removed.

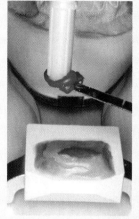 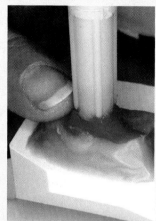

Step 9: Because of the design of the special wax-cutter pin, the lateral anterior guidance angle will be evident as a sharp line running along the bottom edge of the acrylic guide. The edge is marked with a pencil, and any excess acrylic resin may be ground off in front of the line.

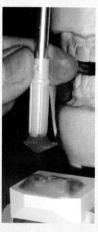

Step 10: One may actually hollow-grind the front surface down to the line to make a scoop-shaped guide, which is excellent for shaving out wax from the fossae.

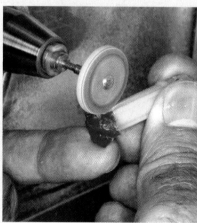

Continued

PROCEDURE   Making the fossa contour guide—cont'd

Steps 11 and 12: To ensure posterior disclusion, the fossa walls must be flatter than the lateral anterior guidance, so the fossa guide angle is flattened on the sides and the tip is rounded to a more opened-out fossa.

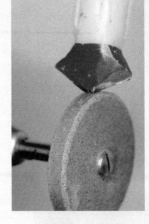
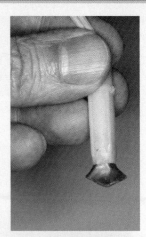

Steps 13 and 14: The fossa guide can be used to contour the wax patterns or as a guide for shaping occlusal surfaces in porcelain. The tip of the guide should be able to touch the base of the fossa without interference from the walls of the fossa. The shape of the special wax-cutter pin will provide for enough thickness of the back of the fossa guide, so that it will be strong enough to use either as a guide to check the carving of the fossae or as a convenient tool to scoop out fossae contours in the wax or the buildup-stage porcelain. If a rubber band is attached through a hole drilled in the handle, the guide can be attached to the articulator for convenience.

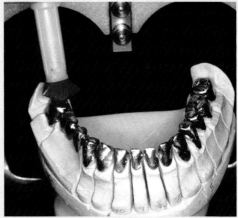
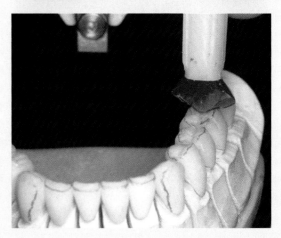

There are three basic rules for using the fossa contour guide.

1. Always hold the handle perpendicularly (Figure 21-9). The cusp-fossae angles were related to the handle when it was straight up and down on the articulator. Tilting the handle would produce an error in the fossa contours.

2. Never destroy a predetermined cusp tip. The depth of the fossae will be limited automatically if this rule is followed (Figure 21-10).

3. Locate fossae in proper relation to cusp tips. A basic knowledge of anatomy is necessary for all techniques. Proper location of fossae ensures saucerlike fossae contours and permits good occlusal form.

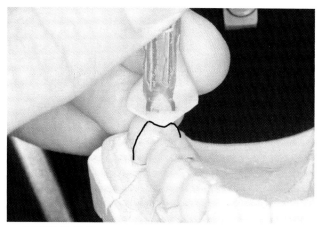

FIGURE 21-10   Relationship of fossa guide to occlusal contour.

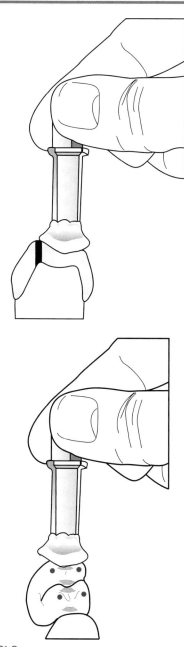

FIGURE 21-9   Position for holding the fossa contour guide properly.

The front of the guide always faces front, and in that position it is correct for either the right or left side. When the handle is held perpendicularly, it exactly reproduces the lateral anterior guidance. Flattening the bottom of the guide will provide extra room for lateral disclusion. Even though the side shift is usually built into the anterior guidance (and consequently duplicated in the fossa contour guide), it is necessary to give a little extra lateral freedom to ensure posterior disclusion.

Modifications in using the fossa contour guide
As long as the base of the fossa is wide enough and the fossa inclines are not steeper than the lateral guidance inclines, supplemental grooves can be placed into the fossa walls and between cusps without fear of creating interferences to the upper lingual cusp. The fossa contour guide can be used before supplemental grooves are placed, or to refine fossa wall inclinations after all occlusal carvings have been completed. Carving the patterns with fairly deep grooves and slightly convex inclines will usually require an opening out of the fossae, but the result is an unusually natural looking occlusal contour, since it simulates normal wear. It is also the way most technicians will prefer because it does not require any change in their carving procedures. It merely adds the simple step of using the fossa contour guide as a scoop to shave away any convexities in the wax or porcelain that interfere with the lateral guidance.

The fossa contour guide can be used in combination with dropped wax techniques and gnathologic mountings. It is especially useful when the dentist does not wish to prepare both upper and lower teeth together. The wax can be built up on the lower teeth to conform to a correct occlusal plane and cusp tip location, and then the guide can be used to modify the fossa contours when necessary. The result will be compatible with the upper gnathologic wax-up, which will be done later.

Finished castings and porcelain occlusals can be checked by the dentist and modified by selective grinding. The fossa contour guide is an easy tool to use. A quick analysis of each fossa can be made when the restorations are received from the laboratory. Fossa walls that are not in harmony with the guide can be opened out by grinding. This is a practical approach because corrections almost always involve taking material away. If inclines are flatter than the guide, the fossa can be deepened to steepen them, provided that there is enough thickness. Fossa walls that are too flat do not constitute an interference, however; and on the lower teeth none of the inclines contacts in function anyway.

If there is any consistency in occlusal contouring errors, it is carving convex or too steep fossa walls. The familiar "Parker House roll" occlusion does not provide room in the lower fossae for the upper lingual cusps. The fossa contour guide enables the dentist or technician to correct this problem.

Carving the marginal ridges

When all cusp tips have been properly located and the fossae correctly placed and contoured, the marginal ridges seem to fall right into place. The most common error noted in marginal ridge contouring is failure to evenly line up the marginal ridges of contacting teeth. Uneven height of adjacent marginal ridges invites food entrapment and often becomes an interference.

The ridges should be contoured to reflect food away from the contact, which means directing it into the fossae. Sluiceways should provide an escape route for the bolus out of the fossae toward the lingual as the stamp cusps crush the food against the fossae walls.

At the risk of being repetitious, I should re-emphasize that no technique will work without a basic understanding of occlusal contours. The procedures described merely provide reference points and guidelines to organize our occlusal form. Remember too that the fossa contour guide is used only when both upper and lower posterior teeth are being restored.

Contouring ridges and grooves

Ridges and grooves give beauty and naturalness to the occlusal scheme. It is the action of ridges and grooves against their opponent counterparts that grasps the food and then crushes, tears, and shreds it as the lower teeth follow their cyclic paths of function against upper inclines. With proper occlusal relationships, it is not necessary for the lower teeth to actually contact the upper teeth in function. The bolus is nearly disintegrated by the time the first tooth contact is made, so the arrangement of ridges and grooves is to permit the cusps to pass close enough to each other to mangle the food between the grooved surfaces without the need for actual tooth contact.

Fairly accurate determination of ridge and groove direction is all that is needed. Extreme preciseness is not required because in cusp-tip–to–fossa contact only the base of the lower fossa contacts the upper lingual cusp. The walls of the fossae never contact, and grooves can be opened out just as fossae are opened out to avoid contact. The only part of any lower posterior tooth that ever needs to contact in any eccentric position is the tip of the buccal cusp, and it can be limited to centric contact only whenever group function is not required.

We must not make the mistake of designing grooves that are slotted so that a cusp can pass precisely through the slot on a given border path. As an example, the walls of such a groove may allow passageway of a cusp in a lateral working excursion, but the groove would not accommodate the cusp in a protrusive lateral path. If we try to provide a groove to accommodate the upper lingual cusp for each path the lower tooth can follow, we would have contiguous grooves starting with a straight working excursion, all the way around through all the protrusive lateral paths, until we come to the border path of the balancing excursion. Thus we would end up with no groove at all. We would have an opened-out fossa concavity, and the walls of the fossa would not clash with the cusp no matter how the lower jaw was moved.

Since this is the effect we are after anyway, it seems practical to simply work out the fossae contours first and then functionalize and beautify the anatomy by placing the appropriate grooves at the working, protrusive, and balancing excursion. There can be no entanglement of cusps in grooves that have been made into inclines that are already out of reach. Other grooves may be added as desired to improve esthetics or to provide more ridges for better masticatory function.

The practicality of actual paths through grooves increases as the difference increases between the lateral and the protrusive anterior guidance angles. A patient with a flat lateral guidance and a steep protrusive guidance could have very definite working excursion grooves that permit passage of prominent cusps because the steep anterior guidance separates the posterior teeth rapidly in protrusive excursions, eliminating the need for opened-out paths except in the flatter lateral excursions. It would be difficult to assess whether there is any advantage of grooves over generally opened-out fossae. There does not appear to be any noticeable clinical difference as far as we can tell.

The direction of any ridge or groove is determined by the path of the lower tooth as it moves with the mandible. Lateral excursion grooves are at right angles to a line drawn from the rotating condyle. The lateral shifting of the mandible may alter the groove direction slightly. However, by the time the lateral shift occurs, the posterior teeth have already been separated by the anterior guidance so that it has no consequence if a correct centric relation is the starting point.

PORCELAIN OCCLUSAL VENEERS

When lower posterior teeth are to have veneered porcelain occlusal surfaces, the same procedures described previously can be used to advantage. Porcelain veneers are much stronger if the veneer thickness is kept fairly uniform. This is also true if the porcelain veneer has a metal base, as it results in the strongest possible porcelain application. It also provides for the best esthetics because there will be no need for thin spots in the porcelain where the opaquer shows through.

UPPER POSTERIOR TEETH

The upper posterior teeth should be the last segment to be restored. It is the fixed posterior segment, and its cusps, inclines, grooves, and ridges are placed and contoured to accommodate the many border movements of the lower posterior teeth. If the upper contours are determined by the paths of the lower posterior teeth, both the form and the paths of the lower teeth should be finalized before the upper teeth are restored (Figure 21-11).

Since the anterior guidance is the major determinant of the paths that the lower teeth follow, it should logically be finalized before the attempt is made at harmonizing posterior in-

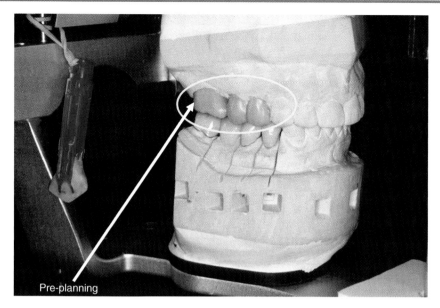

Pre-planning

FIGURE 21-11 Lower posterior teeth should never be restored without relating the occlusion to any planned changes on the upper teeth. By planning the upper corrections before the lower restorations are placed, provisional restorations can be fabricated that properly occlude with the newly altered lower occlusal form. This is part of the concept of preplanning. Note also the fossa guide attached to the articulator by which the dentist can verify accuracy of fossa contours.

clines. When the lower cusp-fossae inclines are then designed to be discluded by the correct anterior guidance and the lower cusp tips are precisely located on an acceptable occlusal plane, upper contours can be refined to any desired degree.

Although it is possible to fabricate upper and lower posterior restorations together, upper posterior restorations should never be fabricated against lower posterior teeth that require correction of their occlusal plane, cusp-tip placement, or fossa contours. If it is absolutely necessary to restore upper posterior teeth first, the lower teeth should be corrected as close to optimum as possible with selective grinding or temporary restorations. It seems most inconsistent to build errors into restorations that are supposed to last for many years.

Preparing Upper Posterior Teeth for Occlusal Restoration

Many restorations are destroyed after they have been cemented in place because of corrective grinding to eliminate excursive interferences. It should never be necessary to grind through any restoration that has been placed on a properly prepared tooth.

When upper posterior teeth are being prepared, they should be checked in all excursions to make certain that there is room for a sufficient thickness of metal and/or porcelain. Too often, preparations are checked in centric relation only, and it is impossible to provide sufficient thickness of the restoration when the tooth moves from its centric position.

If the anterior guidance has not been finalized and the lower posterior teeth are not also in their final form, it is not possible to determine the amount of clearance that is actually available for the upper prepared teeth. For example, if upper fossae inclines are reduced to have clearance in lateral excursions that are guided by an incorrectly steep anterior guidance, flattening the anterior guidance will then bring the

prepared posterior inclines into contact, leaving no room for the restorative material.

Following an orderly sequence of restoration, making certain each segment is correct before proceeding to the next, and checking the clearance in all excursions will guarantee that upper preparations will provide adequate room for the proper restoration of the occlusal surface.

Most Important: Centric Record

Of all the interocclusal records that are made during occlusal reconstruction, the most important one of all is the one for articulating the upper posterior die model. It is the final centric record, and the importance of having it accurate cannot be overemphasized.

Whenever possible, the final centric record should be taken at the correct vertical dimension. Allowing the anterior teeth to contact not only simplifies the record making, but also permits the condyles to seat all the way up into the superior terminal axis position when the record is being made. Taking the centric record at the correct vertical dimension eliminates any error that would have been associated with a missed axis of closure and provides the operator with a means of verifying the accuracy of the centrically articulated casts.

If we are tempted to rush through this important step, we must remember that it takes far longer to grind away all of the carefully placed anatomy on finished restorations than it takes to record the centric position accurately in the first place.

Recording the Border Movements

All of the upper occlusal inclines are related to the border paths that the lower posterior teeth follow. In most patients, we do not want contact against any incline during any excursive movement of the lower arch. We want immediate disclusion of all posterior teeth the moment the mandible moves out of centric relation in any direction. The effect of this disclusion has been meticulously researched, and the principal reason for advocating it is the reduction in elevator muscle activity at the moment of disclusion by the anterior guidance. The disclusion is easily accomplished if the anterior guidance is reasonably steep, or if the condylar paths are healthy and sufficiently disclusive in their angulations. But if the anterior guidance is fairly flat or nonfunctional or if adaptive changes have flattened the condylar paths, the precise recording of border paths becomes more important and more critical.

With normal condylar paths, we can affect posterior disclusion merely by setting the articulator paths flatter than the patient's protrusive movements. Setting the progressive side shift at a greater angle than the patient's will cause disclusion of the balancing inclines. If the lower posterior occlusal surfaces have been contoured with fossae walls that are flatter than the anterior guidance, the upper posterior teeth can be constructed on an articulator, programmed with arbitrarily flatter condylar paths and greater progressive side shift. Disclusion in all excursions will be accomplished rather simply on semiadjustable instruments set in this manner. (See Chapter 22 for a better understanding of simplified instrumentation.)

If, however, it is desirable to have excursive contact on certain inclines, or a near miss of precise dimensions, it will be necessary to follow the lateral anterior guidance paths with preciseness. Upper contours can be planned for group function or a measured miss only if we know exactly the path each lower cusp will be traveling.

For this type of preciseness, both the anterior and posterior determinants of occlusion must be considered although the anterior guidance is the dominant factor. The effect of the border movements of the condyles must be recorded at least to the extent that they can function within the envelope permitted by the anterior guidance. Several methods of recording the border movements will provide acceptable accuracy for completing the upper occlusal surfaces. The important thing to remember about capturing border movements is that it is actually the border movements of the lower teeth that determine upper occlusal contours. It makes no difference whether condylar and anterior guidance determinants are captured directly to then reproduce tooth movements on an instrument, or whether the tooth movements are captured directly at their site, as long as the final upper tooth inclines are in harmony with the functional paths that the *lower teeth* follow.

Supplemental Anatomy on the Upper Occlusal Surfaces

The dentist must decide whether the upper occlusal inclines are to be in group function, partial group function, or total disclusion in excursive movements. Whichever decision is made, it is accomplished by contouring and angulation of the inclines themselves. Supplemental grooves cut into inclines add to the natural appearance and increase the gripping and shredding ability of the tooth surfaces. If the incline surfaces are noninterfering, it will be impossible to create an interference by putting a groove in such a surface. For this reason, it is a logical approach to first develop the incline surfaces according to the type of function desired and then carve into that surface the supplemental anatomy. The grooves are carved smaller than the cusp tips. The tips will just pass over the grooves with no effect on the actual contact through the excursive movement.

LENGTH OF GROUP FUNCTION CONTACT IN WORKING EXCURSION

If we elect to provide group function on the working side, we should be aware that all teeth do not stay in excursive contact for the same length of stroke. As the mandible starts its move to the working side, all of the posterior teeth may contact in harmony with the anterior guidance and the condyle. As the mandible moves further to the side, the first teeth to disengage from contact are the most posterior molars. The disengagement is progressive, starting with the back molar, which has the shortest contact stroke, forward to the canine, which has the longest contact stroke (Figure 21-12).

The molar contact is maintained for only a fraction of the incline surface, whereas the canine contact is often maintained all the way to the incisal tip. The reason for giving the canine such a long contact ride and a progressively shorter contact as we go distally is based on factors of geometry and stress. As the working condyle rotates, the path traveled around the center of rotation lengthens as the distance from the condyle increases. While the canine is traveling the full length of its incline from centric to its incisal edge, the second molar is traveling about half that far. When the canine reaches its incisal edge, the molar still has some incline left on which it could ride out. However, if the molar continued its contact after the canine was disengaged, the stress would no longer be shared by the protective anterior guidance. It would instead be loaded entirely onto the outer incline of the molar and would create considerable lateral torque in the extremely stressful position near the condylar fulcrum (Figure 21-13).

Because of these reasons, the lingual incline of the upper buccal cusps should be contoured to prevent posterior contact from occurring after the lower canine reaches the incisal edge of the upper canine (Figure 21-14). More definitively, the anterior guidance contact should be maintained during all posterior contact in working excursions.

BALANCING EXCURSIONS

The term *balancing excursion* is a remnant of full denture terminology. It originally referred to actual balancing contact to stabilize the dentures on the side of the downward-

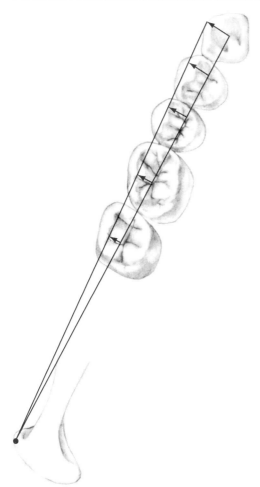

FIGURE 21-12   The length of the contact stroke should be progressively shorter from the anterior teeth back. The molar contact is maintained for only a fraction of its incline surface, whereas contact against the upper canine incline is maintained all the way to the incisal edge.

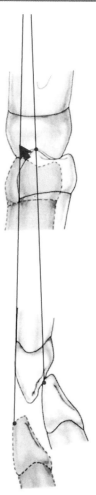

FIGURE 21-13   If molar contact is maintained for the entire incline, the protection from the anterior guidance is lost. The stress exerted against the molar is severe because of its torqueing effect near the condylar fulcrum.

moving, orbiting condyle. It is a part of the three-point contact concept, which for denture stability is a good concept. Many dentists have tried to apply the same concept of bilaterally balanced occlusion to the natural dentition but have abandoned the idea because of the disastrous clinical results. Hypermobility, excessive wear, and periodontal breakdown seem to be the rule rather than the exception, since the posterior teeth succumb to the effects of the so-called balance.

Bilaterally balanced occlusion does not work because there is no way to harmonize the "balancing" inclines of the teeth to all of the variations of muscle force against the unbraced orbiting condyle.

> Balancing inclines must be relieved on all natural teeth regardless of the method used to record the border movements.

The relief can be accomplished rather simply by slight hollow grinding of the buccal inclines of the upper lingual

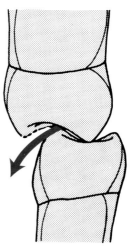

FIGURE 21-14   Upper occlusal inclines should be contoured to disclude in a manner that allows the anterior teeth to maintain contact the longest. The second molar should contact in a working-side excursion for no more than half of its incline length.

cusps between the centric contacts in the fossae and the tips of the lingual cusps.

When the upper restorations are placed in the mouth and the centric contacts have been verified as correct, balancing inclines should be checked with marking ribbon while the mandible is manipulated into firmly guided excursions. The dentist must not rely on the patient to make lateral border movements unassisted. Patient tendency will be to go into a protruded lateral instead of the full border movement. Since balancing incline interferences are so stressful, extra care should be taken to ensure that such inclines are never allowed to contact.

When applied to natural teeth, the term *balancing side* is obviously not a correct connotation. Stuart and Thomas refer to the orbiting condyle side as the *idling side*. The term that seems to be most commonly used now is *nonfunctioning side*. It is certainly a better term, since it correctly indicates a lack of contact.

Regardless of the method used for restoring upper posterior teeth, it will sometimes be necessary to spot-grind slight occlusal discrepancies that result from cementation. Such occlusal corrections should not require more than a few minutes and should not cause mutilation of any occlusal anatomy.

If the occlusion must be grossly adjusted on the finished restorations, one or more of the following errors has probably been committed:

Improper recording of centric relation. The bite record should fulfill all four criteria for acceptability outlined in Chapter 11. Careless recording of the bite records is one of the major sources of error and wasted time.

Errors in mounting. A perfect bite record can be ruined by anything less than extreme care in the laboratory. I believe that this step is so important that in my office it is checked carefully before the case is turned over to the technician.

Improper fit of finished restorations. Castings that do not fit are responsible for a large share of occlusal problems. Casting techniques should be continually checked for accuracy using steel dies. A second die model may also be reserved for careful and gentle seating of the castings by the dentist to check the fit. Precise casting accuracy requires continuous and meticulous attention to many laboratory details. Accuracy in this department cannot be left to chance.

Errors in cementation. Cementation can affect the position of the crown on the tooth. The best we can do is minimize the change. The type of cement, the way it is mixed, the fit of the crown, the taper of the preparation, and many other factors affect the accuracy of this step. The astute restorative dentist is always on the alert for information that can minimize cementation error. Failure to relieve the inner surfaces of crowns is a major cause of cementation errors. Painting the dies with a sufficiently thick layer of die spacer is the most practical method of supplying enough room for cement thickness. It also protects the dies against chipping.

It has been my impression that improper mixing of cements is an all too common error. Mixing too fast or too thick is a sure invitation for raised restorations. There is no substitute for meticulous attention to every detail when you are restoring an occlusion. However, the restoration of the upper posterior teeth is the sequence that can either complement or destroy all of the prior restorative efforts. It is worthy of all the care and skill that might be expended on its perfection.

TYPES OF POSTERIOR OCCLUSAL CONTOURS

There are three basic decisions to make regarding the design of posterior occlusal contours:

1. Selection of the type of centric relation contacts
2. Determination of the type and distribution of contact in lateral excursions
3. Determination of how to provide stability to the occlusal form

For each of the preceding decisions, we have several options from which to choose. Because there are many different arch-to-arch relationships, we must sometimes vary from standardized tooth contours. No one type of occlusal form is optimum for all patients. Nor is only one type of occlusal form correct. There are several ways to satisfy all of the requirements for stability without sacrificing function. So even if stereotyped occlusal contours work well for most patients, the varied problems of stress associated with sick mouths can be better solved by flexibility of form that enables us to vary the direction and distribution of forces. Rather than designing occlusal surfaces on the basis of what they look like, we should instead approach each occlusal surface design to definitively accomplish specific effects.

In the design of occlusal contours, the first decision is where to locate each of the multiple contacts that meet the opposing teeth when the mandible is in centric relation. These decisions are determined when each holding contact is related to how it would direct the occlusal forces. Teeth can withstand tremendous force if the force is directed up or down the long axis of each tooth because when force is directed parallel to the long axis it is uniformly resisted by all of the supporting periodontal ligaments except those at the apex (Figure 21-15). If forces are misdirected laterally, the tooth loses the support of about half of the ligaments that are compressed and puts almost the entire load on the half under tension (Figure 21-16). So the starting point in designing occlusal contours is to shape and locate the centric contacts so that the forces are directed as nearly parallel as possible to the long axis of both upper and lower teeth.

There are many ways to design occlusal contours if direction of forces in centric relation were the only consideration. A perfectly flat occlusal surface contacting another flat surface could be made to fulfill this first requirement, but it would not be a very good design for penetrating or grinding

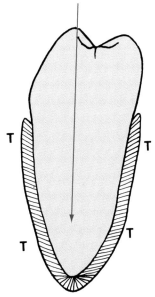

FIGURE 21-15 When occlusal forces are directed axially, all of the periodontal fibers (except at the apex) are in a state of tension *(T)*. Thus forces are resisted equally by fibers around the root.

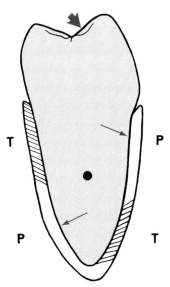

FIGURE 21-16 Lateral forces have the effect of rotating the tooth around a pivotal point within the suspended root. This results in a combination of pressure areas *(P)* and a reduction of tensive resistance by approximately half of the periodontal fibers.

fibrous foods. Proper placement of a sharp cusp against a flat surface could penetrate foods easily and still direct the forces correctly, but a single sharp cusp against a flat surface might lack resistance to the lateral forces that come from the cheeks versus the tongue. The addition of more contacts seems to be an aid to the requirement of occlusal stability, though it is unlikely that any kind of occlusal contour is capable of stabilizing posterior teeth if they are not in horizontal harmony with the neutral zone.

The posterior teeth must do more than penetrate food; they must also be capable of crushing and grinding it. To fulfill these roles, they must be able to work one surface against another in enough proximity to masticate efficiently. To accomplish this, the sharp cusps are broadened at the base and rounded at the tips. The flat surfaces are changed to fossae, and the walls of the fossae are curved and angled to relate to the lateral movements of the mandible as guided by the lower anterior teeth against the lingual surfaces of the upper anterior teeth. Blades are made to emanate from the lower buccal cusps to function in reasonable closeness to the upper inclines.

Our thinking has changed somewhat regarding how closely the lower cusps should function in relation to upper inclines. We once believed a near miss was essential for function, making it mandatory for all inclines to be precisely related to border paths of the mandible. This does not appear to be the case. Patients with fairly flat occlusal contours seem to function as well with a steep anterior guidance that prohibits proximation of cusps in excursive movements. The one essential factor that relates to whether patients are content with function seems to be the number of tooth contacts in centric relation. If a patient complains of inability to masticate properly, we invariably find a lack of tooth contacts in centric re-

lation. This is tested by whether or not a Mylar strip is held tightly by the teeth at the closed position. If centric relation contacts can be re-established, the patient's complaints are almost always satisfied, regardless of how close or how far apart the cusp inclines approximate each other during excursions.

Nevertheless, since it is such a practical matter to restore occlusions so that their fossae walls do relate to the lateral function dictated by the anterior guidance, it is logical to give that benefit to most occlusions that must be restored. It is not practical however for occlusions with very steep anterior guidances because such an occlusal scheme would require fossae that are too deep to be self-cleaning.

In selecting which option to use regarding occlusal contour, we should first determine the desired effect. If the same effect can be accomplished in more than one way, the selection of which option to use would be logically made on the basis of which option can be achieved in the most practical way. We will keep our primary focus on the effect we must achieve and allow the operator to choose the method that is most practical to use on his or her own terms. I will start with defining the choices for centric relation contacts.

TYPES OF CENTRIC HOLDING CONTACTS

Centric relation contact is usually established on restorations in one of three ways:

1. Surface-to-surface contact (see Figure 21-17)
2. Tripod contact (see Figure 21-18)
3. Cusp-tip–to–fossa contact (see Figure 21-19)

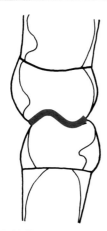

FIGURE 21-17   Surface-to-surface contact.

Surface-to-surface contact

We refer to surface-to-surface contact (Figure 21-17) as "mashed-potato occlusion." It is the form that results if the articulator is simply closed together when the wax on the dies is soft. There is never any valid reason for using this type of contact. It is stressful, and it produces lateral interferences in anything other than near-vertical "chop chop" function.

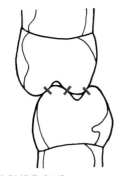

FIGURE 21-18   Tripod contact.

Tripod contact

In tripod contact (Figure 21-18), the tip of the cusp never touches the opposing tooth. Instead, contact is made on the sides of the cusps that are convexly shaped. Three points are selected from the sides of the cusps, and each point in turn is made to contact the side of the opposing fossa. Contacts of the stamp cusps must be made at the brim of the fossa wall so that all posterior teeth can disengage from any contact immediately upon leaving centric relation. Lateral and protrusive disclusion of posterior teeth is essential whenever tripod contact is used because convex lower cusps cannot follow normally concave border paths against upper teeth, which are also convex. This is especially true when the contacts are on the sides of convex cusps. Consequently, if the lateral anterior guidance starts with a near-horizontal path and if rest closure function dictates the need for a "long centric," it would be necessary to use flatter occlusal surfaces and wider cusp tips with the contacts distributed more on the

tips than on the sides of the cusps. Fossa contacts have to be more on ridges and fossa brims than on the walls of the fossa. Some advocates of tripodism do recommend this.

When the working-side condyle translates laterally on a horizontal plane and the lateral anterior guidance permits the front end of the mandible to also move laterally on a horizontal plane before curving down a concave path, there is no way to make tripod contact work if the contacts are on the sides of convex cusps. Allowing the cusps to move through grooves is not practical because contacts aligned on the sides of the cusps to facilitate travel through a straight lateral path groove would interfere with a slightly protrusive lateral path. There is no way to align the contacts around the sides of the cusps to permit the full range of lateral and protrusive paths if the anterior guidance starts out with horizontal paths. This is important to understand because many periodontally involved mouths are best served by such concave anterior guidances.

If tripod contact is to be used with concave anterior guidances, the contacts must be confined to the tip of broad flat cusps. A tripodism of sorts can be achieved if you keep the tips of the cusps wider than the grooves and fossae that they rest against or pass over. This type of pseudotripodism can even be made to function in lateral excursions if the upper cusp inclines are matched to the concave border paths of the mandible. If there is any horizontal movement of the mandible in lateral excursions, convex surfaces simply cannot function against the sides of other convex surfaces without creating stressful interferences.

Tripod contact is difficult to accomplish, but it can be done as long as the anterior teeth are capable of discluding the posterior teeth in all excursions. For patients whose functional movements, anterior periodontal support, arch relation, and tooth position are best served by posterior disclusion, tripod contact can be very comfortable, functional, and beautiful.

Tripod contact should not be used when lateral stress distribution is best served by including posterior teeth into group function to help out weak or missing anterior teeth or when the arch relationship does not permit the anterior guidance to do its job.

With tripod contact, any degree of shifting of any tooth produces an incline interference. Any wear on a centric contact leaves the remaining centric stops for that cusp to be on inclines. Since upper and lower arches are usually restored together, even a minute error in recording or transferring centric relation causes loss of tripodism on all teeth.

Tripod contact is extremely difficult or impossible to equilibrate without losing tripodism and ending up with contacts on inclines. However, this is mostly academic because usually enough counteracting inclines can be kept in contact to maintain a reasonably good direction of force.

If tripod contact is so difficult to achieve and has so many limitations, why is it used? Probably the main reason for the popularity of tripodism is the impression that it is so stable if it is properly done. This certainly has been one of the main reasons for advocating its use. However, there is no scientific evidence that tripod contact is more stable than proper cusp-tip–to–fossa contact. Development of "slides" is common, even among the most meticulous operators.

It should be brought out that some of the real advocates of tripod contact are among the most meticulous operators in our profession. The precise attention that they give to every detail is probably far more responsible for their success than the tripod contact. A precisely recorded centric relation will make the majority of patients very happy even if little else is accomplished, and eccentric disclusion of posterior teeth is always better than posterior interference in excursions. Combined with the clinical observation that most patients can also function quite well with excursive disclusion of the posterior teeth, one can readily see why there are many patients who are very happy with their tripod-contact occlusions.

Nevertheless, I believe that there are no actual *indications* for tripod contact. Although it can be used successfully in a large number of patients, it has definite limitations in many others. It offers no advantages over proper cusp-tip–to–fossa contact, and since it is more difficult to achieve, is hard to adjust, and is limited in its use, we would probably do well to thoughtfully evaluate its practicality.

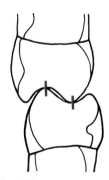

FIGURE 21-19 Cusp-tip–to–fossa contact.

Cusp-tip–to–fossa contact

If cusp tips are properly located in the most advantageous fossae, cusp-tip–to–fossa occlusion (Figure 21-19) offers excellent function and stability with the flexibility to choose any degree of distribution of lateral forces that is warranted. It is the easiest occlusion to equilibrate. Resistance to wear is excellent, since the centric stops are on the cusp tips, whereas if group function is needed in working excursions, contact is on the sides of the cusp tips as they travel along the inclines of the opposing teeth. If disclusion of any tooth is desired in any eccentric excursion, it is accomplished easily by adjustment of the fossa inclines without disturbing the centric holding contacts.

With cusp-tip–to–fossa contact, it is not necessary to restore upper and lower teeth together. In fact, there is no advantage whatsoever to preparing both arches together. Location of cusp tips can be determined with extreme accuracy against unprepared teeth, and cusp height and fossa contours can be established one arch at a time with complete assurance that the contours will be correct.

Location of cusp-tip–to–fossa contacts is decided according to the best interest of each tooth on the basis of direction of forces as near parallel to the long axis of each tooth as possible and stability without interference to eccentric movements.

Cusp-tip–to–fossa contact is not a by-product of any specific technique. It serves the goal of function rather than form. It can be accomplished with simple semiadjustable instrumentation, gnathologic instrumentation, functional path procedures, or a myriad of other instrumentation techniques. The one essential for accomplishing it correctly is an understanding of what we are after. Properly done, it can be beautiful as well as functional and stable.

VARIATIONS OF POSTERIOR CONTACT IN LATERAL EXCURSIONS

As the mandible moves laterally, the lower posterior teeth leave their centric contact with the upper teeth and travel sideways down a path dictated by the condyles in the back and by the lateral anterior guidance in the front. Each lower posterior tooth is limited to these border paths, meaning that they cannot follow a path from centric relation that is any flatter or more concave than the condyles and the lateral anterior guidance permit.

As the lower posterior teeth follow this lateral border path, there are several options regarding their contact with the upper tooth inclines. They may maintain contact with upper teeth, or the cusp inclines may be contoured so that there is no contact at all between any of the back teeth in any jaw position except centric relation. There may be variations in numbers of teeth in lateral contact or in the length of the incline contacts. The reason for bringing any teeth into lateral function is to distribute stress and wear over more teeth. Whether the distribution is beneficial depends on how well it is accomplished and whether it is needed.

To make meaningful judgments about the distribution of lateral stress, we must first distinguish the difference between the rotating condyle and the orbiting condyle. Each side has physical characteristics that are important to understand before an occlusal scheme can be planned with any degree of dependability. In discussing lateral excursions, I divide the movements accordingly into working-side occlusion and nonfunctioning-side occlusion (also referred to as the *balancing side*).

Working-side occlusion refers to the contact relationship of lower teeth to upper teeth on the side of the rotating condyle. The side toward which the mandible moves is the working side. The condyle on the working side can be braced against bone or ligament throughout the working excursion, so it is possible and quite practical to accurately record and restore the posterior teeth to precise working-side border movement contacts.

Nonfunctioning-side occlusion is the side of the orbiting condyle. When the condyle leaves its braced position and slides forward down the slippery incline of the eminentia, it is no longer solidly fixed against the unyielding bone and ligament. Rather, it can move up a little, since the mandible bends slightly under firm muscle pressure. Consequently, tooth contact during nonfunctioning-side excursions should not be allowed. Because of the flexibility of the mandible, it would not be possible to harmonize occlusal contours to all of the variations resulting from the differences in muscle force from light to heavy. Hence we have the rule: *whenever lower teeth move toward the tongue, they should not contact.*

The job of discluding the nonfunctioning side is always the responsibility of the working side. How the working side discludes the nonfunctioning side is an important decision that must be made for each patient. While the teeth on the working side are discluding the teeth on the nonfunctioning side, they must also function as cutters, holders, and grinders.

The dentist must decide how this is done by selecting one of the following choices for working-side occlusion:

1. Group function
2. Partial group function
3. Posterior disclusion

None of these choices is optimum for all cases. Selecting the one that offers the most advantages for each patient is just good treatment planning.

Group function refers to the distribution of lateral forces to a group of teeth rather than protecting those teeth from contact in function by assigning all forces to one particular tooth.

To paraphrase a law of physics, the more teeth that carry the load, the less load any one tooth must carry. We must decide which teeth are capable of carrying how much load and assign the load accordingly. For example, we would not use a loose canine with little bone support to protect strong posterior teeth from contacting in a working excursion. Instead, we would allow the posterior teeth to share the load by bringing them into group function with the canine and the other front teeth on that side.

Group function of the working side is indicated whenever the arch relationship does not allow the anterior guidance to do its job of discluding the nonfunctioning side. The anterior guidance cannot do its job in the following situations:

1. Class 1 occlusion with extreme overjet
2. Class 3 occlusion with all lower anterior teeth outside of the upper anterior teeth
3. Some end-to-end bites
4. Anterior open bite

When you are using posterior group function, the following rule applies: *contacting inclines must be perfectly harmonized to border movements of the condyles and the anterior guidance.* Convex-to-convex contacts cannot be used to accomplish this.

Partial group function refers to allowing some of the posterior teeth to share the load in excursions, whereas others contact only in centric relation. For example, a second molar may be very firm vertically but be hypermobile buccolingually. Such a tooth should touch only in centric relation and be discluded immediately by the other teeth in excur-

sions. A very strong first premolar may work with a moderately weak canine and incisors to disclude a second premolar and molars.

Because of arch relationships, a first and second molar may be the only source of disclusion for balancing-side contact. Group function had better be perfectly harmonized to border movements in such a case, but it can be done successfully. Anterior teeth with postorthodontic root resorption or congenitally poor crown-root ratios should sometimes be harmonized to group function with the working side.

Whether any tooth should share the lateral stresses should be decided on the basis of each tooth's resistance to lateral stress. There is no good reason why such a decision cannot be made on a tooth-by-tooth basis. If a tooth is weak laterally, it should contact in centric relation only. If a tooth is firm and if clinical judgment says that it would be beneficial to the other teeth to let that tooth share the lateral stress and wear, that is what should be done.

Some dentists object to ever having posterior teeth contact in lateral excursions. Strenuous objection to group function usually comes from having had problems with it. Because of the resultant problems, objectors may think that group function is actually harmful. I want to make it clear that problems with group function result from improper harmony of the contacting inclines. Attempts at group function with convex inclines, for example, are invitations to hypermobility. Some patients do change their pattern of function to conform to the restrictive inclines of convex cusps, but it is unpredictable at best. For group function to be effective in reducing stress, the cusp inclines must be in perfect harmony with the lateral border movements of the jaw. Posterior cusp inclines that are not contoured to match the mandibular border movements are discluded if the inclines are opened out too much, or they interfere if any part of the incline is steeper than the corresponding part of the lateral jaw movement. Incline interferences on posterior teeth get progressively more stressful as they get closer to the condyle fulcrum, so a slight interference on a second molar would probably be more stressful than a more noticeable interference on a canine. If this rule of stress distribution is understood, it is quite practical to distribute lateral stress over some or all of the posterior teeth. This can be done effectively by restorative means and by occlusal adjustments of the natural teeth.

Posterior disclusion refers to no contact on any posterior teeth in any position but centric relation. It can be accomplished easily with cusp-tip–to–fossa morphology. It must be accomplished with tripod or surface-to-surface morphology to prevent lateral interferences in any case with centric contact on inclines that are steeper than the lateral border movements of the mandible. It occurs automatically if tripod contacts are distributed on the tips of broad flat cusps or if the lateral guidance angle is steeper than the contacting posterior surfaces, or under both conditions.

In healthy mouths or in mouths with normally strong anterior teeth, it is an excellent occlusion, since normal anterior teeth are quite capable of carrying the whole excursive load, particularly if they are in harmony with functional border movements.

> Posterior disclusion in all jaw positions except centric relation is the most desirable occlusion whenever it can be achieved by an acceptable anterior guidance.

Even some weakened anterior teeth may actually be stressed less by separation of the posterior teeth from contact in excursions. The reason for this phenomenon is the effect that posterior disclusion has on the contractive force of the elevator muscles. The moment complete posterior disclusion occurs in protrusive, the masseter muscle stops contracting, the internal pterygoid muscle stops contracting, and the temporalis muscle contraction is reduced. In lateral excursions, internal pterygoid contraction controls the balancing side.

There are two methods of accomplishing posterior disclusion:

1. The anterior guidance is harmonized to functional border movements first, and then the lateral inclines of the posterior teeth are opened up so that they are discluded by a correct anterior guidance.
2. The posterior teeth are built first and then discluded by restriction of the anterior guidance. This method is backward. Anterior guidance is a proper determinant of posterior occlusal form and thus should be done first. When posterior occlusal form determines the anterior guidance, the correctness of the anterior guidance is a product of chance.

Posterior disclusion can be achieved by two different types of anterior guidance: anterior group function and canine-protected occlusion. Neither is applicable for all cases.

Anterior group function is the most practical method for discluding the posterior teeth when arch relationships and tooth alignment permit it. Anterior group function is beneficial in three ways:

1. It distributes wear over more teeth.
2. It distributes the stresses to more teeth.
3. It distributes stress to teeth that are progressively farther from the condyle fulcrum.

Any one of these considerations would be reason enough to recommend anterior group function, but in addition to its effect on stress and wear, anterior group function is extremely comfortable and efficient. It improves the efficiency of incising movements by providing lateral as well as protrusive shearing contacts.

Despite its advantages, anterior group function is not applicable in all cases. Some arch relationships do not permit the incisors to contact in lateral excursions. Concave anterior guidances permit group function, whereas convex lateral guidances make it difficult to accomplish. When it is impractical to distribute the lateral guidance stresses over several teeth, disclusion of the posterior teeth can be accomplished by use of the canines in one form or another of canine-protected occlusion.

Canine-protected occlusion refers to disclusion by the canines of all other teeth in lateral excursions. It usually serves as the cornerstone of what is called *mutually protected occlusion.* Mutually protected occlusion has been defined in several ways, but the usual connotation refers to an occlusal arrangement in which the posterior teeth contact in centric relation only, the incisors are the only teeth contacting in protrusion, and the canines are the only teeth contacting in lateral excursion. It is an ideal relationship for some patients, is tolerated by some, and is detrimental to others. Clinical judgment should be developed so that canine-protected occlusion is used only when it offers advantages over other occlusal arrangements.

In canine-protected occlusion, all lateral stresses must be resisted solely by the canine. Therefore, the predominant prerequisite for its use is the capability of the canine to withstand the entire lateral stress load without any help from other teeth.

It may seem unlikely that any one tooth could have enough stability to carry such a load over a long period of time without becoming subjected to excessive wear or hypermobility. The fact is that the lateral stresses are minimal if the lingual contours are in harmony with the functional border movements. In other words, lateral stress becomes insignificant if the mandible functions normally within the lingual inclines of the upper canines.

It is impossible to exert excessive stresses against the canines in centric relation because the posterior teeth also resist the stresses in that position, if the occlusion is correct.

In natural canine-protected occlusions, the pattern of function is rather vertical, and so the mandible does not use lateral movements that would subject the canines to stress in that direction either.

The canines actually assume the role more as a guidance that actuates vertical function rather than as a resistor to lateral stress. Any attempt at lateral movement is felt by the pressoreceptors around the canines. *Within limits,* these exquisitely sensitive nerve endings protect the canines against too much lateral stress by redirecting the muscles to more vertical function. As long as the pressoreceptors can keep the muscles programmed to a vertical envelope of function, there is insufficient lateral stress generated to harm the canines.

Some clinicians have reported that the canines have the distinction of being protected by a greater number of pressoreceptor nerve endings than is found around any other tooth. This alleged density of mechanoreceptors is supposed to impart a unique capacity to the canine to redirect any functional pattern that would be destructive. If, for example, a horizontal chewing cycle exerts too much lateral stress against the canines, their special mechanoreceptor protectors would simply change the chewing cycle to a vertical, chop chop function rather than allow harm to come to the canines or their supporting structures.

It is easy to see why such a concept would be popular. If the canines really did have the capacity to change functional movements from horizontal to vertical, it would eliminate much need for concern with occlusal morphology. Good centric contacts are all that would be necessary for posterior teeth, since mandibular movements could be restricted by changing the canines to permit only vertical opening and closing. Some advocates of canine-protected occlusion actually subscribe to such a theory, but further research has failed to substantiate the report that there are more mechanoreceptors around the canines than there are around other teeth. Furthermore, clinical results over a period of time have shown that the canine, just like other teeth, is also subject to the usual problems of excessive lateral stress if it interferes with normal functional movements. Although the canines do have the benefit of normal mechanoreceptor protection, there does not appear to be any valid support for the canine-protection theory on the basis of special sensory capacity to radically alter habitual patterns of function.

However, there are other valid reasons why canine-protected occlusion works well for many patients. The canines have extremely good crown-root ratios, and their long fluted roots are in some of the densest bone of the alveolar process. Furthermore, their position in the arch, far from the fulcrum, makes it more difficult to stress them. In short, they are very strong teeth. If their upper lingual inclines are in harmony with the envelope of function, they are usually quite capable of withstanding lateral stresses without help from other teeth. Many patients have natural canine protection, and if the canines are firm and the occlusion is comfortable, I believe it should be maintained, even if the teeth must be restored.

The natural canine-protected mouth is easily distinguished by convex or very steep lingual inclines on the upper canines. The patient usually cannot move the jaw laterally, even when asked to do so. The chewing cycle is a vertical chop chop. The patient has never functioned laterally and has no need for more than minimal lateral pressure on the closing stroke. If posterior tooth form were brought into group function with such steep inclines, even the slightest shifting of a posterior tooth could subject it to extreme lateral stress because it would be in interference to the powerful closing stroke. The vector of force against a steep incline interference is nearly horizontal, and the stress is further amplified as it gets closer to the condyle. In near-vertical envelopes of function, it is usually better to let the posterior teeth be discluded by the canines if the canine protection is natural and if the canines are firm. If the mouth requires extensive restorative treatment and if minimal changes to the canines would affect anterior group function without noticeably altering the chewing cycle, it would be logical to make that change for the advantages that could be gained. However, changing from canine protection to anterior group function is contraindicated if it would require a major change in the envelope of function or extensive reduction of sound lingual enamel.

For simplicity, canine protection can be divided into two categories:

1. Posterior disclusion by canine inclines that are in harmony with functional border movements
2. Posterior disclusion by canine inclines that restrict mandibular movements within habitual functional border movements

Whether a patient functions normally in vertical chop chop motions or wide horizontal strokes, it is still possible to harmonize canine inclines. If the harmonized canine inclines are the discluding factor for all posterior teeth in lateral excursion, it may be considered a form of canine-protected occlusion. Because of their arch form or tooth arrangement, many patients will be served best by this type of occlusion.

Restrictive canine protection is usually used as an attempt to avoid stressful posterior contact in lateral excursion by forcing the patient into a changed pattern of function. It may result in a reduction of hypermobility of posterior teeth that have been under stress, but then so will proper posterior occlusal form. Restrictive canine protection falls short of the immediate comfort that patients feel with a harmonious anterior guidance. They must get used to the restrictive guidance. Although some patients will change their functional patterns when the canines get sore enough to force them into a chop chop bite, it is an unnecessary irritation to mouth comfort, and the long-term maintainability of such occlusal relationships is very unpredictable. If the canines are stressed into lateral movement, they are no longer able to protect the posterior inclines.

It should be re-emphasized that from the standpoint of comfort many patients can tolerate a change to the more vertical function of a steeper canine rise. The problem is not so much one of comfort as it is of long-term stability. It is far better, whenever practical, to get posterior disclusion from an anterior guidance that is in harmony with the patient's envelope of function.

SELECTING OCCLUSAL FORM FOR STABILITY

Assuming that cusp-fossae relationships are correctly placed for ideal direction of stress, we still must make decisions regarding the number of contacting cusps that are needed for maximum stability under differing conditions. We generally have four basic types to choose from in normal arch relationships:

Type I. Lower buccal cusps contact upper fossae. There are no other centric contacts (Figure 21-20).

If desired, continuous contact can be maintained in working excursions on the lingual incline of the upper buccal cusps, or if disclusion of posterior teeth is desired, it can be easily accomplished by modification of the upper inclines. Disclusion of balancing inclines can be easily accomplished.

This type of occlusal relationship can be very comfortable and can be made to function in a completely satisfactory manner. It is the easiest contour to fabricate when one is restoring posterior teeth because cusp-fossae angles on the lower are not critical.

The only apparent disadvantage to this type of occlusal relationship is its lack of dependable buccolingual stability. Pressure from the tongue can tilt the teeth toward the buccal with very little resistance. Because it lacks the stability that

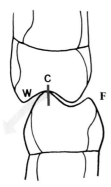

FIGURE 21-20   Type 1. Working-side excursive function is limited to the lingual inclines of upper buccal cusps.

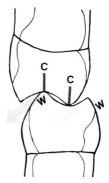

FIGURE 21-22   Type 3. Working excursion contact is limited to the lingual incline of upper buccal cusps and the buccal incline of lower lingual cusps.

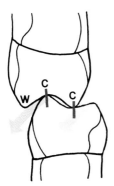

FIGURE 21-21   Type 2. Working-side excursive function is limited to the lingual inclines of the upper buccal cusps. There is no excursive function on any lower incline.

upper lingual cusp contact would give it, more follow-up occlusal adjustment is usually required than is necessary with more stable occlusal contours.

In periodontal prostheses utilizing around-the-arch splinting, buccolingual stabilization is ensured by the splinting itself. It is not necessary to stabilize the teeth with upper lingual cusp centric holding contacts. Lower buccal cusp contact is sufficient to satisfy all needs of the splinted patient. Working excursion contact is an elective that can be used when needed for disclusion of the nonfunctioning side. From the standpoint of either function or comfort, patients seem to be just as happy with only contact of the lower buccal cusp as they are with more elaborate occlusal schemes. Since it is the easiest occlusal form to accomplish and the easiest to adjust, it is an acceptable choice of occlusal form whenever buccolingual stability has been assured by splinting.

Type 2. Centric contact on the tips of lower buccal cusps and upper lingual cusps (Figure 21-21).

The addition of the upper lingual cusps as centric holding contacts contributes greatly to the stability of the posterior teeth. Lateral stress toward the buccal is resisted by the contact of the upper lingual cusps against the lower fossae. Stress toward the lingual is resisted by the lower buccal cusps against the upper fossae. Furthermore, the vector of force against the cusp-tip–to–fossae contacts is directed to-

ward the long axis when the teeth are stressed laterally, because lateral movement takes place by rotation of the tooth around a point within the root.

Lateral excursion contact is limited to the lingual incline of upper buccal cusps, the same as in Type 1. This presents no problem of lateral stress as long as the upper inclines are in perfect harmony with lateral border movements. The return to multiple cusp-holding contacts in each centric closure has sufficient stabilizing effect for maintenance of the occlusion within practical limits. Working incline contact can be discluded when desired by modification of upper inclines.

If the upper lingual cusp is to be used as a holding contact in centric, the inclines of the lower fossae must not be steeper than the lateral anterior guidance. If the upper lingual cusp is to be discluded in all lateral movements, the lower fossae inclines must be flatter than the lateral anterior guidance.

Because lower fossae inclines need only be flatter than lateral anterior guidance inclines, the fabrication of lower occlusal contours is simplified. The lower inclines do not need to be precisely identical to border paths, since they are to be out of contact in excursions.

Contact in working excursions can be accomplished by use of functionally generated path techniques or any other procedure that accurately records lateral border movements.

From every clinical standpoint, the performance of this type of occlusal contour is acceptable. It is comfortable and functional, and because it fulfills all requirements of good occlusal form and can be accomplished with clinical practicality, it is the type of occlusion for which we strive in unsplinted restorative cases when posterior group function is needed.

Type 3. Centric contact on tips of lower buccal cusps and upper lingual cusps (Figure 21-22).

This type of occlusal contour is identical to type 2 except that the buccal incline of the lower lingual cusp becomes a functioning incline.

There is no clinically discernible advantage in making the upper lingual cusps contact in lateral function. There is no recognizable difference in patient comfort or function, and if there is a difference between either long-term stabil-

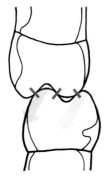

FIGURE 21-23 Type 4. Contact on the sides of cusps and the walls of fossae.

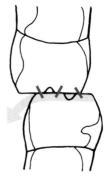

FIGURE 21-24 Centric contact on the brims of fossae and the top of wide cusp tips with no contact in eccentric excursions.

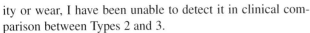

ity or wear, I have been unable to detect it in clinical comparison between Types 2 and 3.

The major difference between this type of occlusal form and Type 2 is the difficulty of accomplishing it. To bring the upper lingual cusps into working excursion contact, the buccal inclines of the lower lingual cusps must be precisely contoured to the exact lateral border movement of both the condyle and the anterior guidance. If the incline is made too flat, it will disclude. If it is made too steep, it will interfere.

Certainly there are methods available to record these border movements accurately and to refine the lower inclines to duplicate them, but unless the additional time, effort, and instrumentation produce an improvement in the result, it is time wasted.

Although complexity of fabrication seems to be the only disadvantage of Type 3 occlusal form, it is reason enough not to advocate it because the result has no clinical advantage over Type 2 occlusal form, which can be fabricated with less complicated and less time-consuming procedures without any reduction in quality.

Type 4. Tripod contact. There are two types of tripod contact: contact on the sides of cusps and the walls of fossae (Figure 21-23) and contacts on the brims of fossae and on tops of wide cusp tips (Figure 21-24).

Contact on the sides of the cusps does not permit any lateral or protrusive movement on a horizontal plane; so if the anterior guidance has been flattened even for a short distance from the centric stops to permit a lateral side shift of the mandible, this type of occlusal form is contraindicated. It is also contraindicated for any patient who requires a "long centric."

It may be used in vertical or near-vertical functional cycles with either canine-protected occlusion or anterior-protected occlusion.

In the cases permitting its use, its performance is clinically indistinguishable from Type 2 or Type 3 occlusions. Like Type 3, its disadvantage comes from the difficulty in fabricating it. Tripod contact is the most difficult of all occlusal forms to fabricate.

Centric contact on the brims of fossae and the top of wide cusp tips with no contact in eccentric excursions

(Figure 21-24) can be made to function with any type of anterior guidance because it permits horizontal lateral movement without interference. It is automatically discluded by any anterior guidance effect other than flat plane; so it cannot be used when posterior group function is indicated.

Since it is essentially a flat occlusal contour and cusp tips do not fit into fossae, it is only necessary to make sure the fossa width is narrower than the width of the cusp tip. Consequently, it is not extremely difficult to fabricate. Elaborate fossa and groove contouring can be accomplished as long as the multiple centric contacts are not disturbed. Even though the contacts may stay the same, it is possible to develop very sophisticated contours within the framework of this type of occlusion.

When posterior disclusion is indicated, this type of occlusal form may be used with the same clinical success as Type 2 occlusal form that has been modified to disclude. It is purely a matter of dentist preference. Patients will not be able to distinguish between the two forms.

SUMMARY

Several types of occlusal form can be used to restore posterior teeth. Whatever contour is selected should be chosen because it:

1. Directs the forces as near parallel as possible to the long axis of each tooth
2. Distributes the lateral stress to maximum advantage in varying situations of periodontal support
3. Provides maximum stability
4. Provides maximum wearability
5. Provides optimum function for gripping, grinding, and crushing

Practicality of fabrication is a factor that should be considered when the type of occlusal form is being selected. If additional time, effort, and expense are required to produce the same clinical result that could be accomplished with greater ease to the patient, the dentist, and the technician, technique orientation has in all probability taken the place of goal orientation.

Chapter 22

Simplifying Instrumentation for Occlusal Analysis and Treatment

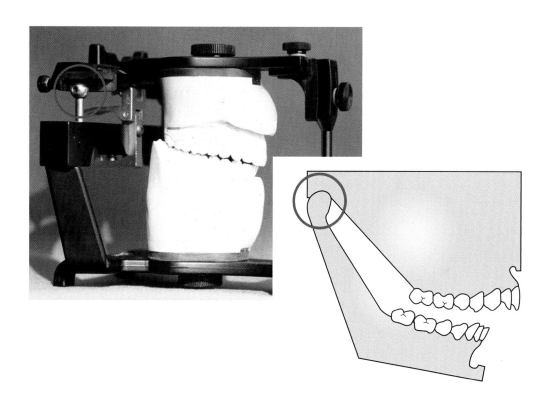

PRINCIPLE

The cost of improperly mounted casts is too high a cost to pay . . . in wasted time, expense, frustration, and lost quality.

THE LOGIC OF SIMPLIFICATION

There was a time when the complexities of fully adjustable articulators and pantographic recordings of condylar paths seemed to be a reasonable requirement for quality occlusal analysis and treatment. As new information regarding the effects of mandibular function or dysfunction on the neuromuscular system has emerged, the requirements for instrumentation have changed. Driving all of those changes is a simple premise: *Determine exactly what the requirements are for a perfected occlusion; then use whatever instrumentation is required to fulfill those requirements.*

Let's review the requirements for a perfected occlusion so we can determine the most logical instrumentation prerequisites for fulfilling each goal. Think first in terms of treatment planning for the following goals as they relate to use of an articulator:

1. Unrestricted access of the condyles to complete seating into centric relation.
2. Nondeflected closure to anterior contact in centric relation.
3. Simultaneous, equal intensity contact of posterior teeth in harmony with completely seated condyles, and centric relation contact of anterior teeth.
4. An acceptable plane of occlusion and incisal plane.
5. An anterior guidance that is in harmony with the envelope of function.

The above requirements for an ideal occlusion must be modified if contact of the anterior teeth in centric relation is not possible. Comprehensive treatment planning for such patients is described in Chapter 38 explaining the different strategies for treating anterior open bites. However, none of these strategies requires more complex instrumentation than what is appropriate for ideal arch-to-arch relationships.

The objectives outlined for ideal occlusion can all be satisfied with the right choice of instrumentation. Once those objectives have been met, the addition of more complex but unnecessary capabilities is not logical. They simply add to the time and expense of achieving the clearly defined goals.

Let's relate each of the stated requirements for an ideal occlusion to the instrument choices available for satisfying these requirements in the most efficient and cost-effective way.

Goal #1: Unrestricted Condylar Access to Centric Relation

The single most important purpose of an articulator is to relate the lower cast to the upper cast in centric relation. To accomplish this relationship and maintain it during any change in vertical dimension, both casts must have the same relationship to the horizontal axis on the articulator that the dental arches have to the condylar axis on the cranium.

> The first requirement for acceptability of an articulator is that it must accurately accept a facebow mounting.

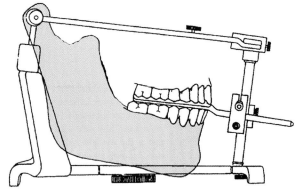

FIGURE 22-1 The facebow relates the upper cast to the same axis position on the articulator as the condyle axis on the patient. When the lower cast is correctly related to the upper cast, the opening and closing arc for each lower tooth will follow the same centric relation path on the articulator as it does on the patient.

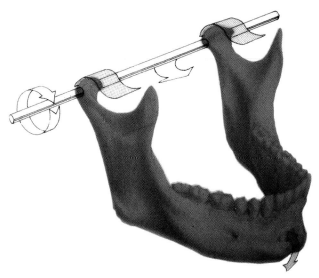

FIGURE 22-2 The horizontal axis of condylar rotation is the most critical of all mandibular movements. The jaw can open and close on this axis without any change of position of the axis (a fixed axis). Thus, if it is duplicated on the articulator, changes in vertical can be made without any error being created. Note that the rotational axis of the condyles can slide forward and down the eminentiae during excursions. But for establishment of equal intensity, simultaneous tooth contact in centric relation, that can only be achieved with the condyles seated and the casts mounted in centric relation.

The rationale and use of the facebow are explained in detail in Chapter 11. A further discussion here is in order because in spite of its importance, use of a facebow is one of the most neglected steps of all procedures required for accuracy in occlusal analysis and treatment. The only explanation for this neglect is a lack of understanding of why it is so important (Figures 22-1 and 22-2).

Reproducing the horizontal axis is the essential first requirement because the accuracy of all other relationships depends on a correct starting point. This most important of all instrument capabilities can be accomplished with the exact same accuracy on any articulator that can accept a facebow recording. This requirement can be fulfilled just as accurately on any

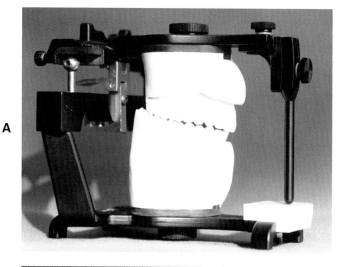
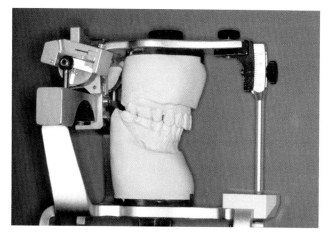
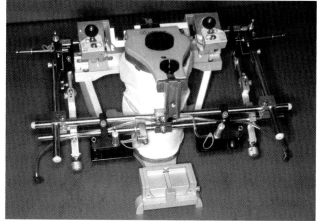
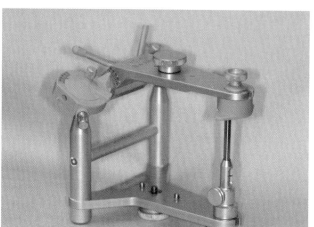

FIGURE 22-3 No difference in centric relation recording. Each of these articulators can accept a facebow recording and can accurately record a correct centric relation for properly mounted casts. **A,** Combi articulator. **B,** Dénar® Mark II Semiadjustable articulator. **C,** Dénar® D5A Completely Adjustable articulator. **D,** SAM articulator. For this first requirement, all of these instruments are equal. There are many other articulators that are equally acceptable for fulfilling this first requirement.

set path, or semiadjustable articulator, as it can be fulfilled on the most complex fully adjustable articulator (Figure 22-3).

Unacceptable instruments

The common use of inadequate articulators is a baffling inconsistency since the basic geometry that it violates is so easy to understand, and the error it produces is so substantial. It is obvious that we cannot open on one axis to record a bite record, and then close on a different axis and still return to the same position. Note the substantial error in the closing arc if the condylar axis is changed as it is on a Galetti articulator (Figure 22-4).

Why Accuracy of the Condylar Axis Is Critical if Changes Are Made in the Vertical Dimension

Many of the most consequential decisions regarding the choice of treatment are directly tied to a change in vertical dimension. Accuracy in the decision process requires knowing exactly how changes in vertical dimension affect the re-

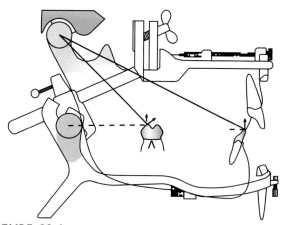

FIGURE 22-4 If restorations are fabricated to a mistaken arc of closure, it would create severe deflective interferences on posterior teeth. Lingual contours on anterior teeth also end up being restored in interference to the normal closing paths.

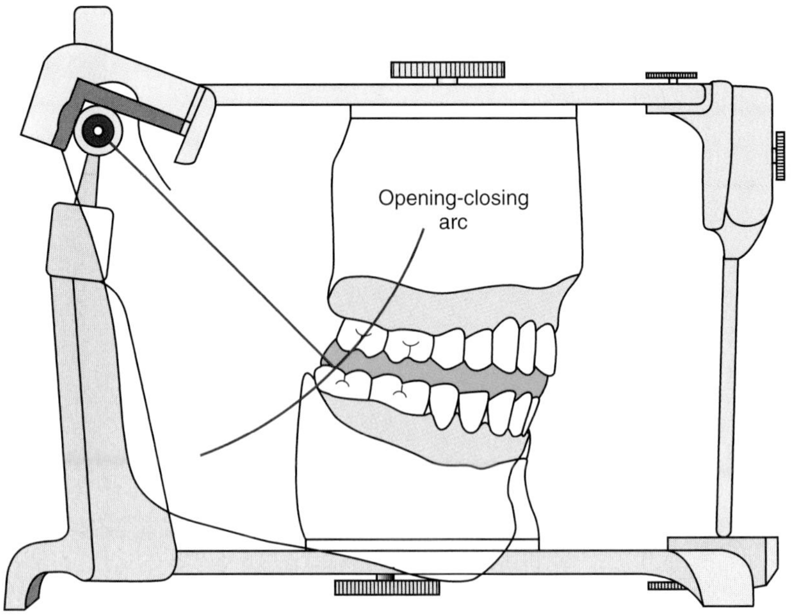

FIGURE 22-5 The first purpose of an articulator is to relate the lower casts to the upper cast in centric relation. If that relationship is to be maintained at different levels of vertical dimension, both casts must also be related to the condylar axis. Note that as the lower jaw opens or closes on a correct centric relation arc, the relationship of the lower arch to the condylar axis is maintained.

Opening-closing arc

lationship of the lower teeth to the upper teeth. These variations of tooth-to-tooth relationships can only be predetermined by knowing the exact path each lower tooth travels as the mandible opens or closes. Even minimal changes in vertical dimension can have a significant effect on where tooth contact occurs. Contrary to what some dentists perceive, the lower arch does not move on a straight up/down path. The lower arch travels *forward* on its closing arc. As the wider part of the lower arch travels forward to the narrower part of the upper arch, it can have a profound effect on buccolingual alignment of lower cusp tips into upper fossae. Differences in vertical dimension from the first point of contact against an interfering incline to the vertical dimension of occlusion (VDO) at maximum intercuspation can amount to several millimeters. With unmounted casts, the position of the condyles is ignored as the casts are just moved around the interfering incline. If the occlusion is finished at that deflected arch-to-arch relationship, it will require one or both condyles to displace every time the teeth close together into maximum intercuspation.

Start with the articulator locked in centric relation

With properly mounted casts locked into a centric relation arc of opening or closing, the best treatment choice can be determined for achieving equal-intensity, simultaneous contacts on all teeth without requiring displacement of the temporomandibular joints (TMJs) to achieve that goal of a perfected occlusion.

If the choice of treatment is equilibration, it can be verified by equilibrating the casts to find out exactly where tooth contacts will occur as the VDO is closed from the first point of deflective contact to a nondeflective closure. If the analysis in centric relation reveals that an increase in VDO will improve the relationship of the lower anterior teeth to the upper anterior teeth, a diagnostic work-up can develop the treatment plan without guessing about its effect on posterior occlusal contacts. The critical point to understand is as follows:

> Correct tooth-to-tooth relationships can be accurately analyzed only at the same vertical dimension as the intended final intercuspal contact in centric relation.

Do not be confused about locking the articulator in centric relation for the initial analysis in treatment planning. This does not mean that occlusions should be *restricted* to centric relation. Nor does it mean that the natural path of closure in patients is restricted to the arc on the locked articulator. The articulator is locked in centric because it is the only way the articulator can hinge open or closed and still maintain the casts in centric relation.

Only when casts are mounted in centric relation with a facebow will changes in vertical dimension not affect the accuracy of arch-to-arch relationships. Centric relation is the starting point of occlusion. It is the arch-to-arch relationship to which all stable holding contacts must be coordinated. This static relationship in centric relation must be established first, before the dynamics of function can be analyzed or determined. This is the first purpose of an articulator (Figure 22-5).

Goal #2: Nondeflected Closure to Anterior Contact in Centric Relation

One of the most important determinations that must be made is how any change in the VDO will affect the anterior teeth, including both the centric holding contacts and the anterior guidance. To determine this accurately, the condylar axis *must* be accurate because the arc of closure is critical to this determination. Remember that as the VDO is opened, the lower incisal edges move back and down from anterior con-

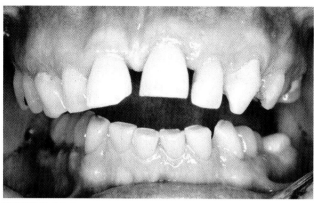

FIGURE 22-6 In this mouth, contact in centric relation is only on the right molar. There would be no way to accurately determine the relationship of the anterior contact without knowing the exact path of closure while both condyles remain seated in centric relation. If casts of this mouth are mounted in centric relation, the best choice of a workable vertical dimension can be established to achieve acceptable anterior contact. Only then can a functional anterior guidance be determined.

tact. As the VDO is closed, the lower incisal edges move forward and up toward the upper lingual surfaces. Many times this anterior relationship is the prime determinant of which vertical dimension is selected for the entire occlusal scheme. Thus it often affects whether the choice of treatment is equilibration, restoration, or orthodontics.

Any articulator that accepts a facebow mounting will satisfy this most important requirement. It hardly seems necessary to mention that use of an acceptable articulator without a proper facebow does not fulfill the requirement. This all too common practice creates a number of problems, including occlusal plane problems.

Goal #3: Simultaneous, Equal Intensity Contacts on All Posterior Teeth

This goal means that posterior tooth contacts should occur precisely in harmony with completely seated TMJs and centric relation contact of the anterior teeth. That is why the condylar axis is so important when determining how best to achieve anterior contact. The question that must be answered early in the diagnostic wax-up is how to get the back teeth out of the way so the front teeth can contact. The finalization of posterior contacts can be completed only when this decision has been made and stable stops have been made possible on the anterior teeth.

To put instrumentation in proper perspective, all of the above decisions regarding anterior and posterior contact are determined with the articulator condyles locked in centric relation. The functional paths that the mandible travels from centric relation cannot be considered until unobstructed access to centric relation has been achieved for both anterior and posterior teeth. Up to this point, there is no need to complicate instrumentation beyond this requirement for an accurate condylar axis (Figure 22-6).

There is yet another important determination that can be made with optimal accuracy without complicating instrumentation. It is the determination of an acceptable occlusal and incisal plane.

Goal #4: An Acceptable Occlusal and Incisal Plane

One of the major considerations in treatment planning is the determination of an ideal occlusal plane, with emphasis on the incisal plane of the anterior teeth. There are very few mistakes that affect esthetics more negatively than a slanted incisal plane. It is a mistake that should never happen if casts are mounted with a facebow and one simple rule is followed: *align the facebow with the eyes.*

There are many ways to unnecessarily complicate instrumentation. Many of these complications involve procedures for facebow use. I suggest that the simplest way to establish a correct incisal plane is to look straight at the patient and visually align the bow so it is parallel with the eyes (the interpupillary line). This can be done with the patient sitting up or lying back. If the facebow is aligned with the eyes on the patient, the mounted casts on the articulator will relate to the interpupillary line. In doing a diagnostic wax-up, the incisal plane is simply aligned with the bench top.

Objections to this simple approach include concerns that the eyes may not be even with a horizontal plane, or that it is too difficult to align the bow visually. I think you will find that neither of these objections is valid. Furthermore, if you follow the rule that whenever any restorative changes in incisal plane are needed, the changes are always made in provisional restorations first. Construction of final restorations should not be started until the provisional restorations are approved by the patient and the dentist. In following this process for hundreds of restorative patients, I have never found that the resolution of any incisal plane problem would have been improved by adding extra procedures. Visual alignment of the facebow with the interpupillary line results in casts that clearly show any discrepancy from an acceptable incisal plane.

Relating the incisal plane to the earholes

The earholes do not always perfectly align with the interpupilary line or the condylar axis. For that reason, some clinicians may object to the use of an earbow to mount casts. It is true that an earbow is not as precise as a facebow that is meticulously aligned with the condyle on each side. The question to ask is "Does use of an earbow cause any problems related to the diagnosis or treatment?" My observation over many years of use is that the earbow is clinically acceptable. Dr. Charles Stuart, one of the "fathers of gnathology" and a strong advocate of hinge axis recordings, developed and promoted use of the first earbows. Today the earbow is used exclusively by almost all of the best restorative dentists I know. Use of the earbow with a mounting jig to correct for the discrepancy between the earholes and the relative position of the condyles is popular because it is sim-

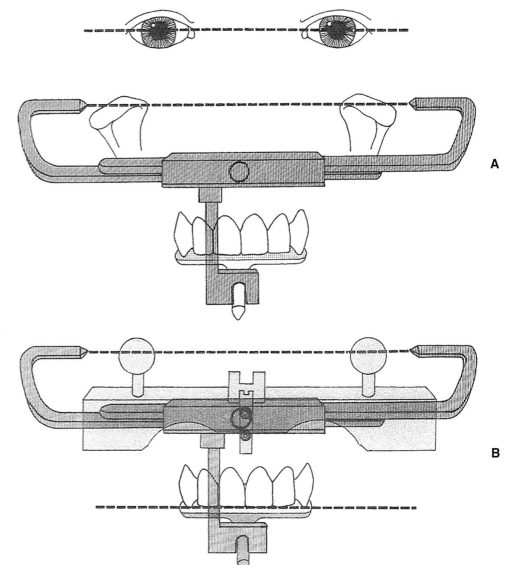

FIGURE 22-7 A, The bow of the facebow should always be observed to make sure it is parallel to the eyes. B, If alignment is correct, the casts will align with the condyles on the articulator. Then the incisal plane can be aligned with the bench top in the laboratory to produce an esthetically pleasing plane in the patient.

ple and effective. I have found no problems whatsoever with its use, even for the most complex restorative problems.

If the earbow is slightly off alignment with the eyes when the earpieces are in the earholes, align the bow with the eyes by slight movement within the earholes. This will ensure that the incisal plane can be related to the bench top, which is the primary goal. The slight variation from a precise intercondylar plane does not have a noticeable effect on the arc of closure at the final stage of the restorative process.

If the restorative procedures outlined in this text are followed, all bite records for the restorative phase will be made at the correct vertical or so close to it that a slightly missed condylar axis will have insignificant effect on the arc of closure from the vertical dimension of the bite record. A misalignment with the interpupillary line, however, can have a noticeable and unpleasant effect on the incisal plane. For that reason, if there is a slight discrepancy between the condylar axis and the interpupillary line, it is usually better to align the bow with the eyes, especially for restorative procedures in-

volving anterior restorations. The same is true whether a conventional facebow or an earbow is used (Figures 22-7 and 22-8).

Setting the Height of the Casts on the Articulator

Setting the correct slant of the posterior occlusal plane is also related to the height of the casts on the articulator, but it is a separate concern. If the casts are related to the condylar axis on the articulator while attached to the facebow, raising or lowering the casts has no effect on the arc of closure in centric relation. It does affect the inclination of the condylar path, which steepens as the casts are lowered, to maintain a set angle with the occlusal plane.

The goal of every mounting, consistent with an accurate relationship of the casts to the condylar axis, is to center the casts between the upper and lower bows of the articulator. The simple reason for this is to make room for mounting plates and

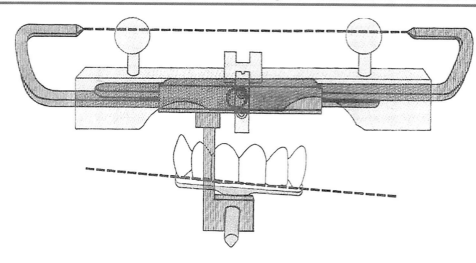

FIGURE 22-8 If an existing plane is slanted in the mouth, alignment of the bow with the eyes will result in a correct view of the slanted plane on the articulator. The diagnostic work-up is then directed at correcting the incisal plane by the best choice of treatment.

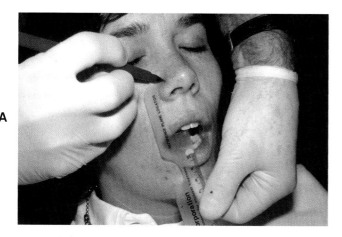

A

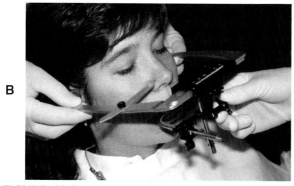

B

FIGURE 22-9 A, Simple measuring guide for locating a spot on the face that can be used as a reference point for setting the height of the earbow. B, This ensures that the casts will be centered between the upper and lower bows of the articulator.

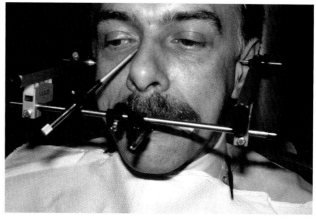

FIGURE 22-10 An intraorbital pointer relates either to the infraorbital notch or to a predetermined spot on the face that can be used as a reference point if a new facebow recording is needed later.

the cast position on subsequent mountings. This is unnecessary if a simple transfer mounting procedure is used in the laboratory. Nevertheless, the use of an infraorbital pointer is effective without being complicated for those who choose it.

Goal #5: An Anterior Guidance That Is in Harmony With the Envelope of Function

As we came to realize that the anterior guidance is the dominant determinant of posterior occlusal morphology, we also learned that the anterior guidance is a completely separate entity. Early gnathologic concepts that the anterior guidance was dictated by condylar paths have been completely discarded. At this point, a review of anterior guidance in Chapter 17 might be helpful because it is an important determinant of the entire occlusal scheme, and accuracy in recording it is critical to any occlusal treatment.

The role of instrumentation

In using any articulator, remember that anterior guidance is a product of functional movements that fall within the outer limits of possible jaw paths. Recording only condylar paths

mounting stone on both the upper and lower casts. On most semiadjustable articulators, the only requirement is to mount the casts in a vertically centered position (Figure 22-9). The traditional way to accomplish this is through use of an infraorbital pointer (Figure 22-10). There is nothing magical about an infraorbital pointer. The infraorbital foramen is just one of several different reference points that can be used effectively to establish a reasonably centered position for the casts. The infraorbital pointer can also be used as a guide for reproducing

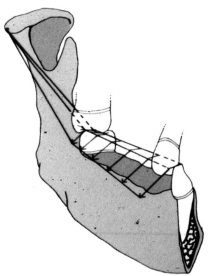

FIGURE 22-11 The path of the lower posterior teeth in working-side function is dictated by the anterior guidance. The anterior guidance is by far the dominant determinant. The paths of the lateral anterior guidance are reproduced by each posterior tooth except that the length of the stroke becomes progressively shorter the closer the tooth is to the condyle. The effect of any condylar side shift is lost because the separation effect from the anterior guidance and the orbiting condylar path occurs first. Studies done at the Dawson Center using functional path models show conclusively that the working-side path of lower posterior teeth follows the same path as the lateral anterior guidances with no evidence of condylar path influence.

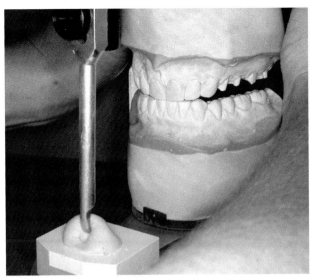

FIGURE 22-12 Incisal pin duplicating the path in the resin material.

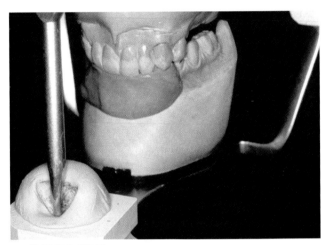

FIGURE 22-13 A completed customized anterior guide table.

does not furnish enough information for the instrument to reproduce jaw movements that are the same as the patient makes in function. The anterior guidance is a separate determinant that must be recorded in addition to condylar paths. It is the combination of anterior guidance and condylar guidance that determines the border path of each lower posterior tooth.

If the anterior guidance is correct in the mouth, the anterior teeth on the articulated casts can dictate the movements at the front of the articulator or can be used to fabricate a customized anterior guide table. But if the anterior guidance is not known, it cannot be determined on the articulator, regardless of how precisely the condylar paths are reproduced.

Anterior guidance must be determined in the mouth before it can be copied at the front of the articulator, just as condylar guidance must be determined on the patient before it can be copied at the back of the articulator. If both the front and rear paths are correctly copied, the path of each tooth between these two determinants will also follow border paths (Figure 22-11).

Recording the anterior guidance

The protrusive path and lateral excursions are recorded in a resin material on a flat anterior guide table. As the upper cast is moved through the protrusive path (Figure 22-12), the lingual contours of the upper anterior teeth guide the incisal pin to duplicate the path in the resin material. When the material hardens, the upper bow of the articulator will follow the same path even if the cast is removed.

The precise paths that were determined on the patient and then transferred to the articulator by casts of the corrected anterior guidance provide perfect accuracy in all excursions for the articulator. As long as the condylar paths are not changed after the guide table is complete, the articulator can be used to precisely duplicate the anterior guidance on restorations (Figure 22-13). The casts of the provisionals are replaced by the master die model for the fabrication phase. The putty silicone index is used to dictate the exact incisal plane as determined in the mouth.

The procedures outlined for precise duplication of a corrected anterior guidance can be accomplished on any articulator that accepts a facebow mounting. In this regard, no one semiadjustable or even set path articulator can claim superiority except for the quality of how well the instrument is fabricated. It is, however, at this point that the condylar path must be evaluated.

The compelling reasons for using complex, fully adjustable instrumentation are no longer valid. Today the simplification of articulator requirements is based on a number of realizations that some of the occlusal premises of the gnathologic era were incorrect.

Precise recording of condylar paths was believed to be essential for conformity with some of the early concepts of gnathology. When it was believed that the condylar paths were the sole determinants of anterior guidance, it was a logical assumption that condylar paths must be precisely recorded. This concept was further enhanced by a belief that occlusal stops should be on the sides of cusps and the walls of fossae to form a tripod of contact around each stamp cusp. The earliest concepts also included a need for bilaterally balanced function on all posterior teeth, and the entire concept was further complicated by an almost religious fervor that insisted the mouth was an unacceptable articulator. Thus all occlusal restorations were to be designed and fabricated according to the precise dictates of a fully adjustable articulator. No corrections were allowed unless they were made on the articulator.

If all the dogmas of early gnathology had been correct, we would indeed need to use fully adjustable instrumentation on all occlusal restorations. But as many of the original beliefs have been proved inaccurate, the exclusive dependence on the condylar path has been diminished to a more realistic use of semiadjustable instrumentation.

The principal changes that have eliminated the original complete dependency on fully adjustable instrumentation include the following realizations.

Bilaterally balanced occlusion is traumatogenic. Because of a normal flexibility of the mandible, there is no way to harmonize the posterior contacts on the balancing side for all degrees of muscle contraction. Thus balancing-side function usually results in unacceptable stress or wear. Because of so many problems of tooth hypermobility, bilateral balancing of occlusions was abandoned many years ago, except for dentures.

Condylar guidance does not dictate anterior guidance. Anterior guidance actually influences occlusal contours more than condylar guidance because it is the principal discluder of posterior teeth in working excursions. Since it must be determined as a separate entity, unrelated to condylar paths, the importance of condylar guidance diminishes whenever the anterior guidance is steep enough to effectively disclude the posterior teeth.

Tripod contact is no more stable than cusp-tip–to–fossa contact. The difficulty of making tripod contacts on the sides of cusps created a need for precise excursive reproduction to align with the fossa walls and to prevent colli-

sions of cusps. As the contacts were moved from the sides of the cusps and the walls of the fossae to the tops of the cusps and the brims of the fossae, the occlusal morphology became arbitrarily flatter and less dependent on precise paths through grooves. Early claims that tripod contacts never needed adjustment were abandoned as it became apparent that tripod contact was not a guarantee of stability.

Complete posterior disclusion by the anterior guidance is the most desirable occlusion. Because of its proved effect on elevator muscle activity, posterior disclusion is the goal of occlusal treatment whenever it can be achieved. This eliminates some major concerns regarding incline paths and ridge and groove directions.

An immediate side shift cannot occur from a correct centric relation. With changes in our understanding of centric relation, the concept of "most retruded" was replaced by "most superior." At the most superior position, the condyles are braced medially, so they cannot travel horizontally toward the midline. This eliminates the concern about immediate side shift and simplifies requirements for instrumentation because without an immediate side shift the lateral anterior guidance is the dominant controlling factor in working-side jaw paths. If fossa-wall angulation on the teeth is related to the lateral anterior guidance, the downward condylar guidance on the balancing side will only add to the disclusive effect.

If the working-side fossa inclines are flatter than the lateral anterior guidance, the posterior teeth will be separated in lateral working excursions before any side shift can take place.

SIMPLIFYING INSTRUMENTATION

Eliminating the need for excursive contacts on the posterior teeth is not a license to ignore condylar guidance. It just makes it possible to simplify instrumentation for most patients because any condylar path that is flatter on the articulator than the path on the patient will result in posterior restorations that disclude the moment the condyle starts down a steeper eminentia in the patient.

Setting the condylar paths flatter on the articulator has neither an effect on centric relation contacts nor any effect on correct anterior relationships as long as it is not changed after the anterior guidance is properly recorded on the instrument.

With new data showing the advantages of posterior disclusion, the goal of most occlusal treatment is to make sure the combination of condylar guidance and anterior guidance can separate the posterior teeth when the mandible moves forward or sideward from centric relation. This treatment goal is further simplified by two different studies involving several hundred patients that showed that for all the patients tested, the minimum horizontal condylar path was 25 degrees. At the beginning of the protrusive path, the average incline is close to 60 degrees. This means that occlusal restorations fabricated on an articulator with 20-degree condylar paths would automatically separate if placed in a mouth with steeper condylar paths. Since almost all patients have condylar paths that are steeper than 20 degrees, this procedure is not as arbitrary as it may seem.

If the joint has been severely damaged by degenerative joint disease to the extent that the normally convex eminentia has been flattened to less than 20 degrees, it would be evident from a routine examination if the examination includes an evaluation of the TMJs and an analysis of wear patterns on the teeth. When upper lingual cusps are worn flat, it is almost certain that both the condyle and the eminence are also worn flat. This is an indication to record the condylar path accurately rather than to use an arbitrary setting. This is especially important if the anterior guidance is also worn flat. If one chooses not to record the condylar paths in such patients, the effect of the flattened path must be accounted for by other methods such as a functionally generated path.

When the anterior guidance is relatively steep, the protrusive or lateral condylar path loses its importance because almost no horizontal function can occur without separation of the posterior teeth by the anterior guidance.

If the anterior guidance is fairly flat, posterior restorations will still be discluded if they are fabricated at the 20-degree condylar setting on the articulator for any patient that has a condylar guidance that is within the normal range of 25 degrees or steeper, as long as the fossa walls on the posterior teeth are no steeper than the lateral anterior guidance and the occlusal plane is correct.

In the determination of what an instrument must do, a proper understanding of the role of the anterior guidance is necessary. In the past, importance was placed on precise recording of the condylar guidance: the anterior guidance was determined arbitrarily. The reverse of this is more logical for the following reasons:

1. *Anterior teeth can maintain contact from centric relation to the end point of function in all excursions.* (All functional excursions do not maintain tooth contact, but the anterior guidance must be able to separate posterior contact through all functional excursions.)
2. *The anterior guidance must be in harmony with the envelope of function, or tooth contact can create stress or wear.* Thus it is important to record anterior guidance correctly. It is also directly related to the neutral-zone stability of the anterior teeth, so an arbitrary anterior relationship will usually conflict with either the neutral zone or the envelope of function.
3. *Posterior teeth ideally contact only in centric relation.* They are in space for all other jaw positions.
4. *The amount of separation by the posterior teeth in excursions does not seem to matter.* Whether the lower posterior teeth just barely miss the upper inclines in function or whether they open and close on a near-vertical path has no discernible effect on function, comfort, or stability.
5. *Since the only requirement for posterior tooth paths is that they miss upper tooth inclines, the condylar path*

can be set arbitrarily flat enough on the instrument to cause posterior disclusion in the mouth. A 20-degree condylar path will accomplish the necessary disclusion on most patients.

How to Tell When an Arbitrary Condylar Path Setting Is Acceptable

Although the use of an arbitrary 20-degree condylar path is practical for most restorative cases, the decision to use a set 20-degree path should never be an arbitrary decision.

First, the requirements for instrumentation may vary depending on whether the articulator is to be used for diagnosis or for fabrication of restorations. If all upper and lower posterior teeth are to be restored, instrumentation can be kept simple because we can control the occlusal plane and the occlusal fossae contours in the restorative process.

Occlusal diagnosis becomes more complex on patients who do not need restorations but who have occlusal plane problems or gross interferences to the excursive paths. For these patients, we need to know how steep the condylar paths are so that we can determine how much occlusal reshaping is required to eliminate the occlusal interferences to excursive paths. If restorations or orthodontics will be required, it should be determined before treatment is started.

Some occlusions must depend almost solely on the condylar path for disclusion of the posterior teeth. An examination of the patient should reveal when a set 20-degree path is not acceptable. More accuracy of condylar path is required when either of the following conditions is noted in the mouth:

1. The anterior guidance cannot disclude the posterior teeth in protrusive or balancing excursions.
2. Severe wear has resulted in loss of upper lingual cusps. This is an indication of an abnormally flattened condylar path.

The condylar path is a critical determinant of posterior occlusal contours in each of the above situations. When the goal of posterior disclusion cannot be accomplished by the anterior guidance, one must rely on the downward path of the condyles to separate the back teeth in excursions. This can occur even with a flat anterior guidance as long as the occlusal plane is acceptable because the occlusal fossae can then be designed with fossa walls that are flat enough to be discluded by the combination of anterior guidance and the actual condylar guidance.

There are several instrument choices for diagnosis and treatment planning of such problem cases. Instruments that can be used effectively for either diagnosis or treatment include the following types:

1. Fully adjustable articulators
2. Semiadjustable articulators
3. Set condylar path articulators
4. Combination (set condylar path or fully adjustable) articulators

Any of the above types of instruments can be used with great success if the operator understands the goals of occlusal diagnosis or therapy. It is strongly recommended that all four types be understood because the selection of an instrument is a very important decision that relates to practicality as well as effectiveness.

The Only Real Difference: Condylar Guidance

The major difference in the various types of articulators is related to variations in how the articulator duplicates the patient's condylar paths. In evaluating any articulator, one should understand that no matter how sophisticated the instrument is, it can still do no more than the following regarding condylar movements:

1. Reproduce the horizontal axis of condylar rotation
2. Reproduce the vertical axis of condylar rotation (Figure 22-14)
3. Reproduce the sagittal axis of condylar rotation (Figure 22-15)
4. Permit simultaneous multiple axes of rotation during condylar translation
5. Reproduce straight protrusive paths of each condyle (Figure 22-16)
6. Reproduce the paths of each condyle during straight lateral excursions of the mandible (Figure 22-17)

7. Reproduce the multiple paths of each condyle during all possible excursions of the mandible between straight lateral and straight protrusion

Although many claims are made regarding complete adjustability of condylar paths, very few instruments are actually capable of reproducing all seven of the above condylar movements without some interpolation.

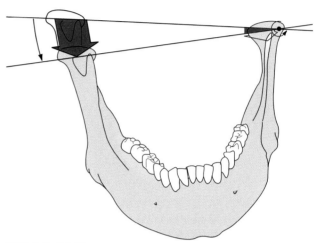

FIGURE 22-15 The sagittal axis of rotation is essential for lateral movement to occur. This is so because the orbiting condyle must move down to enable the working-side condyle to rotate. This results from the design requirement of preventing the lower posterior teeth from moving horizontally toward the midline because to do so would clash with the upper lingual cusps and make the functional purpose of the curve of Wilson not work. Remember also that the mandible cannot move to the left without moving down the canine incline. The downward movement of the orbiting condyle adds to the posterior disclusion effect on the balancing (nonworking) side.

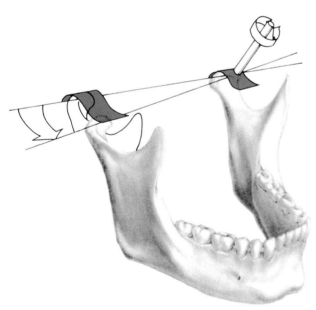

FIGURE 22-14 The vertical axis of rotation can be better visualized when one looks at a composite of rotation because lateral rotation actually occurs around the lateral pole of the rotating condyle. As rotation occurs, the orbiting condyle must travel down the slope of the eminence. The medial pole on the rotating side must also travel down its slope but for a lesser distance. Because the condyles load against inclines, a pure vertical rotation is not possible without being combined with a sagittal rotation of the working-side condyle.

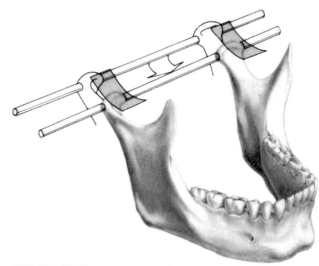

FIGURE 22-16 Straight protrusion can occur only with simultaneous downward movement of the condyles. The condyles are free to rotate at any point on this forward path; so visualize this movement as translation of the horizontal rotational axis.

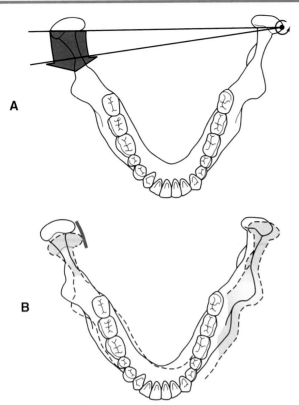

FIGURE 22-17 **A,** The broad arrow represents the path of the orbiting condyle if all movement were confined to a fixed vertical rotation of the working-side condyle. The progressive side shift that occurs as the orbiting condyle is pulled inward along the medial fossa wall is at a greater angle than what would result from an arc around a fixed axis. **B,** This results in a side shift of the working condyle that occurs simultaneously with its rotation. It is important to realize that this side shift cannot occur until rotation has moved the orbiting condyle forward and downward to disengage its medial pole from its bony stop. By the time this occurs, the downward movement of the orbiting condyle and the lateral anterior guidance has already separated the posterior teeth on the orbiting side. If the fossa wall angle on the posterior teeth is flatter than the lateral anterior guidance, the posterior teeth on the working side will also be discluded before the progressive side shift can affect the teeth.

The first six listed movements can be accurately reproduced on most quality gnathologic instruments, but the seventh requirement, recording all the paths between straight protrusive and straight lateral, must be interpolated.

Regardless of how precisely the various condylar movements may be copied on an articulator, condylar movements alone do not give enough information to determine complete occlusal contours. The anterior guidance is far more important in its influence on posterior occlusal form than the condylar path. But the role of the condylar path must be understood because it becomes more important as a diagnostic consideration whenever the posterior teeth interfere with the anterior guidance. In the light of what constitutes a perfected occlusion (the six goals), understanding how the condyles move is also a key to simplifying the selection of a suitable articulator.

The following figures describe how condylar function influences mandibular movements.

HOW DIFFERENT ARTICULATORS RECORD CONDYLAR PATHS

Fully Adjustable Instruments

The term *fully adjustable* refers to the reproducibility of the patient's condylar paths. Any variation from one type of fully adjustable articulator to another will be limited to mechanical variations that affect the ease of reproducing the condylar paths. Instruments may also vary in their quality of materials and workmanship.

Only instruments that can reproduce all condylar border movements, including protrusive-lateral paths, can be truly said to be fully adjustable. Very few can make that claim, and even then there is divergent opinion among instrument buffs about either the importance or the validity of the claims of complete adjustability.

There are two basic methods for recording the condylar paths: pantographic tracings and stereographics. Actually, neither method records the true anatomic contours of the TMJ, and the articulator does not reproduce the anatomy of the joint. It is merely a mechanical equivalent that makes the back end of the articulator capable of going through the same movements that the back end of the mandible follows in function. The condyles on the articulator are not shaped like the irregular condyles in the skull, but they can be made to duplicate the movements of the real condyles. How the paths of the condyles are recorded and mechanically duplicated determines the type of instrument.

Pantographic Instruments

With the almost universal acceptance of posterior disclusion as a desirable goal, the need for pantographic recordings has been all but eliminated. For those who still wish to use it, the use of pantographics has become far more practical since the introduction of the Dénar® pantograph (Figure 22-18). Because of a simplified procedure of using vinyl clutch formers, a central-bearing-point set of clutches can be fabricated in a matter of a few minutes. The clutches are then adapted to the Dénar® pantograph, which traces mandibular movements on tracing plates. The stylus that draws the path lines on the tracing plates is held against the plates by rubber bands, but it can easily be disengaged from the plate when one presses a button that permits air pressure to deactivate each stylus from contact. With practice, a pantographic tracing can usually be achieved within a reasonable chair time of 30 minutes. Some experts can cut that time considerably.

The pantographic technique does have the advantage that goes with the use of a central bearing point. With a properly located central bearing point, all occlusal interferences are disengaged when the condylar paths are recorded. There is no tooth contact during the tracing procedures. Manipulation of the mandible is simpler because of the complete absence of occlusal interferences at the opened vertical.

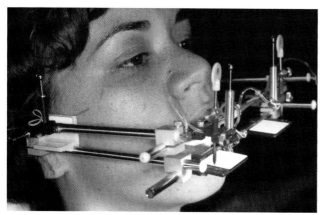

FIGURE 22-18 The Dénar® pantograph.

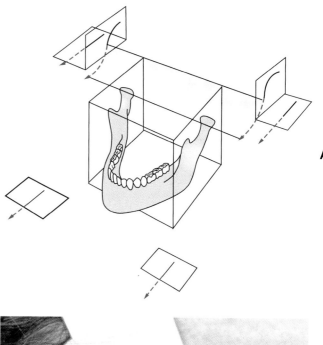

A

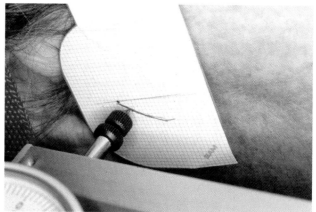

B

Complete preoperative occlusal analysis is possible on models to a more refined degree than is possible with semiadjustable articulators, but there is no real clinical advantage at the preoperative stage, since the analysis of centric contacts, arch relationships, and excursive paths can be accomplished on a semiadjustable instrument with a degree of accuracy that is acceptable for preoperative planning of complex cases.

Errors in mounting are common and easy to make. The slightest movement of either clutch produces a magnified error at the tracing plate. Studies done by Helsing have shown that reproducibility of pantographic tracings is seldom achieved.

Misinterpretation of pantographic tracings

There are two common misinterpretations regarding pantographic tracings. The first misconception is that the tracings represent the actual path of the condyles. Actually, the path that is drawn on the tracing is a mirror image of the condylar path and not the path that the condyle travels. The writing point is fixed to the upper clutch and stays stationary as the recording plate moves with the lower jaw, producing a reversal of the jaw path. Thus a convex eminence is recorded as a concave path (Figure 22-19).

The second misconception is in the interpretation of what appears to be an immediate side shift. This part of the tracing does not relate to a side shift at all. It is the result of the downward movement of the recording plate as the orbiting-(balancing) side condyle travels down the steepest part of the eminence. As the tracing plate moves down, it arcs in a curve around the rotating condyle, but the writing point extends straight down to draw a sideways line (Figure 22-20). The steeper the condylar path, the more the false "side shift" will appear. This supposed shift of the condyle cannot happen if the condyles are in the uppermost position that is medially braced. Furthermore, even severe side shift recordings do not show up in a gothic arch tracing done intraorally.

If the recording plate on the pantograph is aligned parallel with the protrusive path, the extension of the writing

FIGURE 22-19 Typical pantograph results in recordings that are mirror images of the actual path because the recording plate moves with the mandible while the stylus is fixed. **A,** The protrusive path of the recording plate is illustrated *(dotted lines)*. The recording by the fixed position of the stylus against the moving plate is shown *(solid lines)*. A pantographic recording must be interpreted. It does not represent the actual jaw movement. **B,** An axiographic recording tracks the actual protrusive path directly. A pencil attaches to the lower bow to record the mandibular path. The red dot is the centric relation "starting point" determined by a hinge axis recording.

point will be eliminated and the side shift will disappear. Medial-pole bracing is an essential part of anatomic design that is responsible for the "midmost" position of the mandible in centric relation.

It is a mystery why such an easily explained error in pantographic interpretation has been so difficult to dispel.

Stereographic Instruments

One of the simplest "fully adjustable" instruments to use is a stereographic articulator. All border movements can be accurately recorded in three dimensions by means of simple intraoral clutches that are stabilized by a central bearing point.

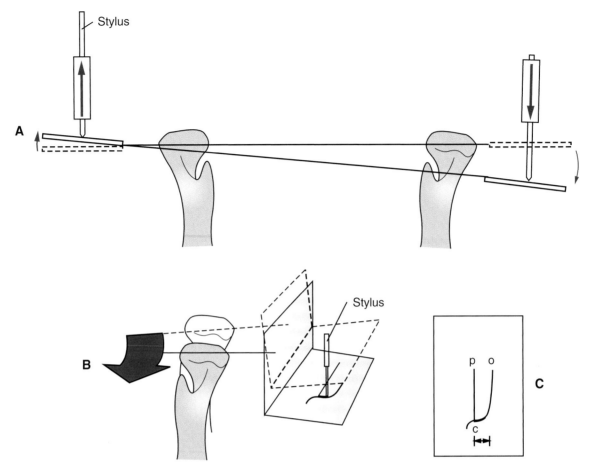

FIGURE 22-20 **A,** A false recording of an "immediate" side shift can result from the downward movement of the orbiting condyle, which moves the recording plate to an angled position. **B,** As the stylus extends straight down to follow the plate, it draws a sideways line from centric relation. The forward movement increases as a condylar path flattens to cause the completion of the pantographic recording. In **C,** the recording shows the protrusive path, *p,* the orbiting path, *o,* and the centric relation, *c.* The little tail that extends forward of the centric relation dot is the back line that occurs during working-side rotation. The *arrow* represents the amount of immediate side shift that is recorded but does not actually exist if the recording is started at centric relation.

The recordings are made by indenting three or four points into doughy self-curing acrylic resin on the surface of the opposite clutch and then moving the mandible through all border movements. Protrusive lateral movements can be included. When the stereographic recording is completed, the acrylic guide paths are allowed to set hard. The condyle paths on the instrument are then made in self-curing acrylic as dictated by the points of one clutch sliding in the indented recordings of the other. Since the three-dimensional recordings were made in the mouth by the paths of the condyles, the procedure can be reversed and the paths in the clutch can dictate the mechanical equivalent of condyle movement on the articulator.

Stereographic techniques have a decided advantage in the use of the three-dimensional recordings. All border paths can be programmed into the condylar guidance, including protrusive-lateral movements. The instrument can be used in combination with customized anterior guidance procedures and all other procedures outlined in this text.

A stereographic instrument is an excellent articulator for fabricating dentures (Figures 22-21 to 22-23). The intraoral clutches are stabilized by the central bearing point, and all recordings are made intraorally within the central area of the bases. This is a decided advantage over pantographic devices, which frequently have a tendency to tilt the denture base with the weight of the external appendages.

Semiadjustable Instruments

What was once considered a shortcoming of semiadjustable articulators is now considered an advantage. The biggest difference between fully adjustable and semiadjustable articulators is that the condylar paths are limited to straight lines for semiadjustable instrumentation. Because of this limitation, these instruments are referred to as *checkbite articulators.* This means that the horizontal condyle paths are set to align with a bite record made at centric relation and another bite record made in the protrusive position. This resultant

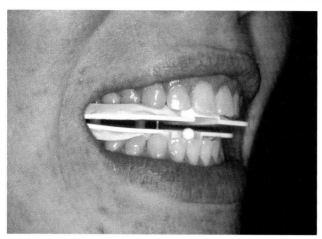

FIGURE 22-21 Stereographic clutches slide through all excursive paths on a central bearing point. Three studs indent and shape doughy acrylic resin. As the jaw moves from centric relation, the condyles are free to follow their unobstructed paths.

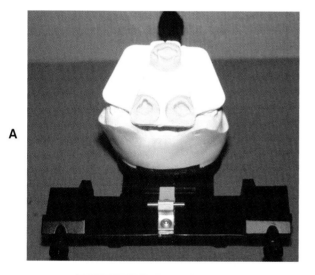

A

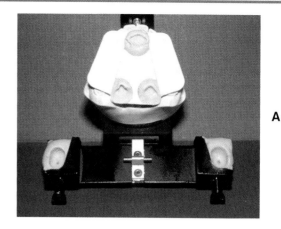

A

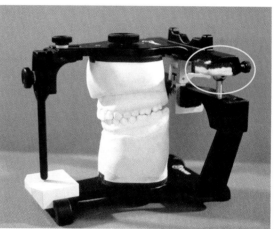

B

FIGURE 22-23 **A,** Condylar paths generated directly into a doughy mix of resin when articulator bows are moved through all excursions while recording studs on the lower clutch track in all three stereographic paths on the upper clutch. **B,** Mounted casts on Combi articulator programmed with fully adjustable condylar paths.

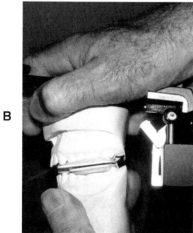

B

FIGURE 22-22 **A,** The clutches fit on casts mounted in centric relation with a facebow. When the studs are positioned in the hard resin recordings and moved through the recorded paths **(B)**, the condyles will track through the same paths as the patient's.

path is a straight line between the two points. Lateral paths are set from the centric bite record plus bite records made in left lateral and right lateral jaw positions. The resultant straight line sets the gradual side shift of the balancing condyle on the articulator.

The advantage offered by the straight-line path in protrusive movement is that it gives a built-in safety factor for the necessary disclusive effect. The condyles follow a convex path on any of the most damaged eminentiae. This convex curve will not be copied on the articulator. Only the two points of the checkbite position will be correct (Figure 22-24, *A*), but the path between the two points will be flatter than the actual convex path. This automatically produces a separation from any restorations made on the straight path when the condyles follow the convex path in the patient (Figure 22-24, *B*).

The progressive side shift of the balancing-side condyle has often been portrayed as following a severe concave path, starting with an immediate side shift before any rotation occurs. This cannot happen if the starting point is at the

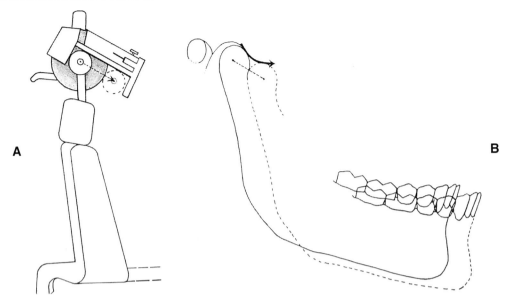

FIGURE 22-24 **A,** Semiadjustable instruments generally follow a straight path. **B,** If the horizontal path is set by a check bite at the beginning and end of a convex path, the condylar path on the articulator will be flatter at the beginning of the protrusive path *(dotted path)* than it is in the patient *(solid path)*. This provides a safety factor because the patient's steeper path will disclude posterior teeth more than the articulator. A convex path on an articulator is never needed because with natural teeth, posterior disclusion in protrusive is always the goal. A condylar path that is flatter on the articulator than it is on the patient is a simple solution to ensuring posterior disclusion on restorative cases.

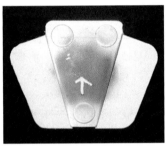

FIGURE 22-25 Gothic arch tracing showing the absence of any side shift from the point of centric relation.

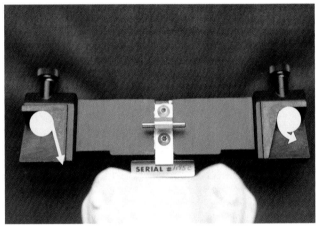

FIGURE 22-26 A simple solution for progressive side shift is to build in a greater angle of the orbiting condyle inward than the patient's condyles can travel. This guarantees clearance of the balancing inclines of the teeth as the mandible moves laterally. All Combi condylar path inserts are designed to accomplish this.

medially braced centric relation. If one will observe numerous gothic arch tracings made by a central bearing point, it will be obvious that the balancing-side condyle follows an arc around the rotating condyle. Never will any side shift be noted on the lateral paths of a gothic arch tracing. In fact, a gothic arch tracing is not even considered correct unless it has a point at the centric relation end (Figure 22-25).

Even if a concave path were followed by the orbiting condyle, straight paths could still be set to follow a path that is angled inwardly more than the most severe progressive side shift. A simple and completely practical procedure is to set all articulators to the maximum progressive side shift possible and leave them that way. This will automatically prevent balancing inclines from contacting for any occlusal schemes that are worked out on such a setting. Furthermore, there are no disadvantages to leaving all articulators at the maximum lateral setting because it takes away nothing that is needed and creates no problems (Figures 22-26 and 22-27).

For many years, all of my articulators have been set only at the maximum progressive side-shift angulation of 15 degrees. I have seen no reason to alter this procedure. Balancing-side contact is never desirable (except for full dentures), and this practice helps to ensure disclusion of all balancing inclines.

For diagnostic studies, one can minimize errors of the checkbite technique by making the protrusive and lateral bite records fairly close to centric relation. The most important part of the condylar path is right after the condyle leaves centric relation, so taking the eccentric bite records within

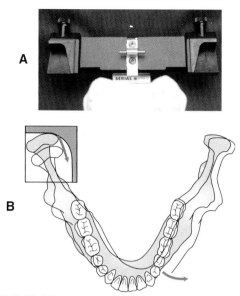

FIGURE 22-27 **A,** Condylar path inserts for the Combi articulator are contoured to provide a more progressive side shift than necessary. **B,** *Red arrow* shows maximum progressive side shift (toward midline) that was observed on more than 600 patients. Compare this with the path on the articulator. This excess clearance guarantees that restorations fabricated on the articulator will have no balancing side interferences in the patient if they have been cleared on the articulator. Simple but totally effective. With the exception of denture patients in which bilateral balance may be desired, there is never a need to take a lateral check bite to record the progressive side shift. On semiadjustable articulators, rotate the vertical alignment to 15 degrees, set it, and forget it.

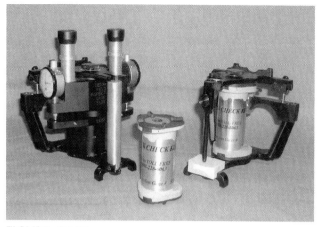

FIGURE 22-28 Dénar® (Water Pik, Inc.) field gauge *(left),* and the Check Key *(right).* Such devices ensure interchangeability of articulators without loss of accuracy.

about 5 mm from centric relation gives greater accuracy where it is needed most. The common practice of taking the protrusive bite record at incisor end-to-end relationship can increase the error in some patients. In patients with severe overjet, this may be too far protrusive. The checkbites should relate specifically to condylar paths for the first few millimeters of separation of the posterior teeth.

Semiadjustable instruments can often be set without the need for any checkbites. If the anterior teeth can maintain contact through the protrusive range in the patient, the condylar paths can be set on the articulator to permit the same protrusive contact. This is easily accomplished by mere steepening of the condylar path until the posterior teeth are just barely separated in protrusive excursions, allowing anterior contact.

If the patient's anterior teeth are separated by the posterior teeth in protrusion, this method cannot be used. This is an indication to use a more precise method for determining the condylar path.

If an arbitrary setting of 20 degrees for the condylar path is being used, it will not always disclude posterior teeth that do disclude in the mouth. If during examination of the patient you observe that the anterior teeth maintain contact through the protrusive range, the articulator paths are easily steepened until the posterior teeth just barely miss in protrusion. It is an advantage for the articulator to have adjustable condylar paths for this reason. The semiadjustable instrument thus

provides the practicality of set 20-degree condylar paths, with the simplicity of easy correction when needed.

New understanding about the benefits of posterior disclusion has made the semiadjustable articulator the standard instrument for any type of occlusal treatment. Setting the condylar path with a protrusive interocclusal bite record can be very close to the actual patient paths but with a slight safety margin that will only add beneficially to the desired disclusive effect.

Working-side excursions need to be related only to the lateral anterior guidance because there is no clinically significant change in lateral angulation from the canine incline back, except for the progressive shortening of the stroke.

Semiadjustable instruments do not record the precise paths of lateral and protrusive condylar movements, but by using any of the above methods, you can adjust the instrument to within a practical degree of accuracy for completely acceptable diagnostic uses. Its use as an instrument for restorative procedures can be more precise. This is because even though the exact condylar paths are not reproduced, the mechanical equivalent of jaw movements can be recorded with as much accuracy as is possible on any available instrument if the instrument's shortcomings are compensated for with the following:

1. Customized anterior guidance procedures (described in Chapter 18). This is necessary regardless of the adjustability of condylar guidances.
2. Simplified fossae contour technique to relate lower fossae form to the anterior guidance (described in Chapter 21).

There are several semiadjustable articulators that fill all the requirements for quality instrumentation. The instruments of choice in my practice for many years have been the Dénar® Combi and the Mark II (Figure 22-28). My reasons for selecting these instruments involve primarily the quality of workmanship and materials used. Because they have ma-

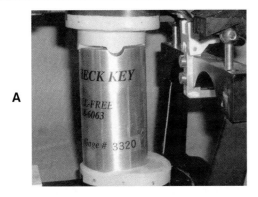

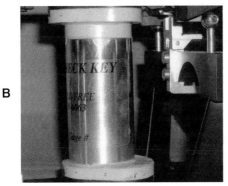

FIGURE 22-29   The Check Key (Comdent, Inc.) is a simplified economical device for maintaining interchangeability of Combi articulators. If the key lock does not fit perfectly **(A)**, the articulator set screws are released and then tightened after positioning the key in the keyway slots **(B)**.

chined parts, they can be interchangeable with the other articulators in the Dénar® system. The use of a simple checking device (Figure 22-29) enables my staff to keep all instruments aligned the same for an extremely practical interchangeability from any Dénar® articulator to another.

Other requirements for an acceptable semiadjustable instrument include the following:

1. Must accept a facebow.
2. Must have a positive centric lock.
3. Must have an adjustable incisal guide pin that permits changes in vertical dimension without moving the position of the pin on the guide table.
4. Must have provisions for a transferable customized anterior guide table.
5. Must permit the casts to be secured by removable mounting rings (preferably magnetic).
6. Must have horizontal condylar paths that are adjustable from 0 degrees to at least 45 degrees.
7. Must have a progressive side-shift path up to at least 15 degrees.
8. Must have an intercondylar width of approximately 110 mm. Adjustability of this dimension is not a critical factor.

Other desirable features for an articulator are the following:

1. Reasonable visibility from the lingual.
2. Easy cleanability.

3. Does not come apart accidentally.
4. Arcon-type condylar guide.

A final feature that I find very desirable is a design that permits easy removal of the upper bow from the lower section. Some clinicians prefer that the articulator not come apart. My preference for being able to remove the upper bow is that it is easier to work with one arch for some procedures without the cumbersomeness of stabilizing an open articulator. It also allows direct line removal of die models from bite records and makes it possible to verify the accuracy of the mounting with greater simplicity.

Set Path Articulators

Because a 20-degree horizontal and 15-degree lateral path works so well for achieving posterior disclusion in the majority of patients, articulators with set condylar paths have become very popular. Such instruments may have all features of an acceptable semiadjustable articulator except that the condylar paths cannot be adjusted. They must be able to accept a facebow for relating the casts to the correct horizontal axis.

The reason for the growing popularity of this type of instrument is solely related to cost. A set path instrument can be purchased for considerably less than an articulator with adjustable condylar paths because the machining of the movable paths is a costly process.

Unfortunately, most set path articulators also have a set anterior guide angle. This is unacceptable. Anterior guidance is never an arbitrary decision regardless of the type of articulator used; so there must be a provision for accepting a customized anterior guide table.

Although a set path instrument may be acceptable for a majority of restorative procedures, it is not adequate for diagnosis on some patients with occlusal plane problems or inadequate anterior guidance. Many patients have needs that require the condylar paths to be considered, and for these patients a set path articulator is not acceptable.

Combination Set Path or Fully Adjustable Instruments

The simplicity of a set path instrument can be enjoyed although it still has the capacity for complete adjustability when needed. This very practical combination can be found in a precisely machined instrument that, despite its much lower cost, fulfills all requirements for quality instrumentation. The Dénar® Combi articulator (see Figure 22-28) provides the option of either set path or full adjustment through the use of precisely machined inserts for condylar guidance and a simplified method for stereographic recording of condylar paths when needed. Through the use of a field gauge or simple key device, these instruments can also be kept aligned, so they can be used interchangeably or even with other instruments in the Dénar® system.

Because of its interchangeability, the Dénar® Combi can be used with set paths as a standard instrument for most restorative needs, but when changes in condylar path are necessary, the casts can either be transferred to a Mark II articulator or the condylar path inserts can be changed to accept a precise border path recording.

The set condylar path insert (Figure 22-30) has a horizontal inclination of 20 degrees, which makes it flatter than the minimal angulation found in healthy articulations. The lateral path is curved to a more medially directed path than the most severe progressive side shift. Use of this insert permits direct fabrication of posterior restorations that will automatically be discluded by all but the most abnormally contoured condylar paths as long as the correct anterior guidance is recorded.

The set condylar path insert can be used as the standard setting for the majority of restorative procedures. With the set path insert in place, the articulator can be used routinely without modification if the following two conditions are met:

1. The anterior teeth in the mouth disclude the posterior teeth in excursions from maximum intercuspation.
2. The posterior teeth on the mounted casts are discluded by the anterior teeth in excursions from maximum intercuspation.

When the above two conditions are met, the instrument can be used for either treatment planning or restorative procedures without altering the set 20-degree path.

For restorative patients, minor alteration of the casts will sometimes be necessary to achieve posterior disclusion on a 20-degree set path articulator. If all posterior teeth are in need of restoration, this should not cause a problem for any patient whose anterior teeth maintain contact during protrusion.

Even if the anterior teeth are separated in the mouth during protrusion, it may not necessarily rule out the simplified approach of set path instrumentation. If anterior excursive contact can be achieved on the casts by occlusal plane corrections that do not require excessive posterior tooth reduction, there are no contraindications to using the set path articulator for patients who require restorations on all posterior teeth.

The adjustable path insert

For the analysis of some occlusal relationships, the set 20-degree path is not adequate. The safest rule for using the adjustable path insert for precise duplication of condylar paths is to use it for occlusal analysis whenever the anterior teeth are discluded by the posterior teeth. However, the following conditions specifically indicate the need for a nonarbitrary condylar path analysis:

1. Protrusive disclusion of anterior teeth when posterior teeth do not need restorations.
2. Restorative cases that would require severe changes to establish an "ideal" arbitrary occlusal plane.
3. Severely worn dentitions, especially when the upper lingual cusps have been worn flat and the anterior guidance is also flat.

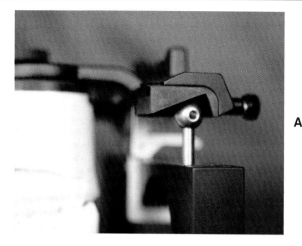
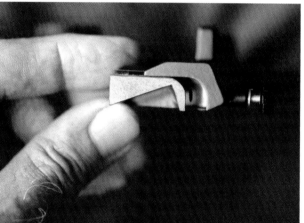

FIGURE 22-30 A, A 20-degree condylar path insert can be used as a set path articulator for many occlusal problems. B, If the condylar path needs to be steepened, the 20-degree insert can be removed and replaced with a different path.

Instrumentation When Posterior Teeth Disclude Anterior Teeth and Posterior Restorative Dentistry Is Not Necessary

For interfering posterior teeth that do not require restorations, the decision to drastically change their shape should not be an arbitrary one. A major purpose of occlusal analysis is to determine how best to achieve posterior disclusion. To accomplish this goal with the minimum amount of tooth reduction, we must take full advantage of the disclusive effect by the condyles. The steeper they move downward, the more they help separate the posterior teeth when the jaw protrudes, and the less reduction of tooth structure will be needed. The only way we can predetermine the amount of occlusal alteration required to achieve posterior disclusion is to know the actual condylar paths.

When posterior disclusion is lacking, it can be achieved by equilibration in some occlusions, or lowering of the occlusal plane at the posterior teeth orthodontically or steepening of the anterior guidance, or a combination of treatment choices. If disclusion is achieved by steepening of the

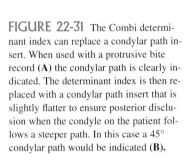

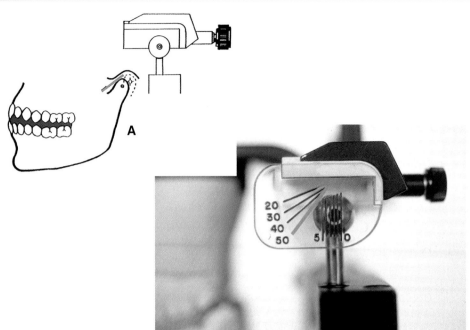

FIGURE 22-31 The Combi determinant index can replace a condylar path insert. When used with a protrusive bite record (**A**) the condylar path is clearly indicated. The determinant index is then replaced with a condylar path insert that is slightly flatter to ensure posterior disclusion when the condyle on the patient follows a steeper path. In this case a 45° condylar path would be indicated (**B**).

anterior guidance, it is possible to create a damaging restriction of functional paths. The determination of how much change is needed for the anterior guidance is dependent on how much disclusive help is possible from the condylar path and how much reduction is permitted for the posterior teeth without destroying too much enamel. *The adjustable condylar path should be used whenever formulation of a conservative treatment plan depends on a pretreatment determination of the precise amount of posterior tooth reduction required to achieve posterior disclusion (Figure 22-31).*

Setting protrusive path on semiadjustable articulators with a mechanical condylar path

PROCEDURE   Setting horizontal condylar inclination

All photographs courtesy of Great Lakes Orthodontics, Ltd., Tonawanda, New York.

With track instruments, the setting of the condylar path requires altering the horizontal inclination until the casts fit perfectly into a bite record made with the mandible protruded.

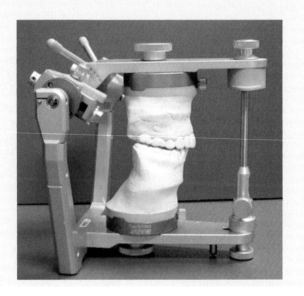

PROCEDURE   Setting horizontal condylar inclination—cont'd

Cast mounted in centric relation to 30 degrees horizontal condylar inclination.

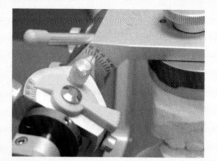

Unlock centric locking hubs.

Loosen condylar inclination screws.

Place protrusive bite between casts.

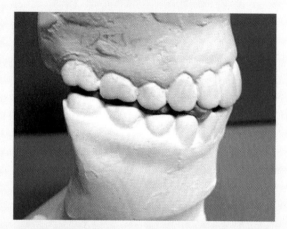

Rotate condylar housing to a point where the models seat perfectly in the wax bite.

Tighten condylar housing screws.

Repeat on the opposite side.

The horizontal condylar housing is now set.

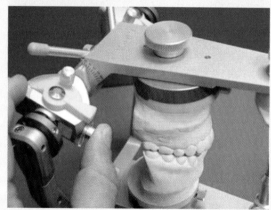

Setting Bennett angulation (side shift)

Loosen Bennett screws.

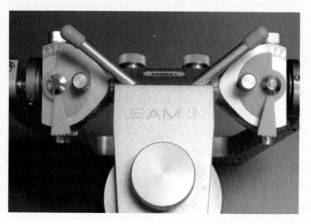

Continued

Unlock centric locking hubs.

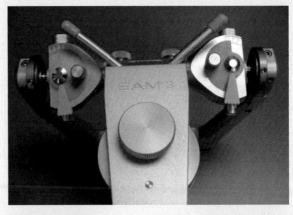

Note: The dentist must remove the standard straight Bennett insert and replace it with a green Bennett insert.

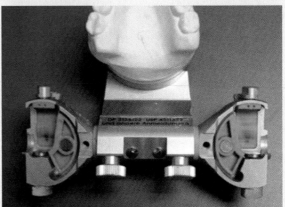

Place the bite with lateral side shift between the models (shift to patient's left sets right insert, etc.).

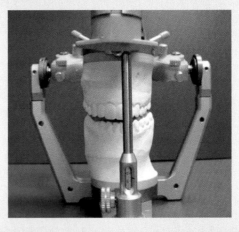

Tighten Bennett screws.

Repeat with the next bite.

The Bennett insert is now set.

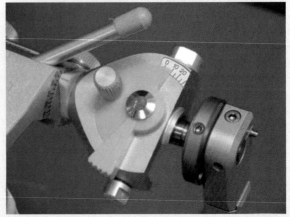

USING INSTRUMENTS TO ADVANTAGE: A SUMMARY

A great amount of time is often wasted on procedures that have little or no value on specific cases. The intelligent use of instrumentation can provide preciseness when it is needed and simplicity when simpler approaches are sufficient to satisfy the actual needs of a given case. By understanding the relationship of condylar movements to specific tooth inclines, you can use the articulator to serve the specific needs of occlusal contouring rather than an overriding concern for precise condylar paths whether they affect the outcome or not.

> A better understanding of the effects of posterior disclusion has simplified demands for precise condylar path recordings.

If posterior disclusion is desired in all excursions, setting the articulator with wider lateral paths and flatter horizontal paths helps to accomplish the disclusive effect. No negative consequences will arise from doing this.

If disclusion in any excursion is desired, the amount of miss is not critical. Variations in disclusive separation do not seem to be discernible as far as function or stability is concerned.

If Group Function Is Desired on the Working Side

If the anterior teeth are not able to achieve the lateral guidance for disclusion of the posterior teeth, the most forward tooth that can contact should be selected to serve as the lateral anterior guidance incline. The working-side posterior inclines should then be brought into group function with the forward tooth. We used to think that this would require precise recording of the condylar paths, but our study of the three-dimensional functional path model showed that harmonizing the upper working-side inclines to the lateral anterior guidance of the most forward tooth that contacts in centric relation will produce group function contact on all posterior teeth that are distal to it. This can be accomplished almost regardless of the condylar path because the condylar path on the working-side has no clinically significant effect on the path of the lower posterior teeth on the working side. The lateral anterior guidance is the dominant determinant.

What was believed in the past was that there was an immediate side shift of the mandible before or during the initial lateral excursion toward the working side. This concept has been clearly disproved and is easily demonstrated on gothic arch tracings, as well as by examination of the anatomy that prevents the medial poles of the condyles from any straight horizontal shift from centric relation.

Articulators that incorporate an immediate side shift into the condylar paths will affect the path from centric relation of the lower teeth on the casts. That path will be incorporated into the occlusal surfaces of restorations when they are

fabricated. This will not create an interference on the restorations. It will cause working side inclines to separate when the restorations are placed in the patient. For this reason, a side shift on an articulator is not suitable for fabricating group function on restorations.

The Dénar® Mark II articulators used in my practice for many years have a mechanical adjustment for incorporating an immediate side shift. Many years ago, we set every articulator at 0° side shift to eliminate all immediate side shifts. This does not eliminate a progressive side shift from occurring, as the balancing-side condyle translates down its protrusive path.

An immediate side shift on an articulator is not representative of true condylar paths. It is thus an unnecessary mechanical addition that adds expense and complexity to the manufacture of instrumentation. The wide choice of semi-adjustable articulators that do not have an immediate side shift can serve the needs of restorative and prosthodontic treatment with no compromise required.

There are many articulators from which to choose. A comfortable instrument that is a quality product should be selected. It is an advantage to determine the type of instrument you wish to work with and then stay with the same type as much as possible. This enables you to standardize your procedures at the chair and in the laboratory. Working with instruments that are interchangeable with each other and with other instruments in a system is a decided advantage.

No articulator should be considered that does not accept a facebow orientation of the casts. The cost of articulators varies widely. It pays to carefully compare quality of workmanship and simplicity of use. Do not be misled that the bigger or more massive an articulator is, the more valuable it is; and recognize that any articulator is only required to do the essential movements described here. There is no reason to complicate instrumentation beyond those requirements.

Simple hinge-type articulators are limited only to movements the patient cannot make. They are a cause of major errors in occlusal contouring and have no value for restorative procedures or occlusal analysis.

Suggested Readings

Bennett NG: A contribution to the study of the movements of the mandible, *Proc Soc Med (Odontol)* 1:79, 1908; reprinted in *J Prosthet Dent* 8:41, 1958.

Levinson E: The nature of the side shift in lateral mandibular movement and its implications in clinical practice, *J Prosthet Dent* 52:1, 1984.

Lundeen H: Condylar movement patterns engraved in plastic blocks, *J Prosthet Dent* 30(6):866-875, 1973.

Ricketts RM: *Orthodontic diagnosis and planning: Their roles in preventative and rehabilitative dentistry.* Denver, 1982, Rocky Mountain Orthodontic.

Solberg WK, Clark GT: Reproducibility of molded condylar controls with an intraoral registration method. Part I. Simulated movement, *J Prosthet Dent* 32:520, 1974; Part II. Human jaw movement, *J Prosthet Dent* 33:60, 1975.

Swanson KH: A new method of recording gnathological movements, *Northwest Dent* 45:99-101, 1966.

Swanson KH, Wipf Articulator Company (TMJ) Articulator Manual, Thousand Oaks, California.

Dysfunction

Chapter 23

Differential Diagnosis of Temporomandibular Disorders

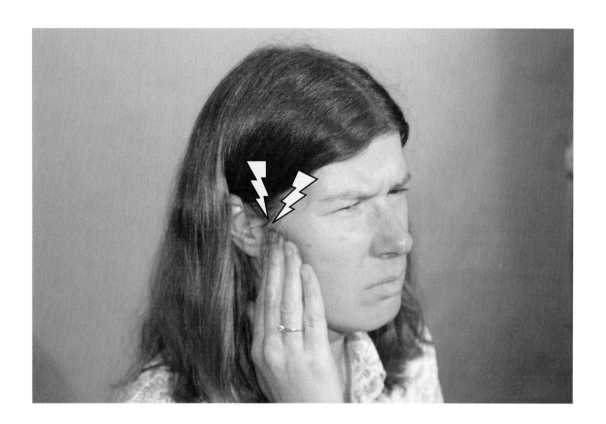

PRINCIPLE

FIRST . . . make a diagnosis.

MAKING SENSE OF TERMINOLOGY

> **Disorder:** A disturbance of function, structure or both.
> —*Stedman's Concise Medical Dictionary*

Temporomandibular Disorder

Temporomandibular disorder (TMD) is any disorder that affects or is affected by deformity, disease, misalignment, or dysfunction of the temporomandibular articulation. This includes occlusal deflection of the temporomandibular joints (TMJs) and the associated responses in the musculature.

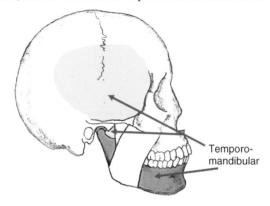

Temporo-mandibular

It is doubtful that any term in the dental literature has created more confusion and more negative consequences than the improper use of the term *TMD*. The term, as used in a profuse amount of literature, in etiologic studies, and in much of dental education, has been in the context of a single, multifactorial syndrome that includes disorders that are unrelated to the temporomandibular articulation and are often even unrelated to any masticatory system consideration. Even when TMD is shown to occur in different forms, or when variations of symptoms are categorized, such categorizations have typically been clustered into a syndrome rather than as distinctly different and specific types of disorders with different etiologies requiring specifically directed treatment.

The definition for TMD that was presented by the National Institute of Health Technology Assessment Conference on Management of TMD (1996) illustrates the terminology problem that must be corrected:

> *"Depending on the practitioner and the diagnostic methodology, the term TMD has been used to characterize a wide range of conditions diversely presented as pain in the face or jaw joint area, limited mouth opening, closed or open lock of the TMJ, abnormal occlusal wear, clicking or popping sounds in the jaw joints, and other complaints."*

As long as this hodgepodge of many different and often unrelated problems is treated as a single disease labeled TMD, the controversy will continue. For this reason, use of the TMD label should be limited to specific disorders of the temporomandibular articulation. These disorders include displacement of one or both joints, misalignment of the disk, various diseases that affect bone or the articular surfaces, and other pathologic disorders, inflammation, or injuries to specific intracapsular structures.

Occlusal disharmony that affects the position of the TMJs, and disorders of the masticatory musculature are also included as specific types of TMDs. The rule to follow is simple and straightforward:

> Never use the term *TMD* without specific classification of the exact type of disorder being discussed, and the structures that are affected.

Craniomandibular Disorder

Craniomandibular disorder (CMD) is any disorder that involves the relationship of the mandible to the cranial base. It may or may not be related to disorders of the TMJ. Thus CMD cannot be considered as synonymous with TMD.

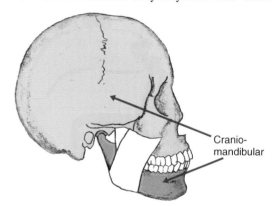

Cranio-mandibular

Common misuse of the term *CMD* has caused great confusion as it is often used as a descriptive term for an entire group of symptoms represented as a multifactorial syndrome. Actually, CMDs include many different disorders with different signs and symptoms, and different etiologies. Each disorder may be multifactorial. Treating CMDs as a syndrome without a differential diagnosis to determine the specific type of disorder is a serious but common mistake that has fostered many misconceptions regarding pain associated with masticatory system structures.

Use of CMD as synonymous with TMD fails to recognize that CMDs can occur in patients with normal, healthy, and symptom-free TMJs.

Masticatory System Disorder

Masticatory system disorder (MSD) is any disorder of the masticatory system structures that is associated with dysfunction, discomfort, or deformation of any part or parts of the total masticatory system. Use of this term should always be accompanied by the identification of the specific structures that are disordered.

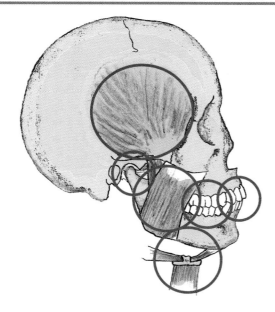

The masticatory system, dentistry's responsibility, includes all of the circled structural components that are common sources of pain. It must be remembered that none of these circled areas is independent of the others. Disequilibrium between parts of the system is a common trigger for pain. The neurologic complex, the vascular system, and the cellular basis for other important structural components are not shown in this illustration, but their significance to pain or dysfunction analysis should not be minimized.

The Glossary of Prosthodontic Terms defines the masticatory system as the organs and structures primarily functioning in mastication.[1] These include the teeth with their supporting structures, craniomandibular articulations, maxilla, mandible, positioning and accessory musculature, tongue, lips, cheeks, oral mucosa, and the associated neurologic complex.

To this definition we will add the vascular complex and the salivary glands, as they are part of the masticatory system and potential sources of orofacial pain.

Evaluation of head, neck, or orofacial pain must include examination to determine if the source of pain is in any masticatory system structures. The strategy for diagnosis depends on an analysis of each part of the system to ascertain if there is deformation or dysfunction.

I strongly advocate use of this terminology (MSD) in combination with labeling of the type and condition of specific structural components being discussed. As an example, MSDs must be differentiated from intracapsular disorders. Even though both types of disorders often occur simultaneously, their etiologies and treatment must be evaluated separately. Nevertheless, because of the almost universal use of the term *TMD* in the literature, we will use that terminology to avoid confusion when describing disorders that specifically relate to the temporomandibular complex.

Readers of the literature should be wary of any attempt to misuse either the TMD or MSD terminology in the context

of a syndrome. Each is a collective term that connotes many different types of disorders that require differentiation.

Getting Specific About Diagnosis

It is axiomatic that you cannot have a stable occlusion with unstable TMJs. Therefore, it is also axiomatic that before extensive occlusal changes are initiated, the condition of the TMJs must be known. Today, more than ever before, the condition of the temporomandibular articulation can be determined with specificity. Furthermore, every type of intracapsular disorder can be classified, and the classification can be verified. The advancement of imaging technology makes it almost impossible for a structural disorder of the TMJs to hide from an astute diagnostician. By matching up specific signs and symptoms with specific structural disorders, the mystery has been taken out of diagnosis and treatment for TMDs.

> The concept of TMD as a "syndrome" of unknown etiology is obsolete.

Improved information about the anatomy and physiology of the TMJs has been combined with new insights into the adaptive capacity of different tissues. Objective analysis has replaced the need for subjective opinions and has encouraged more specificity regarding what is wrong, not only in the joints, but also in the structural elements that relate to the joint. Thus the clinician can design treatment approaches aimed at correcting specific causes in addition to treating symptoms.

The problem with so many of the past treatment approaches is that covering up symptoms without correcting causes allows structural disorders to progress. This is a significant shortcoming of a limited focus on symptomatic treatment because most masticatory system disorders are progressive. The longer the causative factors are ignored, the more damage is done.

Analysis of Orofacial Pain

A narrow focus on pain is shortsighted if it ignores the cause of the pain. Unfortunately, the "syndrome" mentality for describing TMD in all-inclusive terms lumps so many different disorders into the syndrome, it is impossible to be specific about a treatment. For any treatment approach to be effective, it must identify each specific disorder and isolate the factors that either cause the disorder or contribute to its intensity or duration. This approach is not as problematic as it may sound. In fact, the most logical way to simplify any treatment protocol is to first identify what it is that is being treated. *First, we make a diagnosis.*

There is an orderly process for the diagnosis of orofacial pain. That process is just as practical for the general practitioner as it is for the specialist. The process starts with an understanding of the signal that is sent by pain. The definition of pain is "a response to tissue damage." If there is pain within the masticatory system, including the region of the TMJs, the first step in analysis should be to determine *What is the source of the pain?*

The confusion surrounding diagnosis and treatment of TMD is primarily the result of not asking that question. Diagnosis can be simplified by recognition that pain within the masticatory system is almost always a response to some form of structural disorder. In most pain responses, the source of the pain is in the tissue that has been structurally altered, or has been functionally affected by some form of structural alteration. A logical diagnostic process requires a structure by structure analysis to determine which tissues are a source of pain. As examples: Which tooth aches? Which muscles are sore? Which intracapsular structures are painful?

There are exceptions to the source of pain being at the site of pain. It is important to recognize the role of sympathetic sources of pain such as referred pain or complex regional pain syndrome (CRPS). Nevertheless, even the diagnosis of complex pain patterns should be focused on finding a connection between the site of pain and its potential sources. If diagnostic protocols are focused on finding the source of pain, it will become apparent that TMD and other MSDs can be diagnosed and classified with specificity. If that is done properly, it will almost always eliminate a diagnosis of psychosocial stress as a primary cause. That is the diagnosis that too often results from not defining the sources of pain. A search for the source of pain is always a logical starting point.

Analysis of Structural Deformation

It is a mistake to think that TMD is only about pain. Pain is a common symptom of structural deformation, but not all structural deformation causes pain. That is why the differential diagnosis of TMDs must look for signs as well as symptoms.

Signs are commonly found whenever there is disharmony within the masticatory system. Whenever there are signs, there may or may not be symptoms.

Signs usually precede symptoms because some type of structural disorder is almost always responsible for activating awareness of pain or discomfort. Reliance on symptoms alone can allow structural damage to progress unnecessarily. As an example, signs of periodontal disease are observable to a careful clinician long before a patient feels symptoms. Patients are frequently unaware of deep carious lesions until pulpal involvement results in an abscess. Likewise, damage from severe occlusal wear can nearly destroy some dentitions without patients being aware of the consequences. Undiagnosed cracks can become split teeth. Masticatory system tumors can become inoperable, and TMJ deformation can produce severe facial asymmetries if early signs are not diagnosed.

An astute diagnostician can learn much by listening to patients, but will miss much if careful observation and attention to signs is not given the attention it deserves.

> **Key point**
> Signs: Indication of disease or disorder. Signs are objective evidence that is perceptible to the examiner.
>
> Symptoms: Subjective evidence of disease of condition perceived by the patient. Usually expressed as pain or dysfunction.

Observe the mechanism of occlusal disharmony with particular emphasis on how disharmony creates muscle hyperactivity, which in turn focuses its compressive and tensive forces on the intracapsular structures of the TMJs and the teeth. The trigger for muscle hyperactivity is almost always related in some way to deflective occlusal interferences (signs) that activate muscle via the mechanoreceptor sensory system (Figure 23-1). The damage can be intensified by bruxing on the deflective inclines of the teeth. As muscle overloads the joints and the teeth, the weakest link receives the most structural damage (signs), but the muscles are often the primary focus of pain (symptoms). This is the mindset a clinician must have in order to correlate both signs and symptoms and evaluate all factors when making a diagnosis.

Collateral damage

If diagnosis of TMD reveals that the source of pain is primarily in the joints, it is never a reason for stopping the investigation there. If there is deformation in the TMJ structures, there will almost always be signs of attrition, hypermobility, abfractions, or cracks in the teeth; there will virtually always be signs and/or symptoms in the musculature. In occluso-muscle disharmonies, a search for the cause of muscle pain will lead to tooth interferences as the trigger, while the musculature will in turn be the cause of damage to the teeth.

The point that should not be missed is that masticatory system disorders are rarely ever confined to a single structure. There will almost always be collateral effects from disorder in the joints, the teeth, or the muscles. These will be evident as signs or symptoms. Careful observation will usually show that there is a chain of cause-and-effect reactions as one disorder leads to another.

TMDs can be classified in many different ways. For the practicing clinician, the most logical approach to diagnosis is to recognize that the most likely sources of TMD pain or dysfunction can be separated into three broad categories. Each category should be studied in detail to determine if it is a possible source of pain or dysfunction. TMDs can be classified broadly as follows:

1. Masticatory muscle disorders
2. Structural intracapsular disorders
3. Conditions that mimic TMDs

It is imperative that all three classifications be considered when one is evaluating any suspected TMD because combinations of two of all three problems can and do occur. Furthermore, one type of problem can cause or be caused by

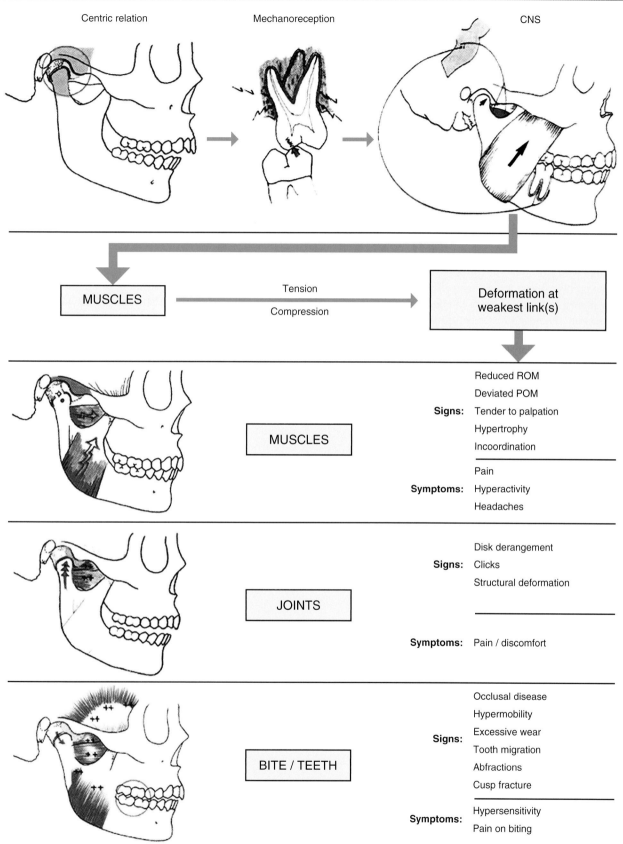

FIGURE 23-1 **Mechanism for deformation.** Occlusal interference to centric relation activates mechanoreceptor sensors in and around roots of teeth that interfere with coordinated muscle action during deflected closure to maximum intercuspation. The results are incoordination and hyperactivity of the masticatory muscles, which in turn activate compressive and tensive forces on the points and the teeth. Deformation occurs at the weakest links to produce signs and symptoms that must be specifically characterized.

a different type of problem. As an example, a disk derangement will almost always be accompanied by a masticatory muscle response. It must be determined whether muscle incoordination activated the disk derangement or vice versa. The role of occlusal interferences must always be evaluated whenever masticatory muscle pain or dysfunction is present because it is so often a factor that must be corrected as part of the treatment for other TMD symptoms or signs.

An in-depth description of the two most common causes of TMD is covered in Chapters 24 and 25. A broader classification is helpful for understanding important interrelationships.

CATEGORIES OF TMDs

In diagnosing the suspected TMD patient, it is essential to determine which of four categories best describes the disorder. The options for treatment, as well as the prognosis, are clearly related to the category of the disorder. More specific classification should be made before the diagnosis can be considered complete; but assigning each TMD to one of the categories in Box 23-1 facilitates discussion and simplifies understanding of the differences in signs, symptoms, and patient response.

Key point
Choice of treatment and results of treatment are clearly related to the category of the TMD.

The classification in Box 23-1 covers most of the TMDs that are commonly seen by the dentist. Further differentiation is needed for each category, but even with that proviso, it may seem that the role of occlusal disharmony is overstated. Clinical experience on properly classified patients

Box 23-1	Categories of TMD
Category 1	Occluso-muscle disorders with no intracapsular defects.
Category 2	Intracapsular disorders that are directly related to occlusal disharmony and are reversible in re-establishing comfortable function if the occlusion is corrected.
Category 3	Intracapsular disorders that are not reversible, but because of adaptive changes, can function comfortably if occluso-muscle harmony is re-established.
Category 4	Nonadapted intracapsular disorders that may be either primary or secondary to occlusal disharmony or may be unrelated.

confirms that occlusal disharmony is a demonstrable factor in selected categories of TMD. By classifying MSDs more specifically, the role of occlusion can be analyzed more accurately to determine when occlusal disharmony is or is not a factor.

The most common source of orofacial pain and dysfunction that can be associated with TMDs is *occluso-muscle pain/dysfunction.* Every practicing dentist should understand its signs, its symptoms, and its possible collateral effects on the teeth, the TMJs, and the musculature. There is hardly an aspect of dentistry that is not related in some way to the cause or correction of occluso-muscle disorders.

Reference

1. The Academy of Prosthodontics: *The Glossary of Prosthodontic Terms.* St Louis, 1968, Mosby.

Chapter 24

Occluso-Muscle Disorders

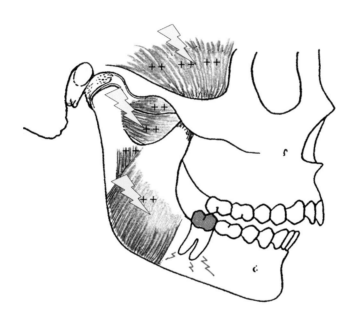

PRINCIPLE

Most temporomandibular disorder (TMD) pain is not temporomandibular joint (TMJ) pain. Most TMD pain is masticatory muscle pain triggered by deflective occlusal interferences.

Occluso-muscle disorder: Discomfort or dysfunction resulting from hyperactive, incoordinated muscle function that is triggered by deflective occlusal interferences to physiologic jaw movements and noxious habits.

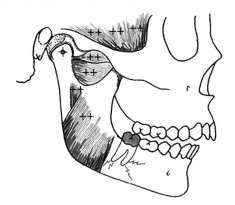

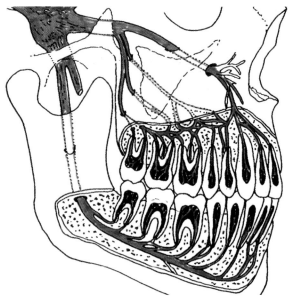

FIGURE 24-1 The effect of occlusal interferences is monitored by one of the most exquisitely innervated sensory systems in the body. Sensory input to the neuromuscular system is programmed via a major allocation of one of the largest cranial nerves. The trigeminal nerve provides an intensive network of reflex responders throughout the periodontal ligaments as well as the innumerable odontoblastic sensory units within the teeth. The system is so exquisitely sensitive that it is capable of responding to the most minute occlusal interferences by activating reflex protective muscle patterns that if prolonged can become a source of myogenous pain.

It is significant that the most common and most correctable cause of orofacial pain is not defined in dental glossaries. Occluso-muscle disorders are, without doubt, the most prevalent cause of orofacial pain. Even in tertiary pain patients, occluso-muscle pain is the most common finding. Occluso-muscle pain is also the most misunderstood and the most ignored of all the masticatory system disorders.

In addition to a variety of painful symptoms in the musculature itself, masticatory muscle incoordination and hyperactivity, triggered by occlusal interferences, can also cause or intensify pain in other structures. Premature or overloaded tooth contact can cause severe pain in teeth, intensify the pain of sinusitis, activate tension headaches (particularly in the temporal muscle region), simulate ear pain because of the proximity of spastic lateral pterygoid muscles, affect the alignment of the disk on the condyle, or cause painful displacement of the TMJs. Pain in muscle that is hyperactivated by occlusal disharmony can be intense enough to obscure the pain of an abscessed tooth or other unrelated pathology (Figure 24-1).

Because occluso-muscle pain often occurs as a separate layer of pain in combination with intracapsular disorders or other pain sources, evaluation for occluso-muscle pain must be a separate step in diagnosis.

It is not possible to fully assess the role of occluso-muscle disorder without *determining first whether centric relation or adapted centric posture can be achieved.* A specific clarification of the position and condition of the jaw joints is the essential starting point for diagnosis.

If any disorder of the masticatory system should be understood by every dentist, it would be difficult to select one that causes more unresolved problems for dentists and patients than *occluso-muscle pain.*

Occluso-muscle pain is not an esoteric disorder. It is a common everyday problem in every dental practice. It is unfortunate that it is so often undiagnosed or misdiagnosed because it is so easy to determine if it is responsible for pain, discomfort, or dysfunction. The signs and symptoms

of occluso-muscle disorder are obvious to any clinician who knows what to look for. Furthermore, an occluso-muscle disorder can be specifically diagnosed, even in the presence of multiple other causes for pain or dysfunction. When there are multiple etiologies, it is practical to differentiate the role of occluso-muscle pain to ascertain if it is responsible for some, all, or none of the pain. The process is logical, practical, and easily learned.

Because occluso-muscle pain always involves the relationship between the TMJs and occlusal contacts, it is necessary to relate occlusal contacts to the completely seated condylar position. So the starting point is always to determine if the TMJs are healthy and capable of complete seating into centric relation or adapted centric posture.

HOW TO DETERMINE IF THE TMJS ARE HEALTHY

Before the occlusion can be evaluated, the TMJs must be evaluated to ensure that they are in an acceptably healthy condition and that the condyle-disk alignment and position is okay. The condyles must be free to go to and from centric relation without discomfort. If there is a problem with either TMJ, it must be resolved to the best degree that is practical before occlusal problems can be resolved. It must be remembered that all occlusal relationships are also relationships with the TMJs. Harmonizing the occlusion to a misaligned joint simply perpetuates a disharmony.

Six ways to verify that the TMJs are healthy

1. Screening history. Every patient should be asked key questions about the TMJs before treating. See the list of questions in this chapter.

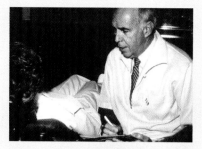

2. Load test. For verification of comfort in centric relation or adapted centric posture. Any sign of tension or tenderness warrants further evaluation. (Review Chapter 10.)

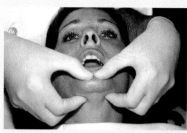

3. Range and path of movement tests. Normal range is 10-14 mm in protrusive. About 10 mm toward right and left. Maximum opening without discomfort is about 40-60 mm.

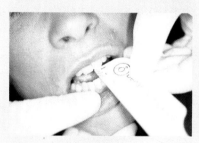

4. Doppler analysis. An intact healthy joint is quiet on rotation and translation.

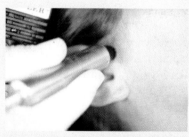

5. Radiography/imaging. Not necessary if other tests and history are negative. Selection of type of imaging should be based on signs and symptoms.

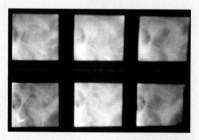

6. Anterior bite plane for muscle deprogramming. Can be used to determine if occlusion is a factor and to determine if an intracapsular disorder is contributing to the pain. If a flat, permissive anterior bite plane does not relieve pain or discomfort at the TMJs, suspect an intracapsular disorder as a source of pain.

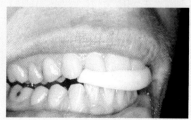

Box 24-1	Chart for Obvious Occlusal-Muscle Disorder		
Load test of TMJs negative		Y	N
Doppler normal		Y	N
Centric relation can be verified		Y	N
Occlusal interferences to centric relation		Y	N
Masticatory muscles tender to palpation		Y	N
Normal radiograph		Y	N

If all answers are YES, suspect that the problem is occluso-muscle disorder with no intracapsular disorder.

A negative history, normal range and path of motion, and negative response to load testing (i.e., zero tension or tenderness) typically indicates no intracapsular TMDs. Complete release of discomfort when an anterior deprogramming splint is in place indicates a probable occluso-muscle disorder.

It is not necessary to use all six methods if no problem is suspected. Specific methods should be selected in response to the patient's history or suspected problems.

If extensive restorative or orthodontic treatment is to be started, Doppler auscultation is recommended, even if other tests are negative (Box 24-1).

Screening History

In your examination, look for "red flags" that are indicative of problems. If you find a red flag, explore it further. There is no need to waste time on areas in which you find no signs or symptoms of any problems. However, do not rely only on what the patient says. You must look for signs (Box 24-2). Remember, signs precede symptoms.

DIAGNOSING OCCLUSO-MUSCLE PAIN WITH NO TMD

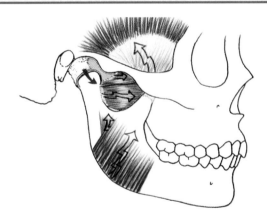

Learning to separate occluso-muscle pain from a TMD is an essential part of differentiating types of pain and can cause diverse side effects such as headaches and neck aches. It is important to examine each aspect of the pain in search of its cause. This can be done effectively by following a six-step procedure outlined in the following box.

Box 24-2	How to Examine Your Patient	
Muscles:	ASK...	Do you have frequent headaches? If so, where and how often?
	ASK...	Do you have any soreness in your muscles? If so, where and when? What causes or relieves the soreness?
Joints:	ASK...	Have you ever been injured? Provide details.
	ASK...	Do you experience any joint noises, pops, or clicks? Do you have any pain or discomfort? Does your jaw ever lock open or closed? Do you have any other joint concerns?
Bite/Teeth:	ASK...	Have you noticed any changes in your bite? Is your bite completely comfortable? Can you bite hard with no discomfort? Does any tooth hurt when you bite?
	Look for...	Any worn teeth, Any broken teeth, Any loose teeth, Abfractions — Show patient
	ASK...	Do you have any bite or tooth concerns?
Esthetics:	ASK...	How do you feel about the appearance of your teeth/smile?

Note: In many patients, esthetic concerns are the result of various forms of occlusal disease. It is helpful to tie in the reasons for esthetic problems with the advantages of correcting progressive destructive disease.

PROCEDURE   Separating occluso-muscle pain from TMJ pain

Step 1: Determine whether any masticatory muscle is involved in the pain. Is the medial pterygoid muscle tender to palpation? The medial pterygoid muscle is diagnostic because it is almost always tender to some degree if there is an occluso-muscle disorder.

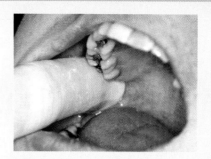

Step 2: Rule out intracapsular problems. Verify that centric relation or adapted centric posture can be achieved. Load testing *must* be negative.

Step 3: Relate the specific muscle pain to the direction of condyle displacement.
a. Find and verify centric relation
b. Locate the occlusal deflection
c. Relate it to the direction of condyle displacement from centric relation
d. Disclude the occlusal factor to test muscle response

An anterior deprogramming device, cotton roll, or aqualizer can be placed to allow complete seating of the TMJs by separating the deflective occlusal interferences.

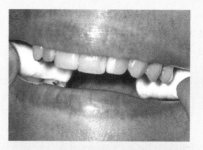

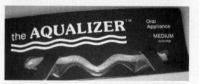

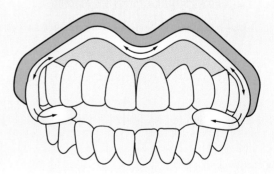

Continued

PROCEDURE   Separating occluso-muscle pain from TMJ pain—cont'd

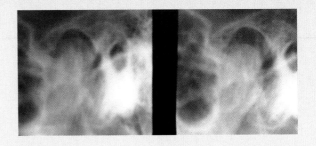

Step 4: Verify the general acceptability of condyle position and condition with TMJ radiographs if warranted.

Note: Precise positioning for centric is not achievable by radiographs.

Comparative transcranial films show the condyle fully seated in centric relation versus the condyle down and forward during maximum intercuspation (right). This relates to comfort in the centric relation position versus muscle pain in the displaced position when the teeth are clenched.

See also Chapter 27 for other imaging options.

Step 5: Rule out pathologic factors as a source of pain.
a. Pulpal
b. Periodontal
c. Soft-tissue
d. Bone
e. Sympathetic and/or referred pain

Even if a definite diagnosis of occluso-muscle pain can be ascertained, it is still important to carefully look for additional sources of pain. A dramatic reduction in pain levels often follows occlusal correction, but that in itself does not rule out other sources of pain. If all pain in the joints and musculature is not eliminated by an anterior deprogramming device or a completed occlusal correction, it is probable that an additional pain source exists and must be located. See Chapters 25 and 26 for diagnosis and classification of intracapsular disorders.

Step 6: Correct the cause of the problem.
a. *Reversibly* with permissive occlusal splint, or
b. *Directly* with occlusal correction
    Options for treatment:
    ○ Equilibration
    ○ Restorative
    ○ Orthodontics
    ○ Surgery

Examine Range of Motion

Two factors limit normal range of motion (ROM):
1. Muscle hypercontraction
2. Joint immobility due to an intracapsular disorder

Observe for smooth, symmetrical, nonlimited movement of wide, left, right, and protrusive openings (Figure 24-2).

General normals: wide   40-50 mm
                    lateral   7-15 mm
                    protrusive 7-15 mm

Maximum rotation only opening ≤ 20-25 mm; wider opening requires translation.

Opening movement that favors one side indicates limited translation of the condyle on that side.

When problems are present, differentiate comfortable versus maximal opening, and ask what the patient feels when opening maximally.

Wiggling movements on initial opening are usually related to disk displacements and attempts to recapture the disk.

Palpating the joints with light fingertip pressure is a good way to check for obvious clicks or crepitus while observing ROM.

What Muscle Palpation Tells Us

The standard screening exam for TMDs includes palpation of the masticatory muscles. Muscle tenderness can almost always be related to hyperactivity of the muscle as a result of overworking it in an incoordinated manner. A muscle is overworked when it is required to constantly hold the jaw in an avoidance pattern during closure to maximum intercuspation. Analysis of which muscles are sore should be related to the direction of mandibular displacement at tooth contact. If the deflective tooth incline relates to the muscles that are tender to palpation, it is an indication of occluso-muscle pain (Figure 24-3).

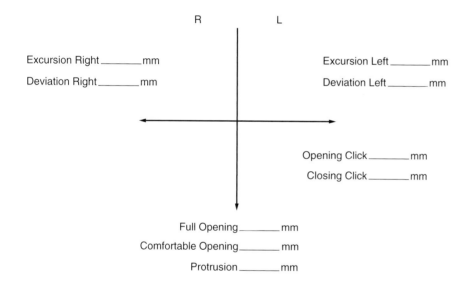

FIGURE 24-2 Range of mandibular motion measurements.

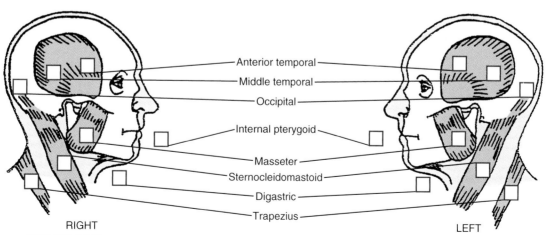

FIGURE 24-3 Standard chart for grading the masticatory muscles for degree of tenderness. This should be part of a routine screening exam on all new patients, especially if occlusal treatment is contemplated or if the patient complains of orofacial pain or discomfort.

MASTICATORY MUSCLE RESPONSES

Internal pterygoid muscle. Palpation of the internal pterygoid muscle has the greatest clinical significance for occluso-muscle imbalance. It is easy to palpate, and it has a direct correlation with the direction of displacement of the
same side condyle. The lateral pterygoid is the main positioner muscle but it is not easily palpated. The internal pterygoid is a dependable diagnostic landmark in that it is almost
always tender to palpation if the same side condyle must displace to achieve maximum intercuspation of the teeth.

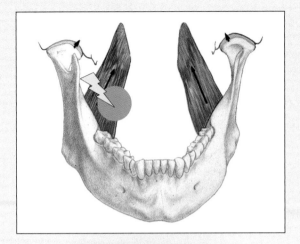

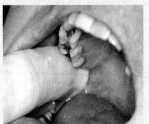

Superficial masseter muscle. Tenderness to palpation almost always indicates some degree of occlusal interference
that requires displacement of the same side condyle to
achieve maximum intercuspation. The muscle may feel
quite enlarged/hypertrophied in strong clenchers and bruxers. Tenderness and restricted opening in the morning are almost certain indications of nighttime bruxing. Occlusal correction may or may not reduce the bruxing, but it almost
always relieves the soreness in the muscle, and it most certainly reduces the damage that strong bruxers inflict on the
dentition.

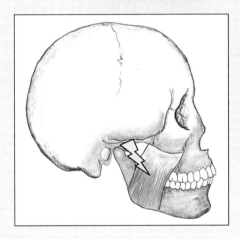

Deep masseter muscle. This muscle pulls the condyles up,
so any deflective incline that requires down/forward displacement of the condyle puts the muscle in direct isometric
opposition to the lateral pterygoid muscle that must act
against it to hold the condyle down the eminentia. It is typically tender when the superficial masseter is also tender.

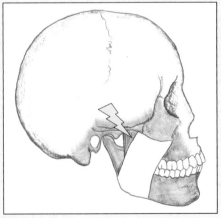

Temporalis muscle. The focus of many headaches that respond favorably to occlusal correction. This muscle is also in direct opposition to the lateral pterygoid. It also has some origination behind the lateral wall of the orbit of the eye, and can be a source of sharp pain behind the eye. Its aponeurosis extends as an innervated sheath to the top of the head, and when inflamed can make the scalp sore to touch. Temporal headaches and pain are some of the most common symptoms related to occluso-muscle imbalance.

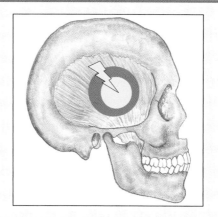

Inferior lateral pterygoid muscle. Any deflective occlusal incline that requires displacement of the condyle to achieve maximum intercuspation is a direct causative factor in lateral pterygoid hyperactivity and tenderness. This is the positioner muscle that pulls the condyle forward every time the mandible leaves centric relation, so even the slightest movement forward always involves the lateral pterygoid muscle. If the mandible is deflected toward the left, the right pterygoid muscle must pull the right condyle forward. Deflections to the right require contraction of the left pterygoid muscle. Forward deflections require contraction of both pterygoid muscles. The most important reason why the lateral pterygoid muscles become a source of pain is because with any forward movement there is also required a downward movement. Thus the inferior lateral pterygoid muscle must hold the condyle down on a slippery, steep incline while all the elevator muscles are pulling up. Centric relation is the only condylar position that permits complete release of the lateral pterygoid muscles during complete closure to maximum intercuspation.

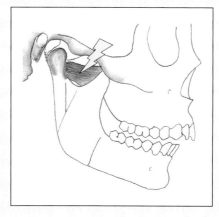

Testing

Palpation of the lateral pterygoid muscle is not practical, but it can be tested effectively to see if it is a source of pain. Have the patient slightly protrude the mandible. Then apply distalization pressure on the jaw to provoke a muscle response. A sore muscle will respond to this test. Bilateral manipulation is also an excellent way to determine if the lateral pterygoid muscles are in protective hypercontraction. Any sign of tension or tenderness on loading indicates either muscle bracing or an intracapsular disorder. This is the perfect indication for anterior deprogramming to differentiate. If there is no intracapsular disorder, the muscle will release.

Superior lateral pterygoid muscle. This is the muscle responsible for keeping the disk aligned during function. It cannot be effectively palpated. However, you will know it is involved if there is a disk misalignment because the disk is held forward if it fails to release contraction when the condyle goes to centric position. A reciprocal click is indicative of hyperactivity or spasm of this muscle. Deprogramming often causes release of contraction and spontaneous reduction of the disk displacement.

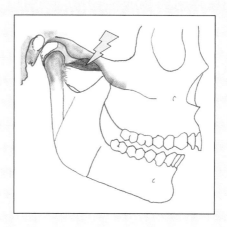

Hyoid area. The digastric and the hyoid muscles are often involved when deflective occlusal interferences cause the mandible to be postured forward to avoid the interferences. Look for protruded jaw position to achieve maximum intercuspation. Many patients develop a forward head posture in response to occlusal deflections and use these muscles as an aid to relieve the lateral pterygoid muscles. You can test this involvement by ascertaining if anterior deprogramming relieves the discomfort. It frequently does.

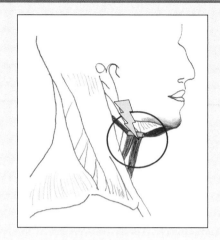

Sternocleidomastoid (SCM) muscle. If this muscle is tender to palpation, evaluate collateral effects from head posture and/or cervical misalignments. Consider referral to a physical therapist for adjunctive evaluation. Be aware that occlusal disharmony is not the only cause for head and neck muscle problems.

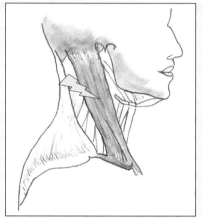

Occipital area. Occipital headaches are commonly associated with occlusal interferences. If tender, look for occlusal interferences to centric relation or excursions. Recognize that this problem may result in combination with head posture and cervical misalignments, or it may be unrelated to occlusal factors. Consider referral to a physical therapist for adjunctive therapy.

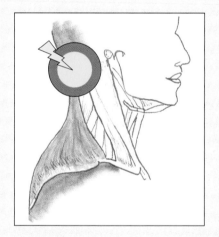

Trapezius muscle. In spite of claims that a form of TMD includes shoulder and back pain, clinical experience indicates that while some pain in this area does disappear when the occlusion is corrected, the result is probably more related to the improvement of head posture that is common when occlusal disharmony is corrected. Cervical misalignment must always be a consideration. Consider referral to a physical therapist.

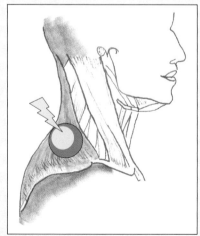

Confirmative Diagnosis

The reason occluso-muscle pain should never be missed as a diagnosis is because the diagnosis can be confirmed by two simple tests.

Test 1: Clench test

If a patient can clench the teeth together and feel tenderness in any tooth when the mouth is empty, this is a positive, dependable test that the tender tooth or teeth are in occlusal interference. Thus the capability for causing occluso-muscle pain is active.

Test 2: Anterior deprogramming test

If separation of the posterior teeth by a flat anterior deprogramming device or even a cotton roll laid across the arch at the premolars relieves the pain, it indicates that the interfering tooth was a factor. This should be further tested however, by firmly clenching against the cotton roll. If there is complete absence of pain on clenching against the cotton roll, you can assume you are dealing with an occluso-muscle problem as the primary source of pain. If clenching on the cotton roll produces discomfort in either TMJ, there is a possibility that an intracapsular disorder is a contributor to the pain. If in doubt, have the patient wear a flat permissive anterior deprogramming device or wear an aqualizer overnight to clarify if an intracapsular disorder is part of the problem. Verify by load testing the joints.

A complete analysis of the TMJs, the muscles, and the occlusion is always in order before a final diagnosis is confirmed, but the two simple tests described above will rarely mislead.

Note: The cotton-roll clench test may require a few minutes of tooth separation to allow release of the lateral pterygoid contraction before firm clenching pressure is applied. Usually 5 to 30 minutes is sufficient.

As simplistic as it may sound, the proper use of a flat, permissive anterior discluder splint is a very reliable aid to diagnosing whether or not occlusal interferences are the cause of discomfort in the musculature. If separating the offending deflective tooth inclines and complete seating of both TMJs is effective in eliminating pain in any of the muscles just described, you may rely on a diagnosis of occluso-muscle pain.

The effectiveness of anterior deprogramming is usually determinable within minutes or hours. If relief is not noticeable with overnight use, either the splint was improperly made (a far too common problem) or there are other causes of the pain that should be evaluated and diagnosed with specificity. If an intracapsular disorder is a source of pain, it should be diagnosed and classified.

If neither an occluso-muscle disorder nor an intracapsular disorder can be affirmed as the source of the pain, it is imperative that other potential causes for pain be explored, including sympathetic pain sources. A last resort is to blame the primary cause of pain on a psychological or emotional etiology. While psychological factors may influence patient responses to pain, a diagnosis of psychosocial factors as the primary source of pain is almost invariably a missed diagnosis.

Suggested Readings

Bakke M, Moller E: Distortion of maximum elevator activity by unilateral tooth contact. *Scand J Dent Res* 67, 1980.

Barker DK: Occlusal interferences and temporomandibular dysfunction. *General Dentistry* Jan-Feb:55-60, 2004.

Belser U, Hannam AC: The influence of altered working-side occlusal guidance on masticatory muscles and related jaw movement. *J Prosthet Dent* 53:406-413, 1985.

Dawson PE: Centric relation: Its effect on occluso-muscle harmony. *Dent Clin NA,* 1979.

Dawson PE: Position paper: regarding diagnosis, management, and treatment of temporomandibular disorders. *J Prosthet Dent,* 1989.

Dawson PE: Temporomandibular joint pain—dysfunction problems can be solved. *J Prosthet Dent* 29:100-112, 1973.

Hannam AC, et al: The relationship between dental occlusion, muscle activity, and associated jaw movements in man. *Arch Oral Biol* 22:25, 1977.

Ingervall B, Carlsson GE: Masticatory muscle activity before and after elimination of balancing side occlusal interferences. *J Oral Rehab* 9:183-192, 1982.

Kerstein RB: Treatment of myofascial pain-dysfunction syndrome with occlusal equilibration. *J Prosthet Dent* 43:578, 1990.

Kerstein RB: Treatment of myofascial pain dysfunction syndrome with occlusal therapy to reduce lengthy disclusion time—a recall study. *J Craniomandib Practice* 13(2):105-115, 1995.

Kerstein RB, Wright N: An electromyographic and computer analysis of patients suffering from chronic myofascial pain dysfunction syndrome: pre- and post-treatment with immediate complete anterior guidance development. *J Prosthet Dent* 66:677-686, 1997.

Kerveskari P, Bell L, Salonen M, et al: Effect of elimination of occlusal interferences on signs and symptoms of craniomandibular disorders in young adults. *J Oral Rehabil* 16:21, 1989.

Krough Poulson WG, Olsson A: Occlusal disharmonies and dysfunction of the stomatognathic system. *Dent Clin NA* 627-635, 1966.

Mahan P: Pathologic manifestations of occlusal disharmony. *J of LD Pankey Institute,* 1981.

Ramfjord SP: Dysfunctional temporomandibular joint and muscle pain. *J Prosthet Dent* 11:353-374, 1961.

Riise C, Sheikholeslam A: The influence of experimental interfering occlusal contacts on postural activity of the anterior temporal and masseter muscles in young adults. *J Oral Rehabil* 9:419-425, 1982.

Schaerer P, Stallard RE, Zander HA: Occlusal interferences and mastication: an electromyographic study. *J Prosthet Dent* 17:438-449, 1967.

Tarantola GJ, Becker IM, Gremillion H, et al: The effectiveness of equilibration in the improvement of signs and symptoms in the stomatognathic system. *Int J Perio Rest Dent* 18:595-603, 1998.

Williamson EH, Lundquist DO: Anterior guidance: its effect on anterior temporalis and masseter muscles. *J Prosthet Dent* 39:816-823, 1982.

Chapter 25

Intracapsular Disorders of the TMJ

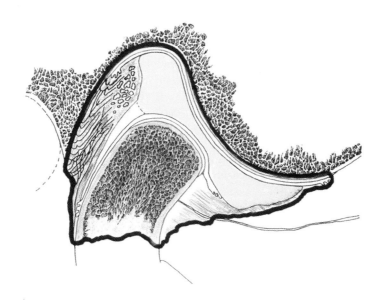

PRINCIPLE

The condition of the intracapsular structure of the temporomandibular joints (TMJs) affects the position of the TMJs. Consequently it affects the jaw-to-jaw occlusal relationship.

INTRACAPSULAR PAIN

The joint capsule is the fibrous sheet of connective tissue that encloses the TMJ. All structures within this capsule are referred to as intracapsular.

> **Intracapsular Disorder of the TMJ.** Any disease, deformation, or disorder that involves the tissues within the capsule of the TMJ.

Many different types of disorders can affect the tissues within the capsule of the TMJ. Deformation of intracapsular structures can produce a variety of different pain symptoms depending on which tissues are affected, the degree and type of damage, variations in compressive or tensive forces applied, and the response to varying levels of pain.

Pain emanating from intracapsular tissues almost always has a recognizable structural explanation. Proper diagnosis requires analysis of each of several intracapsular components to locate specific sources of pain or to rule out deformed but adapted structures if they are not a source of pain.

Diagnosis of a patient with orofacial pain cannot be considered adequate if it does not include a precise classification that defines the condition of the intracapsular structures of the TMJs. Classification based solely on symptoms is not adequate. Neither are incomplete descriptions such as "clicking and popping" that do not specifically define disk condition and alignment for both medial and lateral poles of the condyles.

STAGES OF INTRACAPSULAR DISORDERS

Before treating an intracapsular disorder of the TMJ, one should diagnose the following:

1. Alignment of the disk
2. Cause of derangement
3. Condition of the disk and its attachments
4. Condition of bony structures
5. Level of discomfort and dysfunction
6. Potential for further pathosis and its consequences
7. Potential for correction of the problem through adaptive changes

Many patients can function comfortably with completely displaced disks. There are other patients with almost insignificant beginning derangements who are acutely distressed. Thus the selection of treatment depends not only on the condition of the joint structures, but also on the reaction of the patient to it.

The anticipated prognosis with or without treatment must be related to the choice of therapy. We must determine whether the treatment would be worse than the disease. The age of the patient, the state of health, and the emotional attitude toward the problem are all important considerations in deciding on a course of treatment.

Whenever possible, the safest and most conservative treatment is the adaptive response of the patient in an environment of neuromuscular peacefulness. If damage to the articular parts has not gone beyond the self-repairable stage, treatment will usually consist of correcting structural disharmonies that cause mandibular displacement and its sequela of muscle incoordination. When disk derangements occur, structural disharmonies will be found at both ends of the articulation. Neither the joint nor the occlusion is correctly related, so both must be reoriented to achieve the necessary harmony in the system. There are many conservative ways this can be accomplished for most patients, but in some patients the disharmony is so great that there are no simple solutions. The goal of treatment, however, remains the same, which is to achieve the best possible harmony between the joints and the occlusion, so that there is no mechanical displacement of the mandible and consequently no stimulus for muscle incoordination that overloads both the joint and the dentition.

If damage to the articulation has progressed beyond the capacity for corrective remodeling, treatment may be required to repair the deformities in the joint in order to achieve an acceptable level of stability or relief of pain.

The most significant improvement in the treatment of internal derangements has come from the ability to more accurately diagnose the specific stage of the derangement. Thus treatment can be related to specific causes and effects of a clearly defined problem. The next two chapters relate each stage of disk derangement to the methods for diagnosing it and the corresponding choices of treatment.

The stages of disk derangement usually occur in a fairly consistent sequence that starts with a beginning partial derangement at the lateral pole. From this stage it is progressive, and the degree of damage in the joint is related to time and the intensity of load that the deranged joint must bear because of incoordinated muscle hypercontraction.

The same type of derangement may occur as the result of different causes. If the selected treatment does not correct the cause of the problem, the effects of treatment will not last. The goal of treatment is to return the system to the best level of equilibrium possible so that the requirements for adaptation are reduced to the minimum.

THE PROGRESSIVE NATURE OF DISK DERANGEMENTS

It is an absurd misunderstanding to define temporomandibular disorder (TMD) as a "nonprogressive" disorder. Intracapsular disorders of the TMJs must go through several stages of structural deformation to reach the final stage of bone disease. Recognition of these stages is important for every dentist because it is possible to arrest the destructive effects on many, if not most, TMDs if an early diagnosis is made. Starting with a healthy, properly aligned condyle-disk assembly, the disk becomes misaligned in stages. The stages result from forces that progressively stretch or tear the ligaments that bind the disk to the condyle. As these ligaments are weakened, the forces against the disk cause it to change shape through adaptive remodeling. The changes in the disk are thus the direct result of tensive pull on the disk, and misdirected loading by the condyle. Other than extrinsic trauma, the only source of power for loading the joint in any direction is muscle. Coordinated muscle normally loads the joint intermittently, but incoordinated muscle maintains the contracted force against the joint for prolonged periods of time through clenching or bruxing while simultaneously the incoordinated muscle contraction applies tensive (pulling) forces on the disk. It is the prolonged loading that causes the adaptive changes to occur in both the hard and soft tissues. The shape these tissues assume is a direct result of the amount and direction of the forces applied through the condyle and the disk.

As the disk changes from its normal biconcave shape, its alignment with the condyle becomes less stable until the self-centering concavity is lost entirely and the shape of the disk then becomes itself a major problem. For clarity of understanding and simplicity of communication, the progressive joint changes have been divided into stages. These stages can apply to either lateral-pole derangements or to total condyle-disk derangements. Since most derangements start at the lateral pole, I will discuss that progression first as it occurs in a typical sequence.

Lateral-Pole Disk Derangements: The Typical Sequence

1. Incoordinated contraction of the superior lateral pterygoid muscle applies tensive force to pull the disk forward while elevator muscles pull the condyle back and up. This tends to stretch the posterior diskal ligament and displaces the disk forward.
2. Forward derangement starts at the lateral part of the disk. The disk is still biconcave in shape.
3. The posterior band of the disk starts to flatten under the misaligned load of the condyle's lateral pole.
4. The lateral half of the disk becomes anteriorly displaced in front of the lateral pole of the condyle (reducible).
5. The posterior band thickens and is pushed forward by the lateral pole of the condyle (lateral pole closed lock).
6. The posterior band of the disk is folded into the anterior band at the lateral pole. The two bands may then start to coalesce into a single mass. The medial pole is still seated between the two bands on the medial half, but the disk is rotated medioanteriorly.
7. The disk becomes anteriorly displaced from the medial pole (complete anteriorly displaced disk).

Depending on the amount of distortion of the disk, the derangement may become reducible or nonreducible.

The total disk may become displaced by a similar progression, but other than trauma, it appears to be unusual for simultaneous displacement to occur at both poles. The medial collateral ligament is stronger than the lateral attachment of the disk, but regardless of which ligament gives way first, the causative factors may follow a fairly similar pattern.

An understanding of how adaptive changes relate to the direction and intensity of loading of the joint can be applied to complete disk displacements just as they are to the cause-and-effect sequence of partial disk displacements (Figure 25-1).

To put diagnosis and treatment into the best perspective, let us start the analysis with the healthy joint. The stages of derangement can then start from that baseline.

THE HEALTHY JOINT

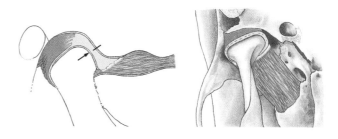

Description

The healthy TMJ is aligned in the center of its disk. Both condyle and eminence are convex and are covered with intact fibrocartilage over a dense cortical bone layer. The disk is firmly attached to the lateral and medial poles of the condyle. The retrodiskal tissues that compose the bilaminar posterior attachment of the disk are intact, and the superior strata exert an elastic pull on the disk.

Methods for Diagnosing

History: Negative
If past symptoms have been observed, they have been corrected satisfactorily. Symptoms of muscle incoordination may be present, even with a healthy joint, and so any muscle problems must be distinguished from signs or symptoms of a true intracapsular disorder.

Clinical observations
Range of motion should be within normal limits. Maximum opening should be in the range of 40 mm or more. Less than a 40 mm opening indicates probable muscle incoordination. Less than a 20 mm opening indicates a possible intracapsular problem. There should be no deviation in protrusive excursions and no restrictions on lateral excursions. There should be no clicks, pops, or grating sounds through the normal range of motion.

Manipulative testing
The joints should be free of any sign of tension or tenderness while firmly loaded by bilateral manipulation. The mandible should be able to hinge freely, protrude, and move laterally while loaded without any sign of discomfort.

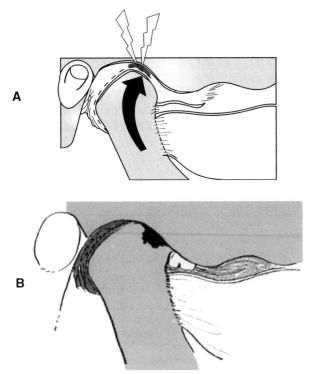

FIGURE 25-1 Painful compression of retrodiskal tissue (**A**) is not treated the same as acute bone disease (**B**), even though both disorders are classified as an intracapsular disorder.

Palpation

Negative at joint. Muscles may or may not be tender to palpation.

Auscultation

A healthy joint is well lubricated with synovial fluids. If its fibrocartilaginous surfaces are intact, it should be noiseless in function. Doppler auscultation of the TMJ produces no crepitus sounds.

Radiographic findings

Condyles are reasonably well centered in fossae on transcranial films. There is a fairly even radiolucent space around the condyles. Both the condyles and the eminence are convex with good cortical bone layer showing.

The use of arthography has been replaced by noninvasive techniques such as magnetic resonance imaging (MRI), but we've learned much about disk alignment and misalignment by observing the joint as it moves through functional ranges (Figure 25-2).

Mounted diagnostic casts

If the TMJs can be positioned into a verifiable centric relation and casts mounted to that position, the occlusion can be related to the physiologic joint position and studied. Problems of malocclusion, muscle incoordination, or excessive tooth wear or mobility often occur before damage to the joint itself, and an occlusal analysis should be done to determine whether correction of the occlusion is needed to reduce the potential for degenerative changes in the joint.

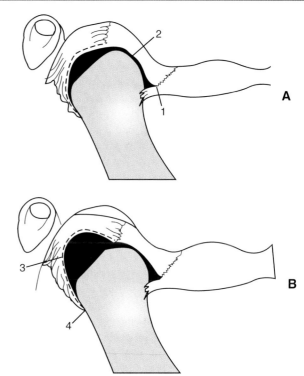

FIGURE 25-2 **A,** Illustration of an arthrogram of a normal joint shows the extension of the dye in front of the condyle limited to 2 to 3 mm. The most anterior boundary of the dye represents the attachment of the superior lateral pterygoid muscle to the disk *(1)*. The filling of the inferior joint space outlines the contour of the underside of the disk. The normal disk has a concave underside *(2)*. **B,** As the condyle moves forward, the disk rotates to the top of the condyle, allowing the dye to bulge out the slackened ligament *(3)* that attaches to the back of the condyle *(4)*.

Treatment

From the standpoint of the joint, there are no contraindications to starting any necessary treatment of the occlusion.

BEGINNING LATERAL-POLE DERANGEMENT

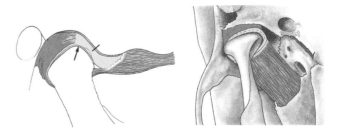

The earliest stage of disk derangement starts with slight anterior derangement of the lateral part of the disk.

Description

At this earliest stage of derangement, the lateral pole of the condyle loads against the lateral half of the posterior band of the disk. The medial pole is still seated properly in the central bearing area between the anterior and posterior bands of the disk. The lateral border of the disk is held slightly forward of its centered position by muscle contraction that creates tension on the lateral diskal ligament as well as the inferior stratum of the bilaminar zone.

Possible Causes

There are at least four ways by which a lateral-pole disk derangement can be initiated:

1. Muscle incoordination
2. Distalization of the working-side condyle in lateral excursions
3. Distalization of the condyle during maximum intercuspation
4. Trauma

The most common cause appears to be muscle incoordination resulting from occlusal interferences, particularly steep incline interferences on second or third molars. But muscle incoordination can result from any occlusal interference. Those that displace the condyle forward are the most commonly found triggers.

Distalization of the lateral pole of the condyle can occur from occlusal incline interferences that force the rotating condyle back as it moves to a working-side excursion. When this occurs, the major part of the force is loaded onto the lateral pole. However, any occlusal relationship that results in distalizing pressure on a condyle can be a factor. When incoordinated muscle hypercontraction pulls the disk forward in resistance to the seating action of the condyle, the condyle-disk alignment is always in jeopardy, and the lateral diskal ligament appears to be the weakest link.

A lateral blow to the mandible can traumatize the lateral pole on the opposite side, injuring the diskal attachment by compression or sudden stretching. A torn ligament does not hold the disk firmly to the condyle, and so the disk is more susceptible to misalignment from incoordinated muscle contraction.

A blow to the jaw can also compress the retrodiskal tissues, causing edema. The swelling behind the disk can exert a forward pressure against the disk. The lateral half of the disk, being less confined by fossa walls, is more easily displaced slightly forward.

Methods for Diagnosing

History

Other than a possible report of trauma, the history is usually uneventful at this stage except for symptoms from muscle incoordination, which can vary from mild to severe. Slight lateral-pole derangements are common in patients with long-standing, undiagnosed TMJ discomfort, but other than an almost unnoticeable, dull click, the joint itself is not generally the specific location of the chief complaint. It is not uncommon for such patients to report multiple attempts at equilibration without ever achieving complete comfort. On these patients it must never be assumed that the equilibration has been accurately performed. Complaints of tiredness in the jaw muscles, headaches, and limitation of opening are not uncommon.

Clinical observations

In early stages of lateral-pole derangement, the range of motion may appear normal, or it may exhibit any of the typical signs of muscle incoordination such as deviation on opening toward the affected side because of muscle hypercontraction or spasm.

Manipulative testing

With delicate bilateral manipulation, a dull, almost imperceptible click may be felt as the jaw is hinged with very light pressure directed through the condyles toward the eminence. After the click occurs, continue to slowly hinge the mandible and test lightly at first for centric relation. If the joint is comfortable and hingeing freely, load it with firm pressure to test it. Maintain the loading pressure as the jaw is hinged and tested through the complete range of motion. At this stage of disk derangement, it is rarely a problem to align the disk on the condyle with correctly done manipulation. If severe muscle spasm accompanies the derangement, it may be necessary to deprogram the muscles by separating the teeth with a cotton roll for a few minutes before centric relation can be found and verified. If the disk is correctly aligned, there will be no sign of tenderness or tension when it is loaded.

Palpation

Muscle tenderness to palpation will almost invariably be observed whenever a disk derangement occurs. It will routinely be related directly to the direction of forced displacement of the mandible from occlusal interferences. At this early stage of derangement, palpation of the condyle is generally unremarkable.

Auscultation

Stethoscopic examination is usually negative because the stethoscope is not sensitive enough to transmit the sound of very early derangements. At this stage the posterior band of the disk is still pliable, and there is no staccato to the sound of the shift in the disk. Doppler auscultation of the TMJ, however, will pick up a fine crepitus sound as the patient opens and closes. The sound produced is similar to rubbing against fine sandpaper. After manipulation into a verified centric relation the joint immediately becomes quiet and reports no sound through the Doppler probe.

Radiographic findings

These are generally unremarkable. At the early stage the joint is still centered, and no adaptive changes can be noticed on lateral transcranial films.

Mounted casts

Casts that are meticulously mounted with facebow and verified centric relation bite record can be expected to show premature occlusal contacts that displace the condyles from centric relation during maximum intercuspation. The forced deviation may be either forward or backward from centric relation. Any occlusal interference that is capable of causing muscle incoordination is capable of causing a disk misalignment.

Diagnostic occlusal therapy

A flat anterior bite plane adjusted precisely to centric relation can be worn by the patient overnight. If all symptoms of discomfort disappear, the disk derangement was caused by muscle incoordination resulting from occlusal interferences.

Treatment

Occlusal correction is indicated to eliminate all interferences to centric relation and to correct excursive pathways. The manipulation into centric relation must be verified to ensure correct disk alignment. The treatment method of choice is selected after analysis of the mounted casts. If interim treatment is needed for some purpose, a full occlusal bite plane can be constructed as a temporary procedure. If a bite plane is used, it should be meticulously adjusted to centric relation, and the anterior guidance on the bite plane should disclude the posterior teeth in all excursions.

Adjunctive treatment for relief of muscle hypercontraction may also be considered, but except in extreme conditions of muscle spasm it is rarely necessary. If a metabolic disorder, nutritional deficiency, or severe emotional stress is related to a lowered resistance to muscle spasm, therapy should be directed accordingly.

Counseling of patients regarding the causes and effects of their disorder is important. The more patients understand about the nature of the problem, the less apprehensive they become. One should start this counseling, however, during the original examination by explaining the symptoms and relating them to the examination procedures.

We have found almost no need for drugs, injections, or any electronic modalities for successful treatment of this stage of disk derangement.

Appliances for positioning the mandible forward are unnecessary and in fact are contraindicated.

Prognosis

The relief of symptoms and the return to coordinated function usually occur rapidly and most often within minutes if all interferences to a verified centric relation are eliminated meticulously enough. The patient should be unable to squeeze the teeth together and provoke any tenderness in the joint if correct alignment of the disk has been achieved in harmony with maximum intercuspation at centric relation.

Recurrence of symptoms is common, and the patient should be told to expect some return of the discomfort until both the joint and the teeth stabilize. Follow-up appointments for further refinement of the occlusion should be arranged. This frequency varies greatly depending on the condition of the dentition, but my experience is that a stable comfort level is usually achieved by the third appointment.

At this stage, any stretching of the posterior attachments to the disk or the collateral ligaments does not cause further problems if the posterior band of the disk is intact, and if all occlusal interferences are corrected. Contrary to earlier belief, the ligaments do not repair themselves once they have been stretched.

PROGRESSIVE LATERAL-POLE DERANGEMENT

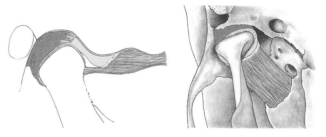

The sequence of deformation progresses to flattening of the posterior band of the disk.

Description

Because of continuous loading of the posterior band of the disk, it is flattened where it has been compressed by the lateral pole of the condyle. The lateral diskal ligament has been stretched, permitting a more medioanterior derangement of the disk, and the flattening of the posterior band also has the effect of lengthening the posterior attachment to let the disk move forward because of the tensive pull of incoordinated musculature.

Possible Causes

The same factors that can cause a beginning derangement at the lateral pole are progressive if not corrected. The flattening of the posterior band is related to the duration and intensity of these same factors (that is, muscle incoordination, distalization of the working condyle in lateral excursions, overload of the condyle during maximum intercuspation, or trauma).

If deflective occlusal inclines are present, they should be considered the primary causative factor of muscle incoordination.

If there is a history of trauma, the derangement may have been initially caused by a torn ligament or by swelling in the retrodiskal tissues. However, normal repair may be hampered by occlusally caused muscle incoordination, and so muscle spasm may be a perpetuating provoker of more serious problems, even though it was not the original cause. Occlusal interference should thus be considered as one of a combination of causes, since it is the principal stimulus for muscle incoordination.

Symptoms

As long as the condyle is still loading the avascular, noninnervated part of the disk, the symptoms will be mostly isolated in muscle. It is doubtful that early flattening of the posterior band will produce pain in the joint itself. Swelling as a result of trauma may produce some intracapsular pain.

Methods for Diagnosing

History
For flattening of the posterior band of the disk to occur, the derangement of the disk must have been present for some time. Careful questioning of the patient may reveal a long history of general discomfort, but at this stage most of the signs will be related to muscle. Tiredness from chewing, inability to open wide, occipital or temporal headaches, or any of the myriad symptoms that muscle incoordination can produce may be reported by the patient. Noticeable clicking may be reported but is generally not yet a principal problem.

Patients frequently report multiple equilibrations done by forcing the jaw back. Try to ascertain why the equilibration was done in the first place. Note the patient's comments about the results. Question the patient about when the symptoms first started. If the onset of problems occurred immediately after restorative treatment, we would suspect the introduction of occlusal interferences.

Ask the patient what time of day the symptoms are most noticeable. If discomfort is greatest in the morning, expect a nocturnal bruxing problem. If the patient has worn a segmental bite plane appliance, you will need to determine if it has caused harm.

Clinical observations
The range of motion may be affected as in muscle incoordination.

Look for occlusal wear facets. Look for thick restorations on the lingual of upper anterior teeth as potential distalizing forces.

In patients with deep overbite, look for possible overgrinding that may have closed the vertical into a wedging, distalizing contact on the anterior teeth.

Manipulative testing
Because the medial pole of the condyle is still centered in the disk, it should be possible to manipulate the mandible into centric relation with minimal difficulty. As the jaw is being delicately eased into centric relation, a soft, muffled click can usually be felt as the lateral half of the disk slips back into its centered alignment. If bilateral pressure is then used to load the joints forward against the eminentiae and the pressure is maintained through excursive ranges, there should be no discomfort.

Palpation
Negative except for muscle, unless pathosis or accidental injury induced the derangement. Then joint tenderness may be found.

Auscultation
Loud clicking generally does not occur until the next stage, but there are exceptions. The click at this stage is usually a soft, muffled sound that is easier to feel than it is to hear. Unguided hinging with Doppler auscultation of the TMJ produces a fine crepitus sound, but such auscultation is quiet with guided, bilateral pressure while hingeing is done in a verified centric relation.

Radiographic findings
These are generally unremarkable.

Mounted casts
Casts mounted in centric relation have, in my experience, invariably shown some occlusal interferences when the disk has been deranged. They should be studied before a treatment approach is selected for correcting the occlusion.

Diagnostic occlusal therapy
If centric relation can be verified, this stage of disk derangement can usually be treated successfully with routine correction of the occlusion. However, whenever changes have taken place in the disk, there may be a corrective remodeling after relief of the incoordinated muscle hypercontraction. These adaptive changes in the disk may slightly alter the position of the condyle in centric relation, thus requiring a corresponding further correction in the occlusion. The potential for joint changes should be considered when occlusal treatment is being planned. Finalization of the occlusion cannot be completed until the joints are stable, and so occlusal splints may be utilized until the stability of the joints can be confirmed (superior repositioning splint).

Treatment
Treatment is directed toward counseling, muscle relaxation, and realignment of the disk. The disk normally aligns automatically when muscle coordination is re-established. Muscle coordination is almost always re-established when the occlusion is corrected to permit undeviated access of the properly aligned condyle-disk assembly to centric relation.

Because the condyle has not yet slipped past the posterior band onto the retrodiskal tissues, inflammation of the posterior attachment is rarely a problem that requires treatment unless it was caused by extrinsic trauma.

Prognosis
If muscle coordination is achieved, the prognosis is excellent. All signs and symptoms seem to be routinely reversible at this stage even though damage to the ligaments is not reversible.

LATERAL-POLE DISK DISPLACEMENT

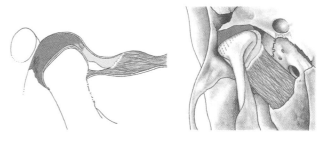

Now the reciprocal click is introduced. It results from a reducible displacement of the disk in front of the lateral pole of the condyle.

Description

At this stage of progression, the lateral diskal ligament and the posterior condylar attachment of the disk have been stretched or torn sufficiently to allow the lateral half of the posterior band of the disk to displace completely in front of the lateral pole of the condyle. The lateral pole of the condyle now rests against the vascular, innervated tissue behind the disk. The medial pole is still positioned in its concavity between the anterior and posterior bands of the disk, but from that point laterally the disk has been deranged anteromedially.

As the jaw opens and the lateral pole translates forward and downward, it clicks past the posterior band and recaptures its position in the central bearing area of the disk. Once recaptured, the condyle-disk alignment is maintained until the final closure, at which point the lateral pole snaps past the posterior band and back onto the retrodiskal tissues.

One should remember that this lateral pole displacement would not occur without help from incoordinated muscle contraction that tightly holds the disk forward, rather than controlling its timed release as the lateral pole moves back.

Possible Causes

Reciprocal clicks result from the same causes that initiated the problem at its start. They are the result of progressive damage that occurs when those causative factors are not eliminated in the earlier stages. The degree of damage may be intensified and accelerated by heavy bruxing or clenching, factors that even a conscientious dentist may not completely control. But what can be controlled are the deflective occlusal interferences that put the teeth in jeopardy and add to muscle incoordination.

Signs and Symptoms

At this stage, there may be some discomfort in the joint itself, and there will almost always be typical signs and symptoms of muscle incoordination, but the chief complaint is often related to a loud, staccato click or pop when chewing. My current opinion is that the louder the click or pop, the more likely it is that it is a lateral-pole disk displacement and not a complete disk displacement. When the disk is held so firmly in place by the medial pole and the confining walls of the fossa at the medial pole, the rigidity of the disk is increased. As the translating lateral pole builds up pressure against the posterior band of the rigidly held disk, it produces a loud pop from the increased friction when it does snap past the thickened posterior band.

Remember that the lateral pole of the condyle must travel forward and downward upon opening even if the medial pole stays on a fixed axis of rotation. The angle of the condylar axis in relation to the horizontal axis of rotation will determine how much the lateral pole must move. The shape of the condyle may also influence the signs or symptoms, and certainly the different possibilities of how the posterior band is shaped or flattened by various degrees of loading from the condyle will affect the way it responds to condylar movement. The posterior band may be flattened to a shape that does not produce a noticeable click. There are endless possibilities of remodeling changes that can occur to both the hard and soft tissues of the joint. I diagnose best when I develop a visualization of what is happening in the joint, based on the signs and symptoms that I can correlate. By observing signs of occlusal wear and relating it to a visualization of how the joint would necessarily respond to the mandibular deviations that such faceted inclines would direct, I can generally get a mental picture of the direct relationship between the signs and the symptoms.

Observing signs and symptoms is also critical from a prognosis standpoint. If there are signs of elevator muscle hypertrophy, I know I am dealing with a habitual bruxer or clencher and I also know the joint is subjected to prolonged heavy loading. Thus, different patients at the same stage of disk derangements may have different requirements for treatment and may have different expectations for a successful prognosis.

Based on the signs and symptoms, try to form a mental picture of what you think is happening to the joint. Then test your tentative hypothesis with different diagnostic methods until a clear pattern emerges.

Methods for Diagnosing

History

This is similar to the earlier stages, except that the patient may have been aware of symptoms longer. The jaw may periodically lock or "go out." Patients sometimes report embarrassment from the pops that occur in the joint during eating.

Clinical observations

Look for the same factors that are evident in the first two stages. Observe the direction of displacement of the mandible as the patient squeezes from the first point of contact. Particularly look for any occlusal configuration that forces the condyle sharply sideward when the teeth are intercuspated.

Manipulative testing

At this stage, the diskal ligaments have become stretched or torn enough to allow the lateral part of the disk to move in front of the condyle. For this reason, the method of manipulation is critical. If the mandible is pushed back, the condyle can easily be forced past a partially deranged disk, completely displacing the disk forward of the condyle. Correct manipulation can, on the other hand, reposition the condyle in the center of the disk. Bilateral manipulation should be done delicately, with the teeth apart. As the jaw opens or moves slightly forward, a click can generally be felt as the lateral pole crosses the posterior band of the disk. As the condyle engages the anterior slope of the posterior band of the disk, upward, forward pressure through the condyle causes the disk to snap back into its centered position.

A characteristic sign of this stage is that the disk is recapturable. Evidence of recapture is the total absence of any discomfort or tension when loaded, as the jaw goes through a full range of motion. There should be no sign of discomfort at any jaw position after the disk is aligned. If upward pressure is applied before the condyle has clicked onto the disk, there should be some evidence of tenderness or tension, especially in lateral excursion away from the affected side. This is diagnostic.

Palpation
With the jaw open, external palpation of the posterior surface of the condyle may elicit some tenderness, but, generally, palpable tenderness is confined to the muscles that always seem to be involved in incoordinated function whenever we find a disk derangement.

Auscultation
Clicks on opening and closing can usually be heard through a stethoscope. On Doppler auscultation of the TMJ, there is a fine crepitus as the jaw opens until the lateral pole crosses the posterior band of the disk, and the joint becomes silent until the lateral pole clicks upon closure as it crosses back over the band. The crepitus sound is then heard again as the condyle rubs against the posterior ligament.

The combination of Doppler auscultation and manipulation is an excellent diagnostic process for lateral-pole displacement. The joint must be both comfortable and quiet while loaded during hinge movements before we can accept a diagnosis of correct disk alignment. Any crepitus indicates lack of correct alignment. By observing where the crepitus occurs in relation to clicks or to discomfort, we can rather clearly visualize what is happening within the joint regarding condyle-disk alignment.

Radiographic findings
Because the medial pole is still centered in its part of the disk, the condyle will appear properly positioned in the fossa on lateral transcranial films. At this stage, we would not yet commonly see remodeling changes in the condyle or the eminence so the joint may look normal with routine radiographic techniques.

Mounted casts
Other than from pathology or accidental injury, I have never seen a condyle-disk derangement initiated in a perfectly occluded dentition. Occlusal interferences can work in two different ways: They can either force one or both condyles distally when the teeth are occluded in maximum intercuspation, or they can displace the condyles forward or lateral to centric relation. Either type of mandibular displacement can be easily missed in the mouth because of tooth mobility, but either type of displacement can cause the muscle incoordination that is necessary for holding the disk forward. Mounted casts permit a three-dimensional analysis of the relationship between the joints and the occlusion. But remember that the accuracy of this analysis is dependent on

the accuracy of the verified centric relation bite record used with a facebow.

It is from the analysis of mounted casts that you decide on the choice of occlusal treatment. If you decide on the use of a bite plane, it can be made on the articulated casts.

Diagnostic occlusal therapy
The disk displacement in this stage is reducible. You must learn whether it will stay aligned in function after you recapture it. The best way to determine this is by use of an anterior bite plane worn overnight. If the disk does not become displaced while the anterior bite plane is worn for one or two days, you can safely assume that it will stay aligned if the occlusion is corrected.

Treatment
If prolonged use of a bite plane is desired, it should include the full occlusion harmonized to a verified centric relation. Do not use any segmental bite plane for more than a few days. Once the diagnosis is confirmed by the anterior bite plane, it is logical to proceed with your selected occlusal treatment. Finalization of the occlusion may not be possible, however, until some remodeling occurs in the deformed disk. If the occlusion is to be restored, equilibration should be done first until a point of stability is reached. This can be done directly or on a superior repositioning splint.

I evaluate the stability by observing the amount of correction needed at intervals of two to four weeks. When minimal or no adjustment is required and the joints are comfortable, the final stage of occlusal treatment can be completed.

Prognosis
If a peaceful neuromusculature can be established, the prognosis is generally excellent. The patient should be checked periodically for any signs of occlusal changes that could trigger a recurrence of the derangement.

LATERAL-POLE CLOSED LOCK

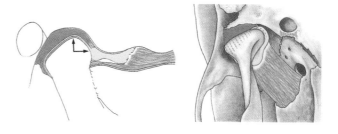

At this stage, the click goes away, but it is not because the joint healed itself. It is because the problem progressed. The lateral part of the posterior band thickens and locks in front of the lateral pole of the condyle.

Description

The disk is rotated medioanteriorly so that the medial pole of the condyle is still between the anterior and posterior bands of the disk, but the posterior band crosses over the condyle diagonally, putting the lateral part of the posterior band in front of the condyle. In a continuous progression from earlier stages, the condyle starts to push the outer part of the disk forward during function. This causes the posterior band to thicken as it is bunched up in front of the forward-moving lateral condyle pole. Proliferation of fibroblasts and chondrocytes forms a progressively thicker mass, which makes it more difficult for the condyle to get across the posterior band and into the central bearing area of the disk. Elevator muscle hypercontraction holds the condyle so tightly against the retrodiskal tissues that they start to thin. The muscle contraction also makes it more difficult for the condyle to release pressure against the back of the raised posterior band to get past it, so it pushes the posterior band and the lateral border of the disk forward.

Possible Causes

Since this stage is the progressive result of the same untreated factors that started the derangement in the first place, the increased severity of the damage to the joint is in direct proportion to the time and intensity of muscular loading of the deranged parts. The changes in the joint are merely adaptive. The tissues conform to the direction and amount of overload. Thus, at least two causative factors will almost always be present as the articulating mechanism breaks down. They are (1) occlusal surfaces that displace the position or alignment of the condyle disk assembly and (2) muscle hypercontraction to overload the deranged articulation.

When one looks at the joint and finds the disk locked in front of the condyle, the erroneous assumption is often made that the anteriorly displaced disk is the cause of the patient's problem. The anteriorly displaced disk is not the cause of the problem. It is the *result* of the problem. Unfortunately, the misplacement of the condyle onto the vascular, innervated retrodiskal tissues now becomes a cause of discomfort as well as a cause of breakdown of the posterior ligament and damage to the disk. However, it is a secondary causative factor that would not have occurred without the primary cause of muscular tension to pull the disk forward, plus overload on a joint that is displaced at maximum intercuspation. This perspective is easier to appreciate if one realizes that there is no loading of the joint when the teeth are apart. When the teeth are together, the condyle must go where maximum intercuspation directs it—or misdirects it. Loading of the joint occurs in that relationship.

Signs and Symptoms

At this stage, discomfort in the joint area becomes a rather commonly reported symptom. Deviation toward the affected side upon opening, plus an aberrant protrusive path, is common. The clicking or popping that occurred in the previous stage has now stopped, or it may be delayed, so the click occurs at a wider opening, in protrusive position, or in lateral excursions to the opposite side.

Any of the signs or symptoms related to muscle spasm such as headache, trismus, or retro-ocular pain may be evident. Generally the combination of pressure on the retrodiskal tissue and the pain of muscle spasm commingle to produce a vague discomfort in the generalized area of the joint and all of its related musculature. In many instances, this combination of pain is further intensified by odontalgia that results from the same muscle-contraction overload the joint is subjected to, applied to the teeth and supporting structures. Thus, although the basic problem may be the same, the symptoms can vary greatly from patient to patient, depending on which tissue or which part of the system cries the loudest, so to speak. The part that hurts the most is not necessarily the part that has the most damage.

Methods for Diagnosing

History

This is similar to previous stages, except the patient may report having had a click that disappeared.

Clinical observations

The protrusive path will generally be irregular because the condyle must move around the enlarged lateral part of the disk. The range of motion is usually limited, but this may be difficult to gauge. Clenching often causes some discomfort in the joint. Look for the same occlusal factors that cause earlier stages of derangement.

Manipulative testing

The jaw may hinge freely, an indication of a normal joint, but testing with bilateral manipulation will cause tension or tenderness when the deranged joint is loaded unless it is completely seated at the medial pole. Even if there is no discomfort when testing at the uppermost hinge position, maintaining the pressure during protrusive or lateral excursion may cause some degree of tenderness as the lateral border of the disk is forced forward ahead of the condyle.

At the early stages of thickening or development of a closed lock, the lateral pole can usually click onto the disk at some point of condyle translation. By using very delicate manipulation, the condyle will not be loaded too firmly to keep pressure on the back of the disk, preventing its recapture. If the disk can be recaptured, pressure should then be applied after the click is felt, to test for alignment (Figure 25-3). Keep the teeth separated, and hinge the jaw a few times while pressure is applied. Place a 3-inch cotton roll between the teeth covering the bicuspids on both sides so that no tooth contact can be made. Then close the jaw into the cotton roll. Verify that the joint is comfortable, and then have the patient squeeze on the cotton roll. If the joint stays comfortable while squeezing on the cotton roll and the disk does not displace with firm clenching, the chances are good

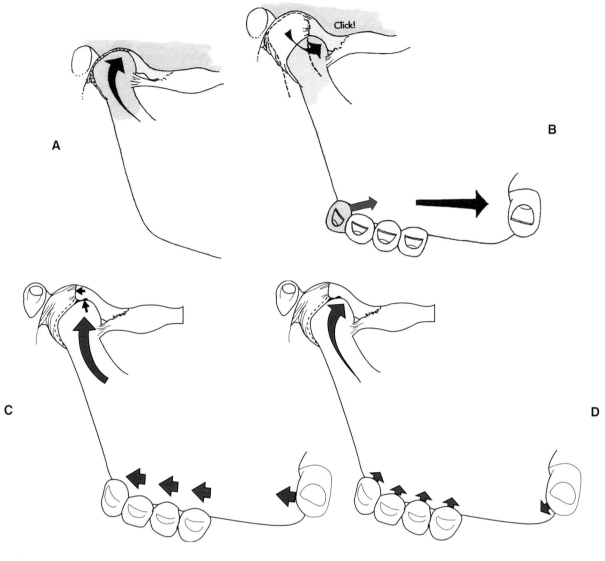

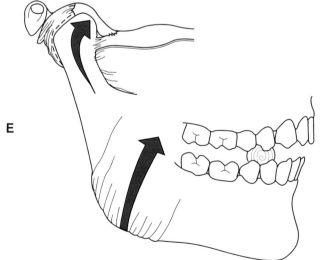

FIGURE 25-3 **A,** Early stage of development of a closed lock. The lateral pole is loaded behind the posterior band of the disk. Elevator muscle hypercontraction locks the condyle against the retrodiskal tissue and the posterior slope of the disk. **B,** Gentle manipulation with the teeth separated encourages the jaw to move forward or laterally, or both, until the condyle clicks onto the disk. Recapture is often helped when the jaw is opened wider during excursions. Bilateral hand position should be maintained, but no pressure is applied until after the condyle clicks back onto the disk. **C,** After reduction occurs, the condyle is gently loaded toward the posterior slope of the eminentia. The pressure is gradually increased in an attempt to lock the disk in a centered position on the condyle. While maintaining forward pressure against the slope, slide the condyle-disk assembly up the slope with gentle upward pressure applied in small increments. Do not load in any direction quickly because it activates muscle contraction. The condyle should push against the posterior band as it goes up to centric relation. **D,** When it feels as though the condyle-disk assembly is against the bony stop (at the medial pole), test the joint for centric relation by loading. Any sign of tension or tenderness indicates that centric relation has not yet been achieved. When the condyle can rotate while loaded with complete comfort, it is an indication that the disk has stayed in line to the centric relation position. It still must be tested to see if it can stay aligned during function. Biting on a cotton roll (**E**) or using an anterior bite plane can be utilized to test.

that the disk has not yet been severely damaged and that occlusal correction will be the treatment of choice.

Palpation

Muscle tenderness will normally be found in the pterygoid complex as well as any of the masticatory muscles that are involved with prolonged contraction. Palpation of the lateral pole via the posterior joint space when the jaw is open often reveals some tenderness.

Auscultation

Doppler auscultation of the TMJ when the disk is displaced will detect different degrees of crepitus that results from the condyle rubbing on the posterior ligament. The greater the breakdown of the ligament or the surfaces of the condyle, the coarser the crepitus.

By listening to the joint through Doppler sound magnification while it is being manipulated, you can easily tell when the condyle clicks onto the disk. If it then becomes quiet during rotation of the condyle in the disk, this confirms that the alignment is acceptable. If at any point the condyle loses its alignment with the disk, the crepitus sounds will recur.

Radiographic findings

Even at this stage of disk displacement, lateral transcranial radiography may show what appears to be a normal joint. Because the medial pole of the condyle is still reasonably centered in its part of the disk, the relationship of the lateral aspect of the condyle may also appear normal.

Mounted cast

As changes in the disk occur, the central bearing area of the disk may be altered in shape so that the condyle does not completely seat, even though we may achieve a realignment of the condyle in the disk. For this reason, the centric relation bite record must be made with extremely careful verification. If any sign of tenderness or tension is present, we cannot consider the bite record as final. Consequently the mounted casts must be related to a tentative treatment position. This position will change slightly as the condyle-disk assemblies adapt to the realignment. As the joint changes occur and the centric relation position stabilizes, new bite records will be needed. Nevertheless, the mounted casts are necessary for determining what must be done to the occlusion to bring it into harmony with the joints, starting with a tentative treatment position when necessary.

Diagnostic occlusal therapy

The anterior bite plane is still the method of choice for determining whether the joint can function comfortably on the disk if there are no occlusal interferences and the disk can be recaptured. If the disk stays aligned and the joint stays comfortable for a day or two, the bite plane should be changed to a full occlusion. It should be equilibrated meticulously to the comfortable joint position and should be readjusted at intervals of two to four weeks until the joint appears stable. At that point, final occlusal treatment can be completed.

Treatment

Even though considerable changes have taken place in the joint, the deformation through this stage is transient. Some derangement of fibers may occur in the disk, but it is still elastic enough to revert to its initial fiber pattern if the load is redirected through the central bearing area. In treating this stage of derangement, special care must be taken to ensure that the entire disk has been recaptured and that it stays recaptured during function. Unless the joint is tested carefully with very firm bilateral pressure, it is easy to be misled about the alignment of the disk because the medial pole can still accept most of the load without discomfort. Doppler auscultation of the TMJ is excellent for verifying that the disk has been completely recaptured. This is because crepitus will be eliminated, or barely audible crepitation will be noticed that probably results from some residual changes in the surface of the disk.

Prognosis

Any disk that is recapturable and will stay aligned in function when tested with an anterior bite plane has a good prognosis if the cause of the derangement is eliminated. If realignment is combined with perfected, nondeviating occlusion, both mechanical displacement and muscle incoordination are eliminated as causes. A continued good prognosis depends on maintaining that relationship.

LATERAL-POLE DISK DISPLACEMENT, NONREDUCIBLE

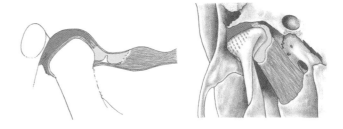

Now it is too late to recapture the disk onto the lateral pole. The lateral part of the posterior band is compressed into the anterior band, obliterating the central bearing area for the lateral pole of the condyle.

Description

The combination of pushing the thickened posterior band ahead of the lateral pole and the damage to the posterior and lateral diskal ligaments from direct loading of the retrodiskal tissues has caused an irreducible displacement of the lateral segment of the disk. As the two raised bands of the disk are pushed together, they coalesce into a single mass. The lateral pole of the condyle can no longer get past the thickened mass; if it could, there would be no concavity for it to rest in. The lateral border of the disk is now severely rotated medioanteriorly, but the medial pole of the condyle is still seated between the anterior and posterior bands of the disk.

Possible Causes

This stage is simply a progressive consequence of leaving the earlier stages untreated. The causes are the same as for the original beginning derangement, compounded by the progressive damage to the ligaments and to the disk. Just as in the previous stage, the adaptation of the disk is a response to excessive loading on the misaligned condyle-disk assembly. Understanding of the cause of this problem requires an understanding of each of the previous stages of derangement. When the progressive nature of the disorder is understood, it will be obvious why early diagnosis and treatment are in the patient's best interest.

Signs and Symptoms

Muscle incoordination is virtually always present at this stage, so one or more of the muscle-related signs or symptoms are usually present. There is generally some discomfort in the joint, and it may range from mild to severe, depending to a large extent on how much the patient keeps the teeth clenched together.

Patterns of occlusal wear or mobility can generally be related to the joint displacement and the muscle incoordination just as they were in the earlier stages.

Limitation of jaw movements becomes a more common sign as the damage progresses.

Methods for Diagnosing

History

The patient may or may not be aware of when the problem started, but in many cases he or she will remember the specific episode that started the acute phase of discomfort. Unfortunately, many acute phases are stimulated by simple dental procedures. Just keeping the mouth open for a prolonged period of treatment causes a loss of muscle memory patterns to maximum intercuspation. Until those engrams are re-established, the jaw will tend to close into a superior axis closure, and the patient will feel interferences that have been there all the time but were not noticed at the engram pattern of closure into maximum intercuspation. When the newly noticed interferences combine with the muscle fatigue from prolonged jaw opening, the result is often acute muscle spasm that in turn intensifies the already advanced stage of the joint disorder. The dentist who may have had nothing to do with causing the major breakdown in the joint gets the full blame for a problem that may have been progressing almost unnoticed for months or years.

The above scenario is avoidable if dentists will follow the advice given repeatedly in this text: Include a screening history and a screening examination of the TMJs as part of the initial complete examination that should be done on every patient. The routine use of Doppler auscultation of the TMJ would easily point out and document that a patient had a TMD before any treatment is initiated. The problem can then be discussed with the patient right away; thus this very common accusation is avoided. Furthermore, the dentist is immediately alerted to a problem that should be diagnosed so that the condition of the joint can be considered in the total treatment planning.

Just as causative factors start early and progress, the complete history does also. This stage is a continuation of that same history.

Clinical observation

One of the most significant observations to make is the path the mandible follows in straight protrusive. To move forward, the condyle may deviate around the thickened mass at the lateral half of the disk. A sudden lateral movement during protrusive movement is usually followed by a return movement back to the protrusive path. Upon opening, the jaw may follow a somewhat figure-S path with deviation toward the affected side.

Manipulative testing

Loading the joint at this stage may or may not produce some degree of discomfort or a feeling of tightness. Oddly enough, the joint may rotate easily during hingeing, giving the appearance of normalcy. If the closed lock has persisted for a while, and the medial pole is still seated on the bearing area of the disk, the joint may accept load testing with no discomfort. This is an indication of successful adaptation (adapted centric posture.)

Palpation

When the jaw is opened, the fingertip can be placed into the indentation behind the condyle. From that position, the posterior aspect of the condyle can be palpated. The finger can also be rolled around onto the lateral pole as the jaw opens and closes so that light pressure is applied to the ligaments behind the disk. This may produce some degree of tenderness if the disk is displaced forward. It may also be possible to feel the aberrant movement of the disk.

Palpation of the masticatory muscles virtually always produces varying degrees of tenderness that relates to the direction of mandibular displacement.

Auscultation

No definite click can be heard at this stage because there is no recapture of the disk. Doppler auscultation of the TMJ produces definite crepitation through hingeing and all excursions but is quiet on rotation. This is a classic finding if the medial pole is still aligned with the disk.

Radiographic findings

At this stage, there is usually little or no displacement of the condyle, so lateral transcranial films may show a normal relationship with the fossa if the medial pole is still reasonably well positioned. The disk derangement can be seen on MRI, which is the gold standard today for accuracy in showing the position of the disk from medial to lateral pole. In spite of this capability, it is generally not necessary to use MRI if it can be determined that the medial pole is aligned with the disk.

Blink mode computed tomography (CT) scan can show serial slices of the disk but does not (as of this writing) show the dynamic positioning in function that can be seen on MRI.

Mounted casts

If adapted centric posture can be verified by load testing, a bite record can be made and the occlusal relationship to the seated TMJs can be studied. Extensive clinical observation and experience with hundreds of patients have given us confidence that a lateral-pole closed lock can be a manageably stable relationship if the disk is still on the medial pole. It is advisable, however, to treat this joint position as tentative and wait for evidence of stability on a permissive occlusal splint before completing any extensive occlusal treatment.

Diagnostic occlusal therapy

Even though we may determine that we are dealing with a lateral-pole displacement, we cannot jump to a conclusion that it must be corrected. Many such derangements result in remodeling of the disk with formation of a new and acceptable bearing area. If the condition has been present for a long time and the adaptive response is acceptable, we may do the best service for the patient by working with that position to quiet the hyperactive musculature. To test such a hypothesis, a full occlusal bite plane can be made at the joint's most comfortable relationship. Careful monitoring of the bite appliance is necessary to keep it adjusted as changes take place in the joint. If the patient can be made comfortable and functional with such an appliance, occlusal therapy can then be finalized on the dentition as needed. The occlusion should still be harmonized to the most superior position of the condyle-disk assembly against the eminentia (adapted centric posture).

Treatment

If the medial pole of the condyle is still positioned reasonably well between the anterior and posterior bands of the disk, the chance for success is very favorable. In fact, today we routinely treat this condition as if it were a normal joint with one exception: The patient is advised that because of existing damage, the possibility of future problems is greater than we would expect from a normal intact TMJ.

At this stage, there are four common reasons why recapture of the complete disk may not be achieved:

1. Muscle spasm or fibrotic contracture of the superior pterygoid may be holding the disk forward and will not release it.
2. The lateral diskal ligament and parts of the posterior ligaments may be torn or too stretched or too weak to pull the disk back.

3. The coalesced anterior and posterior bands may have formed a solid mass that leaves no place for the lateral pole to seat.
4. Any combination of the above.

If the comfort level of the patient is not a problem and the age of the patient and suspected duration of the derangement indicate an acceptable remodeling within the articulation, occlusal therapy appears to be the usual treatment of choice. If a peaceful neuromuscular system can be established, damage in the joint is normally reduced to a level that is quite maintainable by periodic occlusal corrections.

Prognosis

As stated previously, the key to long-term treatment success is medial-pole coverage by the disk. If that can be verified, a perfected occlusal relationship harmonized to adapted centric posture can routinely stop the progression of the disk derangement and provide normal comfort, function, and manageable stability for the long term.

COMPLETE ANTERIOR DISK DISPLACEMENT

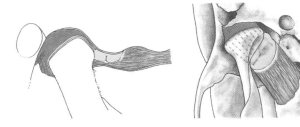

At this stage, the problem gets more serious. The disk is completely displaced forward of the condyle.

Description

The diskal ligaments to the lateral half of the disk have now been torn or stretched far enough to allow severe medioanterior displacement of the disk. As this occurs, more and more of the posterior band of the disk is progressively forced in front of the condyle until the entire posterior band has become anteriorly displaced. The condyle is now loaded entirely on the vascular, innervated retrodiskal tissues. In protrusive movements of the condyle, there is now a progressive tendency to force the disk ahead of the condyle while compressively loading the entire width of the posterior attachments to the disk.

Scapino has shown that the posterior attachments to the disk may respond to this forward thrust by moving the condylar attachment of the posterior ligament up the posterior surface of the condyle through bony remodeling at the attachment site. A response to excessive traction can occur either at the condylar attachment of the posterior ligament or at the temporal bone attachment of the superior strata of elastic fibers. The apparent reason for moving the anchorage of the elastic fibers forward rather than just allowing them to stretch is probably related to the common finding of fibrosis in the elastic fibers of deranged disks. The fibrosis would remarkably reduce the elasticity of the posterior attachment and thus increase the tension on the site of the attachment at the temporal bone.

The forward migration of the temporal attachment does not seem to require bony remodeling as is seen in the forward repositioning of the inelastic collagen fibers that attach the disk to the condyle. This forward attachment of the elastic fibers might also occur as a result of fibrous ankylosis initiated by intracapsular bleeding. Piper reports a fairly common occurrence of such ankylosis or adhesions in the retrodiskal tissues that have been damaged by direct loading from the condyle when the disk is anteriorly displaced.

Variations of Disk Displacements

There are many variations of complete disk displacement. In the early stages, the medial pole is usually reducible even if the lateral pole is not, because at the medial pole the anterior and posterior raised bands are often still intact and separated long after the lateral part of the disk has become irreducibly altered. The separation of the two bands provides a concave bearing area for the medial pole of the condyle just as long and only as long as the condyle can get past the posterior band and into the seating position between the two raised bands. In time, however, the breakdown of the posterior ligament progressively weakens the medial attachment of the disk, just as it has occurred at the lateral pole. So eventually the disk displacement becomes irreducible at the medial pole also. The resultant closed lock of the entire disk is subject to the same progressive changes that have been described for the lateral pole. All of the changes that now occur are dependent on time, intensity, and direction of the load applied through the condyle, tempered by the response of host resistance. It is, simply stated, a matter of adaptive response. The adaptive process can be destructive, or it can be beneficial.

How the disk adaptively responds to different directional loads and functional aberrations affects the type and degree of pathosis. Although complete disk displacements seem to generally follow the progressive stages just described, it is impossible to generalize on either a description of the disk or the exact sequence of derangement that leads to complete displacement. In addition to the variables of muscle hypercontraction and other loading factors, differences in pathosis can vary with age as well as with the wide range of resistance factors that occur from patient to patient. It is not surprising that there are many different configurations of disk displacement and that a description of the condition of the disk is a prime requirement for effective treatment planning.

The most common disk deformities that occur with complete displacement are as follows.

The disk is misshapened but is recapturable by both medial and lateral poles

The posterior band may or may not be thicker than normal. There is no remarkable difference in deformation between the medial and lateral areas of the disk. Displacement of the disk is nearly straightforward. It can become nonreducible, even when the posterior band is of normal thickness. Nonreducible disk derangements that occur without adaptive deformation of the disk are generally the result of sudden accidental injury.

The disk may be folded at the lateral portion but not at the medial bearing area

The flexure usually bends the disk, so the acute angle is on the inferior side, but the disk may fold in either direction. This condition may be reducible or nonreducible, or it may permit recapture of the medial pole only.

The disk is folded through its full width, so the central bearing area is narrowed or is obliterated completely

At this stage, the flexure is still a reversible mechanical deformation, since remodeling has not yet occurred to coalesce the folded segments. Thus, the disk is still capable of adaptive correction if the displacement can be reduced before remodeling changes irreversibly alter it. The disk may or may not be recapturable depending on the amount of damage to the disk or its ligamentous attachments.

The disk has become remodeled so that it is potentially recapturable at the medial pole only

The anterior and posterior bands have coalesced to obliterate the bearing area at the lateral pole. This condition can rapidly become nonreducible.

The disk is nonreducible, and the entire bearing area between the anterior and posterior bands has been obliterated by nonreversible remodeling changes

The above descriptions are related to deformities of the disk itself, but there are further considerations that must be determined before a treatment modality is selected. These determinations involve the mobility of the disk and can be described as hypermobile or hypomobile. A hypermobile disk results from loss of integrity of the ligaments that bind the disk to the condyle and the temporal bone. Disk hypomobility problems can result from several different factors, including adhesions, fibrous ankylosis, muscle hypercontraction, or myofibrositis. Determination of whether the disk is capable of normal translation is of critical importance to the diagnosis and treatment of disk derangements.

Possible Causes for Complete Anterior Disk Displacement

The disk obviously cannot be displaced completely in front of the condyle if all its attachments are intact. There must be some increase in length of the posterior attachments and the collateral ligaments. Other than a sudden accidental injury that stretches or tears those attachments, the process appears to be a rather slow one. Thus, complete displacement of the disk is usually the result of progressive stages of derangement. The early stages, however, may occur unnoticed by the patient, so the displacement may seem to be brought on suddenly by a wide yawn or a routine dental procedure.

Despite the common finding of increased thickness of the posterior band, it has not been correlated with the occurrence of reduction. Disks with no thickening of the posterior band may also be completely displaced and fail to reduce upon opening. This means that the critical element in complete disk displacement is related more to the condition of the retrodiskal attachment tissues than to the disk itself. It is logical to assume that the major deformities to the disk occur after the displacement and are related to time and intensity of load. A severe deformity of the disk is probably a rather reliable indicator that the displacement has been present for a long time.

The potential causes of complete disk displacement are the same causes that initiated the original derangement, compounded by the added factors of progressively damaged posterior attachments and mechanical loading against the posterior border of the disk. It should be remembered that the predominant factor of occlusally caused muscle incoordination that played such an important role in initiating the derangement is still the only intrinsic source of overload to the joint. Muscle incoordination results primarily from occlusal interferences that displace the mandible either forward or backward, so any occlusal deviation can be a causative factor.

Any factor that increases tension or reduces resistance to muscle hypercontraction should be considered as a potential contributing cause. These factors include nutritional or hormonal imbalances, emotional stress, allergies or sensitivities, and reactions to drugs or other chemicals. It is important, however, to distinguish between the actual mechanical displacement of the disk and the patient's response to the displacement. The mechanical displacement may have one set of causative factors. The patient's response may be controlled by a different set of factors that affect host resistance. Although some overlap occurs regarding hypertensive muscle contraction, I do not find hypertension as the initiating cause of disk displacements in a perfectly harmonized occlusion. There appears always to be some mechanical displacement of the mandible either as a direct causative factor or as a stimulus for muscle incoordination that may be intensified by the hypertension.

Once disk displacements are recognized as true mechanical misalignments and not as pure psychological disorders, the search for causes can be more direct and more logical. This is the reason for advocating a thorough enough examination to determine the position and condition of the disk as accurately as possible before speculation is done regarding its cause. Then any factor that could have caused or contributed to the misalignment should be considered, including developmental disorders, injury, habits, or pathologic alteration of any of the parts.

Signs and Symptoms

The principal early symptom in complete anterior displacements is pain in the joint region combined with varying degrees of muscle pain. The patient may be unable to precisely locate the focus of pain because it so often is commingled. At the early stages, the loaded retrodiskal tissues are still vascular and richly innervated, so compression can cause severe pain. As compressive changes occur in the tissues, the normal pattern of vascular retrodiskal tissues may be replaced by a more compact mass of fibers that are almost devoid of the small vessels that were originally present. As the vessels disappear from the bearing area, the pain diminishes. If the adaptive remodeling response is successful, a new avascular bearing pad of fibers that provides a pain-free extension to the disk may be formed. This is often an acceptable substitute for the original correctly aligned disk. From this potential response to displacement, one can see that the symptom of pain can vary from extreme pain to no pain, depending on how the compressed tissues adapt.

Since pain is the most important symptom to consider in determining treatment, it should be evaluated carefully to determine its source. In a large number of patients with complete disk displacements, I have observed the pain almost entirely attributable to muscle incoordination, with little or none in the joint itself. Such patients generally respond well to occlusal therapy.

The principal sign associated with complete disk displacement is clicking. As long as the disk displacement is reducible, a click will be observed on opening as the condyle clicks onto the disk, followed by a reciprocal click upon closing as the condyle slips back off the disk.

When the elastic fibers lose their ability to overcome the forward push of the motive condyle against the disk, the clicks disappear, indicating a closed lock. From that point on, the potential for degenerative joint disease increases.

Methods of Diagnosis

History

When the disk is anteriorly displaced, the history may include a long recital of a series of events that started years before with the placement of a crown or a fixed bridge. It may have started when a dentist adjusted the occlusion and may have progressed through years of unsuccessful attempts to treat the TMJ. If one analyzes such histories, it will become apparent that the beginning of a very high percentage of such problems started with some alteration of the occlusion. From that point on, the progression of symptoms often parallels the progressive stages of disk derangement.

If the history reveals the use of bite splints, the splints should be examined for accuracy. My experience is that very few occlusal splints are in correct harmony with a verified centric relation. Patients also frequently report with positioning devices that do not correctly relate the jaw to an acceptable joint alignment. It is important to evaluate each appliance to be able to understand the results reported in the patient's history.

A complete history should be encouraged, and every rational description should be evaluated to see if it could be explained and related to the current condition. Knowing that disk displacement is at the end of a sequence of progressively deformative derangements, the history can provide many helpful clues regarding the course of the disorder and its effect on the patient.

Clinical observations

On opening, the jaw will normally deviate toward the side of the displacement, sometimes very sharply. If the displacement is reducible, the reducing condyle may suddenly jump forward, bringing the mandible back to a more centered relationship after reduction. If it is nonreducing, the mandible may stay deviated upon opening.

It is often difficult or impossible to move the jaw laterally away from the displaced side, but it moves easily toward the displaced side. If reduction occurs immediately upon opening, the posterior attachments to the disk are still reasonably intact.

If reduction does not occur before the condyle has translated forward about 3 mm (about two finger widths of opening), the posterior attachment may be damaged too badly to recapture the disk and have it stay recaptured during function.

Manipulative testing

If the condyle is loaded with upward pressure against vascular innervated tissue, there will be some response of tenderness or tension. With newly displaced disks, pressure may cause sharp pain. The discomfort must be distinguished from that caused by applied tension against the contracted lateral pterygoid muscle or from pathosis, but any sign of discomfort should alert us to the possibility of disk displacement. Use of other diagnostic tests may be necessary to distinguish between the other possibilities of pathosis, or muscle bracing.

If a disk displacement is confirmed but loading of the joint does not cause discomfort, it is an indication that adaptive remodeling may have altered the retrodiskal tissues to form a new bearing-pad extension of the displaced disk. Even though the disk may be displaced, the new alignment may be acceptable if it permits medial-pole bracing of the condyle. The same may be true in some bone-to-bone relationships if the articulating surfaces of the condyle and eminence have remodeled to hard eburnated surfaces.

Manipulative loading of the joints is an extremely valuable test to determine whether an acceptable level of comfort can be achieved with the present conditions.

Palpation

Finger pressure through the skin depression behind the condyle when the jaw is open will usually provoke tenderness in varying degrees depending on the condition of the posterior attachment. Palpation of masticatory muscles is almost certain to cause a tenderness response in the incoordinated muscles that are involved in the jaw displacement.

Auscultation

Doppler auscultation of the TMJ is an almost foolproof method for determining whether or not the condyle is on the disk. It is also very reliable for determining the precise point of recapture and displacement when the disk is reducible because the reciprocal clicks are audible even when they cannot be heard through a stethoscope.

The character of the amplified crepitus sounds is also diagnostic: The coarser the crepitus, the more there is breakdown of the posterior ligament. Chirping sounds indicate perforation of the ligament. If the chirping is mixed with very coarse crepitus, there is a probability that the posterior ligament has been severely damaged or lost and there is a bone-to-bone articulation.

Ankylosis of the disk would produce opening and closing clicks at the same protrusive position of the condyle. If the disk is not ankylosed but is still reducible, the opening click usually occurs at a more open relationship than the closing click. If the disk is not recapturable, crepitus will be heard for all jaw movements and there will be no click.

Radiographic findings

If the disk is completely displaced, lateral transcranial radiographs usually show the condyle distal to a centralized position in the fossa (Figures 25-4 and 25-5). The space above the condyle is often diminished also, but the diagnosis cannot be based solely on transcranial radiographs because variations in condyle-fossa contour can cause an appearance of displacement when one does not exist. Variations in beam angulation can also distort the apparent condyle position, and so transcranial radiographs should always be used in combination with other diagnostic tests. Nevertheless, transcranial radiographs have great value in many instances, often disclosing important information about the condition of the condyle or eminence such as re-

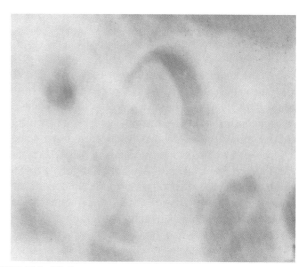

FIGURE 25-4 Transcranial film of a condyle with complete anterior displacement of the disk. Note the distalized position of the condyle in the fossa, and the uneven space showing around the condyle. Compare this with normal joint in Figure 25-5.

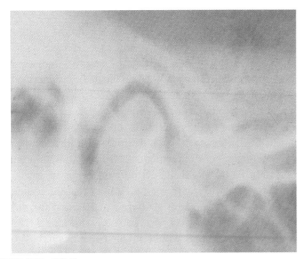

FIGURE 25-5 Transcranial radiograph of a normal TMJ. Note the fairly even space around the condyle. Also note the cortical layer of bone along the eminence and fossa. A picture of normal must be visualized before aberrations can be noticed.

modeling changes at the bony surfaces, degenerative joint disease, or other forms of pathosis.

Arthrography

Although arthrography is rarely used today because of the availability of noninvasive MRI, we learned much about how the disk responds in many different deformative conditions from early studies. Combining arthrography with fluoroscopy, we were able to see the action of the disk during function (Figures 25-6 and 25-7). Through *differential arthrography,* a method developed by Mark Piper, we were able to observe the effect of muscle incoordination on disk alignment. While observing the position of nonreducible disks via the fluoroscope, then anesthetizing the motor innervation to the superior lateral pterygoid muscle, it became evident that muscle contraction played a dominant role in disk displacement. In some TMJs, the disk spontaneously reduced when the muscle was anesthetized.

Magnetic resonance imaging

Today, the unquestioned gold standard for diagnosis of disk derangements is MRI. The consequences of complete disk displacement are too varied to trust to guessing what the condition or position of the disk is. Because of the work of Schellhas, precise procedures for imaging the TMJs make it possible to see the exact position and condition of the disk on both the medial and lateral poles of the condyle. In addition to assessing soft tissues, MRI shows bone marrow changes, disk morphology, mobility, and joint effusion (see Chapter 27).

MRI is typically reserved for complete disk derangements, or when unexplainable pain or dysfunction of the TMJs is present that does not respond to treatment. There is a simple rule to follow in regard to all TMJ problems: *If the joint cannot comfortably accept loading, find out why.* If routine diagnos-

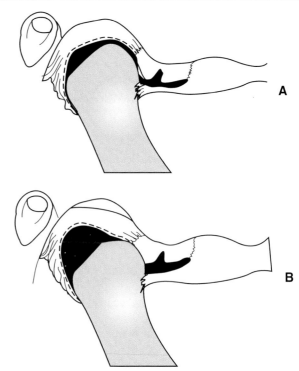

FIGURE 25-6 Early arthrographic studies combined with fluoroscopy show the action of a displaced disk during function. **A,** The dye pattern in retruded position. Notice that the dye extends well forward of the condyle in the inferior joint space and outlines the underside of the disk. The posterior band has been pushed forward, nearly obliterating the normal seating area for the condyle. In **B,** the disk has been shoved ahead of the protruding condyle without reduction. Diagnosis: nonreducible disk derangement. Disk is not bound down and is most likely repairable. In some joints, anesthetizing the superior lateral pterygoid motor-innervation caused the disk to spontaneously reduce.

tic procedures do not reveal the cause of the pain or dysfunction, MRI is recommended. It would be an unwise decision to proceed with extensive occlusal therapy, orthodontics, or restorative treatment in the presence of an undiagnosed TMD.

Please see Chapter 27 for a better understanding of how a magnetic resonance image can be used to determine the relationship of the disk to a correct alignment on the condyle as its image when the disk is misaligned.

Computed tomography

CT is very useful for assessing abnormalities of bone such as ankylosis, dysplasias, growth abnormalities, fractures, and osseous tumors. With the manufacture of head/neck CT scanners, precise analysis of condylar position, contour, and bone surfaces is possible. Structural analysis of the temporomandibular articulation can, today, be as complete as is necessary to arrive at an accurate diagnosis.

New imaging technology offers unparalleled opportunities to examine all of the bony structures in the masticatory system. The NewTom CT scanner (see Chapter 27) facilitates thin 1 mm slices from any direction through the TMJ and other structures. The combination of CT and MRI has opened the door to much better understanding of disorders

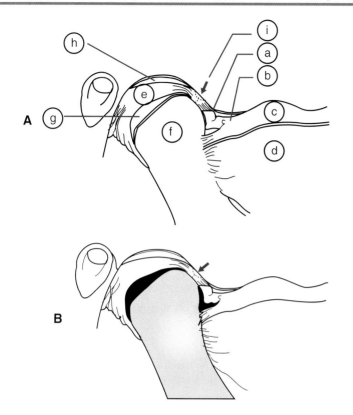

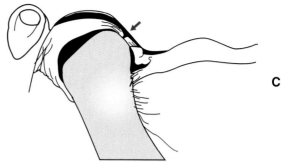

FIGURE 25-7 Arthrogram pattern when there is a perforation in the retrodiskal tissues. Notice how dye leaks through from the inferior joint space into the superior joint space. In this illustration, the disk is folded in front of the protruding condyle. **A,** Orientation of tissues: posterior band of disk, *a;* anterior band of disk, *b;* superior lateral pterygoid muscle, *c;* inferior lateral pterygoid muscle, *d;* posterior ligaments and retrodiskal tissues, *e;* condyle, *f;* inferior joint space, *g;* superior joint space, *h;* perforation through posterior ligament, *i.* **B,** Dye in inferior joint space only. **C,** Leakage of dye through a perforation *(arrow)* in the posterior ligament. Notice how dye then spreads into superior joint space.

in both hard and soft tissues of the masticatory system. Today it is almost impossible for a structural disorder of the TMJs to hide from a knowledgeable clinician.

Mounted casts for complete disk displacement patients
If the disk can be recaptured and can travel with the condyle back to a verifiable centric relation or adapted centric posture, a bite record can be taken at that relationship and the casts mounted with reasonable accuracy for diagnosing occlusal disharmony. In patients with complete disk derangement, the centric relation position, when capturable, should be considered a tentative treatment position because some changes in joint position can occur as the disk alters its shape after being distorted by the displacement and then being returned to a loaded position.

In nonreducible joints that have undergone adaptive remodeling of a disk extension, manipulative testing and imaging may show the new condyle-disk relationship to be acceptable. If the position is comfortable when loaded and if functional excursions are acceptable, that verified position can be used as the correct jaw-to-jaw relationship for mounting the casts.

If a nonreducible disk displacement results in an uncomfortable condyle position that cannot be rectified, mounting of casts to that uncomfortable relationship has limited value. The purpose of mounted casts is to study the occlusal relationship at the fully seated position of the condyles so that harmony between the occlusion and the TMJs can be achieved. If centric relation or adapted centric posture cannot be achieved, a treatment position based on imaging and other

guidelines for determining the most physiologic relationship may be selected. Casts mounted in that relationship may be used for fabrication of occlusal splints made to the tentative treatment position, but final occlusal correction cannot be achieved until adaptation or corrective therapy has repositioned the condyles to an acceptably stable and comfortable relationship. A superior repositioning splint is the appliance of choice when a tentative treatment position is used.

Diagnostic occlusal therapy
Occlusal therapy should always have a specific purpose in mind. Diagnostic occlusal therapy should be designed to test a definitive premise that is related to a suspected or diagnosed condition. In complete anterior disk displacements, the following determinations must be made before a final treatment plan can be selected:

1. Can the disk be recaptured (reduced)?
2. Will the disk translate with the condyle to centric relation?
3. Will the recaptured disk stay aligned in function?

On disks that can be reduced and returned to centric relation without losing alignment, an anterior bite plane can be used diagnostically to see if the disk will stay aligned in function. If the displacement is intercepted early enough before the posterior attachment has been damaged too badly, it is not uncommon to be able to recapture the disk and have it stay aligned in function. When this occurs with the use of an anterior bite plane, a diagnosis of mandibular displacement from occlusion is confirmed as the trigger for disk displacement. If the joint is more uncomfortable with the anterior bite plane, the diagnosis is clear that even though the disk is reducible it will not stay aligned in function. It should then be treated accordingly.

If the disk is irreducibly displaced but manipulative testing shows an acceptable comfort level when the joint is loaded, suspect that remodeling of the vascular retrodiskal tissues has occurred to provide an avascular fibrous extension of the disk. If the joint is comfortable with an anterior bite plane when the disk is known to be anteriorly displaced, the beneficial adaptive response is confirmed and you may proceed with final occlusal treatment as soon as positional stability has been assured at this adapted centric posture (usually through the use of a full occlusal bite plane).

If Doppler analysis of the TMJ has shown a bone-to-bone articulation, confirmed with radiographs and other tests, you may use full occlusal splints diagnostically to see if reasonable joint stability can be achieved by a reduction in muscle hyperactivity. If degenerative joint disease is active from excessive muscular loading, it may be possible to reverse the regressive remodeling with a more peaceful neuromuscular system that reduces the force against the articular surfaces and allows adaptive repair.

If a dentition requires extensive restoration of the occlusal surfaces, equilibration may be used directly rather than using full occlusal splints because any adjustments to natural teeth can be refined if needed in the final restorations.

If a disk is anteriorly displaced but can be recaptured with no more than 3 mm of protrusion and it will not stay aligned with the condyle when translating back to centric relation, or will not stay aligned in function, you may fabricate a diagnostic occlusal splint to see if the alignment can be maintained in a forward jaw position. If alignment of the disk can be maintained in function at the forward jaw position, you can alter the same appliance to see if the condyle and disk can be slowly moved back to centric relation without loss of disk alignment. Such anterior repositioning splints are still advocated by some clinicians, but MRI studies have confirmed that it is extremely rare for the disk to be permanently reduced by this procedure. Anterior positioning splints have no value if the disk is ankylosed or is nonreducible, so determination should always be made before any anterior positioning devices are prescribed.

TREATING COMPLETE DISK DISPLACEMENTS

Treatment Categories

For treatment purposes, the various conditions of complete disk displacement can be categorized into treatment groups:

1. Complete anterior disk displacement
   a. Reducible to function
   b. Segmentally reducible to function
   c. Reducible but not maintainable in function
   d. Nonreducible, repairable
   e. Nonreducible, nonrepairable
2. Posterior disk displacement

By extending the diagnosis to further define the various conditions that exist within the broad group of anteriorly displaced disks, you can target treatment toward specific conditions rather than using a broad-spectrum nonspecific treatment for all displaced disks. The need for this type of specificity becomes apparent in a practice that sees a large number of patients with TMDs. It is not uncommon to see patients wearing anterior repositioning splints for the purpose of capturing ankylosed, nonrepairable, or even nonexistent disks. Such erroneous, empiric treatment has no chance for success. If the exact purpose of the prescribed treatment is not targeted at a clearly defined condition, the diagnosis is incomplete.

Complete anterior disk displacement, reducible to function
Treatment for displaced disks that are reducible to function should have three objectives that must be fulfilled:

1. Recapture of the disk in correct alignment
2. Translation of the condyle to centric relation without loss of the recaptured disk
3. Maintenance of correct disk alignment in function

Since these three goals cannot be achieved out of sequence, the starting point for treatment is always directed toward recapturing the correct alignment of the disk. Complete displacements of the type that are reducible can present two distinctly different conditions that require different treatment formats. From a treatment perspective, functionally reducible disk displacements should be divided into those displacements that are self-reducing versus those that require some form of manipulation or therapeutic intervention to achieve disk recapture.

Self-reducing disk displacements compose the large group of reciprocally clicking joints that click onto the disk upon opening and click off the disk upon closure. But self-reduction of the disk alignment does not automatically mean the alignment can be maintained in function. After reduction is achieved, you still must determine if the disk and its attachments are intact enough to travel with the moving condyle through the full range of function. To test that, you must disengage all occlusal interferences to rule out mechanical displacement. There are three effective ways to quickly determine if the recaptured disk will function in correct alignment:

1. Through cotton roll separation of the teeth
2. Through use of a flat, anterior bite plane
3. Through methods that equalize occlusal pressures while eliminating all incline contacts

The reduction of a disk displacement to function can sometimes be verified on the spot by use of a long cotton roll laid across the arch approximately in line with the premolar area on each side. Sometimes just the separation of the teeth

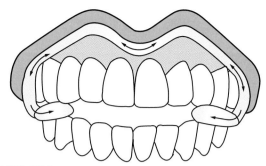

FIGURE 25-8 Aqualizer device is illustrative of a method for muscle deprogramming. Water-filled pads connected for equalization of pressure separate the teeth and thereby eliminate influence from tooth inclines that displace the mandible. The muscles are free to position the condyle in a seated position without interference.

eliminates the muscle incoordination and allows the disk to reduce spontaneously. More likely, it will be necessary to recapture the disk with judicious manipulation and then load the joint with bilateral pressure to verify the position. Pressure is maintained while you hinge the jaw a few times before closing into contact with the cotton roll. If disk alignment is not lost while you are manipulating, release the hands and have the patient close into the cotton. If clenching into the cotton roll does not cause the disk to be displaced, the prognosis is good for treatment with occlusal correction.

The anterior bite plane can be used, as already described, to test the functional stability of the disk alignment for a day or two. Pressure-equalizing devices, such as the Aqualizer™ (Figure 25-8), also permit unrestricted access to centric relation, so they are useful for testing as well as for reduction of muscle hyperactivity.

If the disk is capable of staying aligned in function, it will generally do so once it is recaptured and permitted free access to centric relation. Any of the previously described methods will work to make that diagnosis. However, that diagnosis cannot always be confirmed so easily in the short time a cotton roll or a central bearing point is in place. Minor changes in the newly reloaded disk may help to stabilize the alignment if given more time. If the disk stays reasonably stable but displaces only with rapid or extreme jaw movements, a full occlusal bite plane can be helpful, adjusted precisely to centric relation, with an anterior ramp for posterior disclusion in all eccentric positions.

The patient should also be instructed to make no unnecessary or extreme jaw movements and to wear the splint continuously, even when eating (a soft diet). Stability is usually improved as the disk recontours itself in the improved relationship.

Recapture of the disk to function is often spontaneous once the mechanical reasons for mandibular deviation are corrected or disengaged, but recapturing the disk in some patients is more complex. If the disk displacement has resulted in a closed lock that is held tightly by hypercontracted or spastic musculature, the disk may be prevented from reduction because of the tight loading against its posterior

band. In such cases, reduction may be facilitated by distraction of the condyle away from the eminence to make room for the disk to be pulled back between the two articular surfaces. If enough elastic fibers are still intact to pull the unlocked disk back, the downward distraction of the condyle may be effective. An excellent method for accomplishing this is illustrated in Figure 25-9.

The effectiveness of this procedure is related to how soon it is done after the closed-lock condition began. The sooner the treatment, the better is the chance of reduction to function. The procedure works well on jaws that have suddenly luxated. It is rarely effective on closed locks that have been displaced for extended periods. It should nevertheless be tried on any closed-lock situation because it occasionally will result in reduction of the disk when least expected.

If reduction occurs after an extended period of closed-lock displacement, there will be a separation of the posterior teeth because the thickness of the disk will be added to the height of the condyle. The teeth will erupt back to contact if the disk stays aligned, but the first priority is to make sure disk alignment can be maintained in function. Sometimes a flat anterior bite plane is all that is needed to keep the disk alignment while the posterior teeth erupt. If so, eruption must be monitored carefully so that the anterior appliance can be discarded when enough eruption has occurred to occlude the posterior teeth.

When a full occlusion is possible, it should be equilibrated as needed to prevent a recurrence of mandibular displacement, which could retrigger the disk displacement. If orthodontics or restorative procedures will be required to correct the occlusal disharmony, it will be an advantage to use a full occlusal bite plane to stabilize the joints first (superior repositioning splint). Occlusal treatment cannot be finalized until the joints are stabilized.

Some anteriorly displaced disk problems are caused by distalization of the condyle, although distalization of the condyle is not as prevalent as we once thought. Treatment consists of correcting the position or contour of any contacting surfaces that force the condyle distally during maximum jaw closure. It is not unusual to find that a distalized mandible can be manipulated rather easily into a verifiable centric relation. Often the jaw must first be brought forward a bit with no pressure applied, to recapture the disk. Then after the condyle-disk alignment has been achieved in a slightly protruded position, upward pressure can be used to keep the condyle loaded in the center of the disk while slowly easing both condyle and disk back to centric relation. Now, while maintaining the upward pressure with bilateral manipulation, hinge the jaw a few times but stop short of tooth contact. If the joints are completely comfortable while loaded, maintain the pressure and hinge the jaw delicately to the first point of occlusal contact. Tap lightly a few times against the contact to get the patient used to that position. Then hold the jaw at the first point of contact. Now observe very carefully the direction the mandible slides from first point of contact to maximum intercuspation when the patient squeezes.

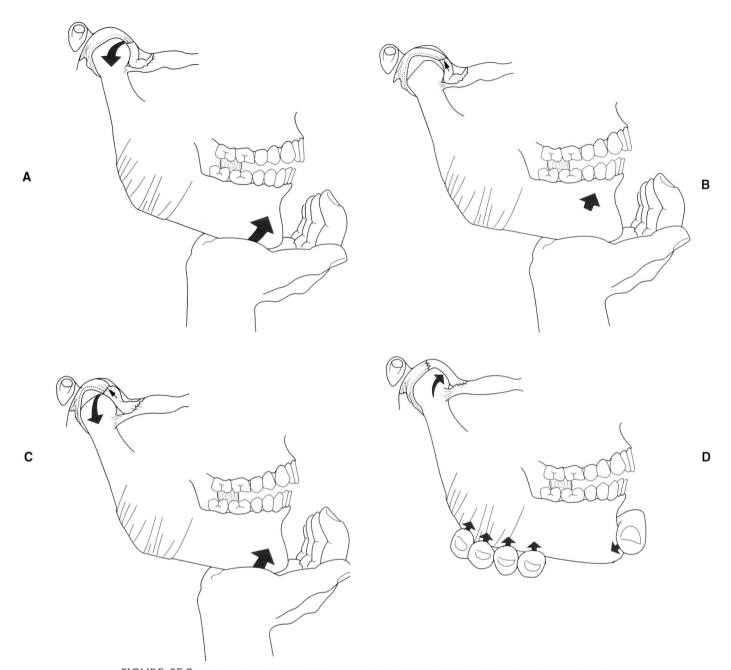

FIGURE 25-9 **A,** Distraction of the condyle from a muscle-loaded, closed lock requires a pivot between the molar teeth and external pressure up at the chin point. This pivots the condyle away from the eminence and provides room for the disk to move back. **B,** When enough space is created, the disk can then be pulled back between the condyle and the eminentia if there is enough tension left in the posterior elastic ligament and if the muscle can release it. Several minutes of distraction may be required. The process will not work if the disk is ankylosed or adhesed. **C,** The disk may snap back into place, or it may slowly extend back. The distraction should be maintained without interruption for best results. **D,** If the disk returns to correct alignment, release of the distraction will not cause discomfort. At that point, manipulation should be used to test for centric relation and also to load the condyles forward toward the eminentiae to help hold the alignment in the concavity of the disk. Teeth should be separated so that displacement is not retriggered. An anterior bite plane can then be used to see if the disk will stay aligned in function.

If the shift tends to distalize either condyle, see if the disk displaces as the tooth-directed distalization occurs. If it does, you are dealing with a true mechanical displacement as the cause of the disk problem. Disks that do not displace until tooth contact occurs have an excellent prognosis for a quick return to function. Treatment must be directed at freeing up the occlusion to allow the mandible a more forward intercuspated position that is coincident with the verified centric relation. This may be accomplished directly with occlusal equilibration, or provisionally with the use of a bite plane corrected to centric relation.

Forward displacement of the condyle

Because the role of muscle incoordination as a cause of disk derangements has been ignored by so many clinicians, the concept of forward displacement of the mandible being related to anterior disk displacement has also been missed. The observant diagnostician, however, will find that the majority of disk derangements do in fact occur with no evidence whatsoever of any distalization of the condyle. When the displaced disk is recaptured and the aligned condyle-disk assembly is moved to a verified centric relation position with the teeth apart, it is not unusual to find, on tooth contact, that the mandibular shift from centric relation to maximum intercuspation is forward. Furthermore, when the mechanical cause of forward displacement is corrected, the disk alignment stabilizes and the tendency for disk displacement is eliminated almost immediately in many of these patients.

When a disk displacement can be reduced to alignment that is retained in function, the patient should be advised to avoid hard foods or wide opening for a few weeks as a precaution against recurrent displacement of the disk because the posterior attachments and the collateral ligaments are obviously stretched to some degree and thus not as protective of the disk alignment as they would normally be. Maintenance of the alignment is not generally a problem if the occlusal harmony is monitored.

With any recaptured disk that has been in a closed-lock relationship, there is the probability of some changes in the disk after the condyle is realigned into its center-bearing area. These adaptive changes may be no more than minor realignment of fiber patterns, or they may involve some adaptive remodeling. However, any changes in the disk will probably result in some slight changes in the centric relation position of the condyles. For that reason, final occlusal treatment should be delayed until the centric relation position appears to be stable. Provisional occlusal correction can be made on a full occlusal splint that is precisely adjusted to centric relation and checked at intervals of two to four weeks. When the need for further adjustment to the bite plane is reduced to minute corrections, or none at all, that is evidence that the condyle-disk alignment has become stabilized. Tooth mobility must also be considered as a factor, and it should be as stable as possible before final occlusal treatment is completed. If extensive restorative procedures are needed, provisional occlusal correction can be accom-

plished directly through equilibration of the teeth or on cemented provisional splints.

The earlier a complete disk displacement can be treated, the better will be the prognosis for maintaining correct alignment. The longer the displacement goes untreated, the greater the chance for irreversible damage to the disk or its attachments. Preserving the integrity of the disk preserves also the synovial lubrication and nutrition that is important to the health of the joint structures.

Complete anterior disk displacement, segmentally reducible to function

A complete disk displacement that can be reduced only to a partial recapture of the disk will almost always be nonreducible at the lateral pole. Treatment will be related to the reasons for nonrecapturability of the lateral part of the disk. These reasons necessarily involve stretching or tearing of the lateral diskal ligament and at least part of the posterior attachments to the disk, and they usually, but not always, include some changes in the disk itself. The most commonly found deformities are related to flexure of the disk with resultant remodeling, which is related to how long the flexure has been occurring and how the posterior band is loaded as a result of the flexure.

If the medial pole can recapture its part of the central bearing area of the disk and then maintain that alignment back to an adapted centric posture, it may be possible to achieve a functional maintainability of the alignment by elimination of all causes of muscle incoordination. Treatment would consist of a muscle relaxation splint made to perfectly coincide with the seated position of the joint. This would have to be considered a tentative position because it would not include proper alignment of the complete disk, but the most important requirement of medial-pole bracing could be accomplished, and this is the essential requirement for achieving a peaceful neuromusculature.

If the medial pole part of the condyle-disk assembly can brace against the uppermost medial part of the fossa, the lateral pterygoid muscle can release its contraction against the elevator muscles. When this can occur, there is no trigger for antagonistic incoordinated muscle contraction.

It appears from our clinical observations that a partially deranged disk has a reasonable chance of remodeling into an acceptable functioning pad for the condyle if we can achieve a coordinated muscle function. If the disk is aligned with the medial pole and is not overloaded by muscle hypercontraction, it serves as a pad to prevent overload on the retrodiskal tissues that are between the lateral part of the condyle and the eminentia. This is sometimes a relationship that stimulates an adaptive response of fibrous remodeling of the retrodiskal tissues combined with a disappearance of blood vessels and nerves from the newly formed pad.

To accomplish the above results, the muscle relaxation splint must be kept in near-perfect harmony with the fully seated joint position of the moment. As joint changes occur, the splint must be adjusted to preserve the harmony between the occlusion and the braced position of the aligned condyle-disk assembly at the medial pole. The muscle relaxation splint must be fabricated so that it fits comfortably and securely. It should have an anterior guidance ramp that discludes all posterior teeth in all jaw positions except adapted centric posture. It should be worn at all times. It is effectively a superior repositioning splint.

The criteria for using this treatment approach are:

1. Medial pole alignment with the disk must be maintainable in function.
2. The level of comfort and function must be tolerable to the patient while wearing the splint.

The patient should be counseled to understand that changes in the joint occur slowly and that patience will be required because many adjustments to the splint may be necessary before the joint returns to a stable relationship. At that point, the splint can be discarded, and whatever occlusal therapy is needed can be accomplished in final form.

Complete anterior disk displacement, reducible but not maintainable in function

Being able to recapture a displaced disk does not necessarily mean it will stay recaptured during function. There are three types of disk problems that may prevent maintaining alignment through the functional range of condylar movement:

1. *Hyper*mobility of the disk
2. *Hypo*mobility of the disk
3. Deformity of the disk

Disk hypermobility results from the disk being too loosely connected to the condyle and the temporal bone attachment. Even though the disk may be recapturable at some point along the protrusive path, damage to the elastic fibers or the ligamentous attachments to the disk allows it to slip out of position as the condyle travels forward and backward on the eminentia.

Disk hypomobility results from the disk being immobilized by adhesions, ankylosis, or muscle spasm. The condyle may move on and off the disk, but the disk cannot move to travel with the condyle.

Deformity of the disk results from either overloading or underloading parts of the disk. Although a prolonged overload or misdirection of forces can cause changes in the shape of the disk, a common factor in disk derangement results from unloading the medial pole. A down-forward displacement of the condyle during intercuspation leaves a void where the medial pole normally fits into a thin concavity of the disk. A correctly aligned condyle-disk assembly, in turn, loads against the reinforced, medial concavity of the bony fossa. When the condyle is held forward down the eminence, the thin, concave bearing area of the disk begins to thicken to fill the space left by the vacated condyle.

The medial pole–bearing area of the disk is normally one of the thinnest parts of the disk, but it can become thickened by several millimeters to a convex shape over a period of time if the condyle is anteriorly displaced by occlusal inclines. The medial thickening can also be encouraged by the medioanterior rotation of the disk as the lateral diskal ligament breaks down.

If the medial part of a thickened, nonreducible disk can be observed through a surgical microscope, it will be evident why it cannot stay aligned with the condyle in function. Surgical thinning of the medial pole–bearing surface of the disk regains a stable concave seat for the medial pole and permits function without displacement.

It is probable that any hypermobile disk that will not stay captured in function will eventually become nonreducible unless treated. We have three treatment choices:

1. Mandibular repositioning
2. Surgical correction
3. Using the patient's adaptive response

Mandibular repositioning splints have one basic purpose: to move the mandible to a position that aligns the condyle with the displaced disk. Mandibular alignment is achieved by relating steeply inclined occlusal surfaces on the splint, so that maximum intercuspation occurs at the position that aligns the condyle with the forwardly displaced disk. The intended effect of this forward repositioning of the condyle is to relieve the retrodiskal tissues from being compressed by the condyle. If the condyle-disk assembly is held in a forward position, it was originally thought that the retrodiskal tissues would heal and regain elasticity. MRI studies show that the retrodiskal tissues develop adhesions and scar tissue that are unstable. Once a very popular clinical approach, anterior repositioning has not produced stable results for the long term. It has also become apparent that fibrotic contracture of the superior lateral pterygoid muscle prevents release of the disk to move back with the condyle.

Corrective surgery can be used to preserve the disk if damage has not progressed too far. Preserving the disk has the advantage of also preserving the nutritional and lubricating effects from the synovial fluids, both of which are preventive for degenerative joint disease.

Surgical correction procedures include the following:

1. Meniscoplasty to reshape deformed disks
2. Release of superior pterygoid muscle contracture
3. Plication to shorten the posterior attachments, which help to hold the disk in place on the condyle
4. Release of an adhesed or ankylosed disk
5. Removal of bony spicules on articular surfaces
6. Correction of pathologic deformities or growth abnormalities
7. Repair of perforations or tears in the posterior and collateral ligaments

Using the patient's adaptive response may be considered if the disk will not stay aligned in function and the posterior ligament is too badly damaged to respond to anterior repositioning. If surgical intervention is ruled out, an attempt can be made to get an adaptive response in the retrodiskal tissues by reducing muscle incoordination to the minimum. A full occlusal splint harmonized to the most comfortable joint position may produce an acceptable result. The patient should be aware in advance that the adaptive response occurs slowly, so patience is required. Repeated adjustment of the splint is required as changes in the joint occur.

The prognosis for adaptive remodeling of the retrodiskal tissues may be more acceptable than one might expect. Before we had a better understanding of the function of the disk, most TMDs were treated without regard for the disk when attempts were made to reduce muscular overload. If the occlusion was maintained in meticulous adjustment long enough, even patients with disk displacements generally improved. There were exceptions, but fortunately they composed a very small percentage of patients. Because of the high success rate enjoyed by some dentists who were extremely proficient at occlusal therapy, there may be some reluctance to consider a surgical approach. New and vastly improved microsurgical techniques enable the specially trained surgeon to repair defects in many joints more directly, and I suspect this can take place with a better long-term prognosis than what can be achieved by adaptation of a misaligned disk. The criteria for advocating surgical correction over more conservative occlusal therapy are based on three decisions:

1. Is the level of discomfort intolerable to the patient?
2. Is the discomfort unrelieved by noninvasive treatment?
3. Is the potential for further pathosis unfavorable without surgical correction?

Unless there is a probability of intolerable discomfort or imminent pathosis without surgical intervention, the conservative treatment of displaced disks is the preferred approach. The reduction of muscle hyperactivity is essential to the success of the surgical approach anyway, so occlusal therapy, usually with full occlusal muscle-relaxation splints, should be attempted before the final decision for surgery is made.

Complete anterior disk displacement, nonreducible but repairable

The options for nonreducible disk displacements are narrowed down to two:

1. Surgical correction or repair
2. Using the patient's adaptive response

Anterior repositioning devices have no value for a noncapturable disk. In fact, they are contraindicated. The purpose of anterior repositioning is to unload the retrodiskal tissues so that they can heal and regain the elastic traction necessary for pulling the disk back with the condyle. We pay a price for anterior repositioning because it produces muscle incoordination. Whenever the mandible is displaced forward of centric relation (even when it is intentional), the combination of lateral pterygoid bracing against elevator muscle contraction occurs. Incoordinated antagonistic muscle contraction has a tendency to develop into muscle hypercontraction. So unless that hypercontraction is directed through the disk, the loading is applied onto the very tissues we are trying to heal. If beneficial adaptive changes are to be encouraged in the retrodiskal tissues, they will occur more

readily with the decreased muscle loading of a peaceful neuromuscular harmony. We do not achieve a peaceful neuromusculature with anterior repositioning forward of medial-pole bracing by bone.

Recapture and repair of a nonreducible disk displacement requires three conditions:

1. The disk must be intact enough to be correctable to a functional state.
2. The disk must be capable of translation (with treatment if necessary).
3. Damage to the posterior ligamentous attachments must be within limits that permit repair.

If the disk is nonreducible, the first treatment decision is whether recapture of the disk is essential for an acceptable level of comfort and function. In some situations, even though a displaced disk could be surgically reduced, adaptive changes that have already occurred make invasive treatment unnecessary. The decision for invasive versus noninvasive treatment should not be based on an "always" or "never" mentality. Both choices should be considered for each patient, and the decision should be made on the basis of which type of therapy will have the best chance of restoring the joint to an acceptable level of comfort without sacrificing functional stability.

Using the level of comfort or discomfort as a criterion for determining treatment has validity only if the cause of the discomfort has been clearly determined. Without question, the cause of discomfort is far more likely to be related to muscle incoordination than it is to intra-articular sources. This point is proved to us repeatedly by the routine success of muscle-relaxation splints, even on patients with displaced disks. More study is necessary, but it appears probable that if we can achieve a level of comfort that is acceptable to the patient, coincidental with a peaceful neuromusculature, we will also achieve adaptive remodeling of the articular structures if treatment is initiated early enough.

Although adaptive remodeling of either hard or soft tissues may make the joint more comfortable, the stability of those remodeled tissues may be tenuous. It does appear that such patients require more frequent refinement of their occlusions in order to maintain comfort because even slight positional changes in the joint create disharmony with the intercuspal relationship. If, however, the treatment is initiated in time to salvage enough of the retrodiskal tissues to form a pseudodisk and prevent a bone-to-bone articulation, the prognosis for long-term stability seems to be quite good.

There are patients with displaced disks who do not respond to muscle-relaxation therapy. Their level of pain in the joint is intolerable, and the source of pain is related to compression of the retrodiskal tissues that are still reasonably intact. If diagnostic analysis clearly depicts a condition that is correctable only by invasion of the joint space, corrective surgery can be accomplished to reposition the disk and repair the ligamentous attachments. This preserves the valuable synovial tissues as well as the disk and the protective fibrocartilage on the articular surfaces.

In addition to the need for meticulous surgical procedures, there is one major requirement for an acceptable success rate in reparative TMJ surgery, that is, the reduction of muscle hyperactivity both preoperatively and postoperatively. Occlusally caused displacement of the mandible must be corrected so that there is harmony between the position of the repaired joint and maximum intercuspation. This is usually accomplished by fabrication of an occlusal splint to harmonize with the tentative treatment position for the joint and then refining of the occlusion on the splint to precisely relate to the repaired joint position. Occlusal equilibration on the appliance should be done immediately after surgery to reduce the tendency for muscle incoordination. This procedure reduces the potential for muscle hypercontraction and its consequent overload on the newly repaired joint structures.

The use of an anterior bite plane is a practical and effective muscle-relaxation splint to use in combination with TMJ surgery for correction of a displaced disk. Eliminating all posterior occlusal stops may seem like an odd way to reduce the load on the joint, but it works very effectively because of the effect of posterior disclusion on elevator muscle contraction. Posterior disclusion causes two of the three elevator muscles to release and thus reduces muscular loading of the joint. The procedure has the added advantage of being easier to fabricate before surgery. Postoperative adjustment is simplified because only the anterior teeth contact. As soon as reasonable joint stability is confirmed, the appliance should be converted to a full occlusal splint to prevent supraeruption of the posterior teeth. Periodic adjustment of the splint should continue until minimal or no adjustment is needed. At that point, final occlusal treatment can be completed if needed.

Complete anterior disk displacement, nonreducible and nonrepairable

The disk may become irreparably displaced because of damage to either the disk itself or the ligaments that attach it to the condyle and the temporal bone.

Destruction of the disk can occur when it is folded, bunched up, or torn so that subsequent loading leads to disintegration or noncorrectable misshaping. Destruction of the diskal ligaments results from tearing or perforations that destroy too much of the ligament to permit repair.

Microsurgical reparative techniques continue to improve. Today there are very few damaged disks that cannot be reshaped and repaired, but there are some that are unquestionably unsalvageable. Most nonrepairable disks are found in older patients, and in many cases the adaptive process will have already changed the contours of the articular surfaces before you see the patient for examination.

How the bony articular surfaces respond to the loss of the disk is the primary determinant for selection of treatment. Examination may reveal any of the three following conditions:

Adaptive remodeling

If the articular cartilage stays intact, the condyle and eminentia can remodel to reshape the articular surfaces so that they conform to functional loading without the disk.

Noninflammatory degenerative joint disease

If the articular cartilage is damaged, the bony surfaces start to break down. There is some evidence that early or slowly progressing degenerative joint disease is noninflammatory and is to some degree self-limiting if the overload is reduced.

Inflammatory degenerative joint disease (osteoarthritis)

Inflammation appears to be a secondary sequela to unstabilized remodeling of bony surfaces that are overloaded.

Gross changes in the articular surfaces can be expected to match the meniscus displacement and its altered shape. If the primary soft tissues change shape, the secondary (bone) tissues adapt. If the primary tissues can be corrected in time, corrective reshaping of secondary tissues can occur as a normal process of adaptive remodeling. If the displaced soft tissues cannot be repaired, the remodeling process continues to adapt the shape of the articular surfaces to conform to the surfaces they load against. The process progresses continuously after the onset of disk displacement. Whether the remodeling process remains a reparative adaptive response or becomes a degenerative disease depends on the combined factors of host resistance and the degree of bruxing or clenching that determines the intensity of load that the bony surfaces must resist. Severe bruxing or clenching when the disk is displaced will most certainly lead to flattening of the condyle and often the eminentia. If the load is greater than the adaptive capacity for conformative remodeling, inflammatory degenerative changes start to occur. Degenerative joint disease varies from patient to patient and is affected by general factors of health, nutrition, and body chemistry changes such as those occurring with hormonal imbalances.

Even in severely flattened condyle and eminentia contours, however, it is possible to have a reasonable degree of stability and an acceptable level of comfort. This depends on the character of the remodeled bone surfaces, which in some instances form very hard smooth surfaces referred to as eburnated bone.

Radiographically, the trabeculas in eburnated bone are densely packed and the articular surfaces have the appearance of cortical bone. The severe flattening of the articular surfaces is evidence that the disk is absent. The bone-to-bone contact of the condyle against the eminentia is evidence on properly angulated transcranial films. Radiographs should be taken in both the superior hinge position and the opened (protrusive) position to observe the comparative condyle position in function (Figure 25-10).

Doppler auscultation of the TMJ for bone-to-bone contact generates a chirping crepitus that often sounds like a gate swinging on rusty hinges. The crepitation can be rather coarse depending on the roughness of the surfaces that rub. If the fibrocartilage that covers the articular surfaces is still present, the Doppler sounds are less coarse, an indication of articular surfaces that are smoother. As those surfaces break down, the sounds generated are more gravelly.

Axiographic recordings present a protrusive path that is often much flatter and less angulated than the typical convex path. This is an important observation because an abnormally flat condylar path may not be able to disclude the pos-

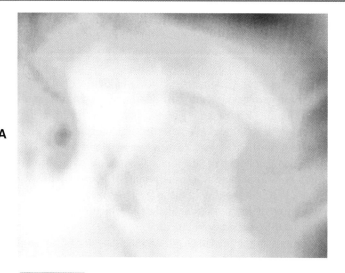

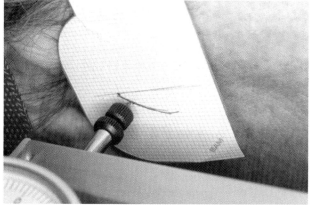

FIGURE 25-10 **A,** Transcranial film of severely flattened condyle and eminence in retruded position. **B,** Axiographic recording of the very flat protrusive path. When the path is flattened, it means that the disk has been completely displaced.

terior teeth in protrusive excursion. Alteration of the anterior guidance may be necessary to prevent posterior occlusal interferences in the functional ranges.

Clinical Observations

The complete displacement of the disk almost invariably leads to progressive flattening of the condyle unless the retrodiskal tissues adapt to form a new pad of fibrous tissue. Flattening occurs as a result of loading the condyle against the eminentia without the biconcave disk interposed to maintain the rounded shape of the condyle. If both the condyle and the eminentia are flattened, it is a sign that the overload on the joint occurs through its range of function. Such a functional overload is particularly damaging to the articular surfaces because without the disk present, the lubrication and nutrition from synovial fluids are also lost. Thus the surfaces of the articulating bones gradually break down, causing a loss of height of the condyle. This loss of height appears to be progressive whenever the disk is lost, and it leads to a further progressive problem of maintaining occlusal harmony.

Because all elevator muscles are behind the teeth, any loss of condylar height causes the upward migration of the condyle to load the most posterior tooth. The damaging effect of such a posterior occlusal pivot is compounded because it separates the anterior teeth and prevents them from fulfilling their job of discluding the posterior teeth in eccentric movements. The result is muscle hypercontraction that overloads both the TMJs and the occlusion. So the joint that is already compromised by loss of its disk is also subjected to the increased loading from the musculature. The problem is progressive because the more the condyle flattens, the more the load is applied to the occlusion.

Perhaps the most dramatic clinical evidence that TMJ problems cannot be separated from occlusal problems can be verified by a consistent observation: Severe wear of upper molar lingual cusps is virtually never seen without also finding commensurate changes in the shape of the condyles or the eminentiae, or both. Nor is severe flattening of the condyle and eminentia observed without directly related occlusal wear. Mongini has shown that changes in condylar shape are directly related to wear patterns in the occlusion and vice versa. If one remembers that maximum muscle contraction does not occur until the teeth are together, it will be obvious that loading of the condyles occurs at that jaw position that relates to maximum intercuspal contact.

Treatment

Because loss of the disk also reduces the nutrition and lubrication to the joint surfaces, it does not seem possible to completely stop all degenerative breakdown on the articular surfaces when the disk is missing. Nevertheless, an acceptable comfort level can usually be achieved with a manageable degree of stability if muscle incoordination can be corrected. The adaptive process can favorably alter even a bone-to-bone relationship in most patients if the nearly continuous loading on the joint can be reduced to intermittent loading with reduced intensity. That is the goal of treatment, and it can usually be achieved by correction of the occlusion to make it noninterfering to the superior hinge position of the condyles.

When the disk is missing, the superior hinge position is determined by bone-to-bone bracing at the medial pole simultaneous with contact against the eminentia. Even in severely flattened condyles, the medial pole of the condyle is still capable of stopping the upward translation of the condyle against the eminentiae. At the bone-braced superior position, the lateral pterygoid muscles can release contraction and allow the elevator muscles to seat the condyles without antagonistic muscle bracing. Even though the disk is missing, muscle coordination can still be achieved if the condyle is free to slide to the superior position without interference from the teeth. The position should be tested for comfort while loading occurs with bilateral pressure. If multiple centric relation stops of equal intensity can be achieved along with immediate disclusion of all posterior contacts in eccentric movement, muscle coordination can be established. Of course, centric relation must be defined differently if there is no disk present. It becomes simply "the most superior position of the condyles against the eminentiae." This position is labeled *adapted centric posture.*

Harmonization of the occlusion may be accomplished provisionally on a full occlusal bite splint, or it may be accomplished directly through equilibration. It is a common misconception that when dentitions have been worn flat, there are no occlusal interferences. If both condyles are positioned on their most superior axis against the eminentiae, there will invariably be premature contacts as well as posterior interferences in eccentric pathways (in untreated patients).

If the condylar path has become too flat to work out lateral or protrusive disclusion of the posterior teeth by equilibration, it may be necessary to restore the anterior teeth to provide a disclusive anterior guidance angle. Equilibration should be completed first to eliminate all centric-relation interferences, and then eccentric excursions should be adjusted as far as possible before the anterior guidance is altered. The steeper anterior guidance will interfere with the extremely flattened envelope of function that the patient has developed, so there will be a tendency to brux against the steeper inclines. This does not create any problems of discomfort as a rule, but it does subject the anterior teeth to lateral forces that could be damaging. The best rule is to steepen the anterior guidance only as much as necessary to adequately disclude the posterior teeth in all excursions, allowing for some eventual wear of the anterior inclines.

The most important occlusal change to make when the disk is irreparably displaced is to provide disclusion of all posterior teeth in all mandibular positions except centric relation. This always involves the anterior guidance as a disclusive factor. The main purpose of this occlusal relationship is the reduction of elevator muscle loading on the condyles. This reduction occurs when posterior teeth disclude. I have found that providing this type of occlusal function noticeably reduces the amount and frequency of postoperative occlusal corrections needed for patients with no disks.

Patients should be made aware that periodic correction of the occlusion will be necessary to keep the neuromuscular system as peaceful as possible. When the disk has been lost, some degenerative changes seem to occur continuously on the articular surfaces regardless of treatment. Maintaining occlusal harmony reduces the changes to a manageable level. An occlusal splint, processed in acrylic resin, is often helpful in reducing the amount of wear on the teeth. It should be adjusted for simultaneous, equal-intensity stops on all teeth in adapted centric posture and for disclusion of posterior teeth in all eccentric positions. Most patients are able to maintain the occlusal surfaces reasonably free of extensive wear just by wearing the appliance at night.

Inflammatory degenerative joint disease (osteoarthritis)

When the load applied through the condyle is greater than the patient's adaptive capacity for remodeling to occur without inflammation, the articular cartilage breaks down,

and soft, vascular tissue invades the articular surfaces. All bearing surfaces may be involved, including the disk if it is still present. The joint may become painful as the loss of the articular cartilage exposes sensory nerves. Condylar height may be lost, sometimes rather suddenly, thereby intensifying occlusal disharmony and its resultant muscle incoordination. I have not seen a single patient with active osteoarthritis of the TMJ who did not present with concomitant masticatory muscle tenderness when palpated.

Bilateral loading of the joints produces a range of discomfort from tenderness to sharp pain. It is usually this response to routine testing of the joints that first alerts us to the possibility of intra-articular pathosis, which then must be confirmed by radiographic methods.

Lesions in the articular surfaces can usually be seen on transcranial films, but a panoramic radiograph sometimes gives a better image. If a lesion cannot be confirmed by either method in a suspected osteoarthritic joint, a submental vertex view may be used to locate it in some instances. The most reliable method, however, for a laminar assessment of the joint surfaces is CT. A TMJ that cannot resist loading without discomfort should be analyzed with progressively more specific methods until the source of discomfort is determined. CT and nuclear magnetic resonance imaging both have value in the search for a verified diagnosis in certain cases and may be selected on the basis of specific need.

The onset of osteoarthritis in the TMJ is apparently more complex than can be explained solely by muscular overload. There appears to be a greater tendency for the disease in females, but at least clinically there also appears to be an increased predisposition for symptoms related to muscle incoordination in women. The role that hormonal imbalance plays could be directed toward disturbances in calcium metabolism that affect both bone and muscle function, so that too could be a factor. The common finding of osteoarthritis occurring unilaterally raises some doubts about a generalized metabolic factor as the principal cause and seems to indicate that host resistance is more of a *contributing* factor. Despite the role that various contributing factors appear to play in the onset of the inflammatory stage, osteoarthritis does not appear to be initiated in the absence of an overload. Furthermore, the reduction of the load on the damaged joint seems to stop the pathosis and stimulate regenerative remodeling. If the disk is intact enough to be repaired or repositioned, the remodeling occurs more rapidly and may even recontour the condyle back to a normal convex shape. The remodeled joint contour depends on the contour of the surface that it functions against; so if the disk is absent, the condyle may adapt itself to a flattened surface, but functional harmony can still be achieved in most instances if muscular overload can be reduced sufficiently.

When active osteoarthritis is observed, the finalization of occlusal surfaces should not be attempted. Until the pathosis is stopped and the defect repaired, the superior axis position cannot be determined with certainty. It then becomes necessary to work with a tentative treatment position. Full

Box 25-1   Guidelines from the American Society of Temporomandibular Joint Surgeons for Temporomandibular Joint and Related Musculoskeletal Disorders

I. Intra-articular (intracapsular) pathology
   A. Articular disk
      1. Displacement
      2. Deformity
      3. Adhesions
      4. Degeneration
      5. Injury
      6. Perforation
      7. Anomalous development
   B. Disk attachments
      1. Inflammation
      2. Injury (laceration, hematoma/contusion)
      3. Perforation
      4. Fibrosis
      5. Adhesions
   C. Synovium
      1. Inflammation/effusion
      2. Injury
      3. Adhesions
      4. Synovial hypertrophy/hyperplasia
      5. Granulomatous inflammation
      6. Infection
      7. Arthritides (rheumatoid, degenerative)
      8. Synovial chondromatosis
      9. Neoplasia
   D. Articular fibrocartilage
      1. Hypertrophy/hyperplasia
      2. Degeneration (chondromalacia)
         a. Fissuring
         b. Fibrillation
         c. Blistering
         d. Erosion
   E. Mandibular condyle and glenoid fossa (see also Musculoskeletal category below)
      1. Osteoarthritis (osteoarthritis, degenerative joint disease)
      2. Avascular necrosis (osteonecrosis)
      3. Resorption
      4. Hypertrophy
      5. Fibrous and bony ankylosis
      6. Implant arthropathy
      7. Fractures/dislocations
II. Extra-articular (extracapsular pathology)
   A. Musculoskeletal
      1. Bone (temporal, mandibular, styloid)
         a. Anomalous development (hypoplasia, hypertrophy, malformation, ankylosis)
         b. Fracture
         c. Metabolic disease
         d. Systemic inflammatory disease (connective tissue/arthritides)
         e. Infection
         f. Dysplasias
         g. Neoplasia
      2. Masticatory muscles and tendons
         a. Anomalous development
         b. Injury
         c. Inflammation
         d. Hypertrophy
         e. Atrophy
         f. Fibrosis, contracture
         g. Metabolic disease
         h. Infection
         i. Dysplasias
         j. Neoplasia
         k. Fibromyalgia
   B. Central nervous system/peripheral nervous system
      1. Reflex sympathetic dystrophy

Excerpted from American Society of Temporomandibular Joint Surgeons website: Guidelines for Diagnosis and Management of Disorders Involving the Temporomandibular Joint and Related Musculoskeletal Structures. For full text please see http://www.astmjs.org/frame_guidelines.html.

occlusal splints offer the best choice for the progressive adjustment of the occlusion as the condyle's position changes during its adaptive remodeling. After the joint stabilizes to a point that requires only minimal occlusal adjustment, occlusal surfaces can be restored. If the disk is absent, the best result that can be achieved will not completely stop all degeneration at the articular surfaces, but it can usually be slowed to a level that allows occluso-muscle harmony to be maintained with minimal periodic occlusal adjustment. Nighttime use of a full occlusal splint can help in this maintenance effort.

The above depiction of intracapsular TMDs is a very "user-friendly" analysis of what practicing clinicians find in everyday practice. Understanding how the variability of disk misalignment affects clinical decisions regarding occlusal diagnosis and treatment is extremely important, and the explanations given will serve clinicians well. It is also recommended that the guidelines prepared by The American Society of Temporomandibular Joint Surgeons (Box 25-1) should be studied on their website for a more complete coverage of specific types and subtypes of TMDs.

Suggested Readings

Chuong R, Piper MA: Open reduction of condylar fractures of the mandible in conjunction with repair of discal injury: A preliminary report. *J Oral Maxillofac Surg* 46:257-263, 1988.
Dawson PE: New definition for relating occlusion to varying conditions of the temporomandibular joint. *J Prosthet Dent* 74:619-627, 1995.
Drace JE, Enzmann DR: Defining the normal temporomandibular joint: Closed, partially open, and open mouth MR imaging of asymptomatic subjects. *Radiology* 177:67-71, 1990.
Farrar WB, McCarty WJ Jr: Inferior joint space arthrography and characteristics of condylar paths in internal derangements of the TMJ. *J Prosthet Dent* 41:548-555, 1979.

Guler N, Yatmaz PI, Ataoglu H, et al: Temporomandibular internal derangement: Correlation of MRI findings with clinical symptoms of pain and joint sounds in patients with bruxing behaviour. *Dentomaxillofac Radiol* 32(5):304-310, 2003.

Heffez L, Jordan S: A classification of temporomandibular joint disk morphology. *Oral Surg Oral Med Oral Pathol* 67(1):11-19, 1989.

Krestan C, Lomoschitz F, Puig S, et al: Internal derangement of the temporomandibular joint. *Radiologe* 41(9):741-747, 2001.

Mongini F: *The stomatognathic system: Function, dysfunction and rehabilitation.* Chicago, 1984, Quintessence Publishing Company.

Piper MA: Microscopic disk preservation surgery of the temporomandibular joint. *Oral and Maxillofac Surg Clinics of North Am* 1:279-301, 1989.

Piper MA, Chuong R: Intraoperative assessment of diskal position using C-arm arthrography during arthroscopic surgery. Presented at the 69th Annual Meeting of the American Association of Oral-Maxillofacial Surgeons. Anaheim, California, 1987.

Rammelsberg P, Pospiech PR, Jager L, et al: Variability of disk position in asymptomatic volunteers and patients with internal derangements of the TMJ. *Oral Surg Oral Med Oral Pathol Oral Radio Endod* 83:393-399, 1997.

Scapino RP: Histopathology associated with malposition of the human temporomandibular joint disk. Part 1. *J Craniomandib Disord* 5:83-95, 1991.

Scapino RP: Histopathology associated with malposition of the human temporomandibular joint disk. Part 2. *J Craniomandib Disord* 5:155-166, 1991.

Schellhas KP, Piper MA, Bessethe RW, et al: Mandibular retrusion, temporomandibular joint derangement, and orthognathic surgery planning. *Plast Reconstr Surg* 90:218-229, 1992.

Schellhas KP, Piper MA, Omlü MR: Facial skeleton remodeling due to temporomandibular joint degeneration: an imaging study of 100 patients. *Cranio* 10:248-259, 1992.

Schellhas KP, Wilkes CH, Fritts HM, et al: Temporomandibular joint: MR imaging of internal derangements and postoperative changes. *Am J Neuroradiol* 1093, 1987.

Wang X, Young C, Goddard G, et al: Normal and pathological anatomy of the TMJ viewed by computerized panoramic arthroscopic images. *Cranio* 21:196-201, 2003.

Chapter 26

Classification of Intracapsular Disorders

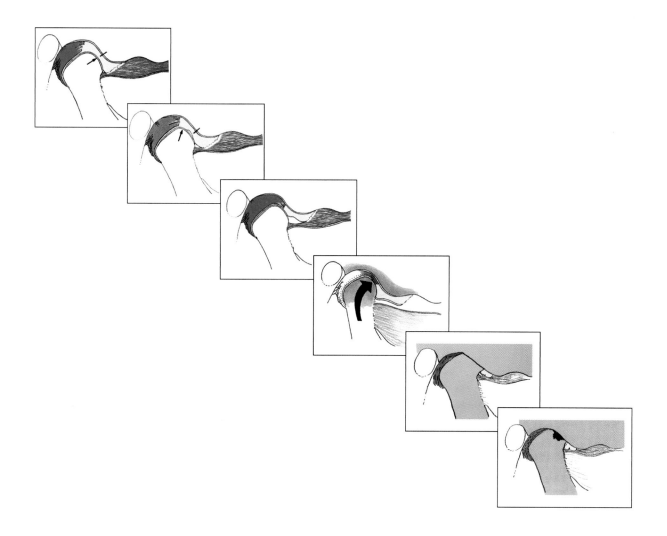

PRINCIPLE

Treatment selection depends on the *specific* classification of the disorder to be treated.

TMJ Piper Classification:	Right:	1	2	3A	3B	4A	4B	5A	5B
	Left:	1	2	3A	3B	4A	4B	5A	5B

Implications: ❑ Stable ❑ Unstable
                  ❑ Immediate concerns _____
                  ❑ Deferrable _____
                  ❑ Optional _____

History: ❑ Neg ❑ Positive for _____

Load Test: Left ❑ Neg ❑ Pain ❑ Tenderness ❑ Tension   Right ❑ Neg ❑ Pain ❑ Tenderness ❑ Tension

Centric Relation: ❑ Verified ❑ Not Verifiable ❑ Adapted Centric Posture

Muscle Palpation: ❑ Neg ❑ Tenderness in _____

Doppler: Left _____ Right _____

ROM: Protrusive _____mm Left _____mm Right _____mm   Path of motion ❑ Normal ❑ Deviates_____

Pain   **Recommend**_____

❑ No Pain _____   ❑ Deprogram muscles   ❑ Occlusal splint

❑ Intracapsular _____   ❑ Transcranial film

❑ Occluso-muscle _____   ❑ Tomogram

❑ Other _____   ❑ MRI   ❑ CT Scan

_____   ❑ Refer for surgical evaluation to _____

FIGURE 26-1 The standard temporomandibular joint (TMJ) segment used in our initial examination of every new patient. This overview of TMJ condition serves as an easy review record as well as a treatment guide for the clinician. More complete details on any problem areas are in order if indicated by the findings on this examination. Analysis following this protocol would prevent many unexpected problems from undocumented pre-existing conditions and missed diagnoses.

PRACTICAL TEMPOROMANDIBULAR JOINT ANALYSIS

To have practical value in clinical practice, a classification system for the condition of the temporomandibular joints (TMJs) must be based on objective findings. It must be simple enough to use that it can be a standard, cost-effective, and time-effective part of every complete examination. In spite of its simplicity, Piper's Classification (Figure 26-1) is complete in all the necessary details for TMJ examination. It is specific in its precise analysis of the intracapsular structures, making it the recommended "gold standard" for research as well as for everyday clinical practice.

Classification of Temporomandibular Disorders

Before any treatment is selected, it is important to classify the specific type of temporomandibular disorder (TMD) into:

1. Occluso-muscle disorders
2. Intracapsular disorders
3. Disorders that mimic TMDs

SYSTEMIZED APPROACH TO CLASSIFICATION

The system we have adopted for intracapsular disorders is the classification by Piper. This classification has become the gold standard, and it is the most practical system for clarifying the exact condition of the TMJs. It describes TMDs in relation to the progressive patterns of deformation in specific intracapsular structures that have a profound effect on occlusion as well as symptoms of orofacial and TMJ pain.

The stages, as described, form a matrix of signs and symptoms that can be determined with specificity by using a series of testing procedures. A diagnosis must be considered inadequate if it merely states that there is a reciprocal click, or if it states that a displaced disk is reducible or nonreducible without differentiation of whether the disk is completely displaced or partially displaced off the lateral pole only.

> In evaluating any TMD, disk alignment on the medial pole and the lateral pole must be evaluated separately.

If the medial pole can maintain an acceptable alignment with the disk, the long-term prognosis is quite good for successfully establishing a harmonious occlusion and a peaceful neuromusculature with complete relief of pain. This favorable prognosis is achievable in most patients even if the lateral pole disk relationship is a closed lock that is not reducible.

Diagnosis of TMDs is not based on observation of a single factor. Proper diagnosis requires a combination of tests that must be related to key questions in the history. The value of Piper's Classification system is that it uses objective tests for evaluating specific structures, so there is no need to rely solely on patients' subjective descriptions of their symptoms. The key to effective diagnosis then becomes a testing process to determine the structural basis for each sign or symptom.

Anatomic and histologic classifications of TMDs provide the most useful mechanism for tracking stages of disease and potential treatment options.

> The classification of TMJ condition directs what you should do for each patient. It guides you in the information you give your patient, and it warns you in advance against starting treatment that could be problematic. Classification of a TMJ condition is an essential part of every new patient examination.

The Importance of Diagnosing Both Medial and Lateral Poles

Disk alignment must be evaluated at both the medial and the lateral poles. In fact, evaluating each pole as a separate factor is one of the most important concepts in diagnosis and selection of treatment. To facilitate a clearly defined decision process, we advocate determining the condition of disk alignment for each pole separately. This tremendously important differentiation is ignored in most of the TMJ literature.

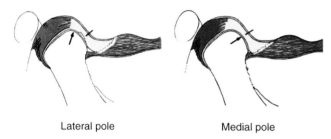

Lateral pole   Medial pole

A typical finding in early disk derangements (Piper Stage II) is a beginning derangement at the lateral pole that can produce a mild, slippery click, while the medial pole is correctly aligned. At this stage, the misalignment is easily treated and is reversible. Harmonization of the occlusion almost always corrects the muscle incoordination and eliminates the click at this stage.

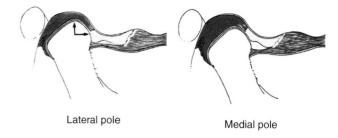

Lateral pole   Medial pole

A more advanced disk derangement problem occurs when the disk is locked in front of the lateral pole but is just at the chronic reciprocal click stage at the medial pole (Piper Stage IV a). At this stage, medial pole reduction often can be accomplished, and even though the lateral pole may remain in a closed lock, the patient will be able to function well and comfortably. If the problem is not resolved at this stage, it will most likely progress to a complete disk derangement.

This condition is almost always associated with occlusal interferences. It typically responds very well to occlusal correction. The stretched ligaments do not normalize, but as long as coordinated muscle function can be maintained by a perfected occlusion, most patients can remain relatively free of clicking.

Piper's Classification

Piper's Classification for intracapsular TMDs relates specific structural disorders to the progressive patterns that routinely occur as TMJs go through stages from health to severe degeneration.

Proper classification of the condition of the TMJs requires an analysis of six structural elements in addition to specific evaluation of pain. The seven structural elements are:

1. Disk alignment. Normal disk alignment positions the disk on the condyle so that all compressive forces are directed through its avascular, noninnervated bearing area. Variations in disk alignment have major implications related to signs and symptoms of TMDs. It is critically important to analyze disk alignment at both the medial and lateral poles of each condyle.

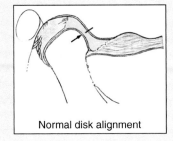
Normal disk alignment

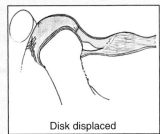
Disk displaced

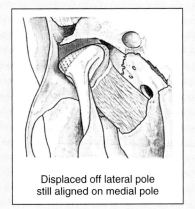
Displaced off lateral pole
still aligned on medial pole

2. Disk shape. The shape of the disk has profound importance. Determining whether the disk is elongated, folded, or deformed into a compressed mass can explain variations in joint signs and symptoms and is often a determinant in treatment selection and prognosis.

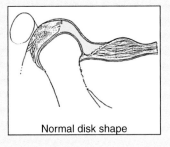
Normal disk shape

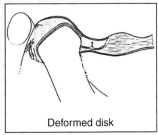
Deformed disk

3. Ligament. It is impossible for a disk to displace unless the ligaments that hold it in place are stretched or torn. Laxity of the ligaments makes disk derangement possible if muscle incoordination is allowed to exert tensive force on the disk. If the disk is not deformed and a peaceful neuromusculature can be maintained, laxity of the ligament is not in itself a sufficient cause for disk displacement.

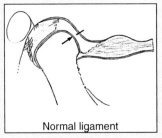
Normal ligament

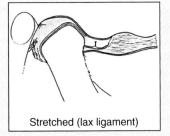
Stretched (lax ligament)

4. Joint space. Analysis of the space between the condyle and the fossa is a simple but effective way to determine if a disk is displaced and to what degree. When this analysis is combined with other diagnostic steps, (history, Doppler, load testing, etc.), imaging can reveal information that is essential to a correct diagnosis.

Note: The "space" between the condyle and fossa is not a void. It is the result of radiolucency of the disk and appears as a dark space on the film that represents the thickness of the disk. If the disk is displaced, the condyle moves higher into the fossa and the space is diminished.

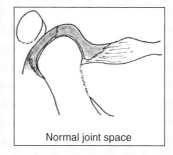
Normal joint space

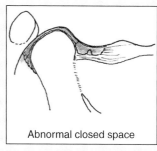
Abnormal closed space

5. Muscle. Analysis of the masticatory musculature results in an amazingly consistent relationship between specific muscle tenderness and specific causes for muscle hyperactivity. There will always be a reason for any muscle to be hyperactive, and the most common primary causes in the masticatory musculature will be either trauma or some form of structural disharmony or deflective occlusal interference. By determining which muscles are tender to palpation and then relating the direction of displacement, a cause-and-effect basis can be found. Even when emotional stress levels are high, or clenching and bruxing is evident, there will almost always be a structural disharmony present that serves as a direct trigger for specific muscle incoordination. The clinician should also be alert for recognition of medical conditions that have a generalized effect on muscle.

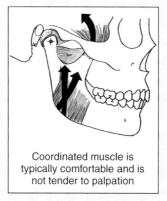
Coordinated muscle is typically comfortable and is not tender to palpation

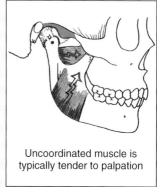
Uncoordinated muscle is typically tender to palpation

6. Bone surfaces. A variety of bone diseases present vastly different symptoms and produce a broad spectrum of signs. These signs may range from mild surface changes on the condyle and eminence to complete destruction of the condyle. While tumors, cysts, and growth disorders are not common, the diagnostician must be forever on the lookout for lesions that can be devastating if they are missed. With the advancement of imaging capabilities, it is unlikely that any disease or deformation of the TMJs could hide from an astute clinician.

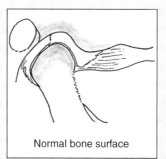
Normal bone surface

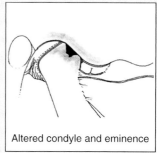
Altered condyle and eminence

7. Pain. Analysis of the type, location, and severity of pain is an essential step in diagnosis of intracapsular disorders. The most important aspect of this analysis is the determination of whether intracapsular structures are the source of any, all, or none of the pain. Compressive loading of the joints in different jaw positions is the most effective way to determine this.

The most common mistake in TMJ pain analysis is failure to focus on intracapsular structures as a potential source of pain. Remember that any response of discomfort or tension when the joints are loaded must be differentiated as to whether the response is from compression of joint structures, from muscle bracing, or both. If pain in the joint region is not affected by compressive loading, sources of pain other than the intracapsular structures must be evaluated until a specific source is located. Any positive response to compressive load testing requires further testing to determine the specific classification of the intracapsular structural condition.

Piper's Classification considers five general stages of intracapsular disorders along with three subgroups of bony alterations (Boxes 26-1 to 26-8).

Box 26-1   Stage I
Structurally Intact TMJ

Many patients are diagnosed as having a TMD who, in fact, have a structurally intact TMJ. Most of these patients are uncomfortable because of muscle pain triggered by deflective occlusal interferences. Some have been injured, and the pain can be emanating from either muscle or from retrodiskal inflammation and edema. Let's look at the way we would diagnose this condition by evaluating the structures involved. Both left and right TMJs must be examined in the same manner.

Disk Alignment . . . Normal at both poles

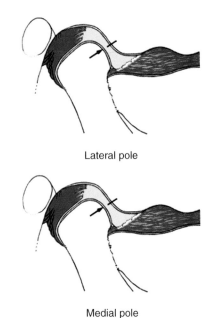

Lateral pole

Medial pole

Diagnosis

History of click	Negative
Load testing	Negative
Doppler	Negative
Imaging	Normal
Range and path of motion	Normal

Note: Load testing may produce tenderness or tension at first because of retrodiskal edema from trauma, or because of lateral pterygoid spasm or hypercontraction. If so, muscle deprogramming should be tried. If trauma is suspected, anti-inflammatory medication may be in order. Load testing will produce no tenderness or tension in an intact TMJ if the lateral pterygoid muscle has fully released.

Muscle palpation. The medial pterygoid muscle will almost always be tender to some degree when palpated, if the same side condyle has to displace from centric relation in order to achieve maximum intercuspation.

Distinguishing characteristics of Stage I. No laxity of ligaments and no alteration of bone surfaces. Therefore, the disk cannot displace. So in patients who do not have retrodiskal edema from trauma, the treatment is focused on eliminating the causes of masticatory muscle hyperactivity with particular attention to complete elimination of any deflective inclines that can activate the lateral pterygoid muscle.

Box 26-2 Stage II
Intermittent Click

This stage is characterized by beginning laxity of the lateral diskal ligament in combination with lateral pterygoid muscle hyperactivity. Disk displacement is reversible if muscle coordination is re-established.

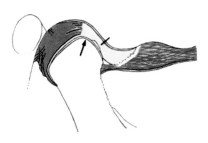

Lateral pole

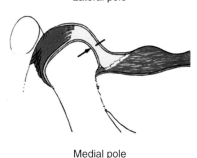

Medial pole

Diagnosis

History of click	Intermittent
Load testing	Negative
Doppler	Possible mild crepitus on translation only
Imaging	Normal
Range and path of motion	Variable
Pain source	Muscle

Implications

Intermittent clicking is evidence of some laxity of the posterior ligament combined with tensive pull on the disk by the superior lateral pterygoid muscle. Because the click is not always present, it is indicative of periodic muscle hyperactivity related to clenching or bruxing. Clicking and temporal headaches on awakening are common findings associated with nocturnal bruxing.

Signs and symptoms at this stage can almost always be completely eliminated by occlusal correction. Since occlusal disharmony is almost always a factor, one should always look for signs of excessive occlusal wear, hypermobility or sensitivity of interfering teeth, abfractions, and other progressive signs of tooth damage.

Box 26-3   Stage III a
Lateral-Pole Click

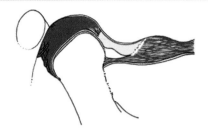

Lateral pole

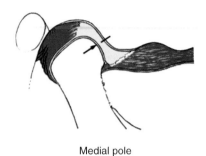

Medial pole

Diagnosis

History of click	Yes (reciprocal)
Load testing	Negative if muscle contraction is released
Doppler	Quiet on rotation; click and crepitus on translation
Imaging (transcranial)	Normal
Range and path of motion	Variable
Pain source	Muscle

Implications

A sure sign of muscle tension on the disk, and elongation of the posterior ligament at the lateral pole. Occlusal correction is usually effective in stopping the click in most III a disk derangements. Since these patients often also have other signs and symptoms including muscle pain and/or signs of tooth wear, instability, or sensitivity, a careful examination of all masticatory system structures is in order. While some of these patients may go for years without progressive damage of the TMJ, many go on to closed locks and an escalation of symptoms.

Box 26-4   Stage III b
Lateral-Pole Lock

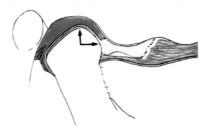

Lateral pole

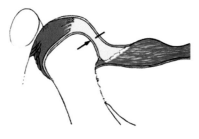

Medial pole

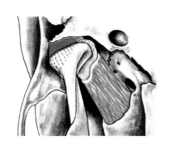

Diagnosis

History of click	Had a click that disappeared
Load testing	Negative when condyles are completely seated
Doppler	Quiet on rotation; crepitus on translation
Imaging (transcranial)	Normal
MRI	Disk displaced off lateral pole only
Range and path of motion	May vary from normal to abnormal paths and restriction of opening
Pain source	Mostly muscle; some retrodiskal compression possible

Implications

Occluso-muscle pain can still be treated successfully. This is the last stage of disk derangement that is treatable with fairly predictable long-term stability of the TMJs. If the occlusion is perfected while the disk still covers the medial pole and adapted centric posture can be verified, we have seen almost no progression to Stage IV. At this stage, surgery (including arthroscopy) is not needed.

Box 26-5   Stage IV a
            Medial-Pole Click

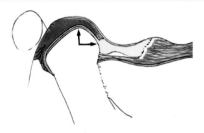

Lateral pole

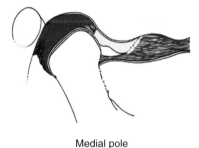

Medial pole

Diagnosis

History of click	Reciprocal click
Load testing	Pain if not reduced; if reduced, can accept loading
Doppler	Click; crepitus on rotation and translation
Imaging (transcranial)	Normal if disk is reduced; space closed if disk is displaced
Range and path of motion	Variable from normal to restricted and deviated
Pain source	Compression of retrodiskal tissue; muscle pain

Implications

This stage is almost always progressive if not treated. Since the disk is still reducible on to the medial pole, occlusal correction is sometimes all that is needed to prevent incoordinated muscle contraction (superior lateral pterygoid) from displacing the disk. If the shape of the disk is not too badly deformed yet, an acceptable result can often be achieved.

The key to conservative treatment hinges on whether adapted centric posture can be determined and then maintained. A full occlusal splint, permissive to ACP, may be effective.

MRI may be justified as a diagnostic step for this stage of intracapsular deformation.

Box 26-6   Stage IV b
Medial-Pole Lock

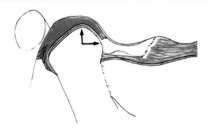

Lateral pole

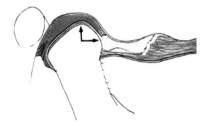

Medial pole

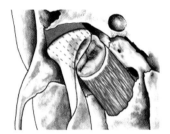

Diagnosis

History of click	Had click that disappeared
Noise	May be none present
Load testing	Tender to gentle loading in early stages
Doppler	Crepitus on all movements
Imaging (transcranial)	Space closed above and behind condyle
MRI	Disk displaced off both poles
Pain source	Compression of retrodiskal tissue; muscle pain

Implications

At this stage, it is very doubtful that the disk can be recaptured and maintained on the medial pole. Progression is a certainty that typically leads to painful loading of the retrodiskal tissues → perforation → osseous changes → loss of condylar height → excessive posterior tooth wear. If the disk displaces medially, there is an increased potential for avascular necrosis. Thus, an MRI analysis and surgical consultation are indicated. Conservative splint therapy may lead to pseudodisk formation and improvement of symptoms, but care in diagnosis is particularly important at this stage.

Box 26-7   Stage V a
Perforation with Acute Degenerative Joint Disease

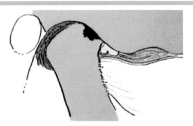

Lateral pole

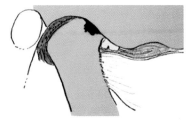

Medial pole

Diagnosis

History of click	May have had an injury; may have had a click that disappeared
Noise	Rough, grating sounds; can be palpated; probably no click
Load testing	Usually painful
Doppler	Coarse crepitus
Imaging (transcranial)	Joint space closed; cortical bone deformed
MRI	Shows extent of marrow death and location and contour of disk
Pain source	Retrodiskal compression; articular surface breakdown; muscle tenderness

Implications

At this stage, permanent irreversible changes in the occlusion are contraindicated. Stability of the TMJs must be achieved to a manageable degree before proceeding with final occlusal treatment.

Specific diagnosis of the type of degenerative joint disease (DJD) is essential, so appropriate imaging is critical.

Use of a full occlusal splint with contact on all teeth at a treatment position for the TMJs is often helpful in reducing discomfort.

Box 26-8   Stage V b
Perforation with Chronic Degenerative Joint Disease

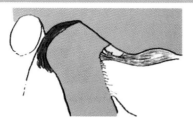

Lateral pole

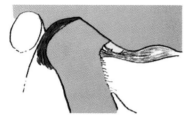

Medial pole

Diagnosis

History of click	Had a click that disappeared
Noise	Palpable crepitus
Load testing	Can usually load with no discomfort
Doppler	Coarse crepitus on all movements
Imaging (transcranial)	Flattened condyle and eminence
Pain source	Usually muscle

Implications

This is the most common progression of TMJ deformation that occurs after complete disk displacement (see Box 26-6, Stage IV b). The bone-to-bone TMJ relationship to the fossae can, in most patients, accept firm loading with no discomfort. This is why a complete history and exam is so essential. In most of these patients, it is possible to achieve adapted centric posture. Occlusal correction can be achieved with the same results as with normal, intact TMJs, but the long-term stability is not the same. Explain to these patients that the problem is manageable but to expect a need for periodic occlusal readjustment to maintain a peaceful neuromusculature.

Piper has expanded the classification system to include all types of disorders of the condylar head including:

1. Condylar hyperplasia
2. Osteochondrosis
3. Osteoarthrosis
4. Osteochondritis dissecans
5. Avascular necrosis

These have importance in relation to occlusal analysis because all of these disorders affect condylar position, which in turn affects arch-to-arch occlusal relationships. It would require a separate text to fully cover the monumental work of Mark Piper in differential diagnosis of the entire spectrum of masticatory system disorders including separate classification systems for specific diagnosis of orofacial pain.

For the purpose of occlusal analysis, I have limited the description of the Piper Classification to the information that every practicing dentist must know and use in daily practice. In addition, I repeat the following classic advice:

> If the TMJs cannot comfortably accept firm loading, find out why.
>
>   Even if the TMJs can accept loading, ensure that they are stable before completing occlusal therapy.

If either of these criteria cannot be fulfilled and solutions are not clear, seek competent consultation with a specialist, and clarify your concerns to the patient.

Suggested Readings

Dawson PE, Piper MA: *Temporomandibular disorders and orofacial pain.* Seminar Manual. St. Petersburg, Florida, 1993.

Piper MA: The TMJ Triad Poster showing progression of TMJ intracapsular disorders. Available from Piper Clinic, 111 Second Ave NE, St. Petersburg, Florida, 33701.

Piper MA: *Therapy for intermediate to advanced TMD.* Seminar manual for course at the Piper Clinic. St. Petersburg, Florida, 2006.

Piper MA: *TMJ diagnostics and basic management.* Seminar manual for course at Dawson Center for Advanced Dental Study, 2002, and at the Piper Clinic, St. Petersburg, Florida, 2006.

Chapter 27

Imaging the TMJs

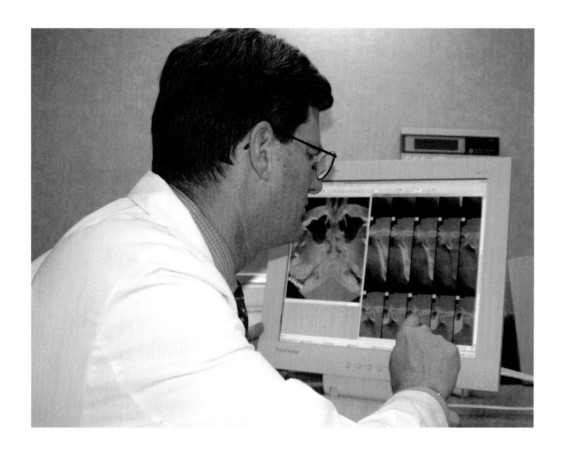

PRINCIPLE

Knowing is always better than guessing.

WHY DENTISTS MUST UNDERSTAND TEMPOROMANDIBULAR JOINT IMAGING

A fundamental tenet in diagnosis and treatment of occlusal problems is that all occlusal analysis starts at the temporomandibular joints (TMJs). This is so because the *position* of the TMJs determines the correct jaw-to-jaw relationship. The *condition* of the TMJs can have a profound effect on the position of the condylar axis, the essential determinant of the correct occlusal contact at complete closure. This is why there is the following inviolate rule:

> If the TMJs cannot comfortably accept maximal loading by the elevator muscles, find out why before initiating occlusal treatment.

Of course if you have read this far in this text, you have heard this rule before. It is repeated because it is one of the most violated rules in occlusal diagnosis and treatment design. It is the reason for recommending load testing on every patient before starting treatment. The rule can be paraphrased: *If you cannot completely load the joints, find out why.* This brings us to the point of this chapter, which is that in many of our patients, we must have an image of the TMJs to learn what is wrong in a joint that cannot pass the load test with complete comfort. The type of image needed to make a correct diagnosis depends on specific signs and symptoms gleaned from a screening history and a screening examination. Patients with a primary complaint of orofacial pain may require a higher level of imaging to establish a diagnosis. Today's dentists should recognize the need and the opportunity to fulfill the role of physicians of the masticatory system. This requires, at the very minimum, an understanding of what TMJ imaging modalities are available and when they should be used.

TYPES OF TMJ IMAGING

As of this writing, there are seven types of imaging procedures that are useful for diagnosis of the health or structural disorder of the TMJs. Selection of the most appropriate method should be based on cost-effectiveness and practicality based on what specific information is needed to determine an accurate explanation for signs and symptoms of the disorder. The choices are:

1. Panoramic radiography
2. Transcranial radiography
3. Tomography
4. Arthrotomography
5. Arthrography with videofluoroscopy
6. Magnetic resonance imaging (MRI)
7. Computed tomography (CT)

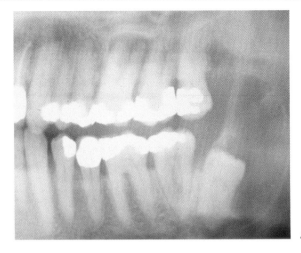

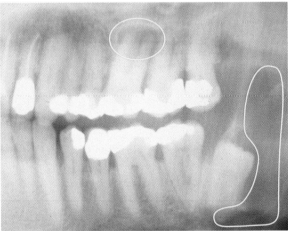

FIGURE 27-1 **A,** Panoramic radiograph of a patient with orofacial pain clarifies the diagnosis of a periapical abscess on the upper first molar, and a large cyst in the ascending ramus (outlined in **B**).

The art and science of imaging is advancing to levels that are beyond one's imagination. With computer enhancement, it is today possible to provide layer-by-layer color images of anatomical sections through the entire body. Such capabilities are opening new opportunities to study functional anatomy and improve diagnostic capabilities. In this text, I have limited the discussion to procedures that are readily available and practical for dental practitioners. The procedures described should serve them well for diagnosis and treatment selection.

Panoramic Radiography

For overall screening for hard and soft tissue lesions of the facial skeleton, the panoramic radiography can be used to show up deviations in the nasal septum and signs of acute sinusitis. It is an acceptable method for observing acute bone deformation and the presence of cysts or tumors in the ascending ramus and the maxilla. It is not the most effective choice for evaluating the TMJs, but it might show gross deformation of the joints. Panoramic radiography is not a good choice for determining the position of the condyles in their respective fossa. However, when they are used as a screening radiograph, they may alert the clinician to a suspected problem that can be studied more thoroughly with a different imaging approach. Panoramic radiography is not a dependable modality for assessment of the articular space, a critical factor in diagnosis of intracapsular disorders.

New developments in technology continue to improve the accuracy of panoramic radiography. With the changes being introduced, it is probable that panoramic radiography will soon achieve a capacity to produce images that may approach a basic CT capability for the TMJs.

Transcranial Radiography

Transcranial radiography is the method most often used for imaging the TMJs. Transcranial radiography is popular because consistently readable images can be achieved economically and with minimum complexity by use of a standard dental x-ray machine.

With the availability of MRI, CT, and the wide range of variable techniques for creating images of the joints in any perspective, there is almost no structural problem of the TMJ that can hide from a persistent diagnostician. Because of these advanced technologies, the use of simple transcranial radiography may seem outdated. There are limitations for transcranial radiography, for sure, but as of this writing, it is still the most practical method for assessing the majority of TMJs radiographically. It should be remembered, however, that transcranial radiography cannot be used to determine centric relation, and although it may be suggestive of certain disk derangements, neither a positive nor a negative diagnosis of disk displacement should be determined solely from transcranial radiography.

Even an image of a perfectly centered, normal-appearing joint is not, by itself, assurance of either alignment or health of the TMJ. Disk displacement can occur without a noticeable displacement of the condyle, and pathologic changes can occur on joint surfaces that are not clearly imaged on transcranial radiographs. Thus a clinical evaluation is an essential preliminary step that must be combined with the radiographic analysis. In fact, the need or purpose of a radiographic examination of the TMJ can be determined only by clinical examination and history.

Indications for transcranial radiographs

Because transcranial radiography can be done so conveniently and economically, it serves as a practical first step for imaging the TMJs when a potential problem is suspected. Even though the image is predominantly of the lateral aspect of the joint, there will be very few structural problems missed, because most of the pathologic changes that occur on the articulating surfaces start at the lateral half of the joint and are visible on a transcranial view.[1-6]

If definite clinical signs or symptoms cannot be explained by transcranial radiographs, more specific imaging methods that will more clearly assess the suspected problem area can

then be selected. If the lateral view shows no recognizable pathosis, it is a logical second step to view the medial aspect of the joint tomographically. Clinical experience has made us aware that this is rarely necessary.

The basic purpose of TMJ radiography is to help determine whether we are dealing with an intracapsular problem or with a purely muscular problem related to spasm or incoordination of the masticatory muscles. If we can ascertain that an intracapsular problem exists, then whatever method is needed should be used to determine the exact nature of the problem so that treatment can be designed that is specific for the pathologic condition. If simple transcranial radiography can answer the questions that must be answered, there is no reason to subject the patient to added expense, inconvenience, or unnecessary radiation.

With the above considerations in mind, transcranial radiography is indicated:

1. When there is a history of joint sounds or unexplained discomfort in the joint region
2. When load testing of the joints produces discomfort
3. When any pathologic or structural changes are suspected

If a screening history is negative and a screening examination produces no evidence of intracapsular problems, there is no need for transcranial radiographs, and they are contraindicated. The use of such films must be triggered by clinical evidence.

Comparison of techniques

There are several different techniques using different types of positioners for relating the head and the radiograph to the direction of the beam. To simplify a comparison, the differences can be confined to the following:

1. How the head is positioned in relation to the radiograph
2. What direction the beam is in relation to the following:
   a. The long axis of the condyles
   b. The radiograph

The most accurate lateral radiographic image of the condyle is produced when the beam is aimed through the long axis of the condyle, perpendicular to the plane of the radiograph (Figure 27-2). Updegrave[1] refers to this as individualized transcranial radiography, as compared to standardized or fixed-angle techniques. Although variations in the direction of the beam can occur either in the vertical or the horizontal angulations, the major difference between individualized versus standardized techniques is the difference in horizontal angulation of the central ray (Figure 27-3).

Omnell and Petersson[2] showed that 47 structural changes could be observed in individualized radiographs, whereas only 19 changes could be seen with a standardized technique. If the wide variety of anatomic differences among individuals is considered, it will be obvious why a standardized fixed-angle technique is unacceptable. Therefore, the method selected should permit alignment of the beam so

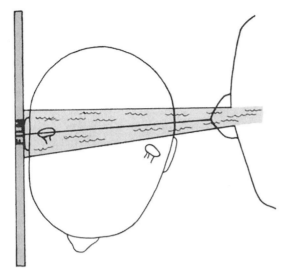

FIGURE 27-2 *Individualized* TMJ radiographic technique. The beam is directed through the long axis of the condyles at a 90-degree angle to the radiograph. In this illustration, there are no controls for accurate repeatability of head position.

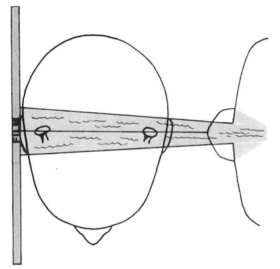

FIGURE 27-3 *Standard (fixed angle)* radiographic technique. Beam is directed at 90 degrees to the radiograph but diagonally across the condyle. This creates distortion of the joint spaces on the image.

that it is as parallel as possible to the long axis of the condyle. With head-holding devices, this beam alignment is usually accomplished by the use of movable ear rods that position the head in relation to the beam.

Vertical angulation alignment

Vertical angulation of the electron beam is changed when the head is tilted laterally. The degree of angulation is controlled when the height of the ear rods is changed (Figure 27-4).

According to research and clinical findings by Buhner,[16] setting the vertical angulation of the central beam at 25 degrees will serve as a fairly consistent average for correct imaging of the superior wall, or the roof of the glenoid fossa

in relation to the Frankfort plane. This angulation is related to the roof of the fossa (not to the condylar head). The space between the condylar head and the roof of the fossa is established by the disk.

According to Farrar and McCarty,[3] a vertical beam angulation of 25 degrees will also minimize superimposition of the petrous portion of the temporal and sphenoid bones over the joint, but this angle will vary to some degree in relation to different head shapes and widths. By moving the ear rod next to the cassette up, the vertical angulation can be increased. Moving the ear rod down decreases the angulation. The vertical angulation on the Accurad head positioner is changed by raising or lowering of the ear plug on the side opposite to the cassette, a range from 21 to 30 degrees, and this range can accommodate almost any patient.

To evaluate the correctness of vertical angulation, the petrous line should be observed on the radiograph. It should intersect the condyle midway between the medial and lateral poles, which should place it slightly above the level of the auditory meatus (Figure 27-5).

The posterior clinoid process should be positioned slightly anterior to the eminentia, level with the superior outline of the fossa. In many transcranial radiographs, the posterior clinoid process is not clearly visible, so it is not always usable as a landmark.

By analyzing a test radiograph, we can determine if a change in vertical angulation is needed. Increasing the vertical angle will position the petrous line more inferiorly. The clinoid process is also lowered. Decreasing the vertical angulation raises the petrous line as well as the clinoid process (Figure 27-6).

All vertical alignments should be made with the Frankfort horizontal plane parallel to the floor. A nasion positioner is used in combination with the ear rods to stabilize the head in that position (Figure 27-7).

This results in an occlusal plane that is slightly lower in front. This relationship must be maintained when the mouth is opened. The normal tendency to tip the head back during opening must be prevented. The use of the nasion positioner combined with two ear rods for positioning the head permits reasonable duplication of head position for comparative radiographs. Thus a comparison can be made regarding the position of the condyle in a comfortable centric relation alignment versus its position during maximum intercuspation. A stable head position also permits accurate reproduction of radiographic records for later evaluation of the joint. The use of reproducible reference points is also essential for making corrections in the angulation of the beam.

Horizontal angulation alignment

To alter the horizontal angulation of the electron beam, move the ear rod on the opposite side from the cassette holder horizontally. By sliding the ear rod left or right, the head must turn, causing the horizontal angulation of the beam to either increase or decrease (Figure 27-8).

When the ear plug is moved forward, the head must turn toward the radiograph. This has the effect of aligning the

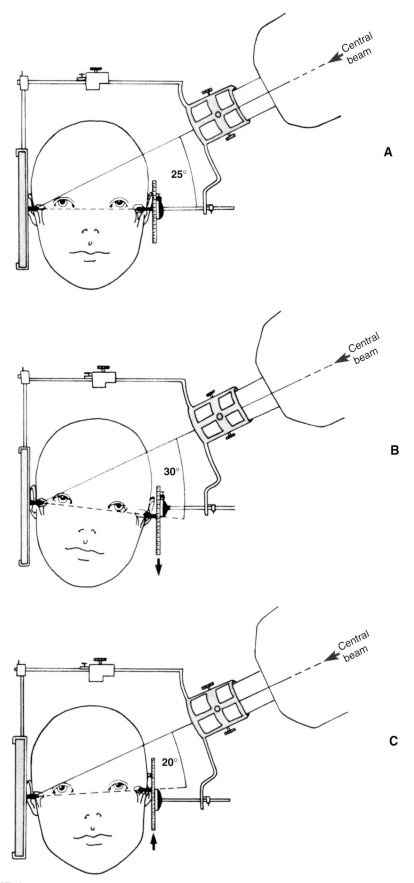

FIGURE 27-4   **A,** Vertical angulation of the beam is altered when the head is tilted laterally. Notice the beam angle when the head is straight. **B,** When the ear rod opposite the cassette is lowered, the chin moves toward the radiograph, tilting the head. This increases the angulation of the central beam. **C,** When the ear rod is raised, opposite the cassette, the chin moves away from the radiograph, causing the beam angle to decrease.

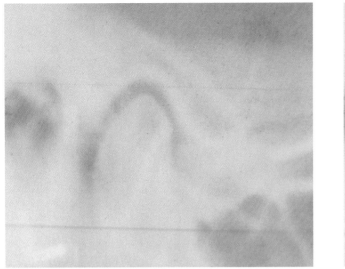
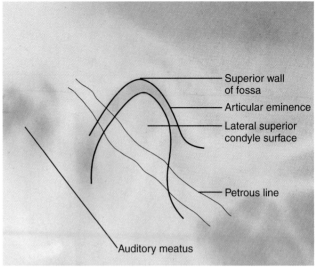

Superior wall
of fossa

Articular eminence

Lateral superior
condyle surface

Petrous line

Auditory meatus

FIGURE 27-5 Proper position of petrous line indicates correctness of vertical angulation. A correct vertical angulation is essential for accurate analysis of the articular space. This is an important aid in determining if the disk is aligned on the medial pole of the condyle.

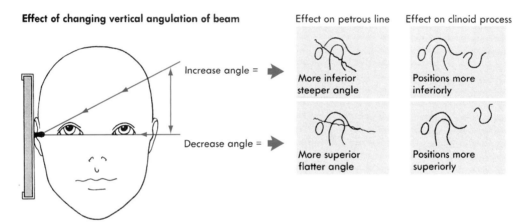

Effect of changing vertical angulation of beam

Effect on petrous line

Effect on clinoid process

Increase angle =
More inferior
steeper angle
Positions more
inferiorly

Decrease angle =
More superior
flatter angle
Positions more
superiorly

FIGURE 27-6 Effects on the petrous line and clinoid process of changing the vertical angulation of the beam.

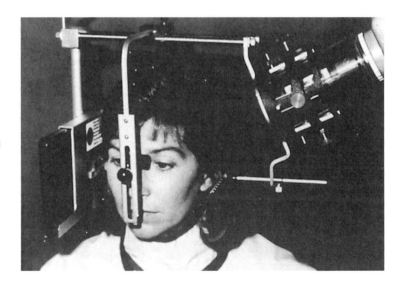

FIGURE 27-7 The Accurad-200 Transcranial System (Dénar®). Head position is controlled by the position of ear plugs and nasion positioner. The head does not move during exposure of three different views. The radiograph is only moved after each exposure. The mandible can move in relation to the fixed cranial base for comparative views of the joint.

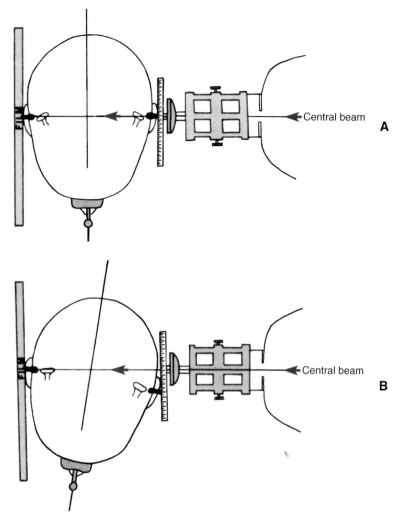

FIGURE 27-8 **A,** Path of the central beam when the radiograph is positioned parallel to the midsagittal plane and the beam is directed at a 90-degree angle to the radiograph. The image results from the beam crossing diagonally across the condyle. **B,** By moving the ear plug opposite the cassette forward, the head turns toward the cassette. This directs the beam through the long axis of the condyle at 90 degrees to the radiograph. The combination of the two ear rods and the nasion positioner provides three points of reference for ease of duplication.

long axis of the condyle with the central beam. It also keeps the radiograph aligned to a 90-degree angle to the rays to provide the least distortion of the image.

The alignment of the head can also be achieved by a combination of horizontal movements of both ear plugs. The important consideration is that the long axis of the condyle should parallel the beam, which, in turn, is at 90 degrees to the radiograph. As long as that is accomplished, the image will have diagnostic value. Simple adjustments to the ear plug positions make this a practical procedure.

The location of the petrous line and the clinoid process is also affected by variations of the horizontal angle. The incorrect horizontal angle can result in superimposition of the clinoid process over the fossa and condyle, or the medial pole of the condyle may be projected into the anterior joint space, and such projection could be misinterpreted as an anterior displacement of the condyle.[4]

The petrous line moves superiorly, and its angle becomes less steep as the horizontal angle is increased. The clinoid process moves more anteriorly as the head turns toward the radiograph and the horizontal angle is increased (Figure 27-9).

By relating the relative position of the petrous line and the clinoid process in a trial exposure, compensation can be made in both vertical and horizontal beam angulations by altering the position of the ear plugs.

If the horizontal alignment of the long axes of condyles is compared with the transmeatal line (frontal plane), the average angular deviance is approximately 13 degrees according to Yale,[17] who studied over 2900 mandibular condyles. He also reported that variations from the frontal plane ranged from 0 to 30 degrees.

The long axis of the condyle generally relates to the ramus at approximately a right angle. In devising a method for

Effect of changing horizontal angulation of beam

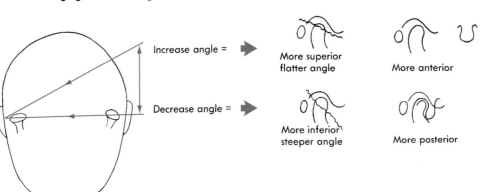

FIGURE 27-9   Effects on movement of petrous line and clinoid process when horizontal angulation of beam is changed.

taking advantage of that relationship, Schier[5] found that if a flat plane is pressed against the side of the face so that it contacts the high point of the zygomas, the gonion, and the lower border of the mandible next to the molars, the long axis of the condyle would be 90 degrees to that plane. Updegrave takes advantage of this relationship by aligning the cassette with that planar base and directs the ray directly through the condyle at the radiograph. A single ear plug is used on the cassette side to position the radiograph.

Use of a transcranial board

Popularity of the transcranial board (Figure 27-10) has grown because of its simplicity. It can be used with a standard dental x-ray, and the image quality is excellent.

The same rules for beam angulation apply, and the same analysis of the image is also used to determine if there is distortion from improper beam direction. The two most useful guidelines are:

1. The earhole on the image should be round.
2. The petrous line should bisect the condyle.

Other considerations

The shorter the radiograph distance from the radiation source, the more distortion occurs in the image. Using a collimated, long cone to lengthen the source-radiograph distance minimizes enlargement of the image of the joint and produces a more readable radiograph.

The use of high-speed intensifying screens permits reduced exposure time and reduced radiation dosage.

Transcranial radiography has definite limitations. It has, however, stood the test of time as a very logical adjunct to a careful clinical examination. Its limitations are more a matter of interpretation than of the radiograph itself and relate to how you plan to use the radiograph. If a transcranial radiograph does not show us what we need to complete a diagnosis, we must proceed to whatever imaging method must be used to provide the needed information.

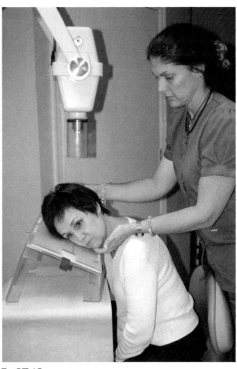

FIGURE 27-10   The TC2000 Transcranial Board from AMD (From American Medical Devices, Inc., San Bernardino, CA.).

Cole[6] has suggested three steps in learning to better interpret transcranial radiographs:

1. First, become intimately familiar with the anatomy of the hard and soft tissues of the TMJ.
2. Next, examine the angle of projection of the electron beam and the image it forms, and be sure you understand them.
3. Finally, practice visualizing the TMJ in three dimensions by studying the radiographic image and remembering that the tissue is "translucent" to an electron (Figures 27-11 and 27-12).

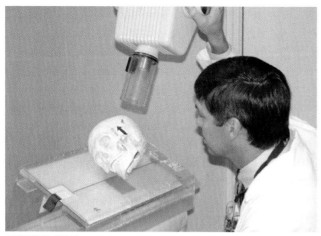

FIGURE 27-11 Practicing beam angulation on a dry skull is an excellent way to learn transcranial radiography.

Standard views of the TMJ

The standardized exposures for transcranial radiographs consist of three views of each joint taken in the following order:

1. Swallow and let the teeth just touch (initial contact)
2. Maximal intercuspation
3. Wide open (maximum joint extension)

We have modified this sequence by taking the first exposure with the teeth closed into a centric relation bite record if a verified centric relation joint position is achievable. If centric relation cannot be confirmed, use the standard sequence.

CT

Tomography provides a better assessment of the medial pole area of the condyle than is possible with transcranial radiography. Breakdown of the articular surfaces can also be shown with slightly improved clarity, particularly at the midpoint of the condylar head and at the medial pole. The critical analysis of articular space is the same as with transcranial radiography.

The cost of tomographic equipment in comparison to transcranial instrumentation is a deciding factor for most practitioners. A practical approach is to incorporate the use of transcranial radiography as a standard screening modality. If a transcranial image does not completely clarify a diagnosis (in combination with other tests), a more advanced imaging modality should be selected (Figure 27-13). This is a reasonable approach as long as the rule is followed to always find out why a TMJ cannot comfortably accept loading. If tomography is readily available, there is no advantage to opt for transcranial radiography as a standard procedure.

Arthrotomography

Arthrotomography is an imaging modality that is typically reserved for specialists in maxillofacial radiography or surgery.

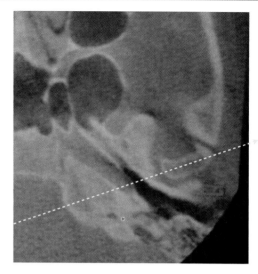

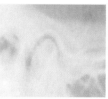

FIGURE 27-12 Correct beam angulation directs the electron beam through the long axis of the condyle to produce a clear image on the radiograph.

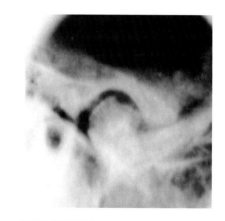

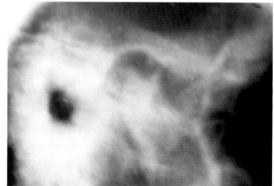

FIGURE 27-13 Tomograms clearly show articular surface deformation of two different TMJs with degenerative joint disease.

TMJ arthrography refers to the injection of a radiopaque contrast medium into the lower joint space followed by radiography. It is primarily used to diagnose the position and condition of the meniscus in relation to the condyle. Abnormalities that can be observed include anterior dislocation of the disk, perforation, degenerative changes, and adhesions.[7-9]

Arthrography with video fluoroscopy

By combining arthrography with videofluoroscopy, it is possible to observe the movement and contour of the disk in relation to the condyle as the jaw opens, closes, and translates. It was through this procedure that much was learned about the action of the disk during subluxation and eventual complete displacement with locking. Wilkes[10] confirmed the accuracy of arthrotomography by comparing the diagnosis with direct surgical observations. Piper[11] developed a procedure termed *differential arthrography,* which demonstrated the effect of lateral pterygoid contraction on completely displaced disks. By observing the locked disk on the fluoroscope, then anesthetizing the motor innervation to the superior lateral pterygoid muscle, spontaneous reduction of the displaced disk occurred in some TMJs. Nonreducible disks that did not respond to the superior lateral pterygoid anesthesia were, on open surgical observation, found to be held forward by fibrotic contracture of the muscle, or by deformation of the disk itself.

Perforations of the disk or the retrodiskal ligament are easily recognized on arthrograms because the contrast medium injected into the lower compartment leaks into the upper compartment.

For some time, arthrotomography was the method of choice for diagnosing soft-tissue derangements of the TMJ. It came into vogue at a time when new insights were needed to explain pain and dysfunction problems of the TMJs. It served its purpose well, but it is an invasive technique that requires meticulous attention to needle placement and other details. There is also some discomfort for many patients. Except for special situations, arthrography has been replaced by advances in MRI. However, it is still a useful procedure for identifying adhesions or in patients in whom the condyle-disk relationship cannot be ascertained by other methods.

▌MRI

MRI has been called the most significant advance in medicine since the discovery of the x-ray. The diagnostic and therapeutic potential of magnetic resonance is unlimited. It has become the "gold standard" for analysis of the TMJs, and it can display subtleties of intracapsular anatomy that in the past could only be seen in dissections in the anatomy lab. It is a noninvasive modality that does not expose patients to radiation.

Its data can be accumulated in slices that can be imaged on whichever selected plane the practitioner needs to visualize.

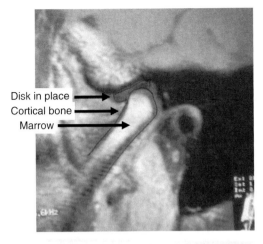

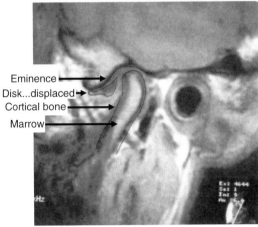

FIGURE 27-14 Magnetic resonance imaging showing the disk centered over the condyle **(A).** Note the image is reversed from typical radiographs. The cortical bone and the disk appear dark. **B,** The disk is clearly visible in front of the condyle. Depending on the depth of the slice, the medial pole can be distinguished from the disk position at the lateral pole.

MRI is particularly useful in determining the position of the disk in relation to the condyle because sagittal cuts can be made at different depths through the condylar head. Thus the medial pole can be clearly differentiated from the lateral pole, one of the most important advantages in diagnosis of intracapsular disorders and a necessary discernment in classifying the condition of the TMJs for Piper's Classification (Figure 27-14).

The use of MRI for imaging the TMJ became a practical process when Schellhas developed special surface coils for focusing the signal on the area of the TMJ. He further outlined the specific process for achieving excellent images of the TMJs[12-14] and correlated his results with clinical, surgical, and pathologic documentation.

As the gold standard for diagnosis of temporomandibular disorders, it is essential for dental practitioners to develop an understanding of MRI. There are significant differences in magnetic resonance images when compared to standard radiographic films. When these differences are understood, the amount of information that can be discerned is worth the effort.

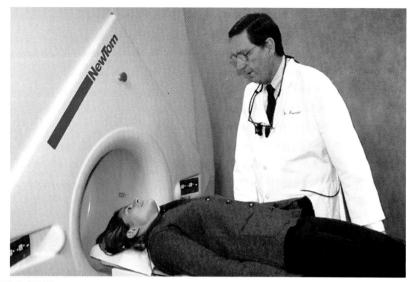

FIGURE 27-15   Preparing a patient for a CT scan in the NewTom scanner designed for head/neck imaging.

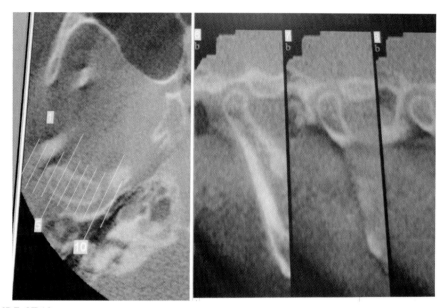

FIGURE 27-16   Progressive slices through the condyle can be viewed to show comparative views from lateral to medial poles. Slices can also be made at different planes. The clarity of the images is excellent.

Another major advantage of MRI is the ability to discern changes in the marrow space of the TMJ. Schellhas and Piper have presented irrefutable evidence of condylar avascular necrosis (AVN) and osteochondritis dissecans (OCD) leading to condylar breakdown and facial skeleton remodeling.[15] The ability to diagnose early stages of AVN is a major contribution toward prevention of jaw asymmetries. It also explains the reason for sudden collapse of some condyles, a clinical observation that for many years was a mystery. MRI enables a clinician to diagnose the various stages of marrow changes from the early stage of edema through necrosis and finally collapse of the cortical bone into the dead marrow space. MRI also shows clearly the location of an anteriorly displaced disk, a factor that can contribute to reduction of blood supply to the marrow. If the disk displaces medially, it has a greater potential for compression of the blood supply that can lead to necrosis of the marrow.

CT Scans

CT is now available for dental office use and it provides for high-quality images of the TMJs from any angulation or plane. The capability to image a thin slice from any plane through the joint structures makes it extremely difficult for a problem to hide from an astute clinician (Figures 27-15 and 27-16).

References

1. Updegrave WJ: Radiography of the temporomandibular joints individualized and simplified. *Compend Contin Educ Dent* 4(1):23-29, 1983.
2. Omnell K, Petersson A: Radiography of the temporomandibular joint utilizing oblique lateral and transcranial projections: Comparison of information obtained with standardized technique and individualized technique. *Odontol Revy* 27(2):77-92, 1976.
3. Farrar WB, McCarty WJ Jr: *Clinical outline of temporomandibular joint diagnosis and treatment*, ed 7, Montgomery, Alabama, 1982, Normandie Publication 90-100.
4. Tucker TN: Head position for transcranial temporomandibular joint radiographs. *J Prosthet Dent* 52(3):426-431, 1984.
5. Schier MB: Temporomandibular joint roentgenography: Controlled erect technics. *J Am Dent Assoc* 65:456-472, 1962.
6. Cole SV: Transcranial radiography: Correlation between actual and radiographic joint spaces. *J Craniomandibular Pract* 2(2):153-158, 1984.
7. Farrar WB, McCarty WJ Jr: Inferior joint space arthrography and characteristics of condylar paths in internal derangements of the TMJ. *J Prosthet Dent* 41:548-555, 1979.
8. Katzburg RW, Dolwich MF, Bales DJ, et al: Arthrotomography of the TMJ: New technique and preliminary observations. *Am J Radiol* 143:449-955, 1979.
9. Dolwick MR, Katzberg RW, Helms CA, et al: Arthrotomographic evaluation of the temporomandibular joint: Correlation with post-mortem morphology. *Oral Maxillofac Surg* 32:193-199, 1979.
10. Wilkes C: Arthrography of the temporomandibular joint in patients with the pain dysfunction syndrome. *Minn Med* 61:645, 1928.
11. Piper M: Differential arthrography. Personal observation.
12. Schellhas KP, Wilkes CH, Hertloff KB, et al: Temporomandibular joints: Diagnosis of internal derangements using magnetic resonance imaging. *Minn Med* 69:516, 1986.
13. Schellhas KP: Internal derangement of the temporomandibular joint: Radiographic staging with clinical, surgical, and pathologic correlation. *Magnetic Resonance Imaging* 7:495-515, 1989.
14. Schellhas KP, Wilkes CH, Fritts HM, et al: Temporomandibular joint: MR imaging of internal derangements and post operative changes. *AJNR* 8:1093-1101, 1987.
15. Schellhas KP, Piper MA, Omlie MR: Facial skeleton remodeling due to temporomandibular joint degeneration: An imaging study of 100 patients. *AJR* 155:373-383, 1990.
16. Buhner WA: A headholder for oriented temporomandibular joint radiographs. *J Prosthet Dent* 29:113, 1973.
17. Yale SH: Radiographic evaluation of the temporomandibular joints. *J Am Dent Assoc* 79(1):102-107, 1969.

Chapter 28

Bruxism

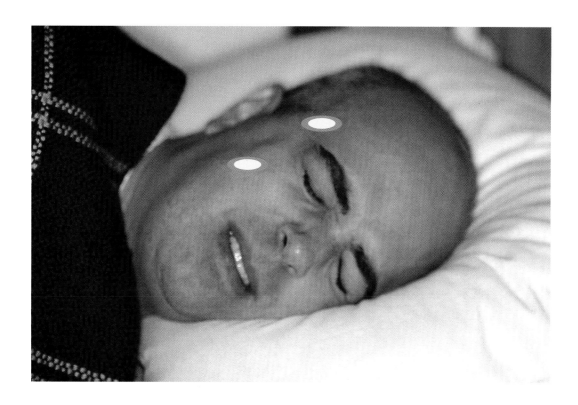

PRINCIPLE

Regardless of the cause, the most effective treatment for the effects of bruxism is perfection of the occlusion.

> **Bruxism:** An oral habit consisting of involuntary rhythmic or spasmodic nonfunctional gnashing, grinding, or clenching of teeth, in other than chewing movements of the mandible, which may lead to occlusal trauma.
>
> — *The Glossary of Prosthodontic Terms*

A common cause for attritional wear, loose teeth, fractured cusps, alveolar exostoses, and muscle pain is the noxious pattern of abnormal clenching and grinding that is referred to as *bruxism*. The relationship between bruxism and psychic stress has been assumed by most investigators[1] as there does appear to be an intensification of masticatory muscle activity during times of stress. Indeed, the Biblical depiction of "gnashing of teeth" was described as a result of extreme stress, an observation that would be folly to deny.

There is a problem, however, if psychic stress is used as the only explanation for bruxism.[1] The problem is that it obscures other factors that are equally important, and eliminates from consideration treatment regimens that may be most effective in either stopping the bruxing or reducing the damage done by it. It is important to recognize that there are different patterns of bruxism and there are different etiologies. Optimal treatment strategies depend on a correct diagnosis that includes both a patient stress profile[2,3] and a precise analysis of the occlusion in relation to the position and condition of the temporomandibular joints (TMJs).[4-6]

CLENCHING (CENTRIC BRUXISM)

Strong clenching of the teeth can be a normal manifestation of increased muscle tonus associated with emotional stress. It also occurs during heavy lifting or other physical demands. Abnormal clenching that occurs when there is no physical or emotional trigger is a form of bruxism (centric bruxism). Habitual clenching usually does not involve noticeable jaw movement, but teeth with deflective premature contacts may be moved or loosened by repeated clenching activity. Patients are rarely aware of their own clenching habit.

Habitual clenching in the presence of deflective tooth interferences often leads to the typical symptoms of occluso-muscle pain.[7,8] Ramfjord and Ash showed that there is electromyographic (EMG) evidence to show a reduction in the level of muscle activity as well as a reduced tendency to clench if all deflective occlusal interferences are eliminated.[9] It is also a common occurrence for hypermobile teeth to tighten following a precisely completed occlusal correction, even if the patient continues to clench. Thus, even though influence from the central nervous system is a factor in habitual clenching that cannot be eliminated in many patients, it should not be a deterrent for occlusal correction. The reduction of pain levels in heavy bruxers is dramatic and consistent when deflective tooth inclines are completely eliminated. Nocturnal EMG studies on my patients who were severe bruxers/clenchers some-

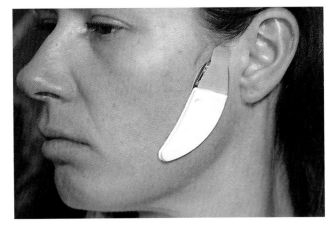

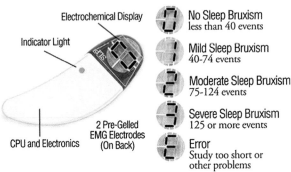

FIGURE 28-1 **A,** BiteStrip™ in place over masseter muscle. The device is held in place during sleep by an adhesive backing. It measures each EMG peak over a period of six hours and then shuts itself off. A score representing the range of bruxing episodes is recorded on the permanent chemical display. **B,** The recording is shown in the display area of the BiteStrip™ as a number that ranges from 0 to 3. Use of the BiteStrip™ makes it possible to compare the level of muscle activity before and after occlusal correction has been completed. (*B courtesy of Great Lakes Orthodontics, Tonawanda, New York. BiteStrip™ manufactured by SLP, Ltd., distributed exclusively by Great Lakes Orthodontics, Ltd.*)

times showed no significant change in nighttime muscle activity after occlusal correction. However, complete relief of symptoms was achieved in each of these patients when there was no intracapsular disorder and other causative factors were ruled out.

Although many patients will continue to clench after occlusal interferences have been eliminated, many will see notable reduction in muscle activity. Today there is a simple way for practitioners to evaluate the extent of excessive jaw muscle activity. A single-use home screening device (BiteStrip™) can be used to measure the existence of either daytime or nighttime clenching and the frequency of bruxism (Figure 28-1).

The role of occlusal interferences as an etiologic factor in bruxing has been a continuous issue for many years. As early as 1901, Karolyi[10] postulated that occlusal interferences were an important factor in combination with psychic influences. He observed that even minor occlusal interferences could be a trigger for grinding habits in neurotic patients. I believe Dr. Karolyi got it right. Occlusal interferences are a potent trigger for bruxing in patients under stress, but they are also a potent trigger for many patients who do not have excessive stress in their lives. And it is certainly true that even the most insignificant-appearing premature occlusal contact can and often does activate high levels of muscle activity that normalizes when the occlusal interference is eliminated.

It seems clear that occlusal triggers are a primary factor in eccentric bruxing. It is also clear that to do damage to the teeth, they must be in the way of border movements of the mandible. A perfected occlusion with posterior disclusion makes excursive contact on posterior teeth impossible to achieve as long as the anterior guidance is stable. The effect is that it leaves nothing to brux except the anterior teeth. Long-term experience has shown that there is no tendency to brux on anterior teeth unless they interfere with the patient's envelope of function. The exception to this is certain types of dystonias from CNS-related etiologies.

Whereas eccentric bruxing can in most cases be reduced or eliminated, successful elimination of clenching is not so predictable.

ECCENTRIC BRUXISM

Eccentric bruxism refers to nonfunctional grinding of the lower teeth against the upper teeth in excursive pathways. If uncontrolled, it generally leads to severe attritional wear of the occlusal surfaces or hypermobility of the teeth and may also contribute to adaptive changes in the TMJs, resulting in flattening of the condyles and gradual loss of convexity of the eminentiae. In severe bruxers, the masseter muscles are often enlarged, sometimes to the point of noticeable changes in facial contour. Bruxism is associated with muscle spasm, split teeth, and fractured fillings. It is the screeching, grating sound in the night that has kept many spouses awake. One of the most unusual aspects of bruxism is that often the one who does it is not even aware of the habit. Habitual bruxers present some of the most difficult challenges in restorative dentistry, and the difficulty increases with the severity of the wear produced.

Etiology

The cause of eccentric bruxism is not completely clear. Although considerable light has been shed on the problem, there are enough unexplained observations to indicate there is still much to learn. One thing seems certain: *There is no single factor that is responsible for all bruxing.* It is also rather evident that *there is no single treatment that is effective for eliminating or even reducing all bruxing.*

There are, however, reliable methods for reducing the *effects* of bruxing, and in the majority of patients it has been my clinical experience that the signs and symptoms of eccentric bruxing seem to disappear completely with the careful elimination of all occlusal interferences. I am still so confident of this result that I ask every patient to report any sign of bruxism because it may be an indication that the occlusion needs refining.

In a 1961 study, Ramfjord[11] found that "some kind of occlusal interference will be found in every patient with bruxism." EMG studies done by Ramfjord and Ash[9] showed that "a marked reduction in muscle tonus and harmonious integration of muscle action follows the elimination of occlusal disharmony."

The results of the research done by Ramfjord and Ash are consistent with many later EMG studies that show a direct relationship between occlusal interferences and muscle hyperactivity, including muscle incoordination. Williamson's[12] classic study showing the effect of eccentric posterior tooth contact clearly relates muscle hyperactivity to occlusal interferences. It further documents the reduction in muscle tonus when the eccentric contacts are removed. If study after study confirms the causal relationship between occlusal interferences and muscle hyperactivity, it would be inconsistent to deduce that occlusal factors play no role as a causative factor in bruxing.

It is also obvious that occlusal interferences can trigger parafunctional jaw movements that were not present before the interference was introduced.[12-16] The consistently observed "erasure mechanism" can be predicted to occur any time the envelope of function is encroached on. Restriction of the anterior guidance, almost without exception, will produce excessive attritional wear on the restricting surfaces. Furthermore, correction of a restricted anterior guidance almost always eliminates the wear problem. Providing a fraction of a millimeter of long centric often makes the difference between excessive wear or no observable wear on the anterior contacting surfaces.

Even in patients with no interferences to centric relation, parafunctional pressure against inclines will most likely occur if the inclines interfere with any functional eccentric jaw movements. Pressure against the restrictive inclines usually causes severe wear, but it may also result in hypermobility of the interfering teeth, or the teeth may be forced out of alignment until they no longer interfere.

Severe wear is a common occurrence in postorthodontic patients whose teeth have been held in functional interference for an extended period by a retainer. Even if centric relation harmony is perfected, eccentric wear will most likely occur against inclines of teeth that are prevented by a retainer from moving out of the position of restricted function. When teeth are prevented by a retainer from adaptively moving into a nonrestrictive alignment, the wear occurs rapidly and often causes severe damage in a short time. The severity of wear in such young postorthodontic patients is abnormal for their age and can only be explained as resulting from parafunctional rubbing. Unless the teeth are moved to a noninterfering functional alignment, the wear will continue even if the worn surfaces are restored. However if the functional alignment is corrected, the wear problem can almost always be predictably eliminated. This consistent clinical observation would indicate that bruxism can be caused by occlusal interferences and can be eliminated, at least in some patients, by correction of the occlusion.

Despite the obvious relationship between occlusal interferences and muscle hyperactivity, it appears that occlusal correction alone may not always be a sure cure for habitual bruxing. Rugh and Solberg[17] showed that habitual nocturnal bruxism continued to occur even after occlusal interferences were removed. By monitoring muscle activity during sleep, EMG recordings seemed to indicate about the same amount of masticatory muscle contraction after occlusal correction as there was before. There was no assurance in this study, however, that the condylar position was in a verified centric relation, or that the occlusal correction was as precise as it needs to be to achieve the results we are reporting.

The time of muscle contraction during sleep appears to fluctuate up in direct relationship to stress-causing stimuli such as an argument before bedtime. Periods of emotional peacefulness seem to result in less masticatory muscle activity.

More research is needed, particularly research that distinguishes between the horizontal rubbing patterns found in the habitual bruxer and the stationary clenching action of many people during sleep. Most studies have measured only the duration of elevator muscle contraction, which may be unrelated to horizontal parafunction. Furthermore, the current studies do not explain why masseter muscle hypertrophy is reversed in some patients after occlusal correction, sometimes to such a degree that facial contour is noticeably changed as the muscles become reduced in size.

To be considered valid research, any studies regarding the effect of occlusal interferences on bruxism must compare the time and intensity of parafunctional jaw movement *with* versus *without* occlusal interferences. This requires meticulous occlusal correction as well as verifiable evidence that all occlusal interferences have been completely eliminated. That includes both noninterference to centric relation and disclusion of all posterior teeth during eccentric jaw paths. Thus proper research protocol would require verification of centric relation as part of the study.

TREATING THE BRUXISM PROBLEM

Despite the controversy that still clouds the cause of bruxism, it is rather clear that habitual elevator muscle hypercontraction has the potential for severe overload on the teeth, the supporting structures, and the TMJs. In the presence of such an overload, damage to some part of the system is almost inevitable. The destructive effects can be reduced by distribution of the load to the maximum number of equal-intensity tooth contacts during intercuspation. Harmonizing those contacts with centrically related condyles reduces the overload on both the teeth and the joint structures and eliminates the trigger for incoordinated lateral pterygoid contraction. Thus, even if the patient clenches, it need not result in prolonged isometric contraction of opposing muscles.

By perfecting the occlusion for a habitual bruxer, full muscle loading occurs only in centric relation when all parts are aligned. Immediate disclusion of all posterior teeth eliminates any potential overload in eccentric positions, and it reduces muscle loading of the joints and the anterior teeth. It is probably this reduction of muscle contraction in eccentric jaw movements that is responsible for the reduction in size of hypertrophic elevator muscles.

To eliminate the signs and symptoms of bruxism, it is particularly critical that centric relation interferences be eliminated with extreme preciseness. This is so because even the slightest premature contact can activate the contraction of the lateral pterygoid muscles and cause incoordinated elevator-muscle hypercontraction. The problem of equilibrating to such preciseness is made more difficult by the slowness of depressed teeth to rebound, and depression of interfering teeth is common in the bruxing patient.

Against teeth that interfere, strong clenching has the effect of compressing the periodontal ligaments. Clinicians now know that rebound from that compressed intrusion can take 30 minutes or longer before the tooth reaches a passive equilibrium in its socket. When a strong clencher or bruxer is being equilibrated, sufficient time for rebound must be provided before the occlusion is finalized or the bruxing trigger may immediately return. Even after careful equilibration, new interferences can easily develop within an hour or less. This may explain why many investigators have reported that their patients continue to grind their teeth even after the occlusion was perfected. The problem of communication that results in this controversy is the same problem that creates such divergent views regarding the causes of TMDs. The difficulty of perfecting an occlusion is not always considered by the investigator, and the so-called occlusal perfection may fall far short of complete elimination of interferences.

If the occlusal therapist does not use precise methods for manipulating the mandible into the terminal hinge position, it will be impossible to achieve an interference-free occlusion, even in centric relation. However, perfection in centric relation alone is not enough. Minute interferences in any excursion can trigger a bruxism pattern, so manipulation of the mandible is again essential to find and mark every incline that interferes with any border movement of the mandible within the limits of a correct anterior guidance.

The bruxism habit may actually be a form of a protective response to occlusal interferences. It could conceivably be nature's built-in mechanism for self-adjustment of occlusal interferences.

For thousands of years before modern man came along with a soft, refined diet, coarse, abrasive foods were the usual daily fare. As proximal tooth contacts wear and the teeth migrate forward, there is a continual need for occlusal adjustment to compensate for the mesial drift. The coarse foods of premodern man were abrasive enough to wear away interfering cusps and inclines when the bruxism mechanism was stimulated by the pressoreceptors around the roots. In effect, a natural "erasure mechanism" developed as a response to occlusal stress, and the coarse diet supplied the grit to adjust the occlusion to within tolerable limits.

This erasure mechanism is still with us, but our modern diet does not supply the grit. So instead of wearing off the interferences, the more frequent tendency is to wiggle the teeth until they become loose.

The excessive wear that occurred from the bruxism patterns of ancient man did not create a severe problem because of the short lifespan. By the time the teeth wore down to the ridges, there was usually little need for them. If the individual lived an unusually long life, the proliferation of the alveolar ridges themselves provided an adequate chewing surface. In modern man, neither loose teeth nor excessively worn teeth are acceptable, and so it is up to the dentist to prevent the results of bruxism.

If we conclude that all bruxism is caused solely by emotional stress, we will have to conclude also that virtually all of our ancestors were emotionally unstable! Coarse diets undoubtedly contributed to a great degree, but it is unlikely that the amount of wear seen on skulls of our early ancestors would have occurred without a considerable degree of parafunction also.

No one would deny that emotional stress could be a contributing factor in bruxism. If muscle tension is increased by stress, the tendency to grind the teeth is also increased, but only if interferences are contactable. A minute interference in a stressed person may trigger bruxism that may cease with either the elimination of the interference or the reduction of muscle tonus when the stressfulness is normalized.

The observable results that are attainable with occlusal therapy do not seem to depend on the psychological state of the patient. We would attempt to adjust the occlusion of a tense person just as quickly as we would treat a relaxed patient. In fact, many patients obviously suffer an increased tension from the malocclusion itself. The concurrent muscle spasm that is so often present in the patient with severe bruxism is often responsible for a considerable amount of facial tension, discomfort, and even pain.

The discomfort from muscle spasm may in some patients be a causative factor in emotional stress rather than vice versa. Results of treatment in a large number of patients seem to indicate that this is the case.

When signs and symptoms of bruxism are observed, a meticulous occlusal examination is in order. Whether occlusal interferences cause bruxism has not been clearly established, but it is very clear that occlusal interferences in a bruxing patient can be extremely damaging.

So regardless of whether the cause is emotional stress or occlusal triggers, the occlusion should be perfected. In fact, the more likely it is that a patient bruxes, the more important it is to keep the occlusion as perfected as possible. The more perfect the occlusion, the less damage can be done to any of the structures of the masticatory system. In addition, overloading individual interfering teeth not only does direct damage to the interfering teeth and their supporting structures, but also the interference causes the additional problem of muscle incoordination during the bruxing.

Whether treatment for bruxism is directed at eliminating the cause or the effects of the problem is at this point academic. It appears that regardless of the cause, the most effective treatment for the effects of bruxism is perfection of the occlusion. This can be accomplished in two ways:

Directly: By equilibration, occlusal restorations, or orthodontics

Indirectly: By occlusal splints

Direct Occlusal Correction

Before alteration of an occlusion is accomplished directly, a careful analysis should be made on mounted diagnostic casts. If it can be determined that the corrections can be made with selective grinding without mutilation of enamel surfaces, equilibration is most often the method of choice. If restoration of posterior teeth will be needed for other reasons, equilibration procedures can be used to correct the occlusion directly even if some enamel penetration is necessary. Even though restoration of the ground surfaces is planned anyway, the occlusion should be stabilized as much as possible by equilibration before restoration.

If there is uncertainty about patient acceptance or operator skill, correction of the occlusion should first be done indirectly by use of a removable appliance. At some point, however, it will be in the patient's best interest to eliminate any appliance that is not necessary and correct the problem directly.

Whenever possible, equilibration should result in multiple equal-intensity stops in centric relation with immediate disclusion by the anterior guidance in all excursions.

Using Appliances

If occlusal splints are prescribed, complete occlusal coverage should be used to perfect equal-intensity centric stops on all teeth against the splint and immediate disclusion of all posterior teeth the moment the mandible leaves centric relation. Disclusion should be accomplished by an anterior guidance ramp built into the occlusal splint.

The occlusal splint has some possible advantages for severe bruxers. Coverage of all teeth in one arch has the effect of diminishing the mechanoreceptive response in the individual teeth that are covered by the splint. The splint coverage may also prevent the minute rebound effect from occurring in teeth that have been intruded. This improvement in stability may better preserve the perfected relationship that is accomplished at equilibration.

A further value of the occlusal splint is to reduce wear that might otherwise occur during nocturnal bruxing. The acrylic splint may become worn but is more easily replaced than tooth structure.

Even though there are obvious advantages in the use of occlusal splints, they are only advantages if they are needed. If there is no evidence of excessive wear or no signs of hypermobility after occlusal equilibration or restoration, there is nothing to be gained by routine use of an appliance.

If the occlusion is perfected, I find that the need for occlusal splints is very limited, and the need is especially reduced whenever I am able to disclude all posterior teeth in all eccentric excursions. For many years, I have almost eliminated the use of nighttime appliances, preferring to keep patients free of any unnecessary prosthesis. I do, however, explain to patients the possibility of needing such an appliance if I notice signs of wear or mobility on routine health maintenance appointments. Up to now, very few patients have showed enough signs to warrant the use of an appliance. Thus, there is no rationale for prescribing appliances for all patients just because they previously had a wear problem.

Appliances can serve a useful function in some bruxism situations as a temporary adjunct to occlusal correction. Acrylic night guards may help to stabilize hypermobile teeth and reduce tendencies to bruxism during treatment. In unusual situations, they may also serve as compromise substitutes for restorative stabilization or correction when such treatment is impractical for financial or health reasons.

The beneficial effect of acrylic resin splints or night guards is the result of occlusal correction in the appliances themselves and the stabilizing effect they have on the teeth. The elimination of signs of bruxism will occur with virtually any technique that eliminates occlusal interferences, either on the teeth themselves or on an appliance that fits over the teeth. If there is no deviation of the mandible required, the muscles can relax and either bruxism tendencies disappear or the corrected occlusion prevents bruxism from doing harm. Please also refer to Chapter 32, "Occlusal Splints."

Use of soft vinyl mouth guards

One of the more difficult bruxism problems to eliminate is in the patient with chronic sinusitis. An occlusion that is perfected one day is off the next day if pressure in the sinuses moves the upper teeth. It is impossible to keep an occlusion refined to a sufficient degree to keep bruxism patterns eliminated when the positions of the upper teeth are forever changing.

A reasonable solution to the problem is to supply the patient with a well-made soft vinyl mouth guard that can be worn at night to cushion the teeth from the effects of transitory occlusal interferences. When the sinusitis subsides, the appliance is not needed.

Caution should be urged to perfect the occlusion during a time when the sinuses are normal. The appliance should not be a substitute for occlusal harmony.

Questioning the patient regarding sinus headaches, postnasal drips, and nasal stuffiness is an important part of the clinical examination. Radiographs should be carefully observed for the presence of extensive sinuses that extend past the roots of the upper teeth (Figure 28-2). It is best to advise the patient in advance of the possible need for such an appliance during sinusitis episodes so that he or she will understand the limitations of treatment.

Stopping the Bruxism Habit When the Occlusion Is Worn Flat

The most difficult bruxism problem to be faced is the patient who has worn the entire occlusion flat and has shortened the anterior teeth into an end-to-end relationship. The effect of bruxism is easy to eliminate if the flat anterior guidance can be maintained, but often such a patient wishes to have the anterior esthetics improved. There is sometimes no way to improve the esthetics without steepening the anterior guidance. A steepened anterior guidance almost always promotes parafunction.

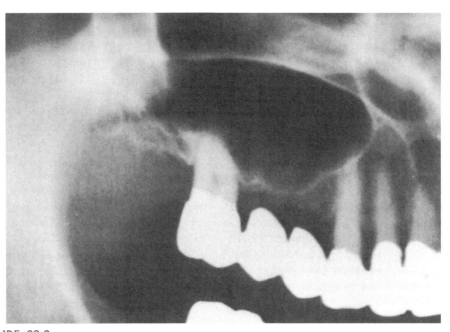

FIGURE 28-2 Pressure from sinusitis can actually move teeth with roots that extend into the sinus. The patient should be aware of the difficulty of stabilizing such teeth in the presence of sinusitis pressure against such root surfaces.

The solution to the problem is at best a compromise. In order to improve the appearance, I will accept a degree of bruxism. The damage from the bruxism can be minimized if the anterior guidance is perfected to disclude all posterior teeth in all excursions while the anterior guidance is kept as flat as acceptable esthetics will permit.

An increased thickness of metal or porcelain should be used to provide more length of wear on the lingual surfaces of the upper anterior teeth, and the patient should be told in advance of the probable continuation of wear. Some splinting may be required to give added stabilization against stress.

A nighttime appliance is indicated whenever there is a restriction of the envelope of function in order to reduce the attritional wear on the anterior teeth. It should have centric relation contact with immediate posterior disclusion.

The anterior guidance should be worked out in the most meticulous manner possible.

Using an Anterior Deprogramming Splint for Severe Clenchers

The arbitrary use of any type of occlusal splint as a standard procedure for all clenching patients is unnecessary, because in most patients appliances are not needed if the occlusion is perfected. However, there are certain patients who will continue to clench, even with a perfected occlusion. These patients may be isolated by complaints about tired masticatory muscles and a feeling of a "closed bite." Dewitt Wilkerson[18] has studied this problem using jaw tracking instrumentation in combination with EMG and JVA (joint vibration analysis). In accord with Glassman's work,[19] he has demonstrated that an anterior deprogramming device reduces elevator muscle contraction force by 80 percent in severe clenchers. Wilkerson also observed that there are three patterns of empty mouth jaw positioning that can be differentiated by jaw tracking while patients go through the following exercise:

1. Rest
2. Swallow
3. Rest again
4. Open

Normal: Comfortable patients

1. Rest: teeth are apart
2. Swallow: teeth contact
3. Rest again: teeth are apart

This patient does not need an occlusal splint if the occlusion is perfected. If muscle discomfort persists after occlusal correction, recheck for missed occlusal interferences or look for other organic causes of muscle discomfort.

Problem: Uncomfortable clenchers

1. Rest: teeth stay in contact
2. Swallow: teeth stay in contact
3. Rest again: teeth stay in contact

In this situation, patients clench continuously, keeping the muscles in an incoordinated hypercontraction. This patient can benefit from an anterior deprogramming splint.

In some patients with occlusal disharmony but no signs or symptoms, Wilkerson found evidence of the following:

Protective tongue pattern:

1. Rest: teeth are apart
2. Swallow: teeth do not contact
3. Rest again: teeth stay apart

This verifies the concept of using the tongue to protect from occlusal interferences. By keeping the tongue between the teeth during swallowing, the occlusal interferences do not have a chance to activate occluso-muscle symptoms.

BRUXISM IN CHILDREN

No one who has ever heard the screeching sounds emanating from a child's bedroom would doubt that children are capable of violent bruxism. Most children grind their teeth at some time or another since occlusal interferences develop naturally during the eruption of teeth. During the mixed-dentition stage, bruxism is common, and some children develop such severe bruxism patterns that they may wear their deciduous teeth flat. There are many theories for explaining why children grind their teeth. The most popular is probably that the child "has worms."

There may be many different contributing factors that increase the tendency to bruxism, but its effects are negligible in the absence of occlusal interferences. This statement becomes academic because all children have occlusal interferences at some time or other. The problem is not generally serious despite the volume of noise that the bruxism generates. A child's resistance to the stress of bruxism is so high that it does not constitute a threat to the dentition.

If the bruxism becomes so severe that it constitutes an irritant in itself, or if the occlusal wear appears to be more extensive than normal, some occlusal adjustment may be in order. Precise refinement is not necessary when a child's occlusion is adjusted, but it is helpful to polish and round all sharp edges and eliminate any gross interferences if the correction can be done without mutilation of a permanent tooth.

Orthodontic appliances may be in order, or some form of bite plane may be used to disengage an offending tooth until other teeth can erupt into contact or necessary corrections can be made. Gross occlusal adjustment usually reduces the bruxism to tolerable limits.

DENTAL COMPRESSION SYNDROME

Occlusal overload that repetitively compresses the teeth also has the potential of compressive forces on the TMJs. The effects of compressive overload have been categorized by McCoy as dental compression syndrome.[20] McCoy lists six major deformations that occur in the oral environment as a result of dental compression. It should be noted that all of the deformations listed by McCoy require that the compressed teeth are in occlusal interference either to centric relation or to excursions.

1. Flattened teeth
2. Exostoses
3. Occlusal dimples
4. Gingival tissue recession
5. Gingival hard tissue fatigue (abfractions). This concept is being contested by other authorities.
6. Restorative material fatigue

> It is important to recognize that as an etiologic factor of any of the above deformations, compression can only reach a destructive level if the posterior teeth can contact before the condyles are completely seated up into centric relation or if they interfere with centric relation contact or any excursive path of a correct anterior guidance.

Prevention of dental compression is always a goal of treatment for the bruxing or clenching patient. It consists of equal-intensity contact at the TMJs, the posterior teeth, and the anterior teeth. This is always the goal of treatment whenever it can be achieved.

Masticatory System Dysfunction and Psychic Stress

Various dysfunctional patterns in the masticatory system are often cited as a cause of bruxism. These dysfunctional patterns are also explained as resulting from psychic stress as the primary etiology of the dysfunction and thus the cause of the bruxism. Ramfjord has pointed out that these theories ignore the facts that "most persons under stress do not develop dysfunctional symptoms and that dysfunctional symptoms in the overwhelming majority of cases will abate by occlusal therapy."[9,10]

Other researchers are in complete agreement with Ramfjord and our own consistent findings.[21-23] Kloprogge and Griethnysen reported that removal of occlusal interferences could lead to instantaneous disappearance of dysfunctional pain symptoms and normalization of the electromyographic jaw muscle contraction pattern.[16] Randow and colleagues[14] demonstrated that dysfunctional disturbances could be reinstated by placement of a single occlusal interference in the same patients that had been relieved of symptoms. The same result was shown by Riise and Sheikholeslam,[13] even when minute interferences were introduced.

In my extensive experience, the bottom line on bruxism is an etiology that must consider the effects of both occlusal interferences and psychic stress. It is the only way we can explain the realities of clinical observation: Some patients with minute occlusal interferences develop dysfunctional patterns with pain, and other patients with major occlusal interferences develop reportable symptoms only when under stress. Many patients with no signs of psychic stress develop symptoms from a variety of occlusal interferences. Regardless of the differences from patient to patient, almost all bruxing patients who do not have intracapsular structural disorders or other tissue damage can be relieved of their pain and dysfunction by very precise elimination of all occlusal interferences. Thus, this is the solid recommendation for patients who are doing damage from bruxing or clenching.

Using Diagnostic Occlusal Splints

Some clinicians have advocated the wearing of an occlusal splint to determine if bruxism is a problem before doing restorative procedures. If the patient wears the occlusal surface of the appliance, it is said to be indicative of a bruxing problem. I disagree with this conclusion because the only way posterior wear patterns can be ground into the splint surface is if the occlusal surface interferes with complete seating of the joints or interferes with anterior guidance in excursions. You cannot wear what you cannot rub. This principle applies to occlusal splints as well as natural teeth.

A posterior occlusion can only wear if it contacts before the TMJs are completely seated up into centric relation. A perfected anterior guidance will immediately separate all posterior contact in excursions. So the key to controlling the damage from bruxing includes an anterior guidance that is in harmony with the envelope of function so its disclusive effect on posterior teeth is maintainable. This is the goal for natural dentitions as well as for occlusal splints. If esthetic concerns for natural teeth result in constriction of the envelope of function, the anterior teeth will wear. In such cases, a nighttime appliance is recommended to reduce anterior wear so the posterior disclusive effect can be maintained.

If an anterior deprogramming device eliminates the bruxing problem, it is diagnostic that occlusal interferences were a trigger for muscle hyperactivity. Correction of the occlusion should eliminate the need for long-term use of the deprogramming device.

It is apparent that occlusal treatment will not stop every patient from clenching or bruxing. But perfected occlusal treatment will almost always reduce the damage done to a maintainable level.

References

1. Levitt SR: The predictive value of the TMJ scale in detecting psychological problems and non-TM disorders in patients with temporomandibular disorders. *Cranio* 8:225-233, 1990.
2. Levitt SR: Predictive value of the TMJ scale in detecting clinically significant symptoms of temporomandibular disorders. *J Craniomandib Disord* 4:177-185, 1990.
3. Levitt SR: Predictive value: A model for dentists to evaluate the accuracy of diagnostic tests for temporomandibular disorders as applied to a TMJ scale. *J Prosthet Dent* 66:385-390, 1991.
4. Levitt SR, McKinney MW, Lundeen T: The TMJ scale: Cross validation and reliability studies. *Cranio* 6:17-25, 1988.
5. Dawson PE: New definitions for relating occlusion to varying conditions of the temporomandibular joint. *J Prosthet Dent* 74:619-627, 1995.

6. Dawson PE: A classification system for occlusions that relates maximal intercuspation to the position and condition of the temporomandibular joints. *J Prosthet Dent* 75:60-65, 1996.

7. Dawson PE: Bad advice from flawed research. *AGD Impact* April:30-31, 1995.

8. Granger ER: Occlusion in temporomandibular joint pain. *J Am Dent Assoc* 56:659, 1958.

9. Ramfjord SP, Ash MM Jr: *Occlusion,* ed 3, Philadelphia, 1983, WB Saunders.

10. Karolyi M: Beobachtungen uber Pyorrhoea alveolaris. *Ost-Unt Vjschr Zahnheilk* 17:279, 1901.

11. Ramfjord SP: Dysfunctional temporomandibular joint and muscle pain. *J Prosthet Dent* 11:353, 1961.

12. Williamson EH, Lundquist DO: Anterior guidance: Its effect on electromyographic activity of the temporal and masseter muscles. *J Prosthet Dent* 49(6):816-823, 1983.

13. Riise C, Sheikholeslam A: The influence of experimental interfering occlusal contacts on the postural activity of the anterior temporal and masseter muscles in young adults. *J Oral Rehabil* 9:419-425, 1982.

14. Randow K, Carlsson K, Edlund J, et al: The effect of an occlusal interference on the masticatory system: An experimental investigation. *Odonto Rev* 27:254, 1976.

15. Brill N, Schubeles S, Tryde G: Influence of occlusal patterns on movements of the mandible. *J Prosthet Dent* 12:255, 1962.

16. Kloprogge MJ, Griethnysen AM: Disturbance on the contraction and coordination pattern of the masticatory muscles due to dental restorations. *J Oral Rehabil* 3:207, 1976.

17. Rugh JD, Solberg WK: Electromyographic studies of bruxist behavior before and during treatment. *J Calif State Dent Assoc* 3:56, 1975.

18. Wilkerson DC: Monitoring "the vital signs" of masticatory system health—a simplified screening for TM problems. *Dent Econ* 83(2):72-73, 1993.

19. Glassman B: The Aqualizer's role. *Dent Today* 21(11):12, 2002.

20. McCoy G: Dental compression syndrome. A new look at an old disease. *J Oral Implant* 5:35-49, 1999.

21. Franks A: Conservative treatment of temporomandibular joint dysfunction. A comparative study. *Dent Pract* 15:205, 1965.

22. Kerstein RB, Farrell S: Treatment of myofascial pain dysfunction syndrome with occlusal equilibration. *J Prosthet Dent* 63:695-700, 1990.

23. Agerberg G, Carlsson GE: Late results of treatment of functional disorders of the masticatory system. A follow up questionnaire. *J Oral Rehabil* 1:309, 1974.

PART III

Treatment

Chapter 29

Requirements for Occlusal Stability

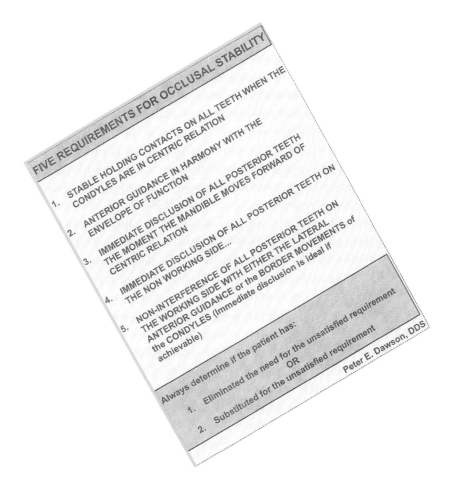

FIVE REQUIREMENTS FOR OCCLUSAL STABILITY

1. STABLE HOLDING CONTACTS ON ALL TEETH WHEN THE CONDYLES ARE IN CENTRIC RELATION

2. ANTERIOR GUIDANCE IN HARMONY WITH THE ENVELOPE OF FUNCTION

3. IMMEDIATE DISCLUSION OF ALL POSTERIOR TEETH THE MOMENT THE MANDIBLE MOVES FORWARD OF CENTRIC RELATION

4. IMMEDIATE DISCLUSION OF ALL POSTERIOR TEETH ON THE NON WORKING SIDE...

5. NON-INTERFERENCE OF ALL POSTERIOR TEETH ON THE WORKING SIDE WITH EITHER THE LATERAL ANTERIOR GUIDANCE or the BORDER MOVEMENTS of the CONDYLES (Immediate disclusion is ideal if achievable)

Always determine if the patient has:

1. Eliminated the need for the unsatisfied requirement OR

2. Substituted for the unsatisfied requirement

Peter E. Dawson, DDS

PRINCIPLE

The requirements for occlusal stability form the framework for all occlusal treatment planning. Learn them.

WHAT A STABLE OCCLUSION "LOOKS LIKE"

There is no visual textbook norm that signifies that an occlusion is stable. Some of the most stable occlusions can appear as serious malocclusions if analyzed solely on the basis of Angle's Classification. Some of the most unstable occlusions appear to be Angle's Class 1 when examined at maximal intercuspation or when observed on unmounted study casts.

Physiologic Malocclusions

Many malocclusions can be maintained in good health and stability and can be completely comfortable. An anterior open bite in some patients may be as stable as an ideal occlusion. Crossbites do not always present a problem of instability, and deep overbites can be among the most stable occlusions. Before any treatment plan is initiated, it is important to determine if an occlusion is stable or unstable, regardless of what it looks like.

There are definite, easily recognizable signs that tell us whether an occlusion is stable or unstable. These signs should become the basis for whether occlusal treatment of any kind is necessary. If a stable malocclusion is esthetically unacceptable, these signs become a cautionary signal to be careful not to turn a stable occlusion into an unstable one. There will always be a reason why an occlusion is unstable, and there will also be a cumulative effect of multiple factors that produce stability. The entire treatment planning process is based on understanding the need for stability as an essential end point for an acceptable treatment result.

HOW TO RECOGNIZE A STABLE OCCLUSION REGARDLESS OF WHAT IT LOOKS LIKE

There are five recognizable signs that an occlusion is stable. All five signs of stability must be evident. If all five signs can be verified, you can count on the occlusion being stable, regardless of what it looks like.

1. Temporomandibular joints (TMJs) are healthy and stable
2. All teeth are firm (Figure 29-1)
3. No excessive wear is present
4. All teeth have stayed in their present position
5. Supporting structures are maintainably healthy

> Observing for the five signs of stability is the best way to avoid overtreatment. It is also the safest basis for making a decision not to alter an occlusion that is stable.

The observation that a malocclusion is stable is not proof that it will remain stable. It does, however, make it practical to avoid doing treatment as long as no signs of instability are observable. The patient should always be advised that there is a

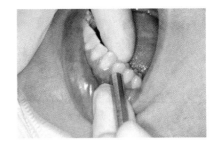

FIGURE 29-1 All teeth should be checked for mobility. It is one of the first signs that teeth are in interference to repeated functional (or parafunctional) jaw movements.

potential for problems in the future and that he or she will be monitored at each recall examination to see if any changes occur that should be attended to. As long as all masticatory structures are staying healthy, there is no need to change anything unless the patient is unhappy with appearance or function.

It is important to remember that *signs precede symptoms.* Careful observation by the dentist is important. Don't wait for the patient to complain. If it is obvious that active problems are starting, search out the cause of the problems and correct it before major damage requires more extensive treatment.

HOW TO RECOGNIZE AN UNSTABLE OCCLUSION REGARDLESS OF WHAT IT LOOKS LIKE

Any one or more of the following signs of instability (Box 29-1) is an indication of problems in the dentition. By looking for these signs, we can get a quick warning that there is something wrong somewhere in the masticatory system. There is almost a certainty that there is some disharmony between the teeth and the movements of the mandible either to and from centric relation, or during excursions.

Box 29-1   Three Signs of Instability

1. Hypermobility of one or more teeth
2. Excessive wear (Figure 29-2)
3. Migration of one or more teeth
   a. Horizontal shifting
   b. Intrusion
   c. Supraeruption

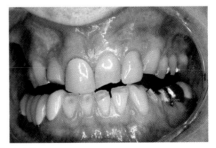

FIGURE 29-2 Wear that has penetrated into dentin is one of the surest signs of occlusal instability. The implication of dentin exposure is a sevenfold increase in the rate of wear.

Signs of instability, in time, will always occur when the teeth are not in equilibrium with muscle (Box 29-2). When teeth and muscle war, muscle never loses.

If any of the five requirements are not in order, the system is not in equilibrium. A system that is not in equilibrium will attempt to regain it through adaptive changes that are often destructive.

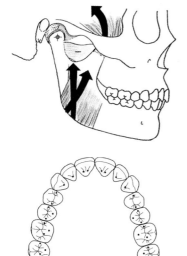
THE FIVE REQUIREMENTS FOR OCCLUSAL STABILITY

There are five requirements for occlusal stability (Box 29-3). They must become a dominant factor in any occlusal analysis, and every occlusion should be evaluated to see whether or not each requirement is fulfilled. The requirements must be used in sequence. They apply to individual teeth or to the entire dentition. These requirements form the matrix for the decision-making process for all occlusal treatment.

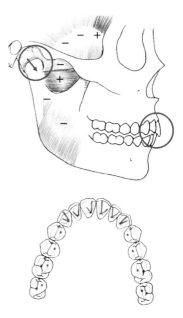

In establishing a stable occlusion, the anterior guidance assumes the key role. The anterior teeth are better able to resist stress than the posterior teeth. This is so because of their relation to the TMJ fulcrum, and the muscle force.

In working with problems of occlusion, the difficulty of each problem directly relates to whether or not an acceptable anterior guidance can be established.

The ideal occlusal scheme as recorded on marking ribbon during closure and grinding in all direction is **lines in front, dots in back.**

How to Use the Requirements for Stability for Treatment Planning

If there are requirements that are not fulfilled and there is no substitute, or if the need for the requirement has not been specifically eliminated, our treatment plan should be designed to:
1. Fulfill the requirement (if possible or practical)
2. Substitute for the missing requirement
3. Eliminate the need

Remember that we apply this treatment plan approach to each requirement *in* **proper sequence.**

Key point
You must determine stability of holding contacts on each tooth *before* analyzing the other four requirements.

The above rules are the basis for all occlusal analysis and treatment planning. The whole concept of *programmed treatment planning* is dependent on understanding and implementing these rules.

Chapter 30

Solving Occlusal Problems Through Programmed Treatment Planning

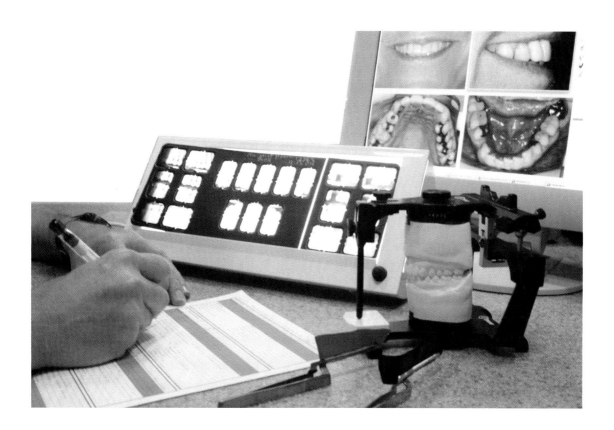

PRINCIPLE

The requirements for stability guide the treatment planning process.

The first treatment goal: Get the mouth HEALTHY

PERIODONTAL	**Classification:** ❏ Healthy ❏ Gingivitis ❏ Mild Perio ❏ Moderate Perio ❏ Severe Perio ❏ Refractory

Implications: ❏ Stable ❏ Unstable
ㅤㅤㅤㅤㅤㅤㅤ❏ Immediate concerns_____
ㅤㅤㅤㅤㅤㅤㅤ❏ Deferrable _____
ㅤㅤㅤㅤㅤㅤㅤ❏ Optional _____

Recommend	❏ **Refer** to: _____
❏ Preliminary mouth preparation	❏ Pocket elimination:_____
❏ Hygiene instructions	❏ Mucogingival:_____
❏ Prophylaxis	❏ Esthetic: _____
❏ Root planing	❏ Crown lengthening: _____
❏ Post root planing evaluation	❏ Furcation barreling: _____
❏ Other_____	❏ Sectioning: _____
Comments: _____	

STRATEGY FOR THE EXAMINATION

There are some critical determinations that must be made in the examination process before a treatment plan for occlusal correction can be initiated. As important as occlusal harmony is to the total plan, it must be put into proper context with the requirements for complete dentistry.

The First Determination

The first concern is always to make sure the mouth is healthy.

The exam process must evaluate the supporting structures to determine how periodontal considerations should be sequenced into the total treatment plan. The determination of whether a tooth is maintainably healthy or can be made maintainably healthy is most often a periodontal decision. Each tooth should be evaluated and recorded on a standardized checklist to determine up front if there are any teeth that cannot be saved and maintained in a healthy condition. Any tooth that cannot be saved should be noted with an *X* on the mounted casts (Figure 30-1). Unsavable teeth should be cut off the cast before any occlusal decisions are made. This process often simplifies treatment planning.

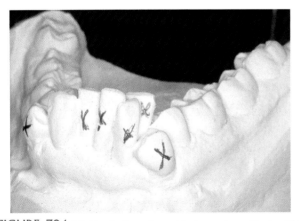

FIGURE 30-1 Marking teeth on the cast that are not savable simplifies treatment planning. At this stage, the decision to remove a tooth is made only on the basis that it is unsavable. After unsavable teeth are removed from the cast, decisions regarding occlusal harmony are determined solely by analysis of the remaining teeth as they relate to the opposing arch in centric relation.

At the initial examination, a tooth-by-tooth analysis should be directed at determining every problem and the implications of not treating each problem in a timely manner (Figure 30-2). The patient should take part in that examination so that each problem or concern is seen and understood. Final decisions are not generally made at that appointment, but tentative decisions should be recorded regarding esthetics, types of restorations needed, and a general appraisal of the direction treatment will go. If there are occlusal problems, no final decisions should be made until mounted casts can be studied and various treatment approaches can be sorted out to determine what would be in the best interest of long-term stability for the patient.

Preparation for Occlusal Treatment Planning

The requirements for stability that guide the treatment planning process must also guide the occlusal examination. That requires verification that the condyles can be positioned in centric relation or adapted centric posture because tooth contacts cannot be accurately evaluated until both the position and condition of the temporomandibular joints (TMJs) are verified. If an acceptable condylar position can be determined at the examination, impressions, bite records, and facebow can be completed at that appointment.

The key questions that must be answered before occlusal treatment can be properly planned are readily noted on the patient's record (Figure 30-3). There are two key questions that should never be left unanswered before occlusal treatment is initiated:

1. Are the TMJs healthy?
2. Can centric relation be verified?

If the TMJs cannot comfortably accept firm loading . . . STOP. Find out why before proceeding with irreversible occlusal changes.

> ## PRINCIPLE
> Accurate occlusal treatment planning requires accurate joint position.

TEETH | **Chief complaint:** _____

Problems: ☐ Decay ☐ Wear (dentin exposed) **Prosthetic:** ☐ Wearing removable partial dtr _____
☐ Mobility/fremitus ☐ Cracks ☐ Splits ☐ Full dentures ☐ upper only ☐ lower only
☐ Periapical abscess ☐ Missing teeth ☐ Crowns/bridges _____
☐ Inadequate restorations ☐ Implants _____

Esthetics: ☐ Acceptable ☐ Could improve ☐ Patient wants improvement Comment _____

Implications: ☐ Immediate concerns _____
☐ Deferrable _____
☐ Optional _____

Dr. Comments: _____

FIGURE 30-2 The checklist form for an overview regarding the condition of the teeth. Further charting should also be done in detail.

TMJ | **Piper Classification:** Right: 1 2 3A 3B 4A 4B 5A 5B
Left: 1 2 3A 3B 4A 4B 5A 5B

Implications: ☐ Stable ☐ Unstable
☐ Immediate concerns _____
☐ Deferrable _____
☐ Optional _____

History: ☐ Neg ☐ Positive for _____
Load Test: Left ☐ Neg ☐ Pain ☐ Tenderness ☐ Tension Right ☐ Neg ☐ Pain ☐ Tenderness ☐ Tension
Centric Relation: ☐ Verified ☐ Not Verifiable ☐ Adapted Centric Posture
Muscle Palpation: ☐ Neg ☐ Tenderness in _____
Doppler: Left _____ Right _____
ROM: Protrusive _____mm Left _____mm Right _____mm Path of motion ☐ Normal ☐ Deviates_____
Pain **Recommend**_____
☐ No Pain _____ ☐ Deprogram muscles ☐ Occlusal splint
☐ Intracapsular _____ ☐ Transcranial film
☐ Occluso-muscle _____ ☐ Tomogram
☐ Other _____ ☐ MRI ☐ CT Scan
_____ ☐ Refer for surgical evaluation to _____

FIGURE 30-3 In this examination form, the most important decisions about the condition and position of the TMJs are organized into a simplified checklist.

If centric relation can be verified, mount the casts using a centric relation bite record and a facebow. The analysis of the mounted casts will also require information observed at the examination appointments for use at the diagnostic work-up. The appropriate questions are listed on the checklist for occlusion (Figures 30-4 to 30-6).

STRATEGY FOR TREATMENT PLANNING

The basis for a programmed approach to treatment planning is an understanding of what makes an occlusion stable or unstable regardless of what it looks like. The requirements for stability form a matrix for decision making that requires evaluation of each requirement in proper sequence. That means that the first priority is to determine if there are stable holding contacts on all teeth when the mandible is in centric relation.

If the mandible can close all the way to maximal intercuspation without having to displace either condyle and there are equal-intensity, simultaneous contacts on all teeth, the first requirement for stability is fulfilled (Dawson Classification Type 1 or 1A occlusion). The treatment planning process can move on to the second requirement for stability. As each requirement is satisfied, the process moves on to the next requirement, always making sure that the correct sequencing is maintained.

The *treatment planning matrix* (Figure 30-7) is an excellent guide for directing the thought process through an orderly sequence of decisions. This process works well for every type of occlusal problem, including complex multidisciplinary treatment coordination.

The *treatment planning matrix* is used in combination with the five options for treatment so that all choices for treatment can be considered for fulfilling each requirement for stability. Treatment choices may also be used to substitute for or eliminate the need for certain requirements (Box 30-1).

OCCLUSION	Dawson Classification: 1 1A 2 2A 3 4

Maxillomandibular ❏ Asymmetry ❏ Retrognathic ❏ Prognathic ❏ Anterior open bite ❏ Posterior open bite

Implications: ❏ Stable ❏ Unstable
❏ Immediate concerns_____
❏ Deferrable _____
❏ Optional _____

First contact in CR or ACP #_____ ❏ Slide to MI ❏ Tooth moves ❏ Direction of slide to MI _____

Anterior contact in CR ❏ yes ❏ no _____

Anterior contact in MI ❏ yes ❏ no _____

Posterior disclusion: Protrusion ❏ yes ❏ no Balancing side ❏ yes ❏ no Working side ❏ yes ❏ no

Occlusal plane ❏ level ❏ slanted ❏ interferes with AG _____

Wear ❏ no problem ❏ slight ❏ into dentin ❏ severe Abfractions _____

Recommend: ❏ Mounted casts ❏ Diagnostic wax-up ❏ Equilibration ❏ Restorative
❏ Refer for Ortho consult to_____ ❏ Surgery Consult to _____

FIGURE 30-4 Checklist for occlusal findings to be used in analysis and treatment planning.

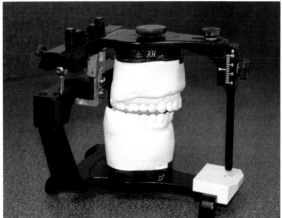

FIGURE 30-5 Casts mounted in centric relation. For accurate occlusal analysis, the condylar axis must be the same on the articulator as the axis on the patient. The jaw-to-jaw relationship must be at centric relation.

Box 30-1   Correction of Occlusal Disharmonies

Five choices for correction
1. Reductive reshaping (equilibration, coronoplasty)
2. Repositioning (orthodontics)
3. Additive reshaping (restorative)
4. Surgical repositioning of segments of the dento-alveolar process without changing the skeletal base
5. Surgical repositioning of skeletal segments in relation to the cranial base

Note: Combinations of choices are frequently necessary.

Three options for treatment
1. Provide the unfulfilled requirement
2. Substitute for the unfulfilled requirement
3. Eliminate the need for the unfulfilled requirement

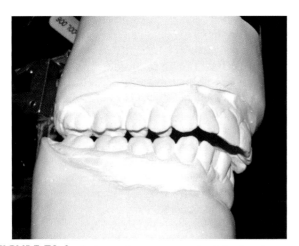

FIGURE 30-6 The first tooth contact at centric relation is at the second molar. If the goal of treatment is to achieve anterior contact in centric relation, the articulator is locked in centric relation while an analysis is done to determine which of the five treatment choices will be best for getting the back teeth out of the way so the front teeth can contact.

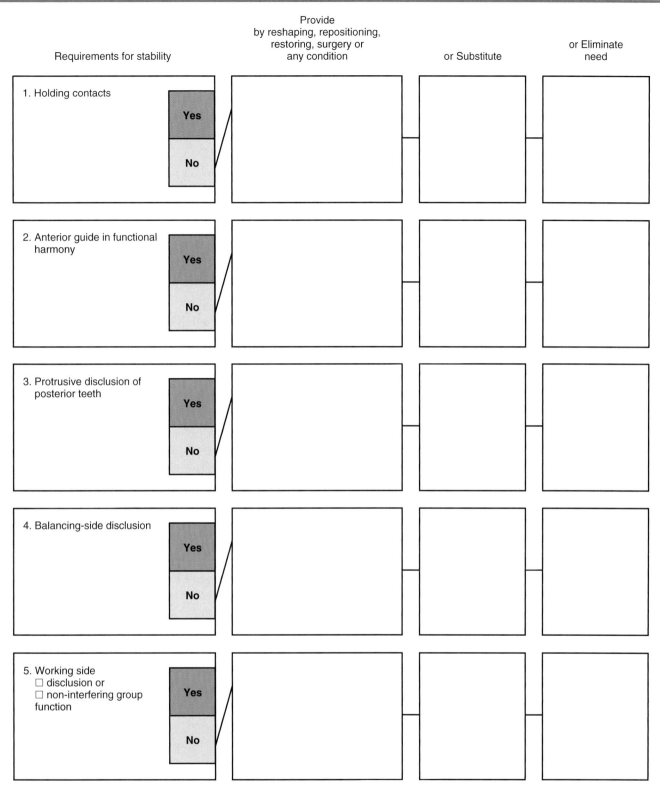

FIGURE 30-7 Treatment planning matrix based on the five requirements for occlusal stability. The treatment planning matrix guides the thought process for treatment design. As each requirement for stability is analyzed in sequence, the examiner determines if any unfulfilled requirement has an acceptable substitute or if the need for that requirement has been eliminated. As each requirement is satisfied, the planning moves to the next requirement. Any of the five treatment options can be selected to solve each requirement.

Treatment Options for Providing Holding Contacts

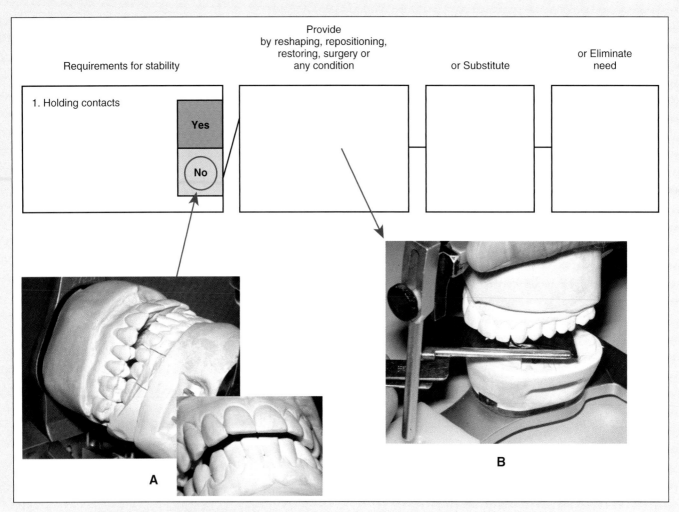

	Provide by reshaping, repositioning, restoring, surgery or any condition	or Substitute	or Eliminate need
Requirements for stability			
1. Holding contacts Yes No			

A, Mounted casts at first point of tooth contact at centric relation. The goal is simultaneous contact. The options for achieving that should be analyzed to determine the best treatment choice. The process eliminates guesswork. **B,** On mounted casts, the premature deflecting contact can be located and marked with articulating ribbon.

First option: Reshape
The casts can be reshaped to determine if it can achieve the goal of equal contact on all the teeth without mutilating too much enamel.

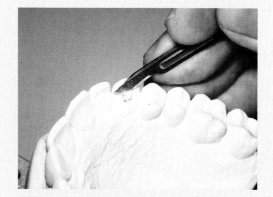

Second option: Reposition
Reshaping helped but could not solve the problem completely, so minor tooth movement combined with reshaping proved to be the best solution.

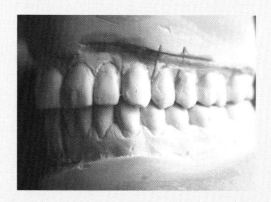

Substituting for Holding Contacts

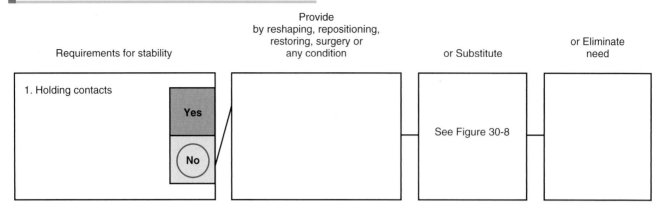

The examination process should always observe the arch-to-arch relationship of the most closed position of maximal intercuspation. If there are teeth that cannot contact at the closed position, there will always be a reason. Teeth erupt until something stops the eruption. The examination must disclose what is preventing teeth from complete eruption (Figure 30-8). In most cases, it will be the tongue posturing between the teeth. The tongue may actually stabilize an open bite by substituting for tooth contact. If this is the case, the teeth should be examined for signs of stability or instability. If the teeth are stable, the tongue is an acceptable substitute.

Other substitutes may be a source of problems. Poorly designed or inappropriate segmental occlusal splints are often a cause of open bites. Other factors include cheek biting, thumb sucking, pipe smoking and pencil biting. Treatment design must consider the cause of the open bite and determine whether it is a stabilizing influence or one that should be eliminated. If a tongue thrust is the *result* of a malocclusion rather than its cause, tooth contact can usually be reestablished (see Chapter 38).

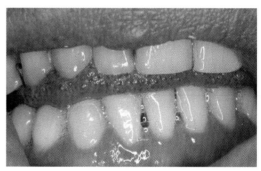

FIGURE 30-8 Open bite stabilized by the tongue.

Options for Anterior Guidance

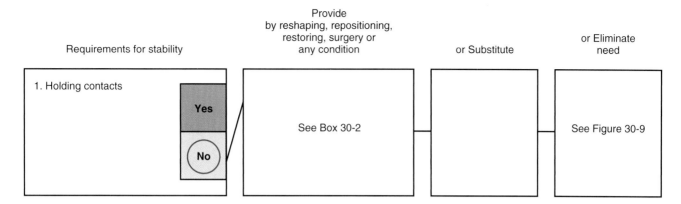

Requirements for stability		Provide by reshaping, repositioning, restoring, surgery or any condition	or Substitute	or Eliminate need
1. Holding contacts	Yes / No	See Box 30-2		See Figure 30-9

Box 30-2   Treatment Options to Consider

- Will reductive reshaping help? (Figures 30-10 and 30-11)
- Is orthodontic repositioning needed?
- Are restorations needed?
- Is repositioning of the dento-alveolar segment needed?
- Does skeletal base alignment need correction?
- Is substitution with an occlusal splint needed?
- Is anterior guidance needed?

Class 3 occlusions that are in an anterior crossbite relationship do not have an anterior guidance, yet they are typically one of the most stable occlusal relationships (Figure 30-9). Class 3 occlusions do not need an anterior guidance to disclude the posterior teeth in protrusive because Class 3 patients don't protrude the jaw. This is an example of eliminating the need for one of the requirements. Other examples are pointed out in the chapters on different occlusal problems.

Substitution as a treatment

The ideal solution for lack of holding contacts is usually *to provide* the contact by one of the five options for treatment. This is not always a viable option. In some instances, providing holding contacts would require such extensive and expensive treatment that it is not an acceptable solution for the patient. In such cases, teeth can often be stabilized by substituting an occlusal splint as an alternative to tooth-to-tooth contact. In many instances, nighttime wearing of an appliance with tooth contact in centric relation is all that is needed to stabilize a dentition and prevent supraeruption of teeth whose alignment does not permit tooth contact at centric relation.

Eliminating the Need for Holding Contacts

The only way (other than substitution) to eliminate the need by the patient for stable holding contacts is by ankylosis. Ankylosed teeth will not erupt even if there is no opposing tooth contact. However, ankylosis is rare so it is not a common solution.

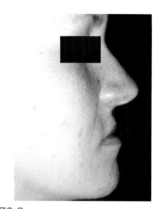

FIGURE 30-9 Is the need for anterior guidance eliminated?

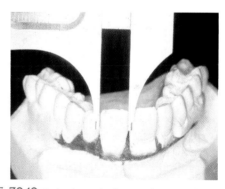

FIGURE 30-10 Reductive reshaping may involve stripping contacts to permit moving upper anterior teeth back to gain contact for an anterior guidance.

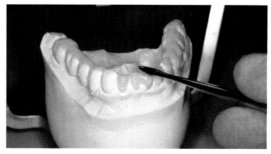

FIGURE 30-11 Additive reshaping may be necessary to achieve contact when there has been severe wear.

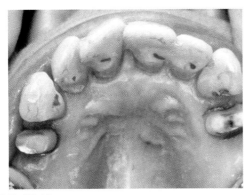

FIGURE 30-12 Stable holding contacts on anterior teeth. The most common cause for instability of anterior teeth is failure to provide axially directed definite stops. Treatment planning should always pay close attention to the stability of the anterior contacting contours.

As a treatment option, splinting can be used to eliminate the need for stable holding contacts. Fixed splinting of teeth that have contact joined to teeth that don't have contact prevents all splinted teeth from supracruption.

Stable Holding Contacts

Remember that tooth contacts must be shaped so they prevent the contacting teeth from erupting. Contacts that do not provide a definite axially directed stop are not acceptable (Figure 30-12). They almost always lead to instability in time.

CHECKLIST FOR FIRST REQUIREMENT ANALYSIS

Analysis #1: Stable Holding Contacts

At maximum closure
- Are there any teeth that do not contact?
- Has the patient substituted for the missing contact?
- Are the teeth that do not contact stable?
- Are there any wear problems?
- Are there any mobility problems?
- Are there any tooth migration problems?
- Did the tongue cause the separation?
- Is the patient a lip biter or cheek biter?
- Is there a segmental occlusal splint?
- Are there any noxious habits?

At centric relation
The same teeth that contact at maximum intercuspation should contact in centric relation.

- Can anterior teeth contact if posterior interferences are removed?
- Are stable stops needed on anterior teeth?
- Are there any wear problems on the lower incisal edges?

Treatment Options

Reductive reshaping (equilibration)
- Can this treatment solve the problem?
- Will the treatment achieve anterior contact in centric relation?
- Will the treatment mutilate good teeth?
- Will the treatment help partially achieve the desired result?

> If indicated, do the diagnostic equilibration on casts. Use clinical judgment regarding the permissible reduction without exposing dentin.

Repositioning (orthodontics)
- Can routine orthodontics reposition the teeth for stable holding contacts? (Observe neutral zone considerations.)
- Would a combination of reshaping and repositioning work better?

> If indicated, move teeth on casts to evaluate orthodontic possibilities. Consult with an orthodontist.

Additive reshaping (restorative)
- Can holding contacts be provided by restorations?
- Do teeth need restorations for other reasons?
- Would restored contours be acceptable regarding esthetics, crown/root ratio, etc.?
- Would a combination approach (e.g., reshaping and/or repositioning) work better?

> If indicated, do a diagnostic wax-up for visualization.

Repositioning dento-alveolar segments
- Are needed corrections too severe to accomplish with simple orthodontics or a combination approach?
- Would a surgical approach be more advantageous?
- Could orthopedic appliances do the job?

Repositioning the skeletal base
- Is the skeletal base the problem?
- Decide which segments are wrong.

> If indicated, do a computer analysis and/or model surgery to position segments correctly. This is usually combined with a diagnostic wax-up. Consultation with an orthodontist and surgeon is in order.

Substitution
- Is a nighttime occlusal splint a reasonable substitute for corrective measures?

Elimination of need for occlusal stops
- Is splinting a viable alternative?
- Would restored contours be acceptable regarding esthetics, crown/root ratio, etc.?
- Would a combination approach (e.g., reshaping and/or repositioning) work better?

Analysis #2: Anterior Guidance

The anterior guidance cannot be accurately determined until all posterior interferences to centric relation have been eliminated. So the treatment plan for the first requirement (stable contacts) must be reasonably in place before decisions are made regarding the anterior guidance. One of the major decisions that must be made in establishing stable holding contacts on the posterior teeth is the determination of a vertical dimension of occlusion. That determination has a profound effect on the relationship of the lower incisal edges to the upper lingual surfaces. The next step is to evaluate incisal edge positions. Review the process described in Chapters 15 to 18 if there is any uncertainty about how to proceed with the anterior segment of the treatment plan. However, some basic questions should be answered from the clinical examination and the study of the mounted casts.

- Are the incisal edges correctly positioned esthetically?
- Are the anterior teeth in a good neutral zone relationship?
- Is there any interference to the lip closure path?
- Do the anterior teeth have stable holding contacts?
- Will the best esthetic result interfere with the envelope of function?
- Does the patient desire a change in anterior esthetics?

> If any changes are to be made in incisal edge position, a diagnostic wax-up should be done on mounted casts. This will be used for fabricating the provisional restorations that can then be refined in the mouth.

Analysis #3: Posterior Disclusion in Protrusive

- Can the anterior guidance separate the posterior teeth in protrusive?
- Is the occlusal plane a problem?

If posterior teeth separate the anterior teeth in protrusive, a protrusive bite record should be made and the condylar guidance should be set on the articulator. This enables you to determine how much correction is needed on the posterior teeth.

Ascertain whether it can be accomplished with any of the following:

- Reductive reshaping of posterior inclines
- Orthodontic correction of occlusal plane
- Restorations
- Surgery

> Equilibration of casts, analysis of occlusal plane, diagnostic wax-up, and model surgery, if indicated, become very important steps in patients who have occlusal plane problems.

Analysis #4: Disclusion of Working and Balancing Sides

If the first three analyses have been done carefully, lateral excursion analysis is usually simple. The key is stable holding contacts, correct anterior guidance, and a correct occlusal plane.

- Do posterior teeth separate immediately in lateral excursions?

If balancing interferences are severe on the articulator, set the condylar path from a protrusive bite record, as the protrusive path of the balancing condyle can be a critical factor.

Note: Working-side contact is permissible on patients who do not have anterior guidance from anterior contact (such as anterior open bites and anterior crossbites.)

MULTIPLE PROBLEMS

Some occlusal problems appear almost insurmountable when we see them for the first time. This is especially so when multiple problems of periodontitis and caries are found in combination with arch relationship problems, destructive habit patterns, and drifted or elongated teeth. Problems of excessive wear on some teeth may be found in the same mouth with elongated teeth. Esthetic problems along with a myriad of other demands for correction of stress direction and distribution may appear unsolvable.

There is one basic rule that must be followed in the resolution of any occlusal problem: *Never start any orthodontic or restorative procedure unless the end result can be visualized.*

Visualizing the result is in effect the setting of a clearly defined goal. Determining this goal of treatment and being able to conceptualize what it must accomplish are the most important factors in treatment design. They are the essence of good problem-solving technique.

The determination of treatment goals must be specific and well defined. The generalized goal of healthy maintainability must be the major criterion for every treatment plan, but it must be applied specifically to each individual tooth and each segment of the occlusion. Problems of maintainability should be carefully searched out by systematic tooth-by-tooth exploration.

A treatment plan should consist of an orderly sequence of procedures that are necessary to:

1. Eliminate pain
2. Eliminate infection
3. Restore all supporting tissues to healthy maintainability
4. Reshape, reposition, or restore the dentition when necessary for optimum maintainability, esthetics, comfort, and function

Too often, the treatment plan is determined before the *problems* have been isolated. The first step in setting up a treatment plan is to diagnose the problems. *Every* problem must be clearly defined, and this requires thoroughness in the examination stage.

It is hard to imagine how a thorough evaluation can be made without properly mounted diagnostic casts and a complete radiographic survey. Knowledgeable dentists would not attempt to plan a treatment without such aids. Models that have been mounted with facebow and centric relation bite record show the terminal hinge interocclusal position at the first point of contact. Occlusal interferences can be eliminated on the models to show what the tooth-to-tooth relationships will be at the correct vertical dimension.

Once tooth-to-tooth relationships at the correct vertical dimension are known, each segment of the occlusion can be evaluated regarding its potential for long-term maintainability. Teeth that are not in a maintainably stable relationship can be studied to determine whether corrections should involve removal, reshaping, repositioning, or restoring. Such corrections can actually be accomplished on the models, and the projected treatment goal can then be assessed for feasibility and correctness. There can be no better way to visualize the goals of a treatment plan than to have an actual model of the projected result.

PROBLEM SOLVING

Problem cases are more easily solved with a programmed approach. Developing an orderly sequence of procedures to use for each new patient is a must. It simplifies the planning of chair time and eliminates confusion for the office staff. Most importantly, though, it enables the dentist to program his or her thinking into sequential patterns. A multiple-problem case loses most of its complexity when individual problems can be isolated and solved one step at a time. In my office, we have found that two visits are essential for treatment planning.

First Appointment

The first appointment with a new patient should be planned to accomplish the following:

1. The patient's complaints are ascertained. The first part of the appointment is listening time. We must find out the patient's problems from his or her own point of view. We must get feelings on esthetics, long-term expectations, and present comfort level. We have to ask questions. An assistant should write down all pertinent information so that the dentist can give undivided continuous attention to the discussion with the patient.
2. Present conditions are charted. There should be a convenient place on every patient record for charting present conditions. It should be kept simple so that it will be used. A cursory examination is all that is needed at this time because the detailed examination will be completed

at the second appointment. Information that is needed includes the following:
   a. *Present restorations.* The general condition of the present restorations should be noted. Specific problems that will obviously need attention should be charted.
   b. *Prosthetics.* Is the patient wearing any prosthetic devices? An appraisal of each appliance should be given. Any patient comments about the prosthetics should be recorded.
   c. *Occlusion.* The type of arch relationship should be noted. Tooth relationships in a manipulated terminal hinge closure should be examined and first point of contact and direction of slide noted. Any patient comments about the occlusion should be recorded.
   d. *TMJ.* Have there been past or present symptoms that could be related to TMJ dysfunction? Such a question should be asked. One of the examination forms for diagnosis of TMJ problems may be used. Palpation for muscle tenderness should be routine.

   The joints should be tested to see if a verifiable centric relation can be determined and to rule out any intracapsular problems. If there is a history of any signs or symptoms or if the examination reveals any abnormalities, we would routinely use Doppler auscultation at this appointment. If further diagnostic tests are needed, they would be recommended.
   e. *Periodontal condition.* A general appraisal of the periodontal condition should be noted at this time. Each tooth should be checked for hypermobility, and any mobility patterns should be noted on the chart at this appointment. Obviously unsavable teeth should be so noted also.
   f. *Oral lesions.* The mouth should be carefully examined for any lesions of soft tissues.
   g. *Caries.* Carious lesions should be charted at this appointment.
   h. *Mouth hygiene.* A general appraisal of the patient's mouth hygiene and attitudes about proper mouth care should be noted.
3. Impressions, bite records, and facebow record for mounted diagnostic models are taken.
4. A radiographic survey is completed. Periapical films of all teeth are essential. Radiographs showing TMJs should be made for evaluation of any joints suspected of possible problems or pathosis.
5. Photographs of the mouth as well as different views of the face are taken.

Purpose of the first appointment. The first appointment is a generalized information gathering session. Enough information must be gained to permit practical study of the radiographs and mounted models before the second appointment. A tentative treatment plan must be formulated from this information, but the final treatment plan should not be accepted until the detailed examination is completed at the second appointment.

The first appointment can proceed in a very orderly manner if it is organized to do so. Impression materials should be measured out in advance, facebow equipment should be ready, and bite-record materials should be on hand.

This appointment is ideally conducted with the patient's participation. By allowing the patient to observe all aspects of the examination in a large hand mirror, we can explain what we find and describe what we are seeing as we examine. By spending more time at the original examination appointment, we find that the treatment explanation is more readily understood and accepted at the second appointment.

Second Appointment

After an evaluation of generalized problems has been completed, it is time to get down to specifics. In most cases, the tentative treatment plan that is worked out on the models is generally correct and requires minimal changes and additions at the final examination appointment. In problem cases, however, an acceptable treatment plan may be formulated only by careful examination at the chair using the combination of radiographs, models, clinical probing, and photographs.

This is the appointment at which each tooth is meticulously examined for any factors that would cause deterioration or prevent its maintenance. At this appointment, a complete periodontal examination should be completed if it is not done at the first appointment (which is my preference). Pockets should be charted and each tooth should be evaluated for periodontal maintainability. If the patient is to be referred to a periodontist, the examination does not need to be quite so definitive, but any area of questionable prognosis should be recorded. The effect of periodontal treatment on the restorative treatment plan should be appraised.

When multiple problems exist, the following programmed approach to problem solving may be used:

1. Each tooth should be evaluated individually. Can it be saved and made maintainable by any procedure? Any special requirements for saving, such as endodontics, hemisection, post coping, and the like, should be noted.
2. Teeth that cannot be saved or maintained should be indicated on the study model and chart.
3. Questionable teeth should be indicated by a question mark being put on the model and chart.
4. The remaining teeth should be evaluated on the basis of stress direction and distribution. It should be determined whether questionable teeth are key teeth in minimizing stress problems. If a questionable tooth offers no advantage for the remaining teeth, it may be a logical decision to extract it. If so, this should be indicated on the model. Questionable teeth should be treated and the results of treatment determined before they are used as key teeth in any restorative plan.
5. Evaluation should be made as to whether remaining teeth would best be served by fixed or removable prostheses or by implants.

6. The problems should be re-evaluated. Sometimes the whole complexion of a case changes when unsavable teeth are removed. Actually doing this on mounted models helps to clarify the process of isolating individual problems. Occlusal problems should be attacked first, and then restorative decisions should be tailored both to the needs of individual teeth and to the occlusal requirements.

DESIGNING OCCLUSAL TREATMENT BASED ON THE REQUIREMENTS FOR OCCLUSAL STABILITY

The requirements outlined for occlusal stability serve as the guideline for planning treatment. If any one of the requirements for stability is not fulfilled, it is almost a certainty that one or more teeth will either become loose, wear excessively, or migrate out of proper position *unless:*

1. The patient provides a substitute for the unfulfilled requirement, or
2. The patient specifically eliminates the need for that particular requirement not fulfilled.

Both exceptions are clinically discernible, and we should always look carefully for either substitutes or factors that eliminate the need for any requirement before we attempt to treat any occlusal problem. We cannot base treatment on appearance of the occlusion alone. We must evaluate every tooth individually to determine if it does or does not have a problem with instability.

The requirements for occlusal stability should be analyzed and treatment planned *in correct sequence.* The first requirement of stable holding contacts for each tooth must be satisfied in the plan before treatment planning for the next requirement of anterior guidance can be properly thought out.

Primary Treatment Objective: Stable Holding Contacts

If the first requirement has not been fulfilled, the analysis should be directed at determining the following:

1. Can we *provide* stable holding contacts for each tooth?
2. If we cannot provide holding contacts, can we *substitute* for the missing contact?
3. If we cannot provide or substitute, can we *eliminate the need?*

The ideal treatment objective is to *provide* the holding contacts, so that is the first priority of our treatment plan. With correctly mounted diagnostic casts, we can analyze the effects of various treatment approaches in regard to accomplishing this goal. If we can't logically accomplish it, we proceed to analyze methods for substitution or elimination of the need.

To determine the best method of solving any occlusal problem, we should analyze as many different methods as possible before selecting a treatment plan. If we apply it to determining the best method for *providing* holding contacts (fulfilling the first requirement for occlusal stability), the sequence to follow in our analysis is as follows:

1. *Reshaping.* Can equilibration or occlusal recontouring reestablish stable holding contacts on teeth that don't have them? If it can do it satisfactorily without our grinding through enamel, we have solved the problem in the simplest manner possible. This is always our first choice of treatment if all needs of the patient can be satisfied by this method.
2. *Repositioning.* Can teeth be moved into correct alignment? Moving teeth is almost always preferable over unnecessary restorations.
3. *Restoring.* If teeth can be reshaped into stable holding contacts by restorations, the decision to use or not use this method can be made logically only by comparing it with other treatment plans. If the teeth would benefit from restorations for other purposes, the decision is easy. If the teeth do not need restorations for other reasons, the alternative methods should be evaluated and pros and cons of each explained to the patient. Factors of treatment time, expense, esthetic considerations, and patient health may influence the occlusion.
4. *Surgery.* If the occlusal problem cannot be resolved by reshaping, repositioning, or restoring the dentition, it may be necessary to reposition parts of the skeletal base to achieve the best overall result.
5. *Combining methods.* Many problem occlusions are best treated by a combined approach to treatment. The sequence is still followed as outlined. Some occlusions can be helped dramatically by judicious reshaping, but optimum occlusal stability cannot be completely achieved without some movement of teeth in combination with the recontoured occlusion. It is not unusual to combine three or even four methods in order to solve some occlusal problems.

Substitution

If stable holding contacts are absent and the patient has not substituted for them by posturing the tongue or lips as a stop for eruption, the *treatment plan* may employ a substitute. An example is an occlusal splint that provides holding contacts when worn at night. The nighttime wear may be all that is needed to prevent eruption of unopposed teeth and may provide a simple alternative to an extensive treatment plan.

Elimination of need

If stable holding contacts are absent and treatment is necessary to stabilize a segment of the occlusion, that stabilization may be accomplished in some instances without either providing contact or providing a substitute. As an example, unopposed teeth can be splinted to teeth that are opposed; thus the need for holding contacts is eliminated.

Selecting which treatment approach to use

For many occlusal problems, the stability of the dentition can be accomplished in several ways. Astute treatment planning, however, requires evaluating all the different possible ways to solve the problem by comparing the methods from several standpoints. Just because we can stabilize an occlusion by complete arch splinting does not automatically make it the correct treatment. We must weigh each alternative from several perspectives:

1. Is it the best plan for achieving a maintainably healthy mouth?
2. Is the cost of the plan reasonable or necessary for the results it achieves? This evaluation may be looked at differently from different patient perspectives.
3. Is the time required to achieve a result logical in comparison with other plans? Again this decision may be different for different patients.
4. Does the health of the patient warrant an extensive treatment plan?
5. Is the prognosis favorable enough to make extensive procedures logical?
6. Is the prognosis, without treatment, unfavorable enough to warrant an extensive treatment plan?

All of these decisions really boil down to making two honest appraisals regarding the proposed treatment:

1. Is the treatment really optimally beneficial for the patient?
2. Would a simpler plan work?

I have a very reliable way for helping me to make every complex decision regarding recommendations for treatment: Would I want the same treatment plan used on me? Would I treat my wife or children in the same way I'm proposing to treat the patient? If I can't honestly answer yes to each of those questions, I don't suggest such treatment for the patient. If the patient must compromise, I try to approach alternative plans that are in line with the best interests and special considerations of each patient. These decisions require understanding of individual circumstances and an empathetic approach to providing the best service possible within the means of the patient and the patient's emotional and intellectual ability to understand it and maintain it.

The treatment planning procedures outlined above should be applied to analyze each of the five requirements for occlusal stability and strategize the best method for fulfilling each requirement, substituting for it, or eliminating the need for it.

Analyzing the anterior teeth

Only after decisions have been made regarding the first requirement of stable holding contacts on every tooth do we then determine the method of choice for satisfying the second requirement of an anterior guidance in harmony with the envelope of function. The evaluation of any anterior guidance must be based on an understanding of the factors that determine anterior tooth relationships. In the following chapters on solving the various problems of occlusion, it will be apparent that working out the correct position and contour of each anterior tooth is the key to solving most of the other problems.

Anterior relationship problems must be solved as a separate entity before we proceed with posterior occlusal problems, unless the posterior teeth must be changed to permit an optimum anterior relationship.

Analyzing the occlusal plane

If posterior teeth interfere with the anterior guidance in any mandibular position, the occlusal plane should be carefully evaluated to determine how it can be corrected. Methods for analyzing the occlusal plane are outlined in Chapter 20. Remember that the front of the occlusal plane starts where the incisal plane ends, so it is essential to have the lower incisal edges correctly aligned with the interpupillary line before the occlusal plane can be determined. Many of the problems we see with poor treatment results are obviously the consequence of restoring posterior teeth without first determining the correct anterior relationships. The sequence of analysis and of treatment is a critical factor that is too often ignored.

Analyzing posterior tooth-to-tooth relationships

After the acceptability of the occlusal plane is either confirmed or corrected, the tooth-to-tooth relationships can be established within those acceptable limits. Within the framework of those limits, a variety of tooth-to-tooth relationships are possible. Many factors influence the type of occlusal contours that are suitable. Whether the problem is a crossbite, an end-to-end relationship, or a posterior open bite, cusp position and contour will need to be decided upon before treatment decisions are finalized. Sometimes the final contours are refined in provisional restorations, but there is always a reason for every cusp-tip position and every fossa contour. Those decisions are more logically made when they are related to the requirements for occlusal stability.

Be certain that whatever occlusal design is used for the posterior teeth, they must not interfere with the disclusive function of the anterior guidance. If occlusal contacts can be positioned in line with the long axes of each tooth so that they meet in simultaneous contact in centric relation with no interference to any anterior tooth contact position, they will probably be at least acceptable. They will, at worst, be adjustable.

Solving restorative problems

Determining the type of restorations to use can be on a tooth-by-tooth basis once the total occlusal scheme has been resolved. The corrected models will show clearly which teeth must be altered by restorations, and the restorative needs of each individual tooth should also be considered. The decision should be made on the basis of what restoration will best serve each tooth and then the choice of restorations evaluated in relation to the combined needs of other teeth. The type of restorations selected should fulfill the needs of strength, protection, and esthetics.

When a comprehensive treatment plan has been completed and a careful re-evaluation of all factors indicates that the plan will produce optimum oral health for the patient, a sequence of treatment should be outlined in writing. Such an order of treatment should be in a prominent place in the patient's record. It has several advantages.

1. It eliminates the need for time-consuming review of treatment every time the patient reports for an appointment. It serves as a ready reference for what has been completed and what is yet to be started.
2. It provides an excellent reference for setting up and reserving appointment times in advance.
3. It aids the staff in preappointment preparations for each office procedure. Auxiliaries always know what procedures to prepare for before the patient arrives.
4. It enables the dentist to present an orderly sequence of treatment to the patient. Patients appreciate an explanation of what they can expect in terms of future appointments. We never attempt a consultation with a patient until we have outlined the sequential order of treatment.
5. It forces the dentist to follow a basic rule of treatment: *Never begin any restorative procedure unless all of the procedures that follow are outlined in advance and properly related to one another.*

An understanding of the principles outlined in Chapter 29 is essential if we are to effectively evaluate any treatment plan. It should be reviewed if necessary and every problem case evaluated on the basis of these criteria. Treatment planning can become the most rewarding challenge in dentistry for the dentist who learns how to search out problems and then find solutions for each problem uncovered.

SUMMARY

Solving problems of occlusion is simplified when one follows an orderly sequence in examination and treatment planning. Only problems that are recognized will be solved. A complete mouth survey must include thorough radiographic analysis, periodontal examination, occlusal analysis on correctly mounted casts, and a systematic tooth-by-tooth search for every factor that could cause accelerated deterioration.

Every problem should be listed. *All possible solutions* for each individual problem should be evaluated. The best solution for each problem should be determined. The result of treatment should be visualized. Corrected models should be used whenever necessary. A sequential, step-by-step procedure for completing the treatment plan in the most orderly manner should be designed.

Finally, the plan should be followed.

Chapter 31

The Diagnostic Wax-up

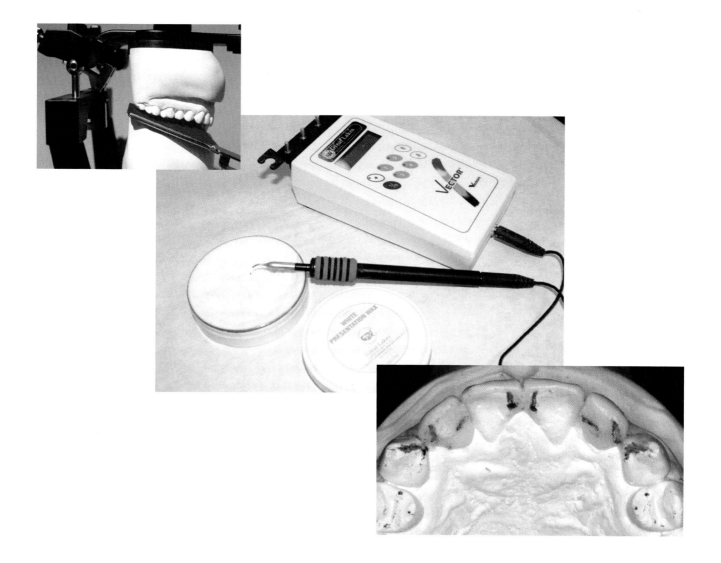

PRINCIPLE

The diagnostic wax-up is the process of converting a programmed treatment plan into a three-dimensional visualization.

THE WAX-UP: THE PROCESS MOST DENTISTS WANT TO SKIP

The diagnostic wax-up should probably be labeled a diagnostic *work-up* because it is the most foolproof way to work up a treatment plan that will result in a three-dimensional visualization of the end result of a "best choice" of treatment. I am convinced that if dentists truly understood all of the benefits of a thoughtfully planned diagnostic wax-up, they would not even consider starting any complex occlusal treatment without first working out the details on mounted diagnostic casts. The diagnostic wax-up is the process by which *programmed treatment planning* is utilized step-by-step to determine the best choice of treatment. It is how we plan the sequence that must be followed to achieve a visualized end result.

Who Should Do the Diagnostic Wax-up?

The answer to this question is influenced by a dentist's perspective of treatment planning and colored by preconceived ideas of hourly productivity. It is also influenced by current skill levels in waxing technique. Waxing technique can be easily learned with electric waxing instruments. What is more important is the understanding of the protocol for decision making in programmed treatment planning. It is this decision tree process that guides even a novice at treatment planning through the sequence of decisions that are best made on mounted diagnostic casts. The dentist is in the best position to utilize this process because key decisions are so often dependent on clinical findings from the patient examination.

So the answer to this question is simple: The ideal person to do the diagnostic wax-up is the dentist who did the complete exam and therefore the one who has an understanding of what the patient wants and needs. This person will be responsible for the end result and must help the patient understand what needs to be done and why. Dentists who learn the necessary skills will find that the benefits from doing their own treatment planning have a huge payoff in case acceptance and higher productivity.

The Purpose of the Wax-up

The purpose of the wax-up is easily distorted. It is not to see how beautiful you can make a set of casts look. The purpose is to see what must be done to fulfill all the requirements for stability. It starts with the first requirement of stable holding contacts on all teeth. An understanding of the first requirement is a good example of why the dentist is in the best position to guide the diagnostic wax-up process. At the examination, the dentist should determine if any requirements for stability are unfulfilled or have been substituted for (such as a tongue substitute for anterior contact). The dentist should have observed the relationship of the upper anterior teeth to the lip-closure path, phonetics, and the

neutral zone. These are important observations that cannot be discerned from diagnostic casts alone but have a profound importance when deciding on the position, inclination, and contour of anterior teeth. Likewise, treatment decisions regarding the height of gingival margins cannot be properly decided on without knowing how much teeth and gum is exposed at high lip position—something that can't be discerned from casts.

As the dentist works through the decision-making process on the casts, remember that it is at this stage that options for treatment must be selected for each requirement for stability.

Selecting the Best Treatment Option

On mounted casts, it is possible to recontour teeth by adding wax to reshape incisal edges or to build up occlusal surfaces. It is also possible to recontour teeth by equilibration or other forms of reductive reshaping. On the casts that show the jaw-to-jaw relationship of the arches in centric relation, it will often be apparent that the best treatment choice is to move teeth into a better relationship. This can be done on the casts. Many problems can be solved using a realistic set of choices. Choices include narrowing teeth (stripping) so they can be moved into a better alignment before restorations are used to complete the perfected esthetics. In the chapters that follow regarding all the different types of occlusal problems, it will be apparent how the process of making treatment decisions on mounted diagnostic casts is such a practical approach.

Extra Advantages

The extra advantages to a well-done diagnostic wax-up include:

1. Working through a clearly defined treatment plan gives the dentist an unmatched level of confidence when presenting the treatment plan to the patient.
2. The diagnostic wax-up is the best visual aid you can use to help the patient understand the goals of treatment. When combined with a set of digital photos of the existing condition, the need for treatment becomes clear to the patient. It also demonstrates the dentist's thoroughness in deciding what treatment is in the patient's best interest.
3. The comparison of unaltered casts with the treatment-planned casts is the perfect aid for explaining to specialists what your treatment goals are. It facilitates co-diagnosis for total clarification of a treatment sequence and opens the door to suggestions for alternative treatment approaches that may better serve the patient.
4. The corrected diagnostic casts serve as models for fabrication of provisional restorations. A putty silicone matrix is made on the corrected casts and can be ready when tooth preparations are completed.

5. If orthodontic tooth movement is indicated, the three-dimensional model of the treatment objective can be used to design the mechanics for moving teeth to a specific new position.

6. Because the jaw-to-jaw relationship is correct on centric relation mounted casts, surgical decisions can be aided regarding movement of dento-alveolar segments or complete arches.

Many of the decisions that can be made in a diagnostic wax-up can only be guessed at with unmounted casts. Dentists who do not take advantage of the benefits of a diagnostic wax-up are typically unaware of the amount of time that is wasted by not having a definite sequential plan for treatment aimed at a predetermined goal.

Diagnostic Wax-ups by the Technician

Many dentists rely completely on a laboratory technician to do the diagnostic wax-up. This misses the primary purpose of using the diagnostic work-up to determine a complete treatment plan. On so many occasions, I have been able to work out solutions that would not have been thought of without the benefit of having examined the patient. Nevertheless there is a place for technician help in refining a wax-up after all treatment decisions have been made by the dentist.

A beautiful diagnostic wax-up by a technician can be impressive to a patient. There is no question that when such wax-ups are used in a case presentation, the acceptance level

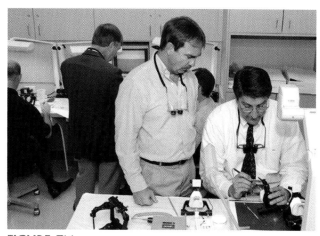

FIGURE 31-1 This class at the Dawson Center is learning to treatment plan on mounted diagnostic casts. Very few dentists have had this type of training, which explains why so many attempt to shortcut the treatment-planning process.

is increased. It is a matter of individual choice whether a technician is used to do the wax-up or to just finalize it after the dentist has made the treatment decisions. I would suggest, however, that the effort made to learn the wax-up process will be well rewarded. We have shown, in hands-on classes at the Dawson Center, that dentists can learn the basic skills in a three-day class (Figure 31-1). They routinely surprise themselves at how competent they become in a short time by understanding some basic principles and the use of good electric waxers.

PROCEDURE   Steps in the diagnostic wax-up

Step 1: *Mount upper and lower casts* with centric relation bite record and facebow. Duplicate the casts to preserve the original conditions.

Step 2: *Verify* the accuracy of the mounting.

Step 3: *Examine the occlusal relationship* on the casts. Note the first tooth contact. Note the relationship of all other teeth when the first tooth contacts at centric relation.

Objective: To achieve centric relation contact on all teeth. However, one should start by determining what must be done to achieve contact of the anterior teeth.

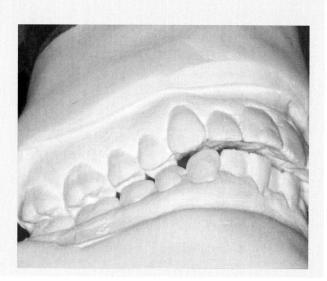

Continued

PROCEDURE   Steps in the diagnostic wax-up—cont'd

Step 4: *Lock the centric latch* when observing the casts. Determine what would be the best choice of treatment to get the back teeth out of the way. Start with equilibration. Can it achieve front tooth contact without mutilating the posterior teeth?

Step 5: *Determine the correct vertical dimension.* Unlock the centric latch and close the teeth into maximum intercuspation. This is the vertical dimension established by the elevator muscles. Lower the incisal guide pin so it touches the guide table.

Step 6: *Return the condyles to centric relation and lock the centric lock.* Observe the incisal pin in relation to the guide table. This will show the amount of closure needed to achieve the same vertical dimension of occlusion (VDO) in centric relation.

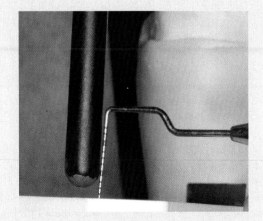

Objective: Occlusal interferences should be eliminated by selective grinding on the casts until the incisal pin contacts the guide plate. At that point, the original vertical dimension will have been re-established in centric relation. If a change in VDO is needed to fulfill requirements for stability, it can be determined now.

Step 7: *Observe the teeth that were reshaped.* If reductive reshaping is mutilative to teeth that do not need restoring, consider one of the other options for achieving centric relation contact on all of the teeth.

Note: Also consider the possibility of the tongue position preventing complete full arch contact.

Step 8: *Remove unsavable teeth from the casts.* From the clinical exam, all teeth that cannot be saved are marked with an *X*. At this stage of treatment planning, do not remove any teeth that can be maintained. That decision should wait.

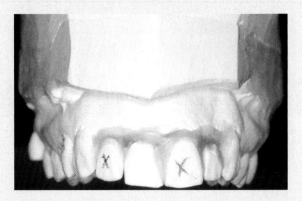

Objective: Removing hopeless teeth from the cast often changes the entire treatment-planning process. It permits use of the cut off teeth in repositioning decisions to achieve holding contacts or improved incisal plane. It also simplifies decisions regarding treatment choices of fixed versus removable prostheses or selection of implants.

PROCEDURE   Steps in the diagnostic wax-up—cont'd

Step 9: If decisions have been made at the exam to use certain types of restorations, mark this on the cast. For example, in the figure the two upper molars have been predetermined to need crowns *(C)*. Also note any teeth that are questionable. If they will not lend anything to the long-term stability of the finished treatment, they can be removed.

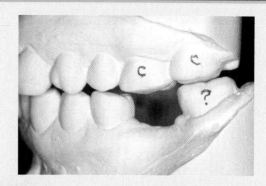

Step 10: Equilibration is the first treatment option to explore.

Objective: To see if anterior contact in centric relation can be achieved by equilibration without mutilating teeth that would not otherwise need restorations.

A, The jaw-to-jaw relationship at the first point of tooth contact in centric relation. Equilibration of the casts **(B)** clearly shows that re-shaping the teeth is a good choice of treatment because contact with the canines is achievable by selective grinding away of the deflective interferences. This also shows that in this mouth, equilibration will not achieve contact on the incisors. The dentist must then refer to the findings at the clinical exam to determine if contact on the incisors has been substituted for. This patient had a tongue thrust, so no attempt was needed to restore contact or move teeth. Esthetics was not a concern, and the anterior teeth displayed no signs of instability. The combination of the clinical exam and the diagnostic work-up on mounted casts enabled the dentist to arrive at a confident decision that equilibration was a good choice of treatment.

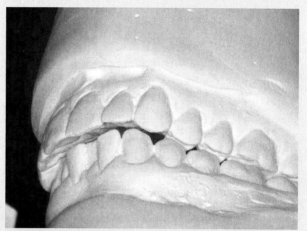

A

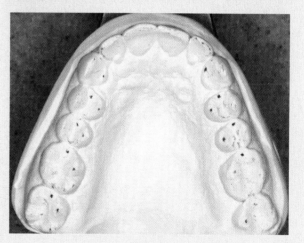

B

Continued

PROCEDURE　Steps in the diagnostic wax-up—cont'd

Step 11: *Examine the plane of occlusion.* If the casts were mounted with a facebow that was parallel with the eyes, the incisal plane and the occlusal plane will relate to the bench top. If the occlusal plane is slanted in the mouth *(yellow line),* it will be slanted on the articulator *(red line).*

Objective: With a true representation of the occlusal plane on the articulator, a treatment choice can be selected that will correct the problem. It is obvious on these casts that simply reshaping or restoring the teeth will not solve the occlusal plane problem. Consultation with a surgeon or orthodontist would be in order.

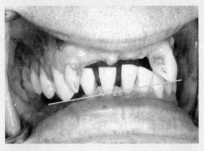

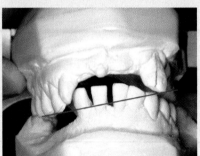

Decisions regarding the occlusal plane are often critical to the planning of the entire restorative process. In the following work-up by Dr. Glenn DuPont, a clear picture of where treatment should lead was established before the first tooth was prepared on the patient.

The lower model, mounted with a facebow and centric relation bite record, permitted occlusal plane analysis in relation to the condyles . . . an important relationship to consider in order to remove the protrusive interference to the anterior guidance.

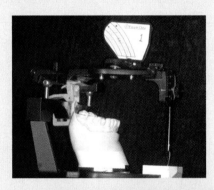

The occlusal plane established by the simplified occlusal plane analyzer (SOPA).

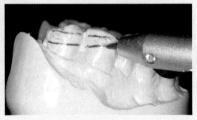

PROCEDURE   Steps in the diagnostic wax-up—cont'd

The model is trimmed back to the established new occlusal plane.

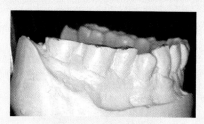

Note how the buccal surfaces have been contoured to move the cusp tip more in line with the upper teeth. The wax-up has been started.

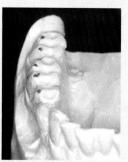

The completed wax-up. These corrected casts are now used to form a putty matrix for fabrication of provisional restorations. They are also the perfect visual aid when presenting the treatment plan to the patient.

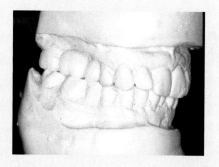

Step 12: *Establish stable holding contacts on the anterior teeth.* This is one of the most important steps in the diagnostic wax-up (work-up). It cannot be determined how it can best be accomplished until the decisions have been made to get the back teeth out of the way of complete closure in centric relation. Refer to the chapters on anterior teeth (Chapters 16, 17, and 18) for details on achieving an ideal anterior relationship.

Objective: Relating the lower incisal edges to an acceptable alignment and contour of the upper anterior teeth.

Unmounted casts do not provide the information needed to fulfill this objective. Anterior contact can only be determined at the correct jaw-to-jaw relationship. That is why casts must be mounted in centric relation. Unmounted casts cause missed diagnoses, wasted time, and unstable restorative results due to missed anterior relationships.

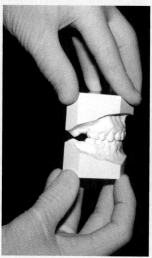

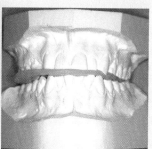

Continued

PROCEDURE   Steps in the diagnostic wax-up—cont'd

Mounted casts permit analysis of the occlusion to determine if contact from centric relation through the range of anterior guidance can be achieved without interference from posterior teeth. This analysis is important because in many cases, anterior contact may be lost when the mandible is permitted to close back in centric relation. Knowing this before equilibration enables the dentist to plan the best way to establish holding contacts on the anterior teeth in centric relation and ensure that the anterior guidance can disclude all of the posterior teeth in excursions. Often this can be achieved with a simple buildup restoration on the canines, but in other patients a better solution may be slight movement of a few teeth.

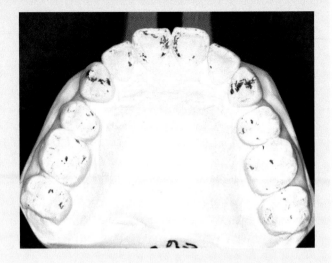

Step 13: *Correct lower incisal edges if needed.* This refers to both position and contour. If the position of the lower incisors does not permit anterior holding contacts, the correction may involve the contour and position of both the upper and lower anterior teeth.

Step 14: *Start with the lower anterior teeth.*

Objective: To establish correct incisal edge contour. That means a definite labio-incisal line angle . . . the leading edge. It also means ideal esthetic contour of the lower incisal edges.

Anterior incisal edges that have worn the leading edge to a slanted contour must be restored to provide a stable holding contact with the upper anterior teeth. It is during this wax-up procedure that some important treatment decisions can be made:

Determine the type of restoration. Can the incisal edge be restored with a laminate, or will full coverage be needed?

Remember that the leading edge of the lower incisors must have a definite labio-incisal line angle.

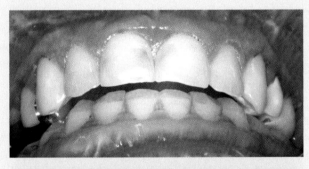

Determine the position and contour of the incisal edge. Can the incisal edge be moved forward or backward if needed to achieve a stable contact? Can it be done by restoration, or must the tooth be moved?

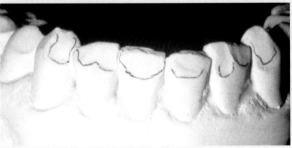

PROCEDURE   Steps in the diagnostic wax-up—cont'd

Determine the type of preparation needed. If the teeth are worn to a thicker incisal edge, should prep reduction be more on the lingual or on the labial to facilitate a normal edge contour in best alignment with the upper?

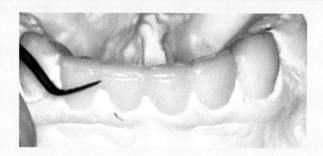

Why start with the lower?

The main reason for starting with the lower anterior teeth first when doing a diagnostic wax-up is that it simplifies the whole wax-up. The range of change in position of lower anterior teeth is minimal compared with the upper anterior teeth. The anteroposterior position of lower anterior teeth has very little flexibility, and their position in the narrow alveolar ridge is quite limited. The height of lower incisors is also within a limited range that is consistent with the height and contour of the occlusal plane. I find it a very useful process to remove the upper cast and just idealize the lower incisal plane and posterior occlusal plane. This is done by any combination of reduction and/or addition of tooth material by grinding on the model and/or waxing contours. When necessary to align contacts, teeth on the model can be moved, but movement forward or backward by lower anterior teeth is limited.

Even though the upper cast is removed for the wax-up of the lower arch, it is nevertheless observed in a centric relation position after the casts are equilibrated so it will be recognized if lower incisal edges must be moved to achieve contact with the upper anterior teeth. At this time some tentative decisions are also made regarding whether the upper anterior teeth will need to be moved to achieve acceptable contact with the idealized position of the lower incisal edges.

Step 15: *Re-evaluate the total occlusion* with the upper cast to see how it can be adapted to occlude with the lower arch. It may require some modification of the lower wax-up, but it is usually a minimal correction.

Step 16: *Establish holding contacts on the upper anterior teeth.* The same five treatment options can be considered to achieve an ideal occlusal relationship.

Objective: The wax-up of the upper anterior teeth is designed to develop your "best guess" for upper anterior position and contour. If there are to be changes in the position of the upper incisal edges, the wax-up will be used to form a matrix for fabrication of provisional restorations. The provisional restorations can then be modified in the mouth (see Chapter 16).

Fabrication of the best-guess contour for the upper anteriors is guided by photographs of the mouth and other clinical observations made at the examination appointment.

Continued

Casts of a patient with a tight neutral zone that positioned the upper anterior teeth with a lingual inclination.

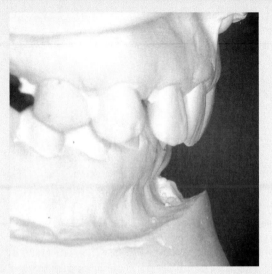

This diagnostic wax-up positioned the incisal edges forward and also made the teeth longer.

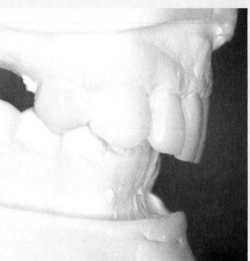

PROCEDURE   Steps in the Diagnostic Wax-up—cont'd

A digital photograph of this patient shows the incisal edges in line with the inner vermillion border of the lower lip. It also shows a lingual inclination of the upper anterior teeth.

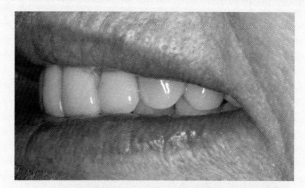

This photograph shows how the provisional restorations made from the wax-up had to be recontoured back to achieve a comfortable lip-closure path and phonetics.

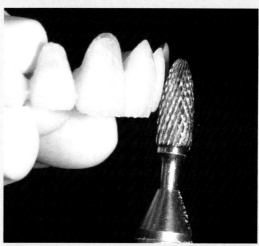

ESTHETIC ANALYSIS ON THE DIAGNOSTIC WAX-UP

The diagnostic work-up has many purposes, not the least of which is the analysis of esthetic considerations. In the following analysis of a patient who was unhappy with the appearance of recently completed anterior bridges, the casts were reshaped to a more esthetic contour for the teeth. It was also used to analyze a defect in the alveolar ridge from the loss of the labial contour by a trauma. Note how Dr. Glenn DuPont planned for a successful result.

Cast of poorly contoured anterior restorations. Note the contour of the pontics where they meet the ridge.

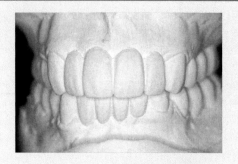

Cast showing defect of lost labial plate of bone that makes it impossible to establish gingival contours on pontics that are esthetically pleasing.

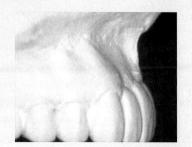

Fill-in of area with pink wax will be used to communicate desired result to the surgeon. A bone augmentation was needed to achieve the planned contour. All guesswork was eliminated.

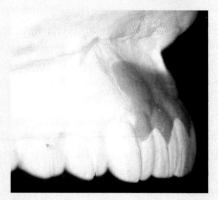

Recontouring of the anterior teeth on the cast will be used to form provisional restorations, as well as explain the treatment goal to the patient and the surgeon.

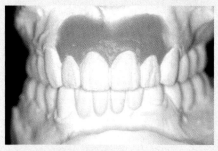

One of the many significant advantages of a diagnostic wax-up is the option of making a preparation guide. A putty silicone index that copies the wax-up can be sliced through in sections one tooth at a time to guide the dentist in preparing each tooth. This ensures that there will be a predetermined amount of room for the restorative materials needed to construct each restoration.

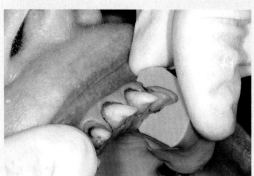

Diagnostic Wax-up: Time Well Spent

The value of the diagnostic wax-up is directly proportional to the doctor's understanding of complete dentistry. If the process is based on the principles of programmed treatment planning (see Chapter 30), there will be an orderly sequence in working through the treatment-planning process. Working with mounted casts to develop a three-dimensional treatment plan is the best way to make treatment decisions that set a framework for start to finish. I am convinced that it is some of the most profitable time a dentist spends because it eliminates so much wasted time once the treatment is started. It gives the dentist confidence that raises the level of doctor-patient communication. It provides the contour for provisional restorations. It is the perfect communication aid for consultations with specialists. It is the best of all possible ways for deciding the best choice of treatment. The learning curve for developing expertise in doing the diagnostic wax-up is exactly the same learning curve for developing expertise in diagnosis and treatment planning. It is truly time well spent.

Chapter 32

Occlusal Splints

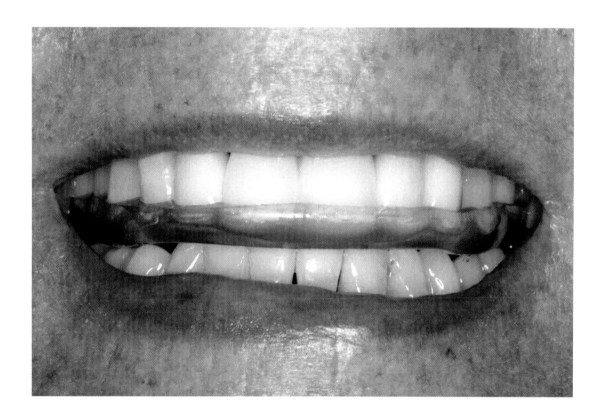

PRINCIPLE

Most occlusal splints have one primary function: to alter an occlusion so it does not interfere with complete seating of the condyles in centric relation.

UNDERSTANDING OCCLUSAL SPLINTS

One of the most useful concepts ever developed for dental patients is the use of a type of interocclusal device that is most often referred to as an *occlusal splint*. In spite of its popularity as the most common "treatment" for patients with orofacial pain related to temporomandibular disorders (TMDs), it is still considered by many as a mysterious treatment that no one really understands. Clinicians who lean toward a psychological explanation for TMDs have explained that any beneficial results from an occlusal splint are most likely a "placebo" effect. Attempts have been made through the literature to show that occlusal splints are no more effective than self-treatment by patients. On the other end of the scale are claims that certain types of occlusal splints are almost magical cures for everything from bruxism to migraine headaches (see Suggested Readings).

The confusion can be easily cleared up by understanding a few facts about how occlusal splints work and when they can be used effectively. Occlusal splints are *predictably* effective if properly designed and accurately fabricated for certain specific problems that are related to occlusal factors. If the fabrication of an occlusal splint is done without an understanding of its very specific purpose, the result will be guesswork. Nondefinitive occlusal splint design may actually help some patients, but it can also do much harm. There is absolutely no reason for guesswork in occlusal splint design.

Types of Occlusal Splints

Every occlusal splint, either by accident or by design, falls into one of two categories. There are only two types of occlusal splints:

1. *Permissive occlusal splints* (Figure 32-1) have a smooth surface on one side that allows the muscles to move the mandible without interference from deflective tooth inclines so the condyles can slide back and up the eminentiae to complete seating into centric relation. The smooth surface can face either the lower arch (as shown) or the upper arch as long as it frees the mandible to slide to centric relation.
2. *Directive occlusal splints* (Figure 32-2) direct the lower arch into a specific occlusal relationship that in turn directs the condyles to a predetermined position. Directive splints have very limited use. They should be reserved for specific conditions involving intracapsular TMDs.

How permissive occlusal splints work

There is no mystery about how permissive occlusal splints work. Most occlusal splints have one primary function: to alter an occlusion so it does not interfere with complete seating of the condyles. This can be accomplished by separation of all posterior teeth, allowing only anterior tooth contact

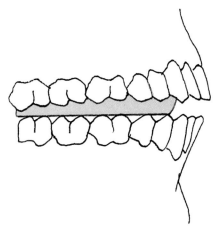

FIGURE 32-1 Permissive occlusal splint. Most occlusal splints are in this category.

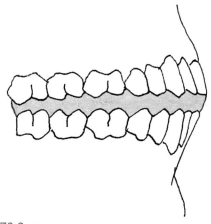

FIGURE 32-2 Directive occlusal splint. These splints are never needed if the TMJs are intact and can accept loading in centric relation.

against a smooth flat surface, or by allowing any segment or all of the occlusal surfaces to freely slide against a smooth surface. As long as the temporomandibular joints (TMJs) are intact and able to comfortably accept loading, any device that permits complete seating of the condyles during clench closure of the mandible will effectively eliminate the need for lateral pterygoid resistance to the elevator muscles. This release of lateral pterygoid contraction is the point at which relief of the discomfort is effected.

Anterior deprogramming splints

Perhaps the best way to illustrate how occlusal splints work is with the simplest type of permissive splint, which is often called an anterior deprogramming splint. If there are no intracapsular structural disorders in the TMJs, a correctly made deprogramming splint is close to 100 percent effective in getting patients comfortable, usually within minutes or hours. In fact, they are so dependably effective that they are an almost indispensable aid in differential diagnosis of many disorders, too often ignored or misdiagnosed, that dentists

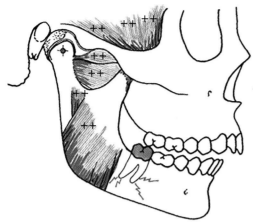

FIGURE 32-3 An occlusal interference such as a high crown or deflective tooth incline activates muscle hyperactivity. Pain is often focused in the masticatory muscles to give the impression of a TMD. A high percentage of misdiagnosed TMDs are occluso-muscle disorders that are readily resolvable.

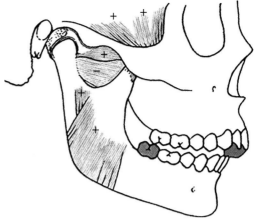

FIGURE 32-4 A permissive (smooth) anterior splint separates the interfering molar from contact, thus permitting the condyle-disk assemblies to seat up into centric relation. This eliminates the trigger for muscle activity and allows the inferior lateral pterygoid muscle to release. Peaceful, comfortable muscle activity resumes quickly. Complete separation of posterior teeth actually causes most of the elevator muscles to completely release contraction.

routinely see in every dental practice (Figures 32-3, 32-4, and 32-5).

Abuse of anterior deprogramming splints. Failure to recognize the simple permissive action of anterior deprogramming splints has led to overuse of flat anterior devices as a substitute for correction of occlusal interferences. Dentists should recognize that such devices can be an important aid in diagnosis of orofacial pain, migraine headaches, and other masticatory system pains; but such devices are not *treatment* devices as much as they are *diagnostic* devices. They are very effective in diagnosing whether deflective occlusal interferences are the cause of occluso-muscle pain (see Chapter 25). Using such devices as treatment over an extended time period may cause intrusion of the covered teeth and supraeruption of the separated teeth. The same is true of any segmental occlusal appliance. When necessary as a device to suppress clenching after perfection of the occlusion, it is possible to manage the stability factor if some basics of occlusal principles are considered.

Use of modified anterior deprogramming devices such as the anterior midline point stop device and the NTI-Tension Suppression System. The popular acceptance of anterior midline point stop (AMPS) devices is understandable because they are very effective in permitting complete seating of both condyles and suppression of clenching. In our many years of successfully using anterior deprogramming devices that included canine contact, we were able to routinely effect a comfortable joint position with release of muscle incoordination. However, it was also routine to find that after 24 hours of wearing such a device, contact on canines would almost invariably be heavier on one side. After adjustment, we could then achieve the "wow" effect of total comfort. Midline point devices that avoid canine contact (Figure 32-6) have an advantage of allowing rotation

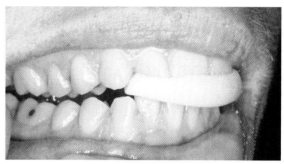

FIGURE 32-5 A simple directly fabricated anterior deprogramming splint allows contact of the lower incisors against a smooth flat surface. As soon as the deflective posterior inclines are separated, the elevator muscles can seat the condyles into centric relation and release the contraction of the lateral pterygoid muscles. This type of splint has been used in my practice for over 35 years.

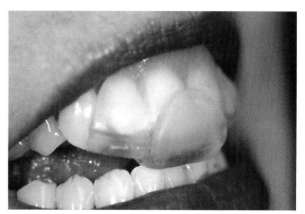

FIGURE 32-6 An anterior deprogramming splint with contact only at the midline. This type of splint was designed by Dr. Keith Thornton many years ago. Many modifications of it are in use today, but the principle of complete permissiveness of condylar movement is the key that prevails.

of the mandible around the anterior midpoint to seat both condyles without interference, so they are a decided improvement over the original design.

Devices such as the NTI Tension Suppression System (NTI-TSS) do reduce voluntary clenching intensity to one-third of maximum, and clinical observation is impressive regarding the rapid relief of muscle hyperactivity on properly selected patients. What we did not realize in past splint fabrication is that canine contact does, in fact, permit an increase in muscle contraction activity over contact at a single midline point stop. This difference is significant enough to warrant its use in diagnosis as well as for clenching suppression in selected patients who continue to clench even with a perfected occlusion.

The important point to consider when using any appliance over an extended period is: Is the appliance necessary? A small percentage of patients will continue to clench (centric bruxism) and some patients will grind (eccentric bruxism), even if all occlusal interferences to centric relation are *completely* eliminated and *immediate* disclusion of all posterior contact in excursions has been achieved. Nocturnal electromyographic (EMG) studies that I have performed convince me that we cannot always eliminate clenching activity regardless of how perfect the occlusion is. But we can, in almost all patients, eliminate the damage it does. Remember that you cannot wear what you cannot rub. Furthermore, only a very small percentage of patients will develop a bothersome degree of muscle discomfort if they have a perfected occlusion, even if they continue to clench. For that select group of patients, a clenching suppression appliance (such as the NTI-TSS) is an acceptable aid for periodic use (as needed) to maintain comfort.

The proper use of any segmental splint is to use it for diagnostic purposes only. If a permissive splint relieves the symptoms of muscle pain and confirms a diagnosis of occluso-muscle disorder, the prudent choice of treatment is either to correct the occlusal disharmony directly, or to extend coverage of the splint to include contact on all teeth. The one exception to this rule is the nighttime use of specially designed anterior deprogramming devices for serious habitual clenchers or bruxers. Separation of the posterior teeth during sleep has a quieting effect on extreme muscle activity and reduces the damage from attritional wear in "delta-stage" bruxers (see Chapter 35). Such devices are rarely necessary in patients with a perfected occlusion, and if a nocturnal appliance is indicated it should in most cases have centric relation contact on all teeth with an anterior ramp for posterior disclusion in all excursions.

If an anterior deprogramming splint does not relieve pain, suspect an intracapsular disorder as a source of the pain. An increase in pain level is diagnostic. Patients should be advised to remove the splint if pain or discomfort in the joints increases. A differential diagnosis should be completed to determine exactly why the TMJs cannot comfortably accept loading. The examination should lead to a Piper Classification before any irreversible occlusal treatment is initiated.

When Occlusal Splints Are Not Necessary

If a screening history and examination reveals no history of problems in the TMJs, including no history of clicking, no discomfort in the joints, and no restriction or deviation of jaw movement, we typically do not suspect an intracapsular disorder. Nevertheless, we *always* load test the TMJs. If firm load testing produces no sign of tenderness or tension in combination with a negative history, it is not necessary to fabricate an occlusal splint prior to restorative dentistry, orthodontics, or equilibration.

When a Pretreatment Occlusal Splint Is Appropriate

If there is doubt about complete seating of the TMJs or if there has been a long-standing intracapsular disorder that has been resolved, such as reduction of a formerly displaced disk, it is appropriate to test the stability of the condylar position by use of a centric relation occlusal splint. Adjustments to the occlusion on the splint may be needed as remodeling of joint structures takes place. When occlusal stability on the splint has been achieved so no further corrections are needed, it is okay to proceed with direct occlusal treatment.

If either the patient or the dentist lacks confidence in the proposed treatment outcome, use of an occlusal splint can confirm that the result will be comfortable when completed. Such use of an occlusal splint prior to irreversible occlusal treatment is appropriate.

Other Advantages of Occlusal Splints

Occlusal splints can stabilize hypermobile teeth and distribute the loading forces over more teeth. Such stabilization can be very beneficial for occlusions in which loose teeth make occlusal correction difficult. As the occlusal forces are better distributed and the mobility is reduced, the occlusal corrections can then be directly completed more successfully.

A common belief among some clinicians is that direct occlusal equilibration does not have the same potential for relief of symptoms as occlusal splints. Based on extensive clinical experience, I would challenge that belief. It has some validity if comparing occlusal splints with incomplete equilibration. Because of the stabilization effect of covering the teeth, deflective contacts lose some potential for activating the mechanoreceptor influence on the musculature when a full coverage splint is in place. If we compare a perfected equilibration result with a correctly occluded splint, there is no difference in patient response. If there are no occlusal interferences to complete seating of the condyles and if all posterior contact is discluded in excursions, an occluso-muscle disorder will be resolved equally as well by contact of teeth against teeth or by contact of teeth against acrylic resin.

PRINCIPLE

If an occluso-muscle disorder can be resolved by an occlusal splint, it can be resolved without a splint by a perfected occlusion with tooth-to-tooth contact.

Potential Problem with Long-Term Use of an Anterior Deprogramming Device

It has long been believed that long-term use of segmental occlusal devices has a tendency to influence intrusion of the covered teeth and allow the uncovered teeth to enlongate (supraerupt). Consistent evidence, demonstrated in this chapter's illustrations, shows that this is exactly what happens, and it happens consistently if the covered teeth are *posterior* teeth. However, careful observation of *anterior* programming devices does not seem to indicate the same result if an anterior splint is worn only at night. A sequence of events commonly occurs with long-term nighttime use of anterior segmental splints: As the deprogramming device allows the condyles to seat more completely, the masticatory musculature becomes coordinated and comfortable. But when the splint is removed in the morning, the previously unnoticed posterior interferences become painfully obvious. Since it is not comfortable to close into only one or two interfering molars, the patient will put the splint back in and keep it in to maintain comfort while the occlusal disharmony persists.

The better option is to correct the occlusion directly so that no appliance is necessary. If long-term use of an appliance is needed (for various reasons such as economics), a full occlusal splint is indicated. If the occlusion on the splint is correct and the TMJs are healthy, the muscles, teeth, and TMJs should be comfortable. Such a correctly made splint can be worn 24 hours a day with no adverse effects.

What Occlusal Splints Will *Not* Do

Occlusal splints *do not unload the joints.* A perfectly made occlusal splint can *reduce the compressive load on the TMJs,* but the joints are always under some degree of loading. It is a common misconception to think that increasing the vertical dimension of occlusion distracts the condyles downward in a vertical direction, taking all loading forces off the TMJs and transferring the load to the teeth. The elevator muscles are between the last tooth and the condyles, so there is no way for contraction of the elevator muscles to do anything other than seat the condyles up (see Chapter 13).

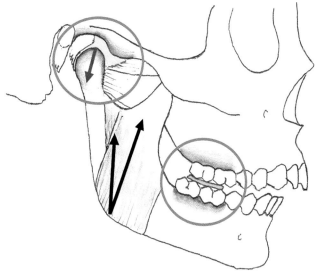

FIGURE 32-7   The fallacy of pivotal appliances. Some advocates claim that posterior bite-raising splints have a pivotal effect and distract the condyles away and down from their sockets *(red arrow).* Since all elevator muscles are behind the teeth, this is not a possible result of contracting elevator muscles *(black arrows).*

The advocacy of pivotal appliances is a baffling concept because it clearly violates basic biomechanics (Figure 32-7).

FABRICATION OF OCCLUSAL SPLINTS

Many occlusal splints fail to achieve a peaceful neuromusculature. Three very common reasons for this are:

1. *The splint does not fit the teeth properly,* so it is uncomfortable or loose, or it rocks in place.
2. *The occlusal contacts on the splint are not in harmony with centric relation.* By far, most of the occlusal splints we have seen have occlusal interferences to centric relation and/or excursions, so they cause displacement of the TMJs and a resultant stimulus to muscle activity rather than a reduction of muscle activity.
3. *An intracapsular structural disorder was not diagnosed,* so centric relation was not achievable.

The most practical way to make a predictably successful occlusal splint is to fabricate the splint on casts mounted in centric relation. The following process is time- and cost-effective.

PROCEDURE   Fabricating occlusal splints on casts mounted in centric relation

Take a verified centric relation bite record.

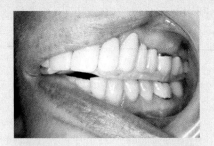

Mount the casts in centric relation with a facebow.

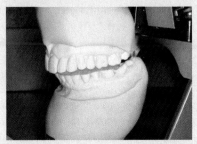

Outline the coverage area of the base.

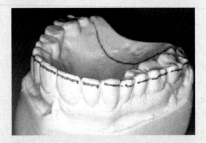

Fabricate a Biostar vinyl base on the cast. (An acrylic or light-cured composite base will also work.)

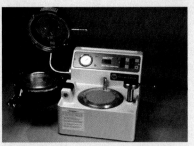

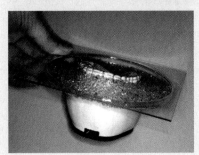

PROCEDURE   Fabricating occlusal splints on casts mounted in centric relation—cont'd

Remove the excess from the base, but do not remove it from the cast.

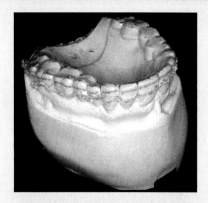

Put the cast and base back on the articulator. Open the pin enough to separate all posterior teeth from any contact with the base. Because the casts were mounted with a facebow, this change of vertical dimension does not affect centric relation.

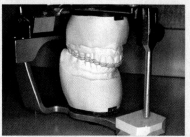

Mix resin (**A**) and position it on the base just behind the upper anterior teeth. Put enough resin to contact and be slightly indented by the lower anterior teeth in centric relation. **B,** Allow the resin to set. Flatten the resin down to the level of the incisor indentations. This surface must be smooth and polished for equal contact of the lower incisors against the resin surface (**C**). The canines may also contact.

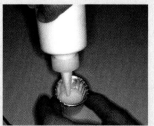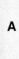

A

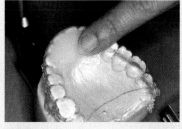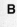

B

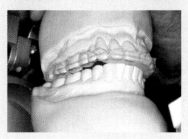

C

Continued

PROCEDURE   Fabricating occlusal splints on casts mounted in centric relation—cont'd

Remove the base and smooth the edges. Remove undercuts into interproximal areas.

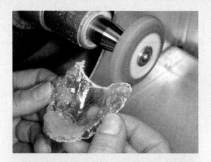

The completed splint should fit perfectly and require almost no adjustment. If done carefully, this indirect method saves a serious amount of chair time.

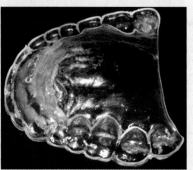

The splint in place may contact all of the anterior teeth in centric relation, but there should be no contact on posterior teeth. Slight adjustment is often needed on the anterior contact area. It should be smooth and flat to permit the condyles to seat into centric relation with no back teeth contact. This is an ideal *permissive anterior deprogramming device* to use. If all tension or tenderness disappears after placement of the splint and there is verification that no posterior teeth are contacting the splint, it is a good indication that the TMJs are in either centric relation or adapted centric posture. It also indicates that the TMJs are not the source of pain. As reliable as this test is, however, a screening history and examination should be consistent with what is indicated by the splint before any final conclusions are made.

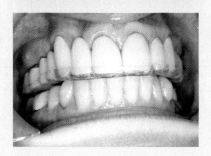

If there is no intracapsular disorder, complete muscle relaxation should occur within minutes or hours. In some cases of severe muscle splinting, overnight use of the splint may be required to release the lateral pterygoid contraction.

If the splint is to be worn for an extended period, contact on the posterior segment should be added for full contact in centric relation and immediate disclusion by the anterior teeth (not shown in this photograph, which shows centric relation contact only).

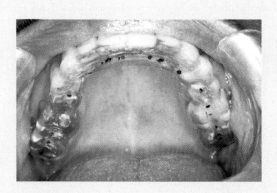

Upper or Lower Splint?

Some clinicians advocate upper splints. Others claim better success with lower splints. The facts don't support any superiority of one over the other. Clinicians should learn to use both upper and lower splints, as there are certain jaw-to-jaw relationships in which one type will have an advantage. The critical factor regarding the effectiveness of any splint, upper or lower, is whether it *completely* frees the mandible to move to and from centric relation. The decision of which type of splint to use should be based mainly on which type will be most comfortable to wear and most unobtrusive esthetically. For many patients, a lower splint is preferable because it interferes less with speech, and flatter anterior ramping is sometimes easier to accomplish without crowding the tongue (Figures 32-8 and 32-9).

Principles of Full Occlusal Splint Design

Whether using an upper or a lower splint, the design must incorporate four main principles:

1. The splint should allow uniform, equal-intensity contacts of all teeth against a smooth splint surface when the joints are completely seated in centric relation.
2. The splint should have an anterior guidance ramp angled as shallow as possible for horizontal freedom of mandibular movement.
3. The splint should provide immediate disclusion of all posterior teeth in all excursive jaw movements from centric relation.
4. The splint should fit the arch comfortably and have good stable retention.

How Long Must the Splint Be Worn?

The splint should be worn until the following requirements are attained:

1. All related pain is gone.
2. The joint structure is stable.
3. The bite structure is stable.

All three of these requirements are related to perfection of the occlusion. Depending on how much remodeling of the TMJs must occur, the occlusion will require follow-up adjustments until the joints stabilize. At that point, it will be evident because further occlusal corrections will become unnecessary.

Occlusal splints for therapy must be worn 24 hours a day except to eat and brush until the occlusion and the TMJs become stable. Stability is determined by three verifications:

1. Elimination of painful symptoms
2. Verification of centric relation by load testing
3. Stability of the bite on the splint over the course of a few days (or weeks if joint damage has occurred)

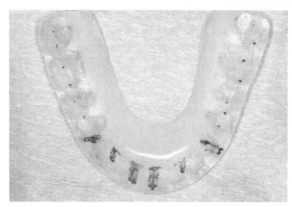

FIGURE 32-8 The ideal occlusal contact on a lower permissive splint. Note the point contacts in centric relation for all posterior teeth but no eccentric contact. The contact during function against the upper anterior teeth is shown *(red lines)*. This splint is advocated by Wilkerson as the preferential design for most patients. Note how flat the pathways for the anterior guidance are.

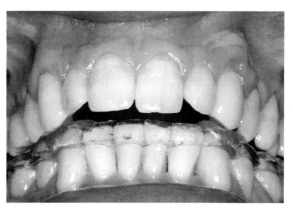

A

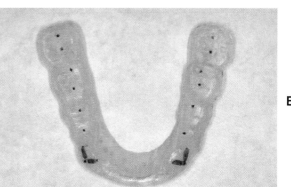

B

FIGURE 32-9 An excellent example of the unobtrusive design for a lower occlusal splint in an anterior open bite patient. **A,** Note that the anterior guidance is confined to the canines. Flatness of the protrusive and lateral guidance contour permits posterior disclusion without a large bulk of material. **B,** Clinical experience seems to be consistent that the flatter the anterior guidance on the splint, the more readily the muscles respond and become comfortable.

For occluso-muscle disorders, these results are usually achieved in a matter of days (not months or years). The average length of splint therapy for occluso-muscle disorders is two to four weeks to achieve a stable occlusion.

What is the next step after occlusal splint therapy?
Successful splint therapy achieves a correct, stable position for the TMJs. It is not a cure for the occlusal disharmony. The common practice of removing the splint without correcting the occlusion is counterproductive, as the original cause of the problem is still present. In time, the uncorrected occlusal interferences will reactivate the problems. The proper next step is to correct the occlusion when the occlusal splint is discarded.

What if the TMJs Are Damaged?

If there has been trauma to the joint, the time required for achieving stability will be longer than required for occluso-muscle disorders. Think of a joint injury as a bad sprain that usually takes about six weeks for recovery. Average length of splint therapy is about six to eight weeks. At first, it may not be possible to achieve complete seating to centric relation because of edema and inflammation in the retrodiskal tissues. If that is the case, the bite record should be made at a *treatment position*. That means the condyle-disk assemblies should be positioned as high up the posterior slopes of the eminentiae as it can move without pain. The bite record should be made at the most comfortable jaw-to-jaw relationship. An occlusal splint can be made on the articulated casts at that position with full occlusal contact, and an anterior ramp for posterior disclusion should be achieved. The contact surface on the splint should be smooth, allowing the muscles to choose the most comfortable jaw position without deflective interferences.

If injury or inflammation has occurred within the capsule of the TMJ, muscle will attempt to protect the joint from compressing the edematous retrodiskal tissue. Use of an anterior deprogramming splint is contraindicated because it increases compressive loading and also activates lateral pterygoid activity to more intense protective contraction.

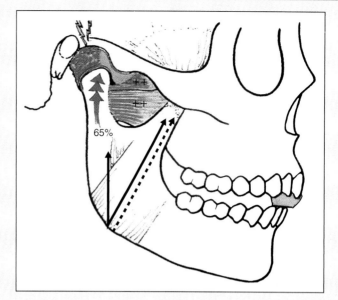

A full-coverage occlusal splint decreases compressive loading of the joint, reduces loading of the joint, and reduces compression of the retrodiskal tissue. Because of the edematous swelling of the retrodiskal tissue, the joints cannot fully seat to centric relation until the swelling is reduced. The smooth surface of the splint allows the mandible to slide back so the condyles can seat as the volume of the retrodiskal tissue decreases. Occlusal adjustments to the splint will have to be made as this occurs.

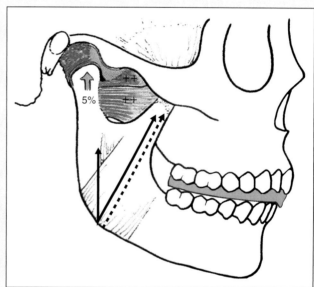

A full occlusal splint in place. Its comfortable relationship with the TMJs was predetermined in the bite record and then fabricated on casts that duplicated the most comfortable jaw-to-jaw relationship.

Note: Posturing the jaw slightly forward *does not unload the joints.* It *moves the condyles down the slopes of the eminentiae* as they come forward. This downward movement makes more room for the swollen retrodiskal tissue up in the fossa behind the condyle. The condyle-disk assemblies remain loaded against the distal slopes of their respective eminentiae.

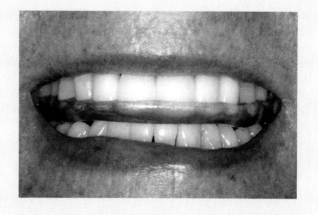

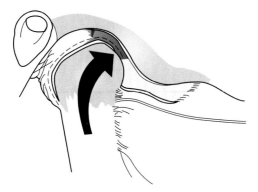

FIGURE 32-10 If the disk is locked in front of the condyle, all of the compressive load is directed onto vascular, innervated retrodiskal tissue. Attempting to recapture a nonreducible disk by a directive anterior repositioning splint is an illogical treatment approach that simply pushes the disk ahead of the condyle as it is moved forward.

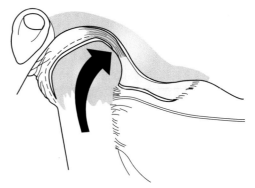

FIGURE 32-11 The retrodiskal tissue includes many undifferentiated mesenchymal cells with the capacity to convert this tissue into fibrous connective tissue to form an extension of the disk (pseudo-disk). Therefore, treatment may be directed at reducing the compressive loading forces to encourage this fibrous conversion. There is no assurance that the treatment will work. If it doesn't work, the tissue will be perforated and a bone-to-bone condylar position will be the result. Either result, however, will usually produce a more comfortable joint in time if the occlusal splint is properly designed.

Anti-inflammatory medication may be prescribed, and a soft diet should be recommended. As the inflammation subsides, allowing the condyles to move up toward complete seating into centric relation, the occlusion on the splint will need to be periodically adjusted. When the condyles reach a solid stop at centric relation, the occlusion on the splint will stabilize. When the patient is comfortable and the occlusion is stable, the splint can be removed and corrections can be made on the teeth directly.

Occlusal splints for TMJs with displaced disks

Some TMJs can adapt to a comfortable position off the disk. When this happens, it is the result of either formation of a pseudo-disk or from bone-to-bone contact of the articular surfaces. In either case, there is a period of time after complete displacement of an irreducible disk when the condyle is loading on vascular innervated retrodiskal tissue (Figure 32-10). During that time, pain is generally a considerable problem in the joint region. It is very important to make an accurate diagnosis with specific classification (Piper IVB) before designing an occlusal splint, because the purpose of the splint is to achieve for an initial time period the opposite effect of complete seating of the condyles. Remember that the goal of permissive splints is to allow the condyles to seat all the way up into centric relation with the disk properly aligned. But if the disk is irreducibly locked in front of the condyle, centric relation is not achievable.

If the disk cannot be recaptured, there are only two options one can choose from:

1. Surgical correction to reposition and attach the disk on top of the condyle
2. Treatment of the occlusion with the condyle off the disk

If the second option is chosen, the goal will be to reduce the compressive force on the retrodiskal tissue with the hope of promoting formation of a pseudo-disk (Figure 32-11). Remember that you cannot unload the joint. The position of the elevator muscles will not permit that. But you can reduce the compressive force on the tissues by a properly made occlusal splint that allows uniform tooth contact as far back toward the TMJs as possible. This is accomplished by the way in which the interocclusal bite record is made.

Taking the bite

The goal in recording a jaw-to-jaw relationship when the disk is locked in front of the condyle is to *gently* manipulate the mandible so the condyles seat as far up as possible but short of being in a painful position. In other words, seat both condyles until some discomfort is felt. Then back off slightly and record the bite at that jaw relationship. Incidentally, bilateral manipulation works very well for this procedure. Record the bite in a wax wafer that covers all posterior teeth (Figure 32-12). Use a wax that is soft for the recording when heated, but is brittle-hard when chilled. This permits the patient to test the position by clenching against the hardened wax to see of the joints are comfortable at that position.

Directive splints

There is never a reason to make an occlusal splint that directs the condyles distally. This can be accomplished automatically by the elevator muscles with a permissive splint. Coordinated elevator muscle contraction always attempts to seat the condyles up into centric relation if there are no obstructions to prevent it. Directive splints are always made to hold the condyles forward.

There is never a need to reposition the mandible forward if correct condyle-disk alignment can be achieved in centric relation and maintained in function.

Anterior repositioning splints should not be considered unless reduction of the disk can be verified. The disk must also be capable of sliding movements. An ankylosed disk will not respond to anterior repositioning splint therapy, nor will a disk that is too badly deformed.

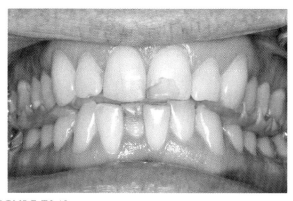

FIGURE 32-12 A bite record made in Delar wax becomes brittle-hard when chilled. By recording the jaw-to-jaw relationship with the condyles as high up in their eminentiae as possible without pain, the relationship can be tested by clenching into the hard bite material. If a firm clench does not cause discomfort, it is the correct record for mounting the casts and constructing an occlusal splint that has maximum tooth contact at this jaw relationship.

A clicking disk is not a justification for anterior repositioning splint therapy. Most clicks are the result of displacement of the lateral half of the disk only with the medial half of the disk still in place. If the medial half of the condyle is covered by the disk, the condyle-disk assemblies can be completely seated into an adapted centric posture. Anterior repositioning is contraindicated. It is also unnecessary since lateral-pole clicks most often disappear with occlusal correction. Those that do not disappear will not present a problem of discomfort if the condyle is completely seated and in harmony with maximal intercuspation.

Indications for an Anterior Repositioning Splint

A disk that is partially displaced so that the condyle has been distalized on the posterior band of the disk may in some unusual situations benefit by moving the condyle forward to a more centered position on the disk. If complete reduction is possible but not maintainable, a directive splint may be used to position the condyle in the disk to prevent it from slipping back past the posterior band. This is rarely necessary because when occlusal interferences to a centered position are eliminated, the superior lateral pterygoid muscle typically releases the forward pull on the disk and allows it to stay centered without the need for a directive splint.

Severe trauma with retrodiskal edema
If the swelling behind the condyle is severe, it may be prudent to hold the condyle forward to prevent compression of the retrodiskal tissue as described earlier in the chapter. If this is done, the patient should be weaned off the splint as early as possible, usually within seven to ten days. Prolonged use of anterior repositioning splints results in ir-

reversible fibrotic contracture of the superior lateral pterygoid muscle, at which point the disk cannot be released back when the condyle goes back to centric relation.

Damaging effects from an anterior repositioning splint
The most avoidable side effect from an anterior repositioning splint is the expense and discomfort of wearing an appliance when it is not needed or when it has no chance for success. If an anterior repositioning splint does not recapture the disk in proper alignment, it can increase damage to connective tissue and intensify the damage to the retrodiskal tissue.

Any anterior repositioning device is an automatic stimulus for muscle incoordination. The protruded relationship of the mandible *requires* lateral pterygoid resistance to elevator muscle contraction.

If the anterior repositioning is maintained over a period of time, the damage can be extensive. Along with fibrotic contracture of the lateral pterygoid muscles, there is a common tendency for adhesions and scar tissue to build up behind the condyles. This scar tissue buildup can be extensive enough to prevent the condyles from moving back to their original centric relation position. When this occurs, it may even be possible to load test with complete comfort against the scar tissue. This creates many problems in the occlusal relationship, and it is not uncommon for these patients to then require extensive orthodontics and/or restorative dentistry to regain a workable bite relationship. The problems do not stop there, however, because the scar tissue seat for the condyles is unstable and the occlusal relationship progressively becomes more malrelated.

Anterior repositioning was a very popular treatment modality for a time, but long-term results have not been good. Today there are very few advocates for the concept. Nevertheless, reports of success still appear in the literature. However, in treating thousands of TMD patients and measuring treatment results by the *criteria for success* (see Chapter 47), we have seen very limited need for anterior repositioning to achieve successful results.

Reports of success with anterior repositioning most often relate to resolution of disk derangements and clicking. But what is not clarified in such studies is whether the disk is completely or partially displaced. Because most clicks result from lateral-pole displacements that respond to occlusal correction, the use of anterior repositioning would be unnecessary even if the click is resolved. Comparative studies also show that centric relation splints are more effective.

SUMMARY

Properly made occlusal splints are an important and practical treatment modality when used for specifically designed purposes. The basis for their utilization should be a clear understanding of how the splint affects the position and condition of the TMJs and/or the suppressive effect on muscle hyperactivity.

Suggested Readings

Ash MM Jr, Ramfjord SP: Reflections on the Michigan splint and other intraocclusal devices. *J Mich Dent Assoc* 80:32-35, 1998.

Boyd JP, Shankland WE, Brown C, et al: Taming destructive forces using a simple tension suppression device. *Postgraduate Dentistry* 7:1, 2000.

Calonico A: *The splint companion.* Bolingbrook, Illinois 2005, Artistic Dental Studio.

Dylina TJ: A common sense approach to splint therapy. *J Prosthet Dent* 86(5):539-545, 2001.

Fosnell H, Kirveskari P, Kangasniemi P: Response to occlusal treatment in headache patients previously treated by mock occlusal adjustment. *Acta Odontol Scand* 45:77-80, 1987.

Greene CS, Laskin DM: Splint therapy for the myofascial pain dysfunction (MPD) syndrome: a comparative study. *J Am Dent Assoc* 84:624-628, 1972.

Kawazoe Y, Kotani H, Hamada T, et al: Effect of occlusal splints on the electromyographic activities of masseter muscles during maximum clenching in patients with myofascial pain-dysfunction syndrome. *J Prosthet Dent* 43:578-580, 1980.

Kreiner M, Betancor E, Clark GT: Occlusal stabilization appliances. Evidence of their efficacy. *J Am Dent Assoc* 132(6):770-777, 2001.

Magnusson T, Adiels AM, Nilsson HL, et al: Treatment effect on signs and symptoms of temporomandibular disorders—comparison between stabilization splint and a new type of splint (NTI). A pilot study. *Swed Dent J* 28(1):11-20, 2004.

Manns A, Valdivia J, Miralles R, et al: The effect of different occlusal splints on the electromyographic activity of elevator muscles. A comparative study. *J Gnathol* 7:61-73, 1988.

Neff P: Trauma from occlusion: restorative concerns. *Dental Clinics of North America* 39(2):335-353, 1995.

Schmitter M, Zahran M, Duc JM, et al: Conservative therapy in patients with anterior disk displacement without reduction using 2 common splints: a randomized clinical trial. *J Oral Maxillofac Surg* 63: 1295-1303, 2005.

Shankland WE: Nociceptive trigeminal inhibition—tension suppression system: a method of preventing migraine and tension headaches. *Compendium* 23:105-113, 2002.

Williamson EH: Temporomandibular dysfunction and repositioning splint therapy. *Prog Orthod* 6:206-213, 2005.

Wood WW, Tobias DL: EMG response to alteration of tooth contacts on occlusal splints during maximal clenching. *J Prosthet Dent* 51:394-396, 1984.

Chapter 33

Occlusal Equilibration

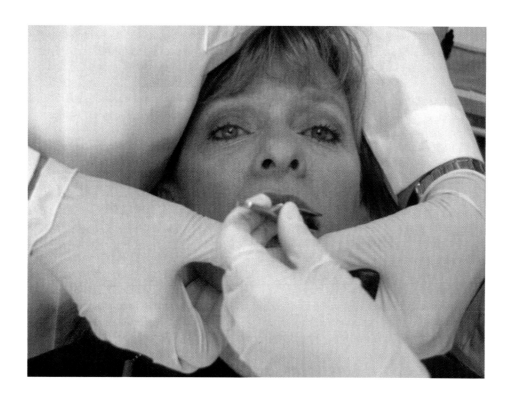

PRINCIPLES
1. Don't equilibrate if the outcome is in doubt.
2. A successful outcome can be determined in advance.

THE IMPORTANCE OF OCCLUSAL EQUILIBRATION

If the importance of occlusion in dentistry were universally understood, no dentist would even consider practicing without a working knowledge of the principles and skills required for successful occlusal equilibration. Whether dentists realize it or not, "adjusting occlusions" is a process that they are expected to do many times a day in any active practice. Correcting an occlusion is typically attempted following placement of a high filling or crown. It is usually done by a guesswork approach of grinding down the restoration until the patient can close into contact with the rest of the teeth regardless of the relationship of the mandible to the maxilla or the position of the temporomandibular joints (TMJs). Such attempts at bite correction are unbelievably crude when compared with a process based on correct equilibration principles. Furthermore, guesswork grinding is almost always more mutilative and unpredictable than the results that can be achieved with a proper equilibration rationale. Proper equilibration on properly selected patients is one of the most predictable services a dentist can perform, and one of the most rewarding.

The advantages of understanding occlusal equilibration principles go far beyond being able to correct a high restoration. The principles of effective occlusal equilibration can only be understood within a context of how the teeth relate to the rest of the masticatory system starting with the TMJs. There is no way to be proficient and predictable in occlusal equilibration without an understanding that the primary purpose of equilibration is to eliminate deflective occlusal contacts that interfere with physiologic function of the TMJs. We'll fall short if we do not understand how the mandibular envelope of function affects the anterior guidance and how the anterior guidance combines with the condylar guidance to dictate ideal occlusal contours on posterior teeth. To understand occlusal equilibration is to understand masticatory system function. Equilibration skills carry over into every facet of occlusal diagnosis and treatment. Without these skills, a significant proportion of everyday dentistry becomes a time-wasting trial-and-error process with limited options for treatment.

Occlusal equilibration is just one of five treatment choices for correcting occlusal disharmony (see Chapter 30). In many patients, it is the most conservative treatment choice. In other patients, it is best combined with other treatment choices. In still other patients, it is inappropriate treatment. If the rules are not understood, we can cause problems that are sometimes serious. But if we understand the requirements for stability and masticatory system equilibrium and then follow a strict rationale for occlusal correction, occlusal equilibration is one of the most predictably successful procedures in dentistry. Without equilibration as a treatment choice, less effective and more extensive treatment procedures, or no treatment, are too often what patients are offered.

ELIMINATING FEAR OF EQUILIBRATION

Many dentists I talk with are afraid to equilibrate because they have been brainwashed to have concerns that any alteration of the occlusion might lead to occlusal awareness or cause temporomandibular disorder (TMD). These fears are constantly reinforced by statements in the literature and by admonitions from clinicians, insurance companies, and even the National Institutes of Health (NIH). Such advice is based on abysmal ignorance of what constitutes masticatory system harmony, and is reinforced by seriously flawed research that treats *TMD* as a single multifactorial disorder rather than a blanket term that includes many different disorders that often have no relationship to occlusion. Without exception, research reports that criticize occlusal correction fail to define the type of TMD being studied; fail to determine (or even attempt to determine) the correct relationship between maximal intercuspation and the position or condition of the TMJs; and routinely fail, to a serious degree, to use proper protocols for correcting occlusal disharmonies.

What must be understood is that occlusal alterations that are not accurately performed, are incomplete, or are done on patients with active intracapsular TMDs can and often do result in more serious signs and symptoms. However, a statement that can be made with complete confidence is:

> If proper equilibration procedures are performed on properly selected patients, the level of predictability is near 100 percent.

There is nothing to fear about occlusal equilibration if it is accurately performed on properly selected patients after proper analysis. There is never a need to even start an equilibration without knowing in advance that the treatment will be successful. Success is assured if all of the rules are followed; this chapter will help you understand the rules. Then you must commit to following them with no shortcuts.

Proper Equilibration: What Does It Mean?

Proper equilibration requires knowing in advance that it will be successful. This statement may cause skepticism, but it is really a practical reality to know in advance if an equilibration is going to result in a comfortable occlusion. For this to have credibility, you must understand that proper equilibration is designed to eliminate all premature or deflective tooth contacts that prevent the condyle-disk assemblies from complete seating in their respective fossa (centric relation) when the jaw closes to maximum intercuspation. For this to be successful, the TMJs must be able to accept firm loading with no sign of discomfort. If the TMJs are disordered so they cannot comfortably accept loading, direct irreversible occlusal changes are contraindicated. But if the TMJs can comfortably accept firm loading, they will predictably be comfortable with a perfected occlusion that is in

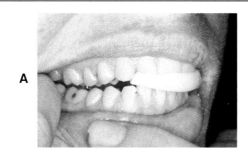

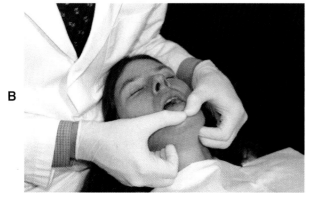

FIGURE 33-1 **A,** An anterior splint that separates the posterior teeth to allow unimpeded loading of the TMJs is an excellent determinant for knowing that the TMJs are not a source of pain or discomfort before occlusal treatment is initiated. This is a short-term test requiring no more than a day or two. **B,** Load testing to rule out intracapsular disorders as a source of pain or discomfort. It is a consistent and dependable observation that if the TMJs can comfortably accept loading they will comfortably accept a perfected occlusion.

perfect harmony with the comfortably seated TMJs. The key to predictability is in knowing with certainty that the TMJs are not a source of pain or discomfort before the equilibration is started. That can be determined with a high degree of accuracy by proper load testing (see Chapter 10). It can be further verified by use of an anterior deprogramming splint (Figure 33-1), a history, and a proper examination.

The examination prior to the equilibration must also rule out disorders that would prevent the musculature from a comfortable, coordinated response. If there is any doubt about the potential for a successful treatment result, it is always possible (and prudent) to verify a response using reversible treatment. This is one of the major advantages of occlusal splints. If this is done, the permissive splint must be made to a perfected centric relation with an anterior ramp for posterior disclusion.

Proper equilibration is selective

It is true that intraoral selective grinding is limited to removal of tooth structure, but that does not eliminate the possibility of *restoring* tooth contours where indicated. It is not an "either-or" concept. It is merely a part of the overall plan to harmonize occlusal stresses. It is the phase of treatment that eliminates only that part of the tooth structure that is in the way of harmonious jaw function. Dentists who believe they must completely restore every patient with an occlusal

problem are guilty of the worst type of technique-oriented tunnel vision. Combining occlusal equilibration with restorative dentistry very often minimizes the restorative needs. Equilibration procedures frequently eliminate the need for restorative dentistry altogether.

Probably the greatest distrust in occlusal equilibration procedures has resulted from observing the results of improper attempts at selective grinding. Doing a poor job of equilibration is far worse than leaving the malocclusion. Improper equilibration actually produces new interferences with which the patient must learn to cope. Mechanoreception of the new interferences can create an occlusal awareness and can trigger extreme discomfort of the teeth, the TMJs, and the masticatory muscles. Proper equilibration procedures do not cause these problems.

Proper equilibration procedures can never harm a patient

If equilibration procedures lead to an "occlusal awareness" or if they force a patient to function where the jaw is not comfortable, the equilibration has been done improperly or, at best, has just not been completed.

Proper equilibration never restricts

Proper equilibration frees the mandible to move wherever and however it wishes to move, consciously or unconsciously. It makes it possible for the muscles to move the mandible to any functional border position without deviation. It eliminates tooth-to-tooth interferences that trigger the "erasure" mechanism of bruxism.

Proper equilibration is stable

There is more to equilibration than just eliminating interferences. Resulting tooth contacts must properly distribute and direct forces for stable maintainability. It may take some time to achieve stability for teeth that have been depressed or moved by occlusal trauma. One of the biggest advantages of occlusal equilibration over immediate restorative correction is that adjustments can keep pace with the movement of teeth as they return to normal equilibrium as depressive stresses are reduced. Restoration should usually wait until maximum stability has been achieved.

EQUILIBRATION PROCEDURES

Equilibration procedures can be divided into four parts:

1. *Reduction of all contacting tooth surfaces that interfere with the completely seated condylar position (centric relation)*
2. *Selective reduction of tooth structure that interferes with lateral excursions.* This will vary as the influence of the anterior guidance varies to accommodate to individual chewing cycles. It will also vary, as necessary, to minimize lateral stresses on weak teeth.
3. *Elimination of all posterior tooth structure that interferes with protrusive excursions.* This must be varied

in arch-to-arch relationships in which the anterior teeth are not in a position to disclude the posterior teeth in protrusion.

4. *Harmonization of the anterior guidance.* It is most often necessary to do this in conjunction with the correction of lateral and protrusive interferences.

There are basic rules to follow for each of these procedures. Taking each procedure separately is a good way to understand the overall goals of equilibration.

Counseling Patients Before Equilibration

Many dentists create problems for their patients and themselves because they do not adequately explain the reason for equilibration and the possible aftereffects. Worst of all, they may fail to adequately study the occlusal relationships in advance and thus mislead the patient into believing that the adjustment requires less tooth reduction than is necessary. It is far better to prepare your patient for more grinding than is needed than to surprise him or her with unexpected reduction of tooth structure.

Proper communication regarding the need for equilibration should be an educational process. It should point out the specific problem as well as the reason for selecting a reshaping procedure over other methods of treatment. Patient understanding and receptivity to the process are usually resolved by the following:

1. *Proper diagnosis* in itself generally prepares the patient. Explain what you are doing as you align the condyle-disk assemblies and test for proper centric relation. Explain why the joints should be comfortable in the seated position and why the teeth should meet properly in harmony with that comfortable relationship.
2. *Point out loose teeth* and relate them to premature contacts or lateral excursion interferences. In the absence of pathosis or injury, loose teeth will always be related to occlusal interferences.
3. *Relate wear problems* to occlusal disharmony with the comfortable joint position. Explain that most excessive wear is an adaptive response that occurs when the teeth interfere with normal jaw movements.
4. *Study the occlusal relationship* on properly mounted diagnostic casts. Demonstrate the conflict between the teeth and the condyles on the articulator. Show how the joints must be displaced when the teeth intercuspate. Explain what must be done to create harmony and distribute forces equally.
5. *Demonstrate on the mounted casts* the amount of tooth reshaping that will be required. If you believe that restorations will possibly be required after equilibration, explain it to the patient.
6. *Tell the patient to expect further adjustments.* There is no sure way to predict the stability of an occlusion after the first equilibration. In my experience, an average

of three appointments is required to achieve an acceptable stability. However, some teeth continue to rebound from a stressed position, requiring more adjustments. Any need for adaptive remodeling of articular tissues could also result in a need for multiple equilibration appointments before stabilizing. The patient should be aware of this possibility before occlusal treatment is started. I prepare my patients to expect multiple adjustments as a possibility.

A cardinal rule that should not be violated is: *Never start an equilibration unless both you and the patient are committed to completing it.*

Locating the Occlusal Interferences

Improper manipulation of the mandible is responsible for most failures in equilibration. You cannot force the mandible into centric relation. Forcing will usually activate stretch-reflex contraction of the lateral pterygoid muscles, causing them to hold the condyles forward of centric relation. Too much pressure on the chin after neuromuscular release can force the condyles down and back from centric relation. For the equilibration to be successful, the condyle-disk assemblies must be free to seat in their most superior positions without any forced displacement when the teeth intercuspate. The centric relation position for each condyle must be confirmed before tooth contacts are marked. Failure to seat the condyles correctly results in imprecise marking of occlusal interferences, so firm pressure should be used to test the position. However, the pressure is not applied until after the condyles have been gently manipulated to the suspected centric relation seat. Loading pressure should be directed to seat the condyles against the eminence while firm upward pressure is also being applied. Distalization of the condyles must be avoided.

Centric relation must be located at the open position before any tooth contact occurs. When it is possible to freely arc the mandible without muscle interference, then apply firm pressure bilaterally. Test for centric relation. Both condyles should be completely comfortable, even when loaded with firm pressure. If there is any sign of tension or tenderness in either joint, equilibration procedures are contraindicated. Unless the posterior teeth need extensive occlusal restoration, a permissive occlusal splint may be used to optimize joint position before equilibration is started.

If centric relation can be verified at the open position, hold the mandible on its uppermost axis and close on that arc by increments of a millimeter or two at a time. Do not jiggle. As the jaw closes and tooth contacts get closer, some resistance may be felt. Just delay for a moment and then start to close again. The patient may help the closure, but loaded pressure through the condyles should not be reduced. Continue a slow opening-closing movement until the first tooth contact occurs. That will be the first interference.

Have the patient feel the first contact. Hold that position for a second and then squeeze. This will determine the di-

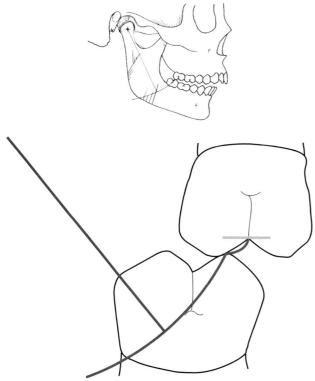

FIGURE 33-2 The condyles must be held firmly on the centric relation axis as the jaw closes to the first point of contact. Note that the mandible cannot close further without displacing the condyles. As the patient squeezes from the first point of contact, the slide from centric relation to maximal intercuspation can be observed.

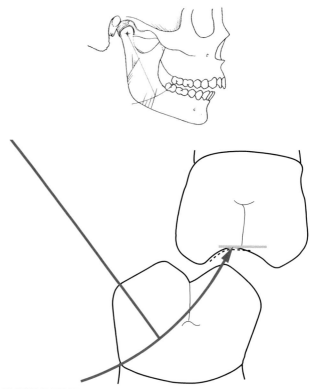

FIGURE 33-3 Equilibration consists of removing the interfering tooth structure that deflects the mandible. Most interferences to the arc of closure displace the mandible forward.

rection and degree of the "slide" from centric relation. The resultant slide must be completely eliminated to allow the mandible to close all the way to maximum intercuspation without any displacement by either condyle from its uppermost axis position.

To mark the interferences, the assistant should insert the marking ribbon on a Miller ribbon holder while the dentist manipulates the jaw with both hands.

Eliminating Interferences to Centric Relation

For simplicity, centric relation interferences can be differentiated into two types:

1. Interference to the *arc* of closure
2. Interference to the *line* of closure

Interference to the arc of closure

As the condyles rotate on their centric relation axis, each lower tooth follows an arc of closure (Figure 33-2). Any tooth structure that interferes with this closing arc has the effect of displacing the condyles down and forward to achieve maximal intercuspation at the most closed occlusal position. Most deviations from the arc of closure require the condyle to move forward. Primary interferences that deviate the condyle forward produce what is commonly called an *anterior slide.*

The basic grinding rule to correct an anterior slide is always MUDL: Grind the *M*esial inclines of *U*pper teeth or the *D*istal inclines of *L*ower teeth (Figures 33-3 to 33-5).

Interference to the line of closure

Line of closure interferences refer to primary interferences that cause the mandible to deviate to the left or the right from the first point of contact in centric relation to the most closed position (Figures 33-6 and 33-7).

The basic grinding rules are as follows:

1. *If the interfering incline causes the mandible to deviate off the line of closure toward the cheek, grind the buccal incline of the upper or the lingual incline of the lower, or both inclines.* The selection of which incline to reduce depends on which adjustment will most nearly place the cusp tip in line with the center of its fossa contact or that will direct the force most favorably to the long axis of both upper and lower teeth.
2. *If the interfering incline causes the mandible to deviate off the line of closure toward the tongue, the grinding rule is: Grind the lingual incline of the upper or the buccal incline of the lower, or both inclines.*

Both rules regarding deviations from the line of closure can apply to any cusp. Remember that the grinding rules refer to inclines, not cusp tips (Figures 33-8 and 33-9).

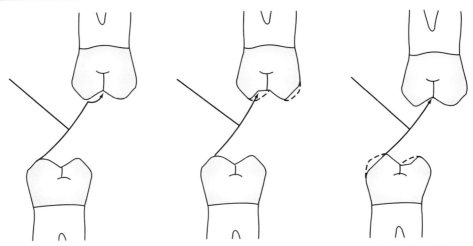

FIGURE 33-4 Interference to the arc of closure: the grinding rule is MUDL: Grind the *M*esial inclines of *U*pper teeth or the *D*istal inclines of *L*ower teeth.

FIGURE 33-5 Note the freedom to close *either* in centric relation or in maximal intercuspation at the most closed vertical.

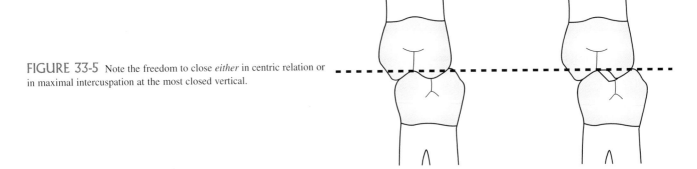

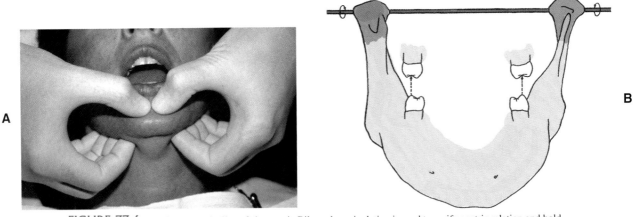

FIGURE 33-6 Interference to the line of closure: **A,** Bilateral manipulation is used to verify centric relation and hold the condyles firmly on the centric relation axis as the jaw closes to the first tooth contact. In a perfected occlusion, the line of closure for each tooth should be a straight line *(as viewed from the front).* **B,** Any deflection off that straight line path is an interference to the line of closure that requires displacement of one or both condyles. The value of bilateral manipulation is apparent when equilibrating because it does not require any intraoral devices that must be removed to achieve tooth contact.

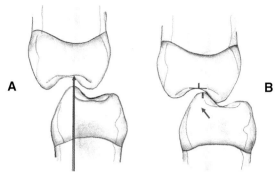

FIGURE 33-7 **A,** Interference to a straight line of closure always shifts the mandible away from the interfering incline. **B,** The purpose of equilibration is to reshape the deflecting surface to permit a straight path all the way to the most closed jaw position at maximal intercuspation.

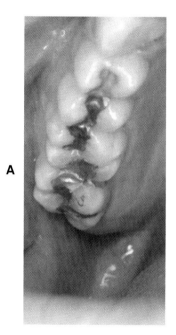

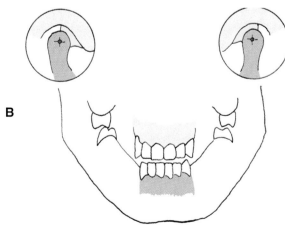

FIGURE 33-8 **A,** A balancing incline interference that would be easily missed if the condyles are not held firmly up on the centric relation axis during closure **(B).** When the condyles are seated, the right molar is the only contact during closure. Squeezing the teeth together shifts the jaw to the right and causes the left condyle to displace.

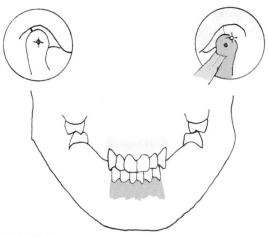

FIGURE 33-9 If the condyles are not held on the centric relation axis during closure, the left lateral pterygoid muscle will displace the condyle to achieve maximum intercuspation. *Biting into a marking ribbon at an unguided closure will miss the interference that is the cause of the occlusomuscle disorder.* The disharmony and the muscle discomfort will persist.

Grinding Rules

Learning where to grind is the key to eliminating mistakes and wasted time. The process can be made a lot simpler by understanding some basic rules.

Rule 1: Narrow stamp cusps before reshaping fossae

This is one of the most important concepts. Understand it and you will multiply your productivity at equilibration. First, what is a *stamp cusp?* A stamp cusp is a cusp that fits into a fossa. In normal occlusions, the stamp cusps are the lower buccal cusp and the upper lingual cusp (Figure 33-10, *A*). In a posterior crossbite, the lower lingual cusp fits into the upper central fossa and the upper buccal cusp fits into the lower central fossa so they are the stamp cusps (Figure 33-10, *B*).

The reason for narrowing the stamp cusps first is because in many deflecting occlusions the cusp tips have worn to a wider contour. If the first reshaping is directed at opening out the fossae to accept bulky stamp cusps, it unnecessarily grinds away more enamel than would be needed to accommodate narrower stamp cusps. If contouring of fossae walls is delayed until stamp cusps have been reshaped, excursive interferences can then be eliminated with less tooth reduction. It also facilitates dividing the reduction of tooth structure more evenly between upper and lower teeth.

Rule 2: Don't shorten a stamp cusp

The goal should be to narrow the thick cusps to reduce mutilation of the opposing tooth. Instead of shortening a stamp cusp, grind the sides of the stamp cusps. Avoid the cusp tip. The cusps should be narrowed on the side that marks when the jaw closes to centric relation contact (Figures 33-11 and 33-12).

Many interferences produce deviations from both the arc of closure and the line of closure at the same time. Upper

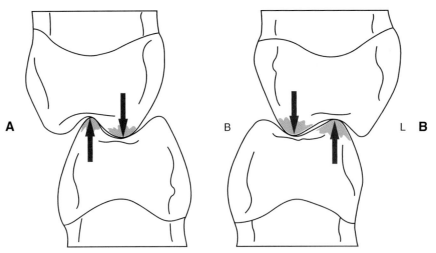

FIGURE 33-10 Stamp cusps are the cusps that fit into fossae. By concentrating on narrowing any stamp cusp that strikes an incline interference before complete closure to maximum intercuspation, there will be no confusion as to whether it is a normal bucco-lingual relationship (A) or a crossbite relationship (B). *B*, Buccal; *L*, lingual.

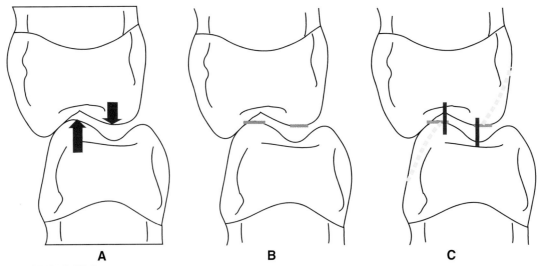

FIGURE 33-11 A, Thick stamp cusps striking an incline interference. B, Grind the sides of the stamp cusps, and avoid the cusp tip. C, The side of the cusp that is ground is the side that marks when the jaw closes to centric relation contact.

teeth are always adjusted on the inclines that face the same direction as the slide. Lower teeth are adjusted by grinding of inclines that face the opposite direction from the path of the slide. This is easy to visualize because of a simple rule:

> Always grind the side of the cusp that marks in centric relation.

The vertical dimension of occlusion after equilibration at centric relation should remain the same as it is in the acquired occlusion before adjustment. If interferences that deviate the mandible forward are eliminated, a "long centric" will be provided automatically unless the vertical dimension is closed. The flat area of long centric will usually be longer than is needed, but the extra length will not generally create a problem.

Tilted teeth

Tilted teeth or wide cusp tips can be adjusted to improve stability as well as to eliminate interferences. If the mark on the upper tooth is buccal to the central fossa, the buccal surface of the lower tooth is ground to move the cusp tip lingually *if the shaping can be accomplished without shortening the cusp tip* out of centric contact. Grinding on the upper teeth only may mutilate upper cusps unnecessarily (Figure 33-13).

If the mark on the upper tooth is lingual to the central fossa and if stability can be improved, the lower cusp tip is moved toward the buccal, and the lower cusp is reshaped by

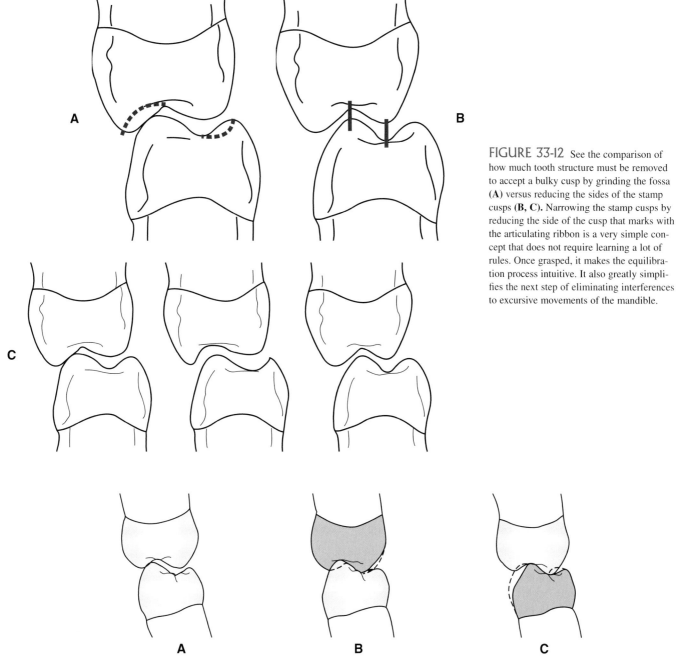

FIGURE 33-12 See the comparison of how much tooth structure must be removed to accept a bulky cusp by grinding the fossa (**A**) versus reducing the sides of the stamp cusps (**B, C**). Narrowing the stamp cusps by reducing the side of the cusp that marks with the articulating ribbon is a very simple concept that does not require learning a lot of rules. Once grasped, it makes the equilibration process intuitive. It also greatly simplifies the next step of eliminating interferences to excursive movements of the mandible.

FIGURE 33-13 **A,** Moving cusp tip by selective grinding. **B,** Grinding upper fossa does not improve cusp tip position and mutilates the upper tooth. **C,** Grinding buccal of lower positions tip in the center.

grinding its lingual inclines to move the contact buccally. This should not be done if it will require shortening of the cusp out of centric contact (Figure 33-14). To grind the upper tooth only may mutilate its lingual cusp unnecessarily without improving the direction of forces.

Influence of skeletal contours

Facial contours that vary the shape of the mandible have a profound influence on the direction of the arc of closure. Because of shape variations, some centric slides that appear to be very long and very devious may be equilibrated with

minimal tooth reduction even though a first impression may lead one to believe that equilibration would require mutilation of the teeth.

Other interferences are frequently missed completely because the deviation from the more vertical closure along steep inclines cannot even be noticed without exceptionally careful manipulation of the mandible so that it can be held with firmness on the centric relation axis while the interfering inclines are being marked.

If the incline that interferes nearly parallels the centric relation arc of closure, a slide from centric may be difficult to

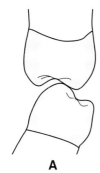 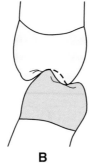 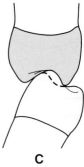

A   **B**   **C**

FIGURE 33-14 **A,** Moving cusp tip by selective grinding. **B,** Grinding lingual of lower tooth positions tip in the center. **C,** Grinding upper fossa does not improve cusp tip position and mutilates the upper tooth.

observe. Such interferences also occur in combination with enough tooth mobility to simply move the tooth rather than displace the mandible. Even such minute, hard-to-find interferences can, however, activate muscle incoordination. It has been a common experience for us to find such interferences in patients who have been unsuccessfully treated with occlusal therapy. The teeth should be dried thoroughly with air, and a fresh marking ribbon should be used to locate the interfering inclines. Firmly tapping the teeth together with sharp taps will produce better marks on steep inclines.

Rule 3: Adjust centric interferences first

It is wise to give first priority to the elimination of all interferences to centric relation closure. There are three reasons for this:

1. *By adjusting centric interferences first, you have the option of improving cusp-tip position.* Most cusp tips are wide enough to permit narrowing toward a more favorable central groove relationship. Better placed, narrower cusp tips require less mutilation of opposing fossae walls when lateral excursions are adjusted.
2. *When cusp-tip position is given first priority, occlusal grinding is more evenly distributed to both arches.* Cusp-tip position is usually improved by narrowing the stamp cusps toward the central groove. Excursive interferences are then corrected by grinding of the fossae walls of the opposite arch. After gross adjustments are made in this sequence, fine contouring can be selectively achieved on either arch.
3. *If cusp-tip contours and position are improved first in centric relation, eccentric interferences can be eliminated with speed and simplicity.*

Rule 4: Eliminate all posterior incline contacts. Preserve cusp tips only.

> If all eccentric contacts on posterior teeth are to be eliminated, any posterior incline that marks in any excursion can be reduced.

Centric stops must be preserved, but all other contacts can be shaped so that they are discluded by the anterior guidance.

If lateral excursions are adjusted first, the option of precise cusp-tip placement is often lost or compromised and the grinding is usually done mostly on upper fossae walls. Although this is an effective way to eliminate interferences, it does not always produce optimum stability. If the posterior teeth are to be restored after equilibration, the sequence is not so important, however, because cusp-tip position can be improved in the restorations.

Lateral Excursion Interferences

The path that is followed by the lower posterior teeth as they leave centric relation and travel laterally is dictated by two determinants:

1. The border movements of the condyles, which act as the posterior determinant
2. The anterior guidance, which acts as the anterior determinant

When lateral excursions are being equilibrated, the mandible must be guided with firm upward pressure through the condyles to ensure that all interferences are recorded and eliminated through the uppermost ranges of motion that can occur at true border paths for both the condyles and the anterior guidance.

If the patient is allowed to mark lateral interferences by unguided excursions, there will be a tendency to slide anterolaterally to the lateral border path. Guiding the mandible with firm pressure during excursions will routinely pick up posterior interferences that are missed with unguided movements. Lateral interferences that can be found only by firm manipulation from a verified centric relation are commonly the interferences that trigger muscle incoordination and excessive muscle loading during clenching or bruxing activity. The elimination of even minute interferences just lateral to centric holding contacts puts an end to many otherwise unsolvable occluso-muscle disorders.

Eliminating Excursive Interferences

Excursive interferences can be divided into protrusive interferences, interferences of the working side, and interferences of the balancing side. Before we understood the rationale for posterior disclusion, it was often recommended to clear balancing interferences first, then working interferences, and finally protrusive interferences. Since both scientific electromyography (EMG) studies and clinical experience have shown conclusively the value of complete separation of all posterior teeth the moment the mandible leaves centric relation, the process of equilibration has been dramatically simplified. There is no reason to complicate it.

The secret to eliminating wasted time is to finalize stable holding contacts before adjusting for excursions.

The ideal pattern of centric relation contacts. Note cusp-tip contacts rather than broad-surface contact. By narrowing the stamp cusps to create a sharper cusp, it not only makes it easier to adjust excursive pathways, it also reduces loading forces on the teeth during chewing.

After this first stage of equilibration has been completed, all excursive interferences can be marked and adjusted without concern for whether the interference is in protrusive, lateral working side, or balancing side. But until all centric relation contacts are established, it is not possible to refine the anterior guidance, which is the key to posterior disclusion.

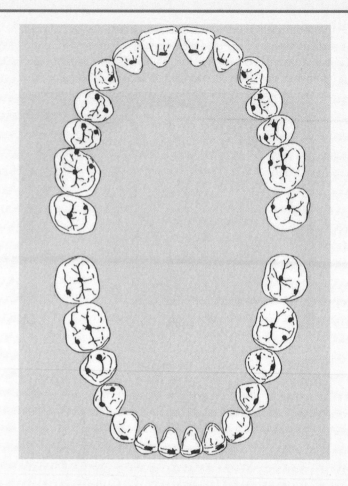

A perfect equilibration by Dr. DeWitt Wilkerson illustrates ideal cusp-tip contacts on the stamp cusps. Notice the size of the contact marks. Even though this patient had a severe slide from centric relation to maximal intercuspation, note the lack of mutilation of enamel.

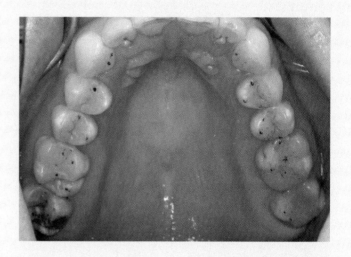

These cusp tips will not have to be touched again as the next phase is completed . . . the elimination of all incline contact in excursions. The goal from here is to confine all excursive contact onto the anterior teeth. In this patient, a tongue pattern prevents the incisors from contacting, so the canines will have to serve as the anterior guidance.

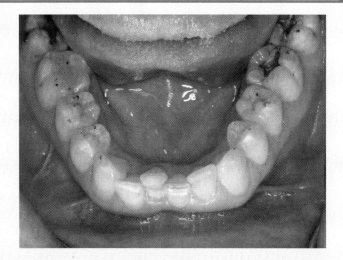

The goal of a perfected occlusion follows the simple formula:

> Dots in back . . . lines in front.

This is the ideal result of marking with a red ribbon while the patient grinds the teeth together in all excursions. Then the patient is manipulated to verify complete seating of the condyles in centric relation and allowed to tap the teeth together. All teeth touch in centric relation. Only the anterior teeth contact in excursion.

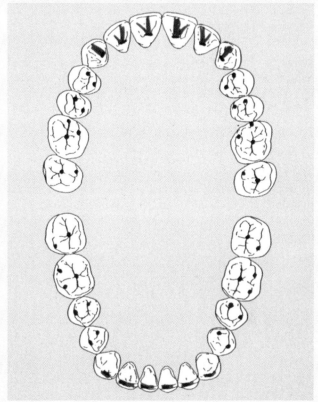

A typical pattern of markings when a red ribbon is placed and the patient is instructed to grind the teeth together. The incline interferences can be on any tooth or teeth, but they are most commonly found on the most posterior teeth. Note the posterior interferences prevent any excursive contact on the anterior teeth. The grinding rule is simple: *Grind all red marks on posterior teeth. Do not touch any black marks.* The process will need to be repeated several times for most patients before the posterior teeth stop interfering with the anterior guidance. As the posterior interferences are eliminated, the anterior teeth start to mark until all red marks are on the anterior teeth and none are on the posterior teeth.

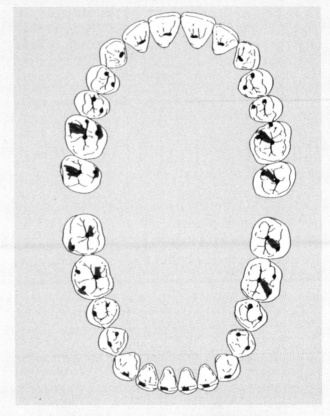

The simple armamentarium for occlusal equilibration: A small diamond wheel stone and a 12-sided football-shaped finishing bur work well for precise reduction and reshaping. Red and black marking ribbons are held in Miller ribbon holders.

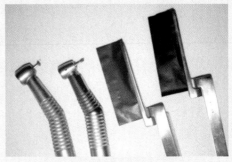

Reduction of the interfering tooth surfaces is confined to areas that are marked with the red ribbon. Black marks are not touched.

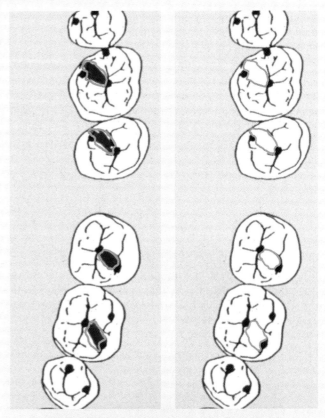

Getting near the final stage of completion but not quite there yet. Marks that might look insignificant can be potent triggers for activating muscle hyperactivity and can prevent the turning off of the elevator muscles that occurs when posterior disclusion is complete. Such interferences can easily be eliminated, and must be, for a predictably successful result.

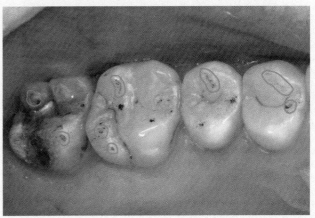

Complete elimination of all posterior excursive contact the moment the mandible leaves centric allows the canine guidance to separate the posterior teeth and shut off most of the elevator muscles. Since the posterior teeth cannot contact in any excursion, it is not possible to generate attritional wear as long as the anterior guidance stays intact and the TMJs remain stable. This is so even if the patient continues to clench or brux.

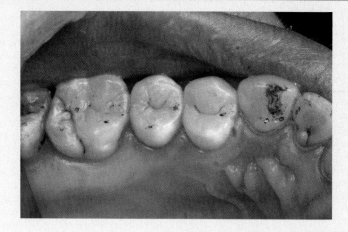

Balancing-side interferences on second molars are among the most commonly missed interferences. Unfortunately they are also some of the most potent triggers for occluso-muscle pain. It is extremely important to keep these teeth dry when marking with fresh ribbon. These interferences are easily missed if the molars have mobility, which they frequently do. At the completion of equilibration, it should not be possible to contact these inclines. Only cusp tips should contact in fossae or at marginal ridges.

PRINCIPLE
You never want balancing inclines to contact.

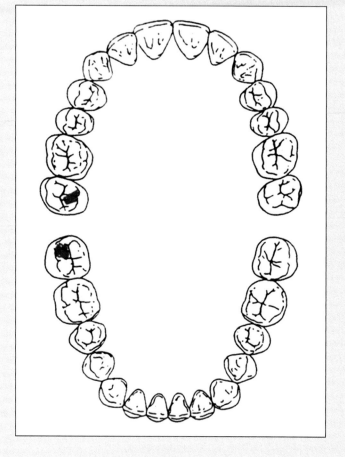

Manipulating to Pick Up Lateral Excursion Interferences

The reason for special manipulation is to ensure that we are moving the mandible all the way out to its anatomic limit (border positions). The patient may not use the full range of freedom, but any interference that prevents the mandible from reaching a border position is a potential trigger for bruxing (and all the damaging results that go with it).

1. Manipulate the mandible to centric relation, and verify centric relation with load testing.
2. Close on the centric relation axis arc to the first point of contact.
   Note: for final refinement of lateral excursions, all centric interferences should be eliminated first.
3. Slide the forefinger around to join the other three fingers on the working side. Use all four fingers to exert upward pressure on the working condyle. Be sure fingers are placed on bone, not into the neck tissue.
4. Use the thumb and bent forefinger to exert pressure toward the working condyle (Figure 33-15).

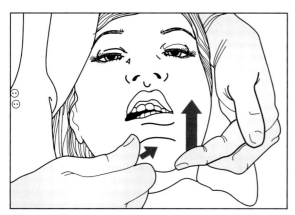

FIGURE 33-15 Directions of pressure *(arrows)* while manipulating the mandible.

5. Ask the patient to let you slide the jaw to the left (or right). It might be necessary to have the patient help, but do not relax the upward pressure through the working side condyle.
6. Have the assistant insert the dry ribbon in the dry mouth to record the interferences. Slide the jaw to the outer border position, and then have the patient squeeze hard back to centric.

Adjusting the Anterior Guidance

You may want to review Chapter 17 as well. The principles for equilibration are the same as those for restorations.

Treatment objective
1. Stable holding contacts on all anterior teeth.
2. Continuous contact from centric to incisal edges on as many anterior teeth as possible in all excursions.
3. Anterior guidance in harmony with the patient's normal envelope of function.

4. Immediate disclusion of all posterior teeth as soon as the mandible leaves centric relation in any excursion.

Different options
Anterior guidance can vary from patient to patient as the interincisal angle varies in relation to the envelope of function. Mutually protected occlusion refers to an occlusion in which the incisors contact during protrusion and the canines contact during lateral excursions. This is also referred to as canine-protected occlusion.

Anterior group function refers to two or more anterior teeth in contact during lateral excursions. Anterior group function can include a canine, a lateral, and both central incisors. In some occlusal relationships, only the incisors contact in lateral excursions.

There is no one type of anterior guidance that is correct for all patients. The more vertical the envelope of function, the more likely you will have canine-only contact in lateral excursions. The flatter the envelope of function (more horizontal pattern), the more likely you will have group function.

Key points
- All interferences to centric relation must be eliminated before the anterior guidance can be corrected. Centric relation (or adapted centric) is the starting point for a correct anterior guidance.
- All posterior interferences to lateral excursions must be eliminated.
- All posterior interferences to protrusive jaw movements must be eliminated.
- As changes are made in the anterior guidance, posterior tooth interferences often come back into contact and must be readjusted so they are discluded.
- If the anterior teeth do not touch during maximal closure because of anterior open bite or overjet, develop the anterior guidance on the most forward upper tooth that can contact in protrusive from centric relation.
- If the anterior teeth cannot disclude the posterior teeth in lateral excursions, consider posterior group function on the working side to disclude the balancing side.

Steps in harmonization of the anterior guidance
Step 1. Establish stable holding contacts on all anterior teeth if possible in centric relation (guided closure).

Step 2. Extend centric contact forward if needed to permit unguided gentle closure into stable stops without striking the lingual incline first. This is done by light tapping from a postural position. Use a red marking ribbon for light postural closure. Then use a black ribbon for centric (guided) closure. If red marks extend onto a fairly steep incline, reduce the incline just enough to permit unguided closure without wedging into the incline before fully closed. This slight freedom is called *long centric.* It never requires more than 0.5 mm of freedom, and about 50 percent of patients do not require it.

Step 3. Equalize contact in the protrusive path. If a single tooth is carrying 100 percent of the forces when the mandible slides forward, reduce the incline as needed to bring more incisors into contact in protrusive. *Note:* Remember that analysis on mounted casts should determine that such corrections are not mutilative. If equilibration would unnecessarily destroy too much enamel, consider other alternatives such as orthodontics.

Step 4. Adjust the lateral anterior guidance as needed to permit smooth, comfortable excursions that do not stress or torque guiding teeth. Observe at contact between the canine and lateral incisor when the jaw slides laterally. Any separation of contacts is a sign of overload.

Reminder: Recheck the posterior occlusion for new interferences when the anterior guidance is altered.

PROCEDURE   Adjusting for protrusive function

As the protrusive path is developed, the guidance is often more continuous on one tooth with separation from contact on the other teeth.

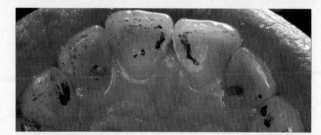

Selective reduction on the guiding tooth should be at the same part of the protrusive path as the skipped section on the other teeth.

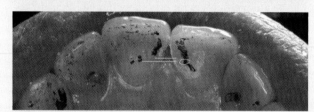

Reduction wipes away the mark to allow contact on the skipped part of the path.

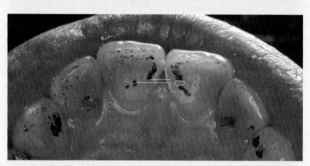

Now, even contact from centric relation to incisal edges is equal on both centrals. Laterals do not contact in protrusive in this mouth. To achieve that would take too much reduction on central incisors. While contact on all four incisors is preferred, it is not always necessary as long as the teeth are stable and there is no fremitus.

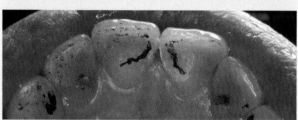

Always recheck to make sure the posterior teeth are completely separated in protrusive.

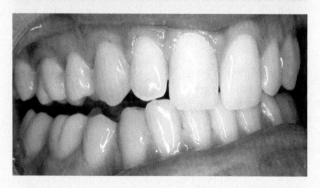

Protrusive Interferences

Only the front teeth should touch in protrusive excursions. All posterior contact should be eliminated in protrusion as soon as the posterior teeth move forward of their centric holding contacts.

The rule for eliminating protrusive interferences is DUML: Grind the *D*istal inclines of the *U*pper or, in some instances, the *M*esial incline of the *L*ower teeth.

In grinding away protrusive interferences, centric stops should be marked with a different-colored ribbon so that they will not be inadvertently ground. The jaw should be positioned in centric relation, and the patient should be asked to "slide forward and back, forward and back." The patient should do the sliding, but the dentist should maintain a firm hold on the mandible to make sure the condyles are staying up against the eminentiae during the movement.

One must look carefully for protrusive interferences because they are often missed. With careful observation, they are frequently found as a little hang-up on a slightly raised marginal ridge. The dentist must also note the linguo-occlusal line angle toward the distal of each upper tooth and also observe the fosse walls in the protrusive pathway. All posterior contact in protrusive interference must be relieved.

Posterior disclusion in protrusion is accomplished by both the anterior guidance and the downward movement of the protruding condyles. With steep anterior guidances, correction for protrusive interferences is usually minimal. Flat anterior guidances rely more on the condyles for disclusion, and the corrections required for protrusive interferences are usually more extensive.

Protrusive interferences are often corrected by some degree of "hollow grinding" of the offending inclines. The concave incline contours are easily discluded by the convex path of the condyles.

A frequent mistake in adjusting occlusions is to assume that the lower buccal cusp tips follow the upper central grooves in protrusion. This would occur only if both sides of the arch were parallel to each other (producing a perfectly square-jawed individual). Most arches taper from back to front so that when the mandible is protruded, the lower teeth follow a straight path forward; this results in the lower posterior teeth moving diagonally across the upper teeth (Figure 33-16). Interferences to this pathway can be easily missed by misinterpretation of the marks as working excursions. Such interferences should be eliminated by concave grinding of the upper distal inclines or the lower mesial inclines. Such inclines are often polished very smooth by wear, and they do not mark easily unless the teeth are dry and the marking ribbon is fresh.

When the arch relationship does not permit the anterior teeth to disclude the posterior teeth, the farthest forward tooth on each side should serve as the discluder of the rest of the posterior teeth in protrusion.

Equilibrating Hypermobile Teeth

All teeth should be checked digitally for any hypermobility when occlusal adjustment is performed. Loose teeth that interfere can easily move out of the way to permit marking stable teeth. The mark on a loose tooth may even be less noticeable than marks on stable teeth. If the firm teeth are ground, the loose tooth is stressed all the more. Each tooth should be checked with the tip of the fingernail contacting the facial surface while the patient closes and goes through all excursions. If there is any noticeable movement in any tooth contact position, the tooth should be held in place with the finger while it is marked.

Occlusions should be checked with both firm and light contact. The use of red ribbon for firm closure and black ribbon for light closure will show whether teeth are moving to permit equal contact at a forced closure (Figure 33-17). The red and black marks should be in the same locations.

If more marks are made on heavy closure than are recorded with light closure, the occlusion is adjusted further by grinding of the marks made with light contact until they are the same as those at firm contact.

THE SECRET OF FINISHING AN EQUILIBRATION

If there are no intracapsular problems and if orofacial pain is the result of masticatory muscle hyperactivity, a perfected occlusal equilibration should completely eliminate all signs of muscle pain, usually by the time the occlusal corrections are completed. If complete relief is not achieved, it is my clinical experience that the equilibration has not been completed. That is to say that occlusal interferences are still present. Most of the time the missed interferences are located on the last molars. The reason such interferences are missed is often because the interfering molars are loose enough to be easily moved by the offending deflective inclines. Thus the loose teeth just depress or move to let the rest of the teeth come together without creating a slide. The secret to complete elimination of all posterior interferences is a simple but highly effective procedure for marking the interferences that too often are missed.

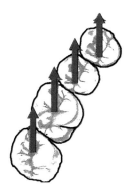

FIGURE 33-16 Because of the shape of most arches, the protrusive path of the lower cusps is diagonally across upper occlusal surfaces. The distal inclines of upper cusps should be carefully observed for protrusive interferences. There should be no contact on posterior teeth in protrusive movements.

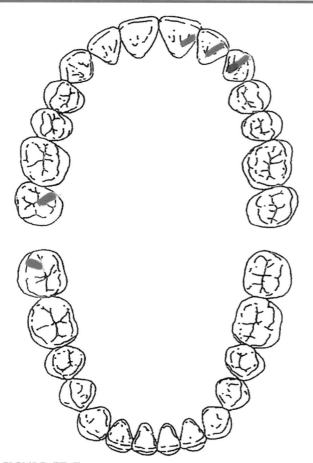

FIGURE 33-17 Typical excursion pattern when molars are hypermobile. When the anterior teeth appear to mark ideally for lateral anterior guidance but muscle hyperactivity is still present, the problem will often be unnoticed interferences on molars that simply move out of the way to allow anterior excursive contact. Make certain that the condyles are completely seated at the start of very firm "chop chop" and grinding jaw movements to pick up such posterior interferences. Be sure the teeth are dry and the ribbon is fresh so marks will show up.

If the patient is not completely comfortable after you think you have completed your equilibration, do the following:

1. Dry the posterior teeth completely; use air, suction, and cotton rolls if needed, but get the occlusal surfaces dry.
2. Use a fresh red marking ribbon. Place it carefully to be sure the entire occlusal surface of the molars is covered. One side at a time is okay.
3. Using bilateral manipulation, find and verify centric with firm upward loading of both condyles.
4. Now, while maintaining firm upward pressure through the TMJs, ask your patient to forcefully chop the teeth together. Urge the patient to "chop chop" as quickly and as firmly as possible.
5. Now, while continuing to hold the condyles up firmly, ask the patient to grind in all directions as firmly as possible.
6. Remove the red marking ribbon and immediately insert a fresh black ribbon. Manipulate to centric and then tap the teeth lightly together in centric only.

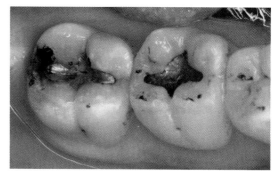

FIGURE 33-18 Marking made on second molar by chopping hard and fast on a black marking ribbon after it was assumed that the equilibration had been perfected. By chopping the teeth together quickly, teeth that are vertically mobile will mark before the tooth has a chance to move. Most equilibrations are stopped short of this important step and fail to achieve complete success.

7. What you will typically find is red marks on cusp inclines that were missed in previous markings. It is common to find red marks covering a major part of the occlusal surface of one or more molars.
8. Grind all surfaces that are marked in red. Do not grind the black mark on the cusp tip or the center of the fossa.

Note: If light tapping on the black ribbon marks only the most distal molar or does not uniformly mark all centric stops, it is an indication that the back tooth needs reduction at the cusp tip (Figure 33-18). Otherwise do not grind centric stops.

Repeat the firm "chop chop grind" maneuver until no eccentric inclines can be marked with red ribbon.

Note: Always keep the teeth dry, use fresh ribbons, and be certain the ribbon is correctly placed.

VERIFICATION OF COMPLETION

Many equilibrations fail to achieve the goal of complete comfort. The reasons for discomfort may be unrelated to the occlusion, or it may be the result of not completely eliminating all occlusal interferences on the posterior teeth. It is not uncommon for teeth to rebound even after a perfected equilibration and thereby reactivate muscle hyperactivity and discomfort. There are two ways to know if there are premature deflective tooth contacts still present: the clench test and using the anterior deprogramming splint.

Clench Test

Ask the patient to clench the teeth together and squeeze firmly (empty mouth). If the patient can feel any discomfort in any tooth, the equilibration is not complete. You may have to stabilize the interfering tooth with your finger while the patient clenches into the marking ribbon to pick up the interference, but you can be sure that an interference is still present.

Be sure the teeth are dry and the fresh marking ribbon is properly placed. Have the patient "chop chop" very firmly and grind in all directions while you load the joints up with bilateral manipulation. There will be an interference there as long as the patient can feel a sore tooth with empty mouth clenching or grinding. This is a very reliable test.

Anterior Deprogramming Splint

If equilibration fails to give complete relief for occluso-muscle pain, the use of an anterior deprogramming splint after equilibration is another reliable test to confirm whether the problem is or is not related to occluso-muscle pain. If the anterior splint completely separates all the posterior teeth, all discomfort will dissipate if the cause of the discomfort is totally related to occlusion. Relief of all discomfort when the posterior teeth can't touch indicates that there were still occlusal interferences remaining and that the discomfort will dissipate when the remaining occlusal interferences are completely eliminated.

I cannot stress enough the importance of leaving minute interferences when equilibrating. I cannot count the number of patients over the years that got only partial improvement from equilibration until those final minute interferences were completely eliminated.

Principle

If an empty mouth clench can make any posterior tooth hurt, the equilibration has not been completed.

EQUILIBRATION ON PATIENTS WITH EMOTIONAL PROBLEMS

Patients with emotional problems may or may not be candidates for equilibration. Many patients' stress-related disorders can be profoundly improved by elimination of painful occluso-muscle incoordination. It has been my experience on numerous occasions that emotional symptoms disappeared when the occluso-muscle symptoms were relieved. The patient who is refused help for a diagnosable problem just because he or she is depressed is often caused greater stress. It may take extra time and extra compassion to help such patients, but good results can be achieved if the diagnosis is accurate and the patient is realistic about the symptoms that relate to occlusal imbalance.

If a patient has unrealistic expectations regarding the effect of treatment, no irreversible procedures should be started. All adjustments to the occlusion should be made on reversible occlusal splints. Only when all symptoms are resolved by the occlusal splints and the patient has a full understanding of the need for occlusal correction of the teeth should direct occlusal equilibration be attempted.

Patients with irrational symptoms cannot be helped by occlusal equilibration, and it should never be attempted on such patients. Unless there is a definite, clearly defined diagnosis that explains the patient's symptoms and those symptoms can be predictably resolvable by definitive treatment, occlusal equilibration is contraindicated.

Regardless of how obvious a causative factor may be or how predictable the occlusal treatment may be, equilibration should not be initiated on any patient with either irrational symptoms or irrational expectations. If there is a definite problem of which the patient is aware and it can be resolved by correction of the occlusion, proper equilibration will not cause an occlusal awareness, even in an emotional patient, as long as the patient is rational.

Occlusal splints are generally the method of choice for resolution of occluso-muscle disorders for patients with possible emotional side effects to treatment. In carefully selected patients who need complete posterior occlusal restoration, direct equilibration may be proper. It prevents the need for wearing an appliance, and the occlusal surfaces are going to be restored anyway.

If there is any question about the position or condition of the TMJs, a diagnostic occlusal splint should be used to verify a favorable response to occlusal correction before direct adjustments are started.

PROPHYLACTIC EQUILIBRATION

There is no need to equilibrate any patient who is completely comfortable and who has no prospects for accelerated wear or periodontal breakdown, or no hypermobile teeth, excessive recession, pulpal sensitivity, wear facets, bruxism habits, TMJ-related symptoms such as popping or cracking in the joint area, tenderness, pain, or headaches. If such patients have no requirements for restorative treatment, there would be no indication for occlusal correction. If equilibrating patients with none of these problems is what is meant by prophylactic equilibration, there would be no reason to endorse the concept.

Unfortunately, finding a patient with occlusal interferences and none of the preceding symptoms is more difficult than most dentists realize. Patients with occlusal disharmony who have "no problems" have in most cases not been examined carefully. There is no reason to postpone treatment until problems are bad enough to become obvious to the patient. Modern dentistry is capable of intercepting and correcting causative factors before the problem requires extensive treatment.

Occlusal stress is a causative factor that accelerates deterioration of oral health. Its correction is usually simple for the well-trained dentist. Correction makes the patient more comfortable and makes the teeth and the supporting tissues more maintainable.

Since proper equilibration cannot harm a patient and has the potential for being so beneficial, what are the objections to correcting an occlusion before damage is apparent?

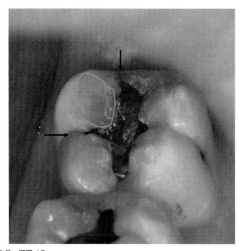

FIGURE 33-19 A typical problem in the making that could be prevented by occlusal equilibration. Note the cracks *(arrows)*. Note the large facet of wear *(circled)*. The wedging effect of high levels of force applied during bruxing is a common etiology for fracturing off cusps. Such force cannot be applied if the incline of the cusp is not in interference. Prevention is the better choice than waiting for the tooth to split.

Dentists who have never seen the results of properly executed occlusal correction have no way to evaluate it and hence have little appreciation for its merits. Similarly, dentists who are not accustomed to thoroughness in examining their patients do not see the need for occlusal corrections because they are not aware that their patients have unhealthy mouths with problems that were caused by occlusal overload.

Dentists who think in terms of optimum oral health will embrace concepts of comprehensive, preventive dentistry. Correction of occlusal trauma is one of the preventive measures that noticeably improves the comfort and maintainable health of the teeth and surrounding tissues. If *prophylactic equilibration* refers to correcting specific problems of stress before the damage is serious, I recommend it. Waiting until after the damage has been wrought hardly seems like a worthwhile alternative. Careful examination is the key to determining whether or not there is a problem that requires correction (Figure 33-19).

CAUTION: One should never attempt to equilibrate any patient unless the problems of occlusal stress are first pointed out in the patient's own mouth. The patient should agree that there is a problem and should understand in advance what will be involved in the treatment.

Dentists who are not totally confident of their expertise in equilibrating should not attempt any form of prophylactic equilibration. The unhappiest patients I see are those who believed they had no problems until the dentist "just started grinding away my good teeth." Improper or incomplete equilibration can cause an occlusal awareness and sometimes even acute TMDs. Such problems are amplified if the patients were reasonably comfortable before the attempted "equilibration."

EQUILIBRATING THE ORTHODONTIC PATIENT

Every orthodontist should learn the principles and techniques of occlusal equilibration. No one can be in a better position to equilibrate orthodontic patients than the orthodontist. Understanding of directional growth factors may eliminate the need for reduction of inclines that will tend to move with growth into more favorable positions.

The orthodontist's appraisal of "rebound" movement of teeth after band removal gives him or her a better sense of timing as to when to equilibrate and how much to relieve certain inclines. The orthodontist is able to make slight corrections in individual tooth position when the alternative would mean grinding through enamel.

We are told by orthodontists who refine their finished cases with equilibration that they tend to constantly improve their orthodontic technique to minimize the need for selective grinding. The careful occlusal analysis that goes with equilibration has made them far more aware of factors of stability, and their results require less retention.

Equilibration should not be used to take the place of correct tooth positioning. Orthodontists who believe it is impossible to position teeth accurately enough to avoid extensive grinding should be aware that many orthodontists are finding it possible and practical to relate the teeth so well that minimal posttreatment spot grinding is all that is required.

Occlusal Adjustment During Treatment

It is permissible to change the shape of cusps, fossae, or inclines during treatment if such changes will benefit stability after the tooth is moved. Nonfunctioning inclines particularly can be reshaped at any time during treatment. Visualizing the final position of any tooth in question can help to determine what changes in shape would be beneficial.

Occlusal Adjustment During Retention

When the bands are removed and a removable retainer is inserted, gross occlusal correction should be initiated. If the occlusion can be corrected in the position of retention, stabilization of the teeth in that position will be enhanced.

If slight movement of any tooth would be beneficial to the occlusal relationship, additional finger springs can be added to the retainer to move the tooth rather than mutilating it with excessive occlusal grinding. When the tooth-to-tooth relationship is as correct as the orthodontist believes it can be, the occlusion should be refined. The combination of occlusal stability and the stabilizing effect of the retainer allows the entire dentition to become quite stable in a greatly reduced time. The alternative of using a retainer to hold teeth in malocclusion is a poor second choice.

EFFICIENCY IN EQUILIBRATION

An extravagant amount of time can be wasted with inefficient equilibration procedures. With well-trained chairside help and a good procedural approach by the dentist, most patients can be equilibrated initially within an hour's time. This means that all interferences to centric relation can be eliminated and all protrusive and lateral excursions can be harmonized.

This does not mean that the resultant occlusion will require no further adjustments. It would be rare to finalize an occlusion to the point of stability in one appointment because stressed teeth have a tendency to move as excessive occlusal forces are reduced. How long it takes the stressed teeth to regain equilibrium with their periodontal ligaments varies greatly after the stress is removed. The occlusal adjustment must be repeatedly refined as the shifting produces new interferences.

At any one appointment, all the dentist can do is to eliminate occlusal interferences for the position the teeth are in at that time. Efficient technique can cut the time required for the initial equilibration and can drastically cut the time required for the subsequent follow-up equilibration appointments.

Role of the Chairside Assistant

Efficient equilibration is a four-handed endeavor because the manipulation of the mandible requires both hands of the dentist.

The assistant has three responsibilities:

1. Keeping the mouth dry so that the ribbon will mark effectively
2. Holding the marking ribbon in place while the dentist manipulates the jaw (Figure 33-20)
3. Keeping the teeth cool while the selective grinding is being performed

For the assistant to be efficient in accomplishing his or her responsibilities, he or she must learn to effectively alternate three implements in concert with the procedures of the dentist: the marking ribbon, the evacuator suction tip, and the air syringe.

One of the secrets to rapid equilibration is to work in a dry mouth. Letting the teeth get wet prevents the ribbon from marking adequately. The combined use of vacuum evacuation and a stream of air soon dries up all but the worst salivator. We have found very little need for chemical anti-sialagogues if we have efficient assisting. Drying the teeth with a cotton roll leaves a thin film that reduces the effectiveness of the marking ribbon. The continuous stream of air on the occlusal surfaces in combination with the vacuum during grinding procedures keeps the teeth cool and dry. The marking ribbon can then be inserted immediately when the grinding is completed for each previous marking.

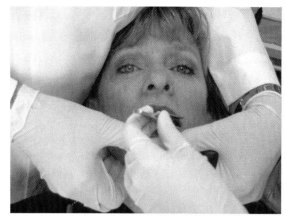

FIGURE 33-20 Since bilateral manipulation involves both hands, the chairside assistant must place and hold the ribbon while the dentist taps the teeth together in centric relation guided closure.

All equilibration procedures except the final check for long centric interferences can be accomplished with the patient in a supine position. The dentist and the assistant can be seated comfortably. The dentist should have easy access to the handpiece. The assistant holds two implements and lays the third on the patient's chest or on the bracket table. (In the supine position, patients do not object to having instruments laid on the napkin near their left shoulder. It is the most convenient place for the assistant.)

Hand and head signals can be used for rapid communication with the assistant. A nod of the dentist's head means to insert the ribbon. Hand positions can be worked out to show where to place the ribbon. Raising the thumb means to take out all instruments so that the occlusion can be checked. Voiceless communication is not only faster, it is a more relaxing way to work.

ARMAMENTARIUM FOR EQUILIBRATION

For Marking Interferences

Ribbons
The most efficient way to mark interferences is to use very thin film impregnated with different colors of ink. The material of choice for me is AccuFilm®. The thinness of the film prevents it from smudging around the sides of cusps and permits it to mark only surfaces that contact. It must be changed after several markings because the ink is lifted off the film by the pressure of the contacts and transferred to the teeth.

Ribbon holder
AccuFilm® (Parkell Inc., Edgewood, NY) and other types of thin marking ribbons are best held in place with a holder. The Miller ribbon holder is excellent. Several holders should

be loaded with two colors so that time is not lost at the chair replacing worn ribbons.

Marking paper

Marking paper is not generally the best material for marking interferences because the ink rubs off too easily and smudges. If the paper is not too easily penetrated or torn, it is acceptable as long as it is not too thick. Thick papers do not confine the marks to the first interference. They tend to also mark any inclines that are as close to contact as the thickness of the ribbon. For that reason, I sometimes use a thicker paper for marking balancing inclines for which I want more separation.

Waxes

Thin sheets of dark-colored wax can be placed over the occlusal surface of the teeth in one arch. The opposing teeth are then tapped gently into the wax until it perforates. The perforations represent interfering contacts. They are then marked with a pencil and then reduced, with the usual rules for grinding being followed. The procedure is repeated until the perforations are in the right spots.

Wax is an excellent material for finding interferences on sharp-line angles that are often difficult to pick up by other methods. As a routinely used material, however, it is not recommended because it requires an excessively large amount of time, compared with the use of marking ribbons.

Pastes, sprays, and paint-on materials

A variety of materials are available that can be painted or sprayed onto tooth contact, and then the material is perforated so that the contact areas are made visible. The use of such materials can be extremely accurate because the film thickness is so thin.

COMPUTER-ASSISTED DYNAMIC OCCLUSAL ANALYSIS

One of the most innovative systems for quantitative occlusal analysis was developed by Maness. Through a menu-driven software system, the T-scan® II system from Tekscan (Boston, MA) uses a sensor unit that records occlusal contacts on a thin Mylar film and relays the information to a computer. Through analysis of the occlusal contacts, it is possible to determine the sequence and timing of which teeth contact and with what degree of comparative force. Comparisons can be made for occlusal contacts in centric relation versus maximal intercuspation.

The T-scan® II system is practical in that it allows direct real-time recordings of occlusal contacts to be shown on a monitor during any phase of functional jaw movements. It also allows the operator to record contacts at any jaw relationship either on the monitor or on a printout. A special value of the system is that it provides immediate information that is understandable for the patient regarding stressful oc-

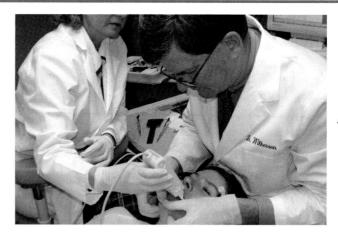

A

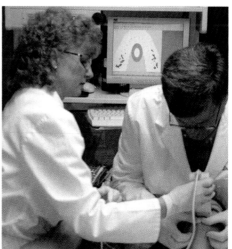

B

FIGURE 33-21 The assistant holds the sensor unit in place as the dentist manipulates to centric and verifies that the joints are completely seated in centric relation. While the dentist maintains upward loading through the jaw joints, the patient or the dentist can tap. The contacts can be seen directly on the computer screen or can be printed. This instrumentation has been continuously improved since its inception and has furnished excellent data regarding the importance of minute interferences in centric relation. It has also documented the importance of immediate posterior disclusion as an effective goal for achieving peaceful coordinated musculature.

clusal contacts. The hard-copy printouts are also valuable as a permanent record. A three-dimensional representation of the occlusal contact data is shown by use of columns that emanate from each contact point. The height of the column indicates relative timing of the contact or relative force (Figure 33-21).

The T-scan® II system is so simple to use and provides such clearly defined quantification of both time and force sequence of contacts that it appears to have promise as a practical method for use in routine occlusal analysis and treatment. Posttreatment results can also be clearly recorded for the patient's permanent record.

With the availability of precise methods for quantifying occlusal contacts, it has become all the more important that dentists understand the importance of multiple equal-intensity contacts and develop the skills for correcting oc-

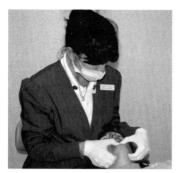

FIGURE 33-22 Joanne Schultz, RDH, has been trained to check for occlusal interferences at every hygiene appointment.

clusions to such a precise end point. It should be remembered that no instrumentation can take the place of the operator's judgment. Such instruments have little if any value without that judgment and the equilibration skills that go with it (Figure 33-22).

LONG-TERM OCCLUSAL STABILITY

One of the most commonly heard criticisms of occlusal equilibration is that it does not last. We are told that even the most precisely done occlusal correction always redevelops a new "slide" from centric relation to maximum intercuspation.

It is true that some apparently perfected occlusions do redevelop varying degrees of a slide. In my experience, those are by far the exception. If the occlusion is once corrected to the point of stability, patients remain amazingly stable. Retrospective analysis of my equilibrated or restored patients has shown that post-op redevelopment of interferences is a rarity. Every patient is checked for both tooth hypermobility, and interferences in centric relation and excursions at every hygiene visit. Patients who have not been re-equilibrated for 10 to 30 years still have stable occlusions, with only rare exceptions requiring minimal correction.

Historically, such stability has not always been the norm. In earlier years (prior to 1965) when I was shoving the jaw back into the most retruded position, readjustment of occlusions was a common necessity. Long-term stability has been achieved with attention to the following:

Equilibration Procedures in a Nutshell

1. Find and verify centric relation or adapted centric posture (ACP). Rule out intracapsular disorders.
2. Mount casts with a facebow and a centric relation or adapted centric bite record.
3. Analyze casts to make sure that equilibration is the best choice of treatment.
4. Eliminate all deflective inclines that interfere with complete closure in centric relation or ACP.
5. Verify simultaneous contact on both posterior teeth and anterior teeth if arch alignment permits.
6. Verify that maximum intercuspation occurs in perfect harmony with centric relation or ACP.
7. Eliminate all excursive contact on posterior teeth. The only posterior tooth contact is in centric relation or ACP.
8. Refine anterior guidance for all excursions (may need to do more reduction of excursive inclines on posteriors as anterior guidance is altered).
9. Recheck posterior teeth while *firmly* clenching and grinding. There should be no contacts on inclines.
10. Verify dots in back . . . lines in front.
11. Test the results. If an empty mouth clench can cause any sign of discomfort or pressure in any posterior tooth, the equilibration is not completed.

---

1. Determining *and verifying* a stable centric relation using bilateral manipulation
2. More preciseness in recording the uppermost position of the TMJs
3. Changing from group function to posterior disclusion in all excursions
4. Better understanding of the importance of anterior guidance in harmony with the envelope of function and the neutral zone
5. Correcting occlusions to cusp-tip–to–fossa relationships
6. Careful observation and correction of hypermobile teeth that interfered without causing a slide
7. Meticulous clearance of molar interferences including those at heavy clenching and grinding movements
8. Continuing to refine occlusions until stability of the TMJs was verified and tooth rebound was complete
9. Never starting an equilibration without finishing the job

Chapter 34

Neuromuscular Dentistry: Bioelectronic Instrumentation

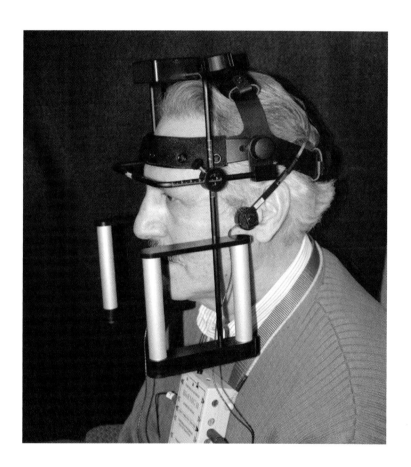

PRINCIPLE

Even accurate data collection can mislead if its interpretation is based on wrong assumptions.

EXAMINING THE RHETORIC

For the past few years, many dentists searching for answers regarding occlusion have been confused by an intense campaign to discredit centric relation dentistry. For those who understand centric relation and have a reasonable grasp of the role of how occlusion affects the neuromuscular system, it is not a problem to separate facts from commercially driven rhetoric about neuromuscular dentistry (NMD). Dentists who have not had an adequate education on principles of occlusion, however, are often swayed by assurances that NMD is the cutting edge that replaces "old fashioned and outdated concepts." Such claims are seriously misleading. It is important that we differentiate the proper use of bioelectronic instrumentation from its use to promote a clinical agenda that has serious flaws.

It is unfortunate that the term *neuromuscular dentistry* has been taken out of its proper context to promote concepts that are in such clear violation of the true meaning of what Ramfjord[1] and others have advocated as the primary goal of all occlusal therapy: *a peaceful neuromuscular system.* The principles advocated in this text have been routinely subjected to very rigid and very specific *criteria for success* (see Chapter 47). The results of NMD as advocated by its principal proponents cannot pass those tests. It is important to understand why, so let's take an objective look at NMD and point out the specific reasons for rejecting it as a replacement for centric relation dentistry.

It Is Not the Instrumentation, But How It Is Used

Advancements in electronic modalities have been impressive, and there are many applications that have value in diagnosis and treatment of occlusal problems. In my former practice, electronic instrumentation is being used to advantage in several different ways. The important thing to realize is that electronic instrumentation cannot change physiological or biomechanical principles. It can help us measure and record. The use of sophisticated electronic instrumentation has value, however, only when used to achieve realistic goals of treatment based on the *requirements for occlusal stability* (see Chapter 29). It is important to realize that regardless of how accurately data may be collected, it is the interpretation of the data that is critical. The problem with NMD as it is being promoted is not with instrumentation. The problem is with misinterpretation based on some seriously flawed concepts.

Centric Relation versus the Claims of NMD

Dentists who understand the physiologic and biomechanical reasons for centric relation will not be misled. Unfortunately, it is the unusual dentist who graduates today with a workable knowledge of occlusion and the temporomandibular joints (TMJs). Without this solid basis for clinical decision making, dentists can get their patients (and themselves) into some costly problems. NMD warrants serious scrutiny before accepting it as an alternative to centric relation dentistry. The conflict in philosophy and concept is too important to ignore.

The label of NMD has quite an appeal because it appears to be in synch with the "peaceful neuromusculature" that has been advocated by Dawson,[2] Ramfjord,[3] Mann and Pankey,[4] and others for many years. But don't be fooled by the label. As long as NMD[5] is limited by its promoters to a clinical process that denies the importance of centric relation, and advocates jaw relationships that are potentially problematic, one should be aware of its shortcomings.

Part of the appeal of NMD is its use of electromyography (EMG) to measure muscle activity. There is nothing wrong with this. The problem lies in misinterpretation of the data. We have learned much of what we know about muscle coordination versus incoordination from extensive use of EMG research.[6-10] However, there is a tremendously important difference in EMG studies that include needle electrodes into the separate bellies of the pterygoid muscles versus the use of the surface electrodes on the skin to determine the maxillo-mandibular relationship. One of the most critical requirements for centric relation is the timely release of the inferior lateral pterygoid muscle during closure. Lateral pterygoid activity cannot be measured by surface electrodes and is not a consideration in NMD.

And what is wrong with using biomedical instrumentation for relaxation of muscles? There is nothing wrong with it. We have used transcutaneous electrical neural stimulation (TENS) for releasing muscle spasms and hyperactivity for many years, although simpler methods are just as effective, less time-consuming, and do not require expensive equipment. What is highly erroneous is the conclusion that electronic stimulation of the masticatory muscles determines the correct jaw relationship. The concept as explained by Dickerson is that "the comfortable position of the mandible is determined by muscles, not joint anatomy." But that is not a true picture of how muscles function. Sophisticated EMG studies show that how the condyle-disk assemblies relate to the glenoid fossae during tooth contact has a profound effect on masticatory muscles. Disharmony between the occlusion and the joint anatomy is a major cause of masticatory muscle pain and dysfunction.

The major flaw in NMD is its denial of centric relation.[11-13] This is based on electronic muscle stimulation that recruits the lateral pterygoid muscles into contraction while determining the jaw-to-jaw relationship. This results in a down and forward posture for the TMJs[14-16] and automatic occlusal interferences that require displacement of the TMJs to achieve maximum intercuspation. This down and forward position for the TMJs is actually advocated as the correct jaw relationship for NMD occlusion.[11]

The second major flaw in NMD is its reliance on a rest position as programmed by electronic instrumentation, as the starting position for determining maximal intercuspa-

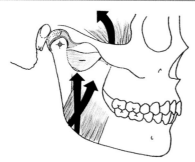

FIGURE 34-1   **The goal:** *Coordinated* muscle is assured if maximum intercuspation is coincident with centric relation. EMG studies confirm this.[2,7,8,10] Clinical experience with thousands of patients confirms that it is predictably comfortable.

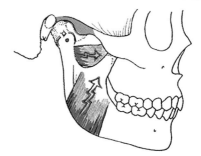

FIGURE 34-2   The result of NMD forward posturing as established by Myomonitor recording of condyle position. The lateral pterygoid muscle must oppose elevator muscle contraction during every closure. EMG studies with needle electrodes confirm this.

tion. This routinely results in a forward postured jaw position at an increased vertical dimension.

Increasing the vertical dimension based on electronic instrument determination of a rest position[11] is unscientific at best. The vertical dimension of occlusion is determined by the repetitive contracted length of the elevator muscles. At rest, the teeth are not in contact. Use of the longer resting length of muscle to influence or determine the vertical dimension of occlusal contact can lead to unnecessary overtreatment. Unfortunately, it is being used by some to justify complete coverage of all the teeth in patients who could be better served by conservative dentistry at their correct vertical dimension.

The increased vertical dimension that is so often advocated by NMD proponents also results in anterior teeth that are too long for a natural appearance. It also puts those teeth at a stress disadvantage because of the inappropriate alteration of crown-root ratios.

Problems associated with NMD are related to both the shortcomings of the instrumentation and the misinterpretation of data collected. The most serious problem is the inability of the advocated instrumentation to record an accurate centric relation. Jaw tracking that shows the condyles moving down and forward as the jaw opens are consistent with what we can easily observe clinically, but misinterpretation of those data by Myotronics advocates has resulted in the serious error of making the teeth occlude in a protruded relationship. This creates a variety of potential problems because coordinated muscle activity repeatedly pulls the condyles back and up into centric relation during jaw closure. Let's review what happens and the consequences of NMD jaw positioning (Figures 34-1 and 34-2).

The effect of having to displace the TMJs down the slope of the eminence to make the teeth fit is always directed at muscle. Extensive studies by Gibbs and Lundeen show that even when teeth are aligned to intercuspate with a forward-postured mandible, the elevator muscles repeatedly pull the joints up into centric relation during jaw closure.[6] Teeth that interfere with complete seating of the TMJs are in interference every time the patient clenches. This directs the heaviest loading on the most posterior teeth, which is a major

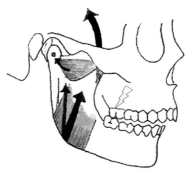

FIGURE 34-3   If the TMJs must be displaced downwardly to achieve intercuspation, heavy posterior contact overloads the teeth every time the elevator muscles pull the TMJs up into centric relation. Patients, directed by mechanoreceptor protective reflex responses, then tend to protrude the mandible to avoid the posterior interferences. The condyles have to move down to get forward, which takes the load off the posterior teeth. However, that often causes heavy contact against the anterior teeth. Dentists often misinterpret this and grind the front teeth when what is needed is to eliminate the deflective interferences on the posterior teeth.

cause of excessive occlusal wear, fractured teeth, and tooth hypermobility if the occlusion is not in harmony with the uppermost joint position (Figure 34-3).

An example of this misconception is the concept advocated by Dickerson and Jankelson in their explanation of anterior faceting: "Doesn't anterior wear suggest the masticatory muscles are trying to free the mandible from posterior entrapment by the maxilla?"[13] Clinical evaluation and treatment on thousands of occlusal problems is clearly in disagreement with this rationale.

A very important point to remember is that whenever you see heavy contact and wear on anterior teeth, always look first for deflective inclines on the posterior teeth that drive the mandible forward during closure. This is by far the most common cause of anterior wear and overload. If there are no interferences to centric relation at maximum intercuspation, look for premature contact of the anterior teeth during centric relation closure and examine for a restricted envelope of function (anterior guidance).

MAKING SENSE OF THE LITERATURE

The scientific literature has been very clear in its opposition to some of the major claims of NMD. Dentists who are searching for factual information should be wary of relying on claims of superiority that are routinely published in non-refereed promotional publications.

Analysis of the Literature

A partial review of the literature may illustrate how statements should be analyzed. Recognize that statements in the literature are not always correct, so keep an open mind and use references as a starting matrix for further analysis. The key to good analysis is in asking the right questions and then doing further literature search to compare with statements by the author. Let's use as an example the following statement published in a nonrefereed journal.[13]

"A physiologic jaw trajectory has now been scientifically determined, eliminating the need to use less accurate manual position in establishing an occlusal position."

Remember that in a nonrefereed journal that is published as promotion, the author is not held accountable for statements made, so special scrutiny is in order.

Questions you should ask:

1. Has jaw trajectory tracking really been scientifically determined as accurate and beneficial for determining the jaw-to-jaw relationship?
2. Is manual manipulation really less accurate?
3. Does the instrumentation being promoted determine a reproducible, unique position?

Let's examine references that have no commercial interest in the product. We'll turn to unbiased research studies in peer-reviewed journals.

The literature search reveals:

"Myomonitor centric registration does not result in a reproducible or unique mandibular position"[14]
"Bilateral manipulation showed the most consistent reproducibility of mandibular centricity"[15]
"Bilateral manipulation had the lowest random method error in all dimensions; the Myomonitor had the most errors"[16]
"Mandibular movements of symptomatic subjects could not be differentiated from those of normal subjects using four of the tests advocated by Myotronics, Inc."[17]

Recent Research

In one of the most extensive studies of bioelectronic diagnostic instrumentation done jointly at three universities and published in a peer-reviewed journal,[18] the results reported are consistent with what we have observed clinically over a period of years. This study supports the contention of many clinicians and researchers that the American Dental Association (ADA) does not have sufficient scientific evidence to warrant its seal of approval on certain bioelectronic devices including those promoted by NMD advocates. Some quotes from the study are as follows:

"The American Dental Association has approved several devices as aids in the diagnosis of temporomandibular disorders. Concerns remain however about their safety and effectiveness."
"These devices have not been shown to have stand alone diagnostic value and, when tested, they have demonstrated unacceptable sensitivity and specificity levels."
"The only gold standard for temporomandibular disorder is a global clinical examination performed and a thorough history taken by an expert examiner."
"There is considerable concern about the safety and effectiveness of these approaches."

Unfortunately, many of the objections to bioelectronic instrumentation are based on the distorted claims of NMD promoters. Use of the instrumentation to support concepts that encourage overtreatment or wrong treatment should be criticized. However, an open mind should be encouraged regarding when the instrumentation can have value.

Clinical Concerns

There are some major concerns regarding the long-term effects from NMD results. One of the most obvious problems occurs because coordinated masticatory muscles generate a vector of force that pulls the condyles up into centric relation when heavy clenching and bruxing occur during sleep. The mandible must fulcrum around the most posterior teeth to achieve complete seating of the joints, putting excessive overload on the molar teeth. This problem, which is what is produced by following the down-forward condylar position advocated by NMD, is exactly what proper equilibration attempts to correct. Correction of an occlusion to permit complete centric relation seating of the condyles during maximum intercuspation is so routinely successful, it hardly seems reasonable that a concept that puts the interferences in place could be credible (Figure 34-4).

Accuracy of jaw-to-jaw relations

An argument against NMD that has never been answered is the consistent finding that the Myomonitor does not produce a unique or repeatable position for the condyles.[14-16] The only way we can predictably eliminate deflective inclines on crowns, bridges, or implant prostheses is to work with casts that are *precisely* related in centric relation. A bite record that produces a different jaw relationship every time it is recorded falls far short of what is needed for predictably successful results. Advocacy of a down-and-forward condylar position by NMD advocates is a serious mistake that is the cause of many problems with comfort, excessive over-

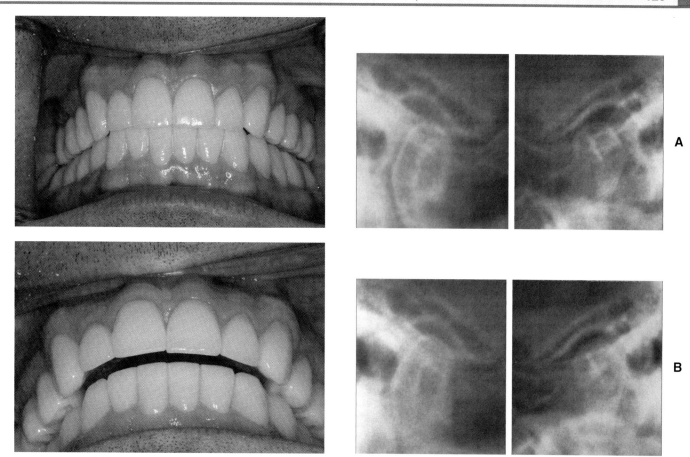

FIGURE 34-4 Classic example of Myomonitor centric as advocated by NMD leaders. **A,** Maximal intercuspation position for complete mouth reconstruction by NMD advocate. As shown in radiographs taken at maximal closure, down-forward displacement of both TMJs is required to achieve this relationship. The patient was extremely uncomfortable with muscle pain and sore teeth. This down-forward condyle displacement is exactly as advocated by NMD leaders in lectures, courses, and literature. **B,** Occlusal relationship when the TMJs go to centric relation. Note how the anterior open bite results from pivoting around the last molar as the elevator muscles pull the condyles up. An occlusal splint made to allow complete seating to centric relation produced complete comfort. Note centered condyle position on TMJ radiograph made at the comfortable centric relation jaw position. Correction of this NMD occlusion requires remaking the restorations.

load on posterior teeth, and a tendency in the long term toward instability.

Muscle Recruitment: A False Argument

One of the most consistent claims by NMD advocates to justify the "neuromuscular position" is that it results in the greatest degree of muscle recruitment possible. Proponents of the neuromuscular position claim that patients are able to chew better when restorations are built in such a power position for the musculature. Generating a greater clenching force in the neuromuscular position is exactly what you don't want during nocturnal episodes of bruxing and clenching, especially with molars in interference to the fully seated joint position.

It is true that there is less muscle recruitment in centric relation. The goal of a perfected occlusion is actually to have the lateral pterygoid muscles shut off during maximal closure to tooth contact. NMD activates (recruits) the lateral pterygoid muscles along with increased electrical activity in all of the elevator muscles, which is exactly what Williamson, Mahan, and others demonstrated when posterior occlusal interferences were present.[7,9]

The ability to chew food is never an issue with a perfected occlusion. The primary concern with an NMD occlusal relationship is not just that muscle hyperactivity is stimulated. It is that it is stimulated to produce nonaxial forces at the most susceptible power point of the entire occlusion, the molar teeth. This is particularly problematic in implant prostheses because implants cannot tolerate nonaxial forces without damage.

It is nonaxial loading that destroys bone around implants and damages fixtures, breaks screws, and causes restorations to fail. The increase in the vertical dimension of occlusion that occurs with the use of the Myomonitor in the recommended NMD position results in an unfavorable crown-root ratio for implants or restored teeth. Coupled with increased muscle forces and nonaxial loading, it is an unnecessary added risk for failure.

NMD CRITICISM AGAINST CENTRIC RELATION

The rhetoric denouncing the use of centric relation has been profuse and unrelenting in nonjuried publications and especially in promotional type journals. Constant attacks against centric relation are an almost daily fare on the Internet along with claims for the superiority of NMD. Informed dentists can readily separate the false rhetoric from the facts. That is why it is so important to understand the true rationales that undergird the requirements for stability. It is also important to understand why some of the most prevalent NMD arguments against centric relation are based on misinformation and lack of experience in treating patients with occlusal disorders.

NMD position: Centric relation is repeatable but not necessarily comfortable.

Centric relation perspective: The condyle-disk assemblies in centric relation are comfortable. That is why load testing is used to verify that centric relation has been accurately achieved. It is diagnostic that if the joints are not completely comfortable when loaded, they are not in centric relation.

NMD position: Manipulating techniques have proven invalid when using EMG and jaw-tracking instrumentation.

Centric relation perspective: Quite the opposite is true. EMG studies have repeatedly confirmed that when maximal intercuspation is in harmony with centric relation, muscle activity is coordinated and a resting level of muscle activity is resumed immediately when the teeth separate. Tracking the jaw to a confirmed centric relation while simultaneously recording EMG status of the masticatory muscles while tooth contact is recorded on a T-scan provides evidence for the importance of the centric relation/occlusion relationship. If occlusal interferences to a manipulated closure to centric relation are present, there is an increase in electrical activity and a delay in returning to a peaceful level of muscle activity when the teeth separate.

NMD position: Even teachers of centric relation techniques claim that few dentists can master this procedure.

Centric relation perspective: That is not what our experience has been. At our Dawson Center, classes of 20 dentists typically locate and verify an accurate centric relation by the end of the first morning. They verify repeatability with needlepoint preciseness using multiple bite records and recordings on a Centri-Check instrument. With further practice, the procedure becomes progressively easier (see Chapter 11).

NMD position: Even if a dentist is trained to do this, it (centric relation) is not necessarily a functioning physiologic position.

Centric relation perspective: Casts mounted in centric relation consistently show that on teeth that can touch in centric relation, facets of wear always extend all the way to centric relation. If the jaw doesn't function in centric relation, how do wear facets form on teeth that interfere with centric relation? The main purpose of smooth permissive occlusal splints is to permit the musculature to move the mandible without restriction to whatever condylar position is dictated by coordinated muscle action. When free to do so, muscles always seat the condyles in centric relation during closure (see Chapter 6). Learn the meaning of *coordinated* muscle activity.

NMD position: What medical doctor ever manipulates a joint in a so-called seated position when treating an injury or pathologic joint problem in the orthopedic medical profession? None.

Centric relation perspective: Load testing of joints is a standard orthopedic procedure for orthopedic physicians. The load testing process always starts with gentle compression, and if no tenderness results, gradual increments of increased compression are applied. Load testing is one of the most reliable tests for determining if the source of pain is in the joint structures. This diagnostic information is critical in the analysis of TMJ-related pain (see Chapter 10).

ACCEPTABLE INSTRUMENTATION

As advances in electronics make bioelectronic instrumentation more accurate and more practical, there will be a stream of new sophisticated ways for measuring masticatory system function. At this point, some old and some new devices do have merit as long as they are used in a context of understanding the tried and true principles of diagnosis. Some of the most useful methods are as follows:

Doppler auscultation

Developed by Dr. Mark Piper,[19] Doppler auscultation has become a standard diagnostic device for determining the condition of the intracapsular structures so that a classification of joint condition can be determined. It is highly accurate, especially for determining the degree of disk derangements. There is a learning curve to becoming competent in its use.

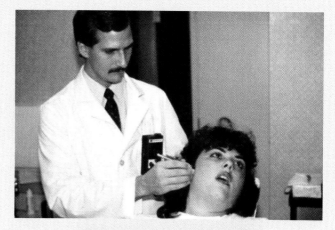

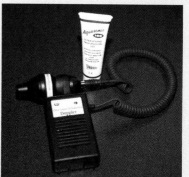

Joint vibration analysis (JVA)

This instrument measures vibrations within the joint that are characteristic of different changes that occur when deformation has taken place. Like the Doppler, there is a learning curve to become competent in its use. However, it has the advantage of producing a visual image of the recording and permits a permanent hard-copy record. It does not rely on sound but records the wavelengths of different types of vibrations. It can be paired with other devices to synchronize the vibration analysis with jaw-tracking and EMG recordings.

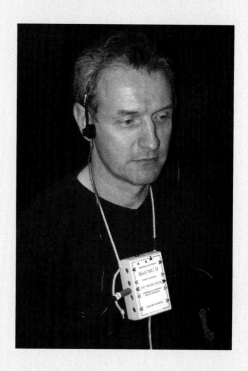

T-Scan II® computerized occlusal analysis system

First introduced by Maness and others in 1984 as the T-Scan I system, the new version from Tekscan (Boston, MA) has become one of the most practical measuring instruments for precise analysis of occlusal contacts.[20] The T-scan can be synchronized with the Biopak Electromyography recording system to simultaneously record and play back the effect that occlusal contacts have on muscle function. However, the use of the T-scan alone has value as a precise recorder of occlusal interferences and as a guide for determining when occlusal treatment has been completed.

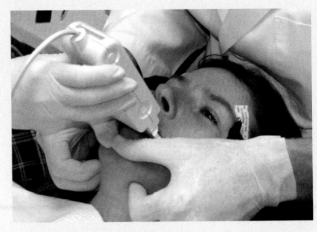

A T-scan recording showing heavier contacts on the left side as evidenced by the taller column where the heaviest contact occurs.

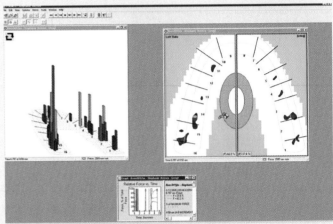

A more balanced occlusion as noted by the red marker on the midline and the fairly even heights of the columns. It should be clearly noted that it is still essential to properly manipulate the jaw to centric relation and hold the joints in the seated position when closing the jaw to record tooth contacts.

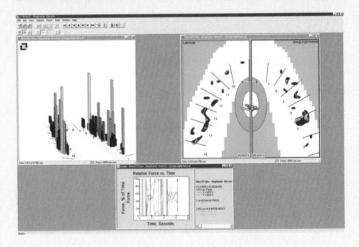

Kerstein[21] has used the T-Scan to demonstrate the tremendous importance of immediate disclusion when the mandible moves from centric relation. He has measured the variation in muscle responses as well as myofascial pain symptoms as disclusion time is shortened. This is excellent documentation for the importance of the occlusal concepts recommended in this text and is in agreement with other research studies.

Electromyography

The BioPak Electromyography Recording System has made recording EMG a practical diagnostic tool in the dental office. Much of what we have learned about occlusion and the effect it has on muscle coordination, incoordination, and hyperactivity has been learned through EMG studies. While there is a great variation in EMG studies from simple skin surface electrodes to elegant studies,[22,23] using needle electrodes into single motor units of muscle, useful information can nevertheless be gleaned from surface EMG recordings. Ramfjord[24] showed that muscle responses during swallowing were adversely affected by occlusal interferences, and the muscle incoordination was quickly converted to coordinated function when the occlusal interferences to centric relation were removed. He also demonstrated that in a harmonious occlusion the electrical activity of the muscles quiets down almost immediately after a clench is released whereas with occlusal disharmony muscle activity is prolonged after the teeth are separated.

EMG studies recorded in our practice as well as numerous sophisticated studies using eight-track EMG recordings are absolutely in agreement with the concepts presented in this text: If we can get precise harmony between the occlusion and intact TMJs, we can get "happy muscles."

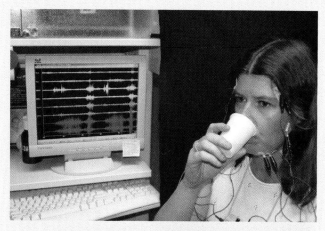

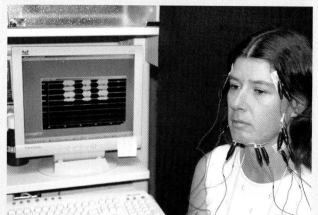

Jaw tracking

The combination of jaw tracking and JVA offers some interesting insights into the timing of joint deformations in relation to jaw movements. The Biopak system has made it possible to coordinate these recordings with relative ease once the learning curve has been mastered.

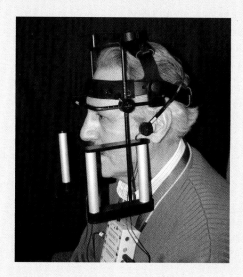

Commentary

If one is under the impression that any or all of the bioelectronic devices will impart expertise in occlusal diagnosis or treatment, it is a false assumption. The devices described above measure specific factors, all of which are important in regard to total masticatory system harmony. The data will be meaningless and possibly even misleading for a clinician who does not have an in-depth understanding of the anatomy, physiology, and biomechanics of the masticatory system.

An accurate requirement for using bioelectronic instrumentation would be a global understanding of differential diagnosis of TMDs. A dentist who does not have a clear understanding of Piper's Classification of intracapsular TMDs will not have a logical basis for interpreting the data that this equipment is capable of producing. The starting point for diagnosing TMDs and for understanding differential diagnosis of occlusal disorders is to first learn how the masticatory system functions in health and in disorder. Then there will be a logical basis for understanding what is being measured and what it means.

SUMMARY

No instrument, electronic device, or automated system of any kind can supersede the necessity of understanding how the masticatory system functions or dysfunctions. Clinicians who do not know how the masticatory system works will not know what is wrong when it isn't working properly regardless of the type of instrumentation available to them.

The only acceptable standard for diagnosis of occlusal problems is a thorough examination and history performed by an examiner who understands the biomechanics of mandibular function and what is required to achieve harmony between the TMJs, the anterior guidance, the posterior teeth, and the corresponding responses of the masticatory musculature.

As improved bioelectronic instrumentation becomes available to add to an already impressive choice of instruments, smart clinicians will use devices that are cost-effective and accurate to help them in their clinical evaluation. They will not use such instruments to invent clinical methods that are in violation of proven scientific principles and knowledge of masticatory system harmony.

References

1. Ramfjord SP, Ash MM: *Occlusion,* ed 3, Philadelphia, 1983, WB Saunders,
2. Dawson PE: *Evaluation, diagnosis and treatment of occlusal problems,* St Louis, 1989, Mosby.
3. Ramfjord SP: Dysfunctional temporomandibular joint and muscle pain, *J Prosthet Dent* 11:353-374, 1961.
4. Mann AW, Pankey LD: Oral rehabilitation. *J Prosthet Dent* 50: 685-689, 1983.
5. Radu M, Mirandici M, Hottel T: The effect of clenching on condylar position: A vector analysis model. *J Prosthet Dent* 91(2):171-179, 2004.
6. Gibbs CH, Lundeen HC: Jaw movements and forces during chewing and swallowing and their clinical significance. *Advances in Occlusion,* Boston, 1982, John Wright-PSG, Inc.
7. Williamson EH, Lundquist DO: Anterior guidance: Its effect on anterior temporalis and masseter muscles. *J Prosthet Dent* 34:816-823, 1982.
8. Sheikholeslam G, Mollar E, Louis I: Postural and maximal activity in elevators of the mandible before and after treatment of functional disorders. *Scan J Dent Research* 90(1):37-46, 1982.
9. Mahan PE, Wilkinson TM, Gibbs CH, et al: Superior and inferior bellies of the lateral pterygoid muscle EMG at basic jaw positions. *J Prosthet Dent* 50(5):710-718, 1983.
10. Schaerer P, Stallard, RE, Zander HA: Occlusal interferences and mastication: An electromyographic study. *J Prosthet Dent* 17(5):438-449, 1967.
11. Chan CA: Identify a physiologic mandibular rest position—the key to taking an accurate bite. Part II, *LVI Visions*: Las Vegas Institute for Advanced Dental Studies.
12. Chan CA: Centric relation—time tested ignorance. *LVI Visions*: Las Vegas Institute for Advanced Dental Studies, 2000.
13. Dickerson WG: The truth about centric relation. *LVI Visions* 8(6): Las Vegas Institute for Advanced Dental Studies, 1999.
14. Carlson J: The mandible and centric relation. *LVI Visions*: Las Vegas Institute for Advanced Dental Studies, 1999.
15. Dickerson WG: Why neuromuscular dentistry? *LVI Visions*: Las Vegas Institute for Advanced Dental Studies.
16. Roblee RD: The determination of the accuracy and reproducibility of six maxillomandibular relation techniques. Thesis, Baylor University, 1989.
17. Feine JS, Hutchins MO, Lund JP: An evaluation of the criteria used to diagnose mandibular dysfunction with the mandibular kineseography. *J Prosthet Dent* 60:374-380, 1980.
18. Baba K, Tsukiyama Y, Yamazaki M, et al: A review of temporomandibular disorder diagnostic techniques. *J Prosthet Dent* 86(2):184-194, 2001.
19. Dawson PE, Piper MA: Temporomandibular disorders and orofacial pain. Seminar Manual. St. Petersburg Center for Advanced Dental Study, 1993.
20. Maness WL: Force movie. A time and force view of occlusion. *Compendium* 10:404-408, 1989.
21. Kerstein RB: Treatment of myofascial pain dysfunction syndrome with occlusal therapy to reduce lengthy disclusion time—a recall study. *J Craniomandib Pract* 13(2):105-115, 1995.
22. Murray GM, Phanachet I, Uchids S, et al: The role of the human lateral pterygoid muscle in the control of horizontal jaw movements. *J Orofacial Pain* 15(4):279-292 discussion; 292-305 review, 2001.
23. Phanachet I, Whittle T, Wanagaratne K, et al: Minimal tonic firing rates of human lateral pterygoid single motor units. *Clin Neurophysical* 115(1):71-75, 2004.
24. Ramfjord SP: Dysfunctional temporomandibular joint and muscle pain. *J Prosthet Dent* 11:353, 1961.

Chapter 35

Solving Occlusal Wear Problems

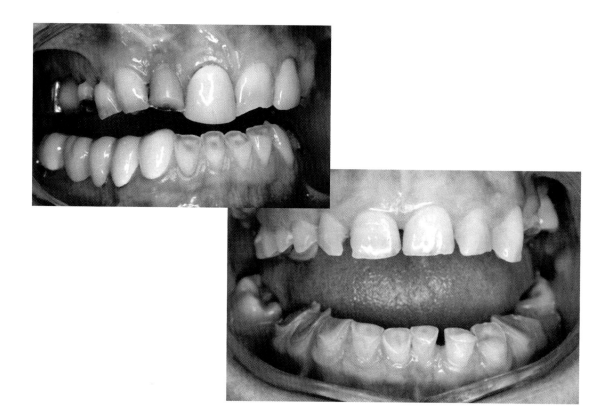

PRINCIPLE

Occlusal wear occurs seven times faster when dentin is exposed. "Watching it" doesn't help.

IMPORTANT CONSIDERATIONS

Severely worn dentitions present one of the greatest challenges in dentistry. Yet the treatment planning process for severe wear can be simplified if the rules for *programmed treatment planning* are precisely adhered to in correct sequence, starting with verification of stable, completely seated temporomandibular joints (TMJs).

Before discussing the specifics of treatment planning, there are six observations that should be understood:

1. Severe wear does not cause a loss of vertical dimension of occlusion (VDO).
2. Severe wear does not eliminate all deflective occlusal interferences (even if the occlusal surfaces appear to be flat).
3. Severe attritional wear can only occur if upper teeth are *in the way* of lower teeth during functional or parafunctional movements of the mandible.
4. Severe attritional wear is not caused by bruxing or clenching unless teeth are in the way of mandibular movements. Teeth cannot wear if they cannot rub.
5. Posterior teeth cannot wear (from attrition) if posterior disclusion is perfected and the anterior guidance is stable.
6. Do not steepen or restrict the envelope of function except as a last resort. Any restriction of the anterior guidance can result in wear, mobility, or movement of the anterior teeth and a loss of the critical disclusive effect on posterior teeth.

The goal of treatment for all severe wear patients is posterior disclusion the moment the mandible moves from centric relation . . . discluded by a perfected anterior guidance.

IDENTIFY THE CAUSE OF THE WEAR

Types of Wear

The four types of wear are attritional wear, wear from erosion, abrasive wear, and wear caused by toothpaste abuse. The paragraphs that follow describe the types of wear in detail.

Attritional wear

This is wear caused by rubbing tooth surfaces of the lower arch against tooth surfaces of the upper arch. Attritional wear cannot occur if lower teeth cannot rub against upper teeth that are in the way. If there is attritional wear on posterior teeth, it is certain that they are in interference with either the completely seated TMJs or/and the anterior guidance. Intracapsular TMJ disorders that result in a shortened ramus height put the molars into interference and contribute to excessive wear.

If the cause of wear is attritional, all worn surfaces can be contacted during centric relation closure or during excursions to and from centric relation. If a worn surface cannot be contacted by opposing teeth, the wear is caused by something other than attrition. The most likely cause is erosion from chemical action.

Wear from erosion

This is the result of chemical action on tooth surfaces. The most likely possibilities include:

1. *Carbonated beverages* that are very acidic. Always ask about consumption of carbonated soda drinks, which have an acidic pH approaching that of battery acid.

Abrahamsen has listed "coke-swishing" as the second major cause of wear from erosion.[1] This refers to the habit of swishing carbonated drinks back and forth in the mouth to reduce the uncomfortable sensation of carbonation in the throat. This diagnosis can be confirmed when the wear patterns on the hand-articulated casts do not coincide and when cupping or cratering with sharp enamel edges is present. Amalgam restorations will be raised above the eroded surface. The molars are the prime location of the cupping effect.

2. *Gastric esophageal reflux disease (GERD).* The reflux of highly acidic gastric excretions may be a cause of dissolution of enamel. Loss of enamel does not follow any occlusal contact surfaces and is more pronounced around the molars. It varies according to sleeping positions but is most likely found on the lingual surfaces of molars. Restoration to resurface corroded areas is quite effective if the restorations are extended into the gingival sulci.

3. *Regurgitation.* Projectile vomiting is a potent cause of wear from erosion. The pattern of wear is diagnostic as it is most noticeable on the upper anterior segment. The wear extends all the way to the gingival margin on the lingual surfaces. The lower anterior teeth are not involved because they are protected by the tongue. Upper or lower posterior teeth are often affected, primarily on the palatal surfaces. Abrahamsen has pointed out that cupping or cratering is quite common.[1] If amalgam restorations are present, they will be elevated above the eroded tooth surfaces.

The typical pattern of wear from regurgitation is a classic diagnostic sign of bulimia, a psychological disorder that is characterized by self-induced vomiting. Every attempt should be made to get professional help for a patient who exhibits these signs. It is my experience that such patients are often resistant to recommendations for such help, but gentle concern for the patient's welfare seems to be the best approach.

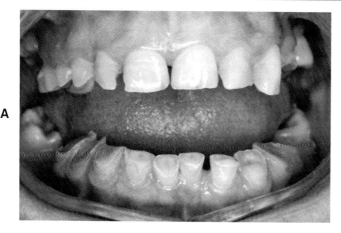

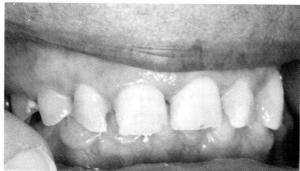

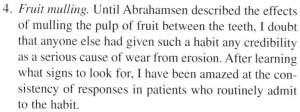

FIGURE 35-1 **A,** Severe wear at first appears to be a form of chemical damage. Analysis of the occlusion shows that all worn areas are reachable by excursions of the mandible. **B,** The patient had no habits of using any erosive or abrasive materials. The diagnosis is a form of enamelogenesis imperfecta that made the teeth uniquely susceptible to attritional wear. Restoration of the dentition with full coverage on all teeth resulted in a long-term successful result. However, because the wear was allowed to progress to such a severe degree, the restorative process was made more complex and more costly, and required surgical crown lengthening that would have been unnecessary if treatment had been started earlier.

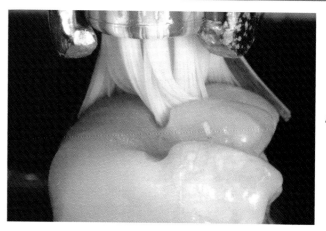

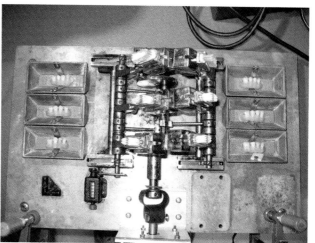

FIGURE 35-2 **A,** Deep noncarious cervical lesions with sharp line angles resulted solely from brushing with toothpaste. Research by Dr. John Dzakovich showed that no wear was produced while brushing without toothpaste.[2] **B,** Brushing machine used by Dr. Dzakovich to duplicate work by Dr. W.D. Miller. Horizontal brushing strokes on embedded teeth routinely produced lesions that are identical to what has been described as abfractions. No lesions were produced when toothpaste was not used.

4. *Fruit mulling.* Until Abrahamsen described the effects of mulling the pulp of fruit between the teeth, I doubt that anyone else had given such a habit any credibility as a serious cause of wear from erosion. After learning what signs to look for, I have been amazed at the consistency of responses in patients who routinely admit to the habit.

Look for cupping or cratering with abraded enamel edges on both upper and lower posterior teeth. The wear is about equal on both arches, and abraded enamel edges are peripheral to the cups or craters. Abrahamsen has listed fruit mulling as the third major cause of wear from erosion. It is often observed in vegetarians who are heavy bruxers.[1]

Abrasive wear

Abrasive wear is typically seen in tobacco chewers as a result of grinding the teeth with an abrasive material between the occlusal surfaces. It can cause occlusal wear even in a perfected occlusion.

The wear patterns can sometimes be confusing. I have seen bizarre wear patterns in patients who eat a lot of seeds and break the seeds open between their anterior teeth, forming a deep *V* between the central incisors.

The rule is simple: If the worn surface cannot be contacted by the opposing teeth, look for abrasive wear from some habitual use of an abrasive substance. Or look for a chemical cause of erosive action on the enamel surface (Figure 35-1).

Toothpaste abuse

The abrasive effect of toothpaste is a far greater cause of wear than previously realized. Abrahamsen and Dzakovich have shown clearly how much damage can be done on any enamel surface by vigorous brushing with toothpaste (Figure 35-2).[1,2] The use of a toothbrush without toothpaste does not produce any noticeable wear. It is significant that a study of skulls from periods before toothpaste or toothpowder was introduced does not show any signs of abfraction lesions or other effect that match the wear produced by toothpaste.

Apparent Closed Bite Due to Wear

A popular misconception about severely worn dentitions is that patients have lost their VDO and that it must be restored. This belief is reinforced when patients complain about needing more support for relief of muscle fatigue. Many patients feel that they have lost their VDO because of the strained feeling they have when they hold their teeth together. The most closed position is *always* a strained relationship because all of the elevator muscles are in a state of contraction when the teeth are together. The muscle fatigue is further intensified if there are occlusal interferences to centric relation because the clenched position must be resisted by incoordinated and prolonged contraction of the lateral pterygoid muscles.

Facial profile should not be determined with the teeth clenched. Correct, natural facial height occurs with the teeth apart. It occurs at the resting length, not the contracted length of the elevator muscles. The teeth should not be in contact when the jaw is at the postural position that determines lip/face contour. One of the most persistent concepts regarding treatment of severely worn dentitions is that any increase in the VDO must be tested with provisional restorations "to see if the patient can tolerate" the increase in VDO. This is an unnecessary step because comfort is not a criterion of whether the VDO is correct. Comfort is unrelated to the determination of an acceptable VDO at maximal intercuspation. The comfort level is unaffected within a wide range of vertical alteration if the condyles have unrestricted access to centric relation. So there is no need for testing an increased VDO to see if a patient can tolerate it when restoring a severely worn occlusion.

What is more important regarding a changed VDO is the effect such a change has on the relationship of the anterior teeth. Increasing the VDO too much may result in anterior teeth that are too long. Remember also that opening the bite results in arcing the lower incisors back as well as down. This change in the horizontal relationship between upper and lower anterior teeth may be a solution to some problems and a detriment to others. Establishing the VDO that is most beneficial to the anterior teeth is one of the primary objectives in working with mounted diagnostic casts.

If the resolution of a severe wear problem requires changes in the incisal edge position or the steepness of the anterior guidance, the provisional restorations for the anterior teeth should be tested in the mouth until both the dentist and the patient are satisfied with the results. If the process is followed for determining the functional matrix for anterior teeth (Chapters 15 to 18) the time required for testing is greatly reduced as all contours and inclination of the anterior teeth are determined without having to guess. Just remember that the diagnostic wax-up is just a "best guess." Until the provisional restorations are refined in the mouth, the final details for the anterior guidance and esthetics will typically be compromised.

Severe anterior wear may result in a loss of anterior facial dimension. If anterior wear occurs because of forwardly displaced condyles, the VDO at the anterior teeth may close. This is so because the condyles must move down as they are displaced forward by posterior interferences. The VDO is established by the repetitive contracted length of the elevator muscles at maximal intercuspation. As the condyles are allowed to go back to centric relation, they also move *up*. This shortens the dimension of the elevator muscles. Thus the anterior segment can be opened at least 2 mm for each 1 mm of upward condylar movement to centric relation without interfering with the contracting length of the elevator muscles. Refer to Chapter 13, and make sure you understand how condylar position affects the vertical and horizontal relationship of the anterior teeth. It is often the key to achieving the best choice of treatment for severe anterior wear.

How Wear Occurs

All occlusions wear to some degree. The parabolic contours of the cusps were designed to permit the maximum amount of wear without penetrating into dentin. Even the proximal contact surfaces of teeth wear as the result of rubbing against each other during function (attritional wear). So physiologic wear results in both shortening the vertical length of the teeth and narrowing the horizontal width of the teeth. If the masticatory system is kept in equilibrium, the occlusal wear compensates for the normal proximal wear and the minimal loss of enamel will be of little concern. In a balanced masticatory system with a normal diet, the dentition can stay intact for a long lifetime. The teeth should outlast the body.

To understand problems of occlusal wear, one must understand how the adaptive process compensates for wear. Built into the design of the system are two adaptive processes for maintaining the following:

1. VDO
2. Tight proximal contacts

The VDO is maintained even when rapid abrasive wear occurs. As the occlusal surfaces of the teeth wear, the dentoalveolar process elongates by progressive remodeling of the alveolar bone. The increase in vertical length of the alveolar process matches the loss of occlusal height, so the VDO of lower facial height is maintained at a constant dimension throughout adult life unless the teeth are lost.

The horizontal dimension of length around the arch is shortened by several millimeters during life. The proximal wear is compensated by a constant forward pressure that keeps the contacts close together. Not unlike the vertical stabilizing factors, it is part of the adaptive process for maintaining the equilibrium of the parts of the masticatory system.

These adaptive processes continue to function throughout life. They are beneficial if all parts of the system are correctly interrelated. They may contribute to the destruction of the dentition if the interrelating parts get too far out of functional harmony.

Because elongation of alveolar bone matches the amount of occlusal wear, restoration of severely worn teeth is not simply a matter of restoring lost tooth structure. To do such restoration results in an increase of VDO that may actually intensify the problem in some patients. Analysis of a severe wear problem should take into consideration how normal muscle function would move the mandible if there were no barriers from interfering teeth, either vertically or horizontally. In other words, an analysis should be made of mandibular function to determine how and why any part of the dentition is in interference with any jaw movement. The treatment plan should then be directed toward alteration of the dentition so that it is in complete conformity, with no interference to any functional jaw position or excursive movement. Very often the wear patterns themselves are the key to determining the functional pathways of the mandible.

In analyzing any dentition, we should make a distinction between physiologic wear and excessive wear.

Physiologic wear is normal. It results in progressive but very slow loss of convexity on the cusps, accompanied by flattening of cusp tips on the posterior teeth and loss of mamelons on the anterior teeth. Some facets of wear may be found, but they should be minimal in length and depth. Physiologic wear must be evaluated according to age, habit patterns, and history of the wear. It should not result in premature deterioration of the dentition to the extent that it would require correction.

Excessive wear refers to any level of occlusal wear that can be expected to require corrective intervention in order to preserve the dentition. Excessive wear results in unacceptable damage to the occluding surfaces, and it may destroy anterior tooth structure that is necessary for acceptable anterior guidance function or for esthetics.

Excessive attritional wear is diagnostic. It is dependably related to tooth surfaces that are in direct interference with the functional or parafunctional movements of the mandible. Tooth structure that is not in the way of jaw movements will not be worn excessively.

Excessive wear can be stimulated either at the site of a direct interference to jaw movement or at the end point of a slide. Severe anterior wear is often the result of a posterior interference that displaces the mandible forward into a pressured contact of the lower anterior teeth against the upper lingual inclines. Lateral displacement of the mandible may also result in stressful contact against posterior tooth inclines at the end of a slide. The wear on the inclines that stop the slide is often more severe than the wear on the inclines that cause the displacement. This will be particularly so if the displacement forces lower teeth into a wedging contact with steep upper inclines.

TREATMENT PLANNING FOR WEAR PROBLEMS

Treatment for any excessive wear problem should be designed to accomplish six things:

1. Equal-intensity contacts on all teeth in a verifiable centric relation.

2. An anterior guidance that is in harmony with the patient's normal functional jaw movements.
3. Immediate disclusion of all posterior contacts the moment the mandible moves in any direction from centric relation.
4. Restoration of any tooth surfaces that have problem wear through the enamel.
5. Counseling, so that the patient understands that normal jaw posture keeps the teeth apart except during swallowing. Advice: "Lips together, teeth apart."
6. Nighttime occlusal splint if habitual nocturnal bruxism persists after occlusal correction.

Determining what treatment is necessary to correct an occlusal wear problem depends directly on what changes are necessary in the dentition to make it conform to the first four goals.

Relating the Combination of Anterior Guidance and Condylar Guidance to Occlusal Wear

Because successful reduction of most wear problems requires the separation of all posterior teeth in all jaw positions except centric relation, the analysis of any severe wear problem must focus on how that goal can best be achieved. Thus both the anterior guidance and the condylar guidance must be analyzed because posterior disclusion depends on a combination of anterior guidance and condylar guidance, and it is very common to find that either or both guidances have been severely flattened whenever extensive occlusal wear has occurred.

If the anterior guidance is worn flat, the downward path of the condyles must be relied on for separating the posterior teeth in excursions. If the normal convexity of the eminentiae is intact, the condyles must travel down when the jaw moves forward, so posterior disclusion can be worked out even with a flat anterior guidance. But if the condylar guidance has been flattened also, that disclusive effect is not available.

Observation of posterior wear patterns will indicate whether flattening of the eminentiae has occurred because such flattening does not occur without simultaneous wear of the upper lingual cusps. On the other hand, flattening of upper lingual cusps cannot occur with normal condylar paths because lower posterior teeth cannot move forward or toward the midline without moving downward unless the eminence is flattened. This is so even with a zero-degree anterior guidance.

If only the anterior teeth are worn flat, it is an indication that acceptable posterior disclusion can be achieved without the anterior guidance being steepened.

If both the anterior and the posterior teeth are worn flat, it is a probable indication that posterior disclusion must be accomplished by steepening of the anterior guidance.

The exception to the above rules may occur when there is a severe curve to the occlusal plane so that the plane slants up in back, making it nearly parallel with an undamaged condylar path. When the occlusal plane at the molars parallels the condylar path, the posterior teeth may be worn flat, but that problem can usually be corrected when the occlusal plane is lowered in back without the anterior guidance being steepened.

It is always advantageous to work out the disclusion of the posterior teeth without steepening the anterior guidance if it is possible to accomplish it, because steepening the anterior guidance restricts the existing envelope of function and triggers further parafunctional bruxing. It is my consistent observation that when a patient with a horizontal envelope of function is forced to function more vertically, there is routinely an attempt to regain the more horizontal function by wearing away the steeper anterior inclines, by loosening the anterior teeth, or by moving them out of the way. The instability of a steepened anterior guidance often goes unnoticed because it does not generally cause any discomfort to the patient.

Regardless of whether a steepened anterior guidance may cause increased wear of the anterior teeth, it may still be the only option for posterior disclusion if the condylar path has been flattened.

The analysis of the condylar path is critically important in severe occlusal wear problems for two reasons:

1. To determine how much help can be expected from the condylar path for discluding the posterior teeth
2. To determine whether the condylar path will be stable after occlusal correction

Because the health and alignment of the condyle-disk relationship are so critical to the long-term prognosis for occlusal wear treatment, an analysis of severe occlusal wear should include a determination of whether the disk is intact and aligned during function. Displacement of the disk eventually leads to loss of condylar height by flattening of the condyle and eminence. This, in turn, perpetuates the occlusal wear problem by repetitively re-creating an interference with the most posterior teeth on the side of the displacement, which in turn causes muscle incoordination and elevator muscle hyperactivity (Figure 35-3). For this reason, *patients with irreducible disk derangements must expect a continuing need for repeated occlusal corrections, done periodically to compensate for the continuing loss of condylar height from progressive breakdown of the articular surfaces. Patients should be informed of this in advance.*

It appears that the wear problem from a displaced disk can be minimized for both the damaged joint and the occlusal surfaces when a perfected occlusion is provided. Maintaining that perfected occlusion should especially be considered an important follow-up step whenever synovial fluid flow to the articular surfaces is disrupted by a displaced disk. The wear problem is generally manageable but may require replacement of restorations in less time than normal wear would require.

Analysis of the condylar path can be accomplished in the following ways:

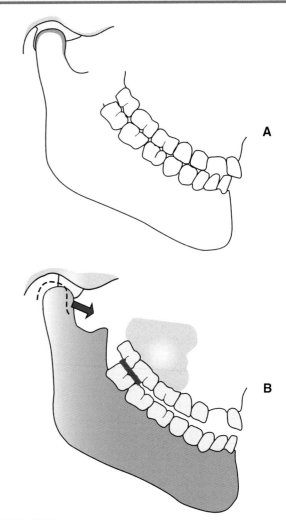

FIGURE 35-3 If the occlusal plane at the posterior segment is steeper than the condylar path and the anterior guidance, it is an interference to the protrusive path that is a potent cause of wear on the posterior teeth including wear on the upper lingual cusps. **A,** Centric relation; **B,** Protrusive.

1. *Clinical observation.* If the anterior guidance can disclude the posterior teeth in protrusive excursions, there is no condylar path problem. If the anterior guidance cannot disclude the posterior teeth, further analysis of the condylar path should be made by one or more of the following methods.
   a. *Protrusive checkbite* at the incisal edge-to-edge position, for setting the condylar path so that its effect can be analyzed on semiadjustable instrumentation.
   b. *Pantographic, axiographic, or stereographic recording* of the condylar path for precise analysis. (All methods are described in Chapter 22.)

Analysis of the occlusal plane can be more critical when the condylar path is known. Even a severely flattened condylar path will most often have some angulation downward. As long as the occlusal plane at the molars is flatter than the condylar path, it can be discluded, even by a zero-degree anterior guidance. Analysis of the occlusal plane is critical when severe posterior wear is being evaluated. There are two ways to increase the eccentric separation of the posterior teeth by alteration of the occlusal plane:

1. Flattening a curved occlusal plane
2. Lowering the occlusal plane in back

Either of the above procedures can increase posterior disclusion without requiring an increase in anterior guidance steepness as long as the posterior half of the occlusal plane is flatter than the condylar path and the fossa-wall angulation is flatter than the anterior guidance.

Analysis of the anterior guidance must relate to the existing paths of function after wear has occurred. Even though functional movements were originally more vertical, they become more and more horizontal as the teeth are abraded. Once a more horizontal envelope of function has been developed, the flattened anterior guidance cannot be steepened without the probability of triggering more wear against the anterior teeth. Thus a tobacco chewer who has worn the occlusion flat will attempt to regain the flattened pathways if they are restricted by a steepened anterior guidance.

Some parafunctional wear against anterior teeth can be corrected without triggering a recurrence of the wear. If the anterior wear occurred primarily as a result of posterior interferences that are still present, the anterior surfaces can often be restored with a good prognosis after the posterior interferences are eliminated.

Diagnostic Wax-up

Analysis of a worn anterior guidance cannot be made accurately until all posterior interferences have been eliminated. This is best done on mounted diagnostic casts. After the casts have been equilibrated, a diagnostic wax-up of the anterior teeth should be done. The wax-up should recontour the anterior teeth to the flattest possible guidance consistent with maintaining correct incisal edge position. The first analysis should be at the most closed VDO. Four primary questions should be answered by the diagnostic wax-up of the equilibrated casts in the following order:

1. Can the lower incisal edges be correctly contoured?
2. Can a definite holding stop be provided for each lower incisal edge against its upper lingual surface?
3. Can the upper incisal edges be corrected or maintained without interference to the existing neutral zone or lip-closure path?
4. Can an anterior guidance be worked out between the established centric stops and the upper incisal edges?

The above questions should be analyzed first at the most closed VDO of the equilibrated casts. If the anterior relationships can be worked out without increasing VDO, that is ideal. If VDO must be increased to accomplish an acceptable anterior relationship, it should be increased only as much as necessary. A goal of treatment is to reduce requirements for adaptation to the minimum, and this is done best

by maintenance of the existing VDO. However, there should be few if any problems resulting from a slight increase in VDO if a perfected occlusion is achieved at the increased VDO.

The next step in analysis is to determine the effect of the waxed-up anterior teeth on posterior disclusion. The key questions to resolve are as follows:

1. Can the anterior guidance (as waxed) disclude all posterior teeth in all excursions?
2. If the anterior guidance cannot disclude the posterior teeth, can the problem be resolved by changes in the posterior segments?

Failure to answer the above questions early in the diagnostic analysis is probably the major cause of failure in the treatment of wear problems. Disclusion of the posterior teeth in all excursions is an essential element of successful treatment. It must be thought out in advance because if steepening the anterior guidance is the only way to provide posterior disclusion, it must be accomplished as the first restorative priority. It may be a reasonable treatment choice to increase the VDO to allow for a flatter anterior guidance.

Testing the Treatment Plan with Provisional Restorations

After an acceptable anterior relationship has been waxed up, it still must be refined in the mouth. A matrix should be made for construction of the provisional restorations in acrylic resin after the teeth are prepared.

When anterior wear is severe, it is best to complete all refinements on both arches of anterior teeth before either segment is cemented. Upper and lower provisional restorations are usually placed, and all adjustments are made before the lower segment is copied. The lower anterior restorations should be completed in final form, but they should not be cemented until all functional excursions have been verified against the upper temporary restorations. The anterior guidance should be checked carefully at this stage to make certain that posterior disclusion is effective and that the upper contours conform with the lip-closure path and phonetic requirements. At that point, the lower permanent restorations can be cemented, and the upper anterior restorations can be finalized. Care should be taken in the laboratory to duplicate incisal edge positions and guidance contours that were worked out on the provisional restorations.

If splinting is not required, it may be practical to complete the upper and lower anterior restorations before the posterior teeth are prepared. The posterior teeth will, of course, have to be equilibrated as part of the preliminary mouth preparation before finalization of the anterior guidance either in the provisionals or in the permanent restorations.

If the posterior teeth are prepared at the same time as the anteriors, the provisional restorations can be made for the full arch. The anterior guidance can still be worked out in the normal manner, and the posterior teeth can still be adjusted so that they are discluded by the anterior guidance on the temporary restorations. The entire occlusal scheme can thus be worked out provisionally in this manner before any final restorations are fabricated. It then becomes a matter of reproducing all the guidelines that were determined in the mouth. This can be done in the laboratory with precise accuracy if all the guidelines are communicated.

If the provisional restorations are full arch splints, the posterior segments can be sectioned through the distal canine contact and removed. An impression of the anterior segment in place can then be made. A centric relation bite record can be made on the posterior teeth at the correct VDO with anterior contact. This same bite record can be used to articulate both the master die model and the cast of the anterior provisionals in place. From these two articulated casts, the customized anterior guide table can be fabricated as well as an index for incisal edge position.

The secret to success in solving severe wear problems is definitely keyed to working out the correct anterior guidance. If posterior disclusion can be achieved with an anterior guidance that is in harmony with the envelope of function, the prognosis will be excellent.

If the anterior guidance must restrict the envelope of function in order to disclude the posterior teeth, the result will still be acceptable and patient comfort can be good, but a varying degree of progressive wear can be expected on the anterior teeth. A nighttime occlusal splint can be used to reduce wear from nocturnal bruxing.

If it is necessary to steepen the anterior guidance, the posterior teeth should be monitored periodically for any signs of excursive interferences as the anterior guidance is flattened by recurrent wear. The same monitoring is especially important if an irreducible disk derangement is present because of potential loss of condyle height.

PROCEDURE   Solving severe wear problems

Severe wear on a patient with a very steep envelope of function and a tight neutral zone. The severe wear on the lower anterior teeth is the result of restricting the envelope of function by poorly contoured restorations on the upper anterior teeth. Note the slight lingual inclination of the upper anterior teeth. This should be maintained in the new restorations to conform to the very strong neutral zone.

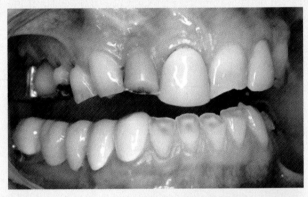

Step 1: Casts mounted in centric relation make the starting point obvious. The lower anterior teeth are waxed up to establish definite labio-incisal line angles. This wax-up is easily done and is typically made a little thicker and longer than needed. This makes it easier to shape the provisional restorations in the mouth as needed for non-interfering centric relation holding contacts.

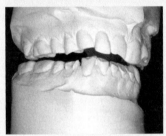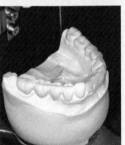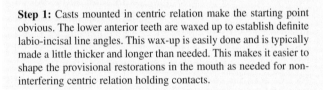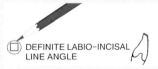

DEFINITE LABIO–INCISAL LINE ANGLE

PROCEDURE   Solving severe wear problems—cont'd

Step 2: The lower teeth are prepared, and the provisional restorations are placed.

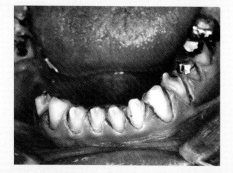

Step 3: The provisionals were formed from a putty matrix that was made to duplicate the diagnostic wax-up. Minor changes can be made at this stage, and the upper arch can be equilibrated to allow complete closure in centric relation as planned in the diagnostic wax-up.

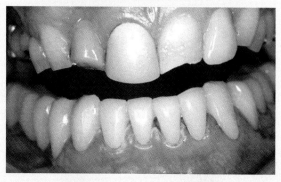

Step 4: A, New impressions are taken of the upper arch and the provisionals in place. This makes it possible to refine the upper wax-up for copying in the upper provisional restorations after teeth are prepared (**B**).

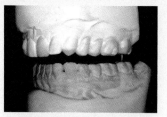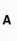

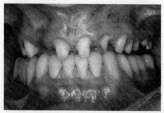

Step 5: After placement of the upper provisional restorations, both upper and lower arches can be refined for best anterior guide function and esthetics. The final restorations are not started until the provisional restorations are approved.

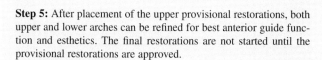

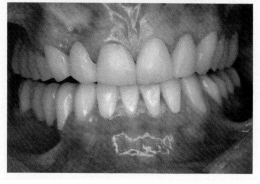

Continued

PROCEDURE   Solving severe wear problems—cont'd

Step 6: An index made on a cast of the lower anterior provisional restorations is used to communicate exact details to the technician.

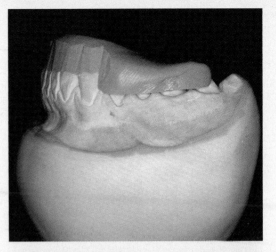

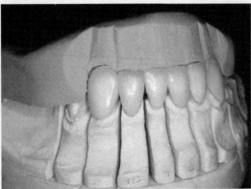

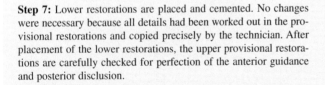

INCISAL EDGE POSITION

☐ FOLLOW E/O CAST
☐ COPY CAST OF TEMPS
☐ COPY CAST OF ORIGINAL

Step 7: Lower restorations are placed and cemented. No changes were necessary because all details had been worked out in the provisional restorations and copied precisely by the technician. After placement of the lower restorations, the upper provisional restorations are carefully checked for perfection of the anterior guidance and posterior disclusion.

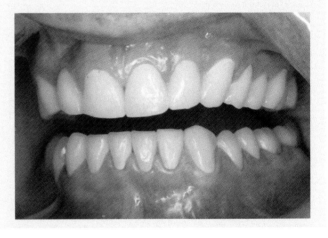

PROCEDURE   Solving severe wear problems—cont'd

Step 8: After verification of the correct anterior guidance, the upper provisional splint is sectioned and the two posterior segments are removed so a centric relation bite record can be made at the correct VDO with anterior teeth in contact.

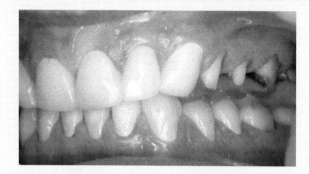

Step 9: The cast of the approved provisional restorations is mounted in centric relation. A putty index is made to communicate precise incisal edge position and contour to the technician.

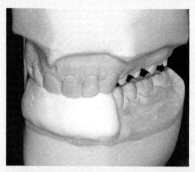

Step 10: A customized anterior guide is made to communicate precise details of the anterior guidance to the technician.

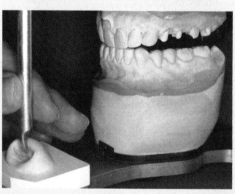

Step 11: This is then copied into the final restorations, eliminating all guesswork. Ceramic contouring is related to the matrix.

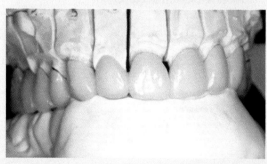

The final restorations are in place.

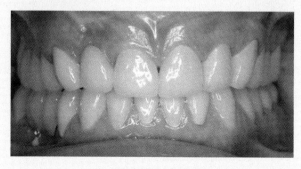

Restoring Severely Worn Posterior Teeth

Restoration of the posterior occlusion is dependent on determination of the correct anterior guidance first. In the analysis of various types of occlusal wear, the focus should be directed first to the anterior teeth. The posterior teeth must be fitted in between the anterior guidance and the condylar guidance, but they must not interfere with either one. Thus the establishment of stable holding contacts is the primary goal of the posterior occlusion.

With long-term wear, the posterior teeth are sometimes abraded nearly to the gumline. There are generally four choices for treatment of such severely worn teeth:

1. *Pin-retained all-gold restorations.* The use of parallel pin retention permits restorations of the exposed dentin without significant increase in VDO. This is not always esthetically acceptable in the anterior segments.
2. *Increase in the VDO.* An increase in the VDO may improve the esthetic result, but in some patients it can lead to excessive stress. Although increasing the VDO may be the best choice for some patients, it is contraindicated if the alveolar bone is sclerotic and the masticatory muscles are hypertrophied.
3. *Crown-lengthening procedures.* It may be necessary to surgically expose enough tooth structure to provide retention and esthetic contouring.
4. *Pulp extirpation and endodontic post and coping construction.* This choice can provide retentive form when needed. It may also require an increase in VDO. Pulp extirpation may also be combined with crown lengthening to provide improved esthetics and retention without increasing the VDO. New information on reduction of mechanoreceptor protection of pulpless teeth makes this choice the treatment of last resort. It should be avoided if at all possible.

Retentive Preparation for Severely Worn Teeth

It is often possible to restore shortened teeth with surprisingly good esthetic results, especially if the lip line covers the cementoenamel junction. Retention is jeopardized whenever the restoration can rotate off a tooth. Preparing with opposing, near-parallel walls prevents rotation and provides maximum retention (Figure 35-4).

When Should Occlusal Wear Be Restored?

All occlusal wear does not need to be restored. Even penetration into dentin may not need treatment. If the cause of the wear can be eliminated through equilibration so that worn surfaces are no longer subjected to parafunctional contact, exposed dentin may remain intact for years. Whether the worn surfaces should be restored depends on the answers to the following questions:

1. *Will treatment be complicated by delay in restoring the wear?* Often the same type of restoration would be possible without compromise even if more wear occurs. In such cases, there is no need to rush treatment, especially if there is a chance the wear problem has been corrected by the improved occlusion.
2. *Is restoration necessary to control sensitivity?* Exposure of dentin produces different responses in different patients.
3. *Is restoration required to satisfy esthetic desires?* Worn teeth can be unsightly. Matching restorations to look like adjacent worn teeth severely limits the esthetic result that could be achieved. The patient should always be informed of the options.
4. *Is it relatively certain that restorations will eventually be required?* If so, the patient should be fully informed about the probable time frame, and the condition should be monitored on a regular basis if the patient elects to delay.

Conservative Correction of Lower Incisal Wear

When incisal wear penetrates through the enamel, the softer dentin begins to cup, leaving an elevated ring of unsupported enamel rods. This leads to chipping away of the enamel and makes the incisal edges unsightly and rough.

A preventive measure that seems to help considerably in stabilizing the incisal edges while improving the appearance is to bond composite resin into the cupped-out dentin area

FIGURE 35-4 **A,** Preparation for retention on short teeth is often inadequate because it provides no resistance to rotation off the prepared tooth. **B,** Retention can be increased greatly by preparing in steps so that opposing walls are nearly parallel. This prevents the restoration from being rocked off.

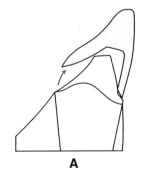

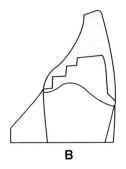

A   B

(Figure 35-5). If the resin is bonded to the ring of acid-etched enamel, it adds to the dentin bond and prevents the destruction of loose enamel rods.

Dentin bonding agents have further enhanced this procedure, and more wear-resistant resins have also helped. However, the incisal edges do not function on the composite resin except in end-to-end relationships. Instead, most functional contact occurs against the enamel ring. As long as this procedure is performed before the enamel ring has been destroyed, the prognosis is good enough to make the procedure recommended over the unnecessary use of full coverage (Figures 35-6, 35-7, 35-8).

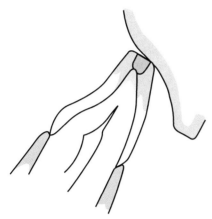

FIGURE 35-5 If cupped incisal edges are recontoured with resin bonded to the enamel ring, the resin prevents wear on the dentin but is not subject to occlusal wear because most of the function occurs against the enamel contact. Dentin bonding agents have made this procedure even more practical.

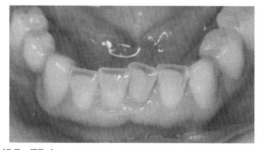

FIGURE 35-6 A common wear problem on lower incisal edges: Cupping occurs when dentin is exposed. If the enamel ring is intact, bonded composite works well.

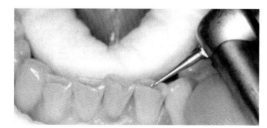

FIGURE 35-7 Clean out enough dentin to expose the enamel ring. A ½-round bur is ideal.

Severe Anterior Wear That Results in an End-to-End Relationship

Badly worn teeth that have drifted into an end-to-end relationship present a real restorative challenge. It is difficult to lengthen the appearance of the upper teeth without opening the bite or severely steepening the anterior guidance. This usually calls for a compromise that permits the lower incisal edges to move forward on a fairly flat guidance and then progress into a steeper incline as gradually as possible by way of a concave pathway (see Figure 35-9).

To make the concave contour possible, it is usually necessary to restore the worn lower teeth with full coverage, to narrow the broad incisal edges from the labial, and to position the incisal edge lingually. By moving the incisal edges lingually, we can lengthen the lower incisors to provide some overjet for the upper teeth. With sufficient overjet, the upper incisors can then curve down from the cingulum centric stop, providing more length for the upper anterior teeth. Both esthetics and function are improved by such a procedure.

It should be remembered that even though the esthetics and function are improved by the above process, the envelope of function will still be restricted from its flattened pathways. It will usually be necessary to either splint the upper restorations or provide a nighttime retainer to prevent movement. The nighttime retainer can include full occlusal coverage to reduce wear on the steepened anterior inclines.

Common Option: Reshape

Severe incisal wear results in thick, round lower anterior teeth (Figure 35-9, *A*). In order to restore to a normal incisal edge contour, more tooth structure must be removed than the thickness needed for restorative material. If the incisal edge needs to be moved lingually, most of the reduction for the preparation should be on the labial. If the incisal edge needs to be moved labially, most of the reduction should be on the lingual (Figure 35-10). The best place to make these deci-

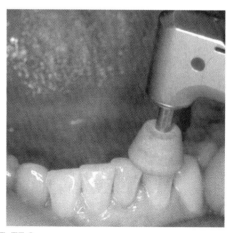

FIGURE 35-8 Composite bonded and polished. The main objective is to preserve the enamel leading edge.

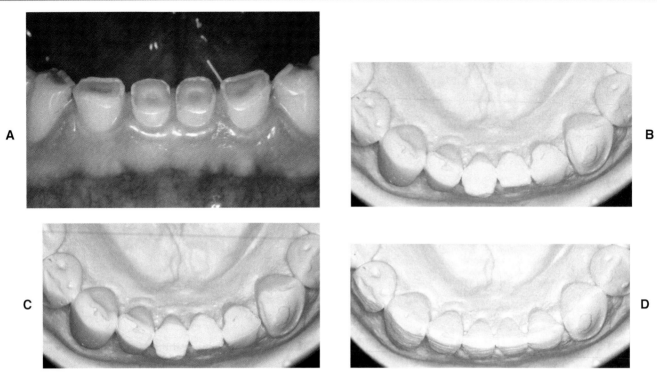

FIGURE 35-9 **A,** Severe incisal wear shortens the teeth and results in a thick, round edge. The alveolar process elongates to match the loss of tooth length. Crown lengthening is often necessary to achieve an acceptable ferule for needed crown retention. **B,** Cast of the lower arch showing the thickened incisal edges that had gradually moved into an end-to-end relationship with the upper anterior teeth as the overbite relationship was worn flat. **C,** Plan for reshaping the incisal edges to a more esthetic contour that also moves the edges back to allow for an anterior guidance overlap. **D,** Casts are shaped back before wax-up is done to work out the ideal relationship with the upper anterior teeth. Corrected casts show the desired end point of restorations. Preparation for restorations will require further reduction.

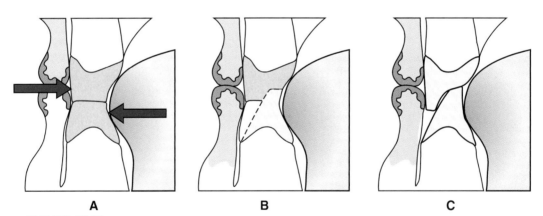

FIGURE 35-10 **A,** As the incisal edges are worn flat, the tongue presses the lower teeth forward while the lips press the upper teeth backward. This is the compressive nature of the neutral zone that results in an end-to-end anterior relationship. **B,** By removing more of the labial surface of the thick incisal edge, the incisal edge can be recontoured more to the lingual. By reductive reshaping of the lingual part of the upper anterior teeth, the lower incisal edges can also be lengthened. **C,** More length can then be added to the upper incisal edges to form an overbite relationship that also re-establishes an anterior guidance capable of posterior disclusion. The added length of the upper anterior teeth improves the esthetics without increasing the VDO.

sions is on mounted study casts in centric relation (see Figure 35-9, *B* to *D*).

The problem that may arise whenever a flat anterior guidance is changed to a more restrictive one is that patients will almost always press and brux against the restricting anterior tooth surfaces. For that reason, it is often prudent to fabricate a nighttime appliance for protecting the anterior guidance surfaces. A full occlusal splint with centric relation contact on all teeth, and a ramp for posterior disclusion is in order.

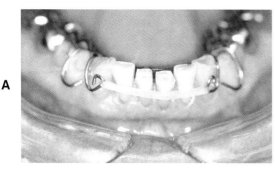

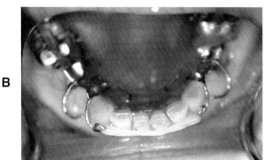

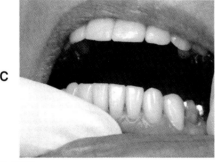

FIGURE 35-11 **A,** Lower incisors that had migrated too far forward to permit an acceptable anterior guidance are narrowed and then repositioned back with a simple appliance that uses a rubber band to move the teeth. **B,** Note that the lingual plate on the appliance was precontoured to stop each anterior tooth when it reached the position worked out on the diagnostic casts. This is a very simple way to move lower anterior teeth. **C,** Finished restorations copied provisional restorations on which all the final contours were established for both upper and lower anterior teeth before proceeding with final restorations. Because of the severity of the wear and the need for narrowing the teeth, the restoration chosen was full-coverage.

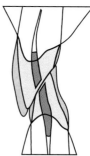

FIGURE 35-12 When severe wear occurs on both contacting surfaces, correction sometimes requires a choice of either devitalizing the teeth or increasing the VDO. Devitalizing a vital tooth is never the treatment of choice if opening the VDO can be achieved without compromising other treatment decisions.

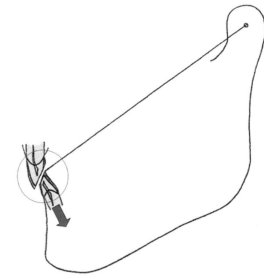

FIGURE 35-13 Increasing the VDO on an anterior wear problem does two things: It opens space vertically, and it opens space horizontally because of the opening arc around the condylar axis. This provides room to restore worn surfaces on the labial of the lower incisors or the lingual of the upper incisors. The same effect is achieved when deflective posterior occlusal interferences are equilibrated if it allows the condyles to seat further back in centric relation.

Another Option: Reposition

Lower anterior teeth that have migrated forward as both upper and lower incisal edges are worn flat may have to be moved lingually and then reshaped in order to establish an acceptable relationship for anterior guidance and esthetics (Figure 35-11).

Severe Wear on Labial of Lower Teeth and Lingual of Upper Teeth

If the contacting surface enamel is worn severely on both the upper and lower anterior teeth, there is sometimes no room to restore the surfaces back without either invading the pulp or increasing the VDO (Figure 35-12). Invading the pulp is rarely the best choice.

This type of problem is usually treated by opening the VDO. As the mandible swings open, the lower anteriors arc away from the worn surface contact (Figure 35-13), providing room for restorative materials that are necessary regardless of the treatment selected.

Treating the problem in this manner generally has a good prognosis if the increased VDO is kept to a minimum and if stable holding contacts are provided for the anterior teeth.

Care must be taken to reinforce the incisal edges with sufficient thickness to prevent fracturing thin unsupported porcelain. There is generally no problem working out the anterior guidance because in this type of wear the envelope of function is quite steep.

All details of the anterior relationship should be refined in provisional restorations, which are then copied in the laboratory. Care should be taken to avoid interference with a

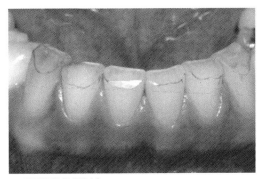
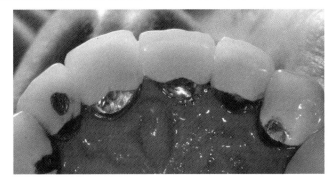

FIGURE 35-14   Note how lower incisal wear patterns match up with the poorly contoured upper restorations that interfere with functional jaw movements. Attempts to restore either arch without correcting the opposing contours are a serious yet all too common mistake.

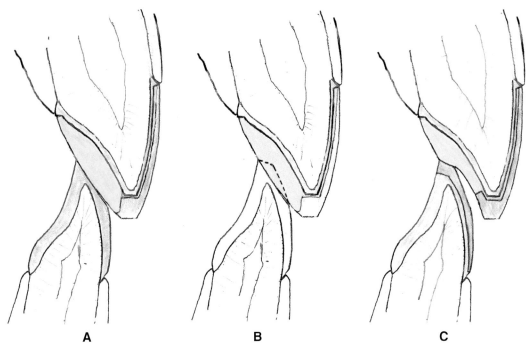

A   **B**   **C**

FIGURE 35-15   **A,** Severe labio-incisal angle wear caused by bulbous lingual contours on upper restorations. This is one of the most common causes of lower anterior wear. There are no holding contacts, and the lingual contours interfere with the envelope of function—a certain cause of many problems. **B,** The upper lingual surfaces must be recontoured to accommodate the lower incisal edge. **C,** Laminate restores the lower leading edge. New correctly contoured restoration is on the upper.

tightly restricted neutral zone and lip-closure path, which usually are present with this type of wear.

All interferences to centric relation should be removed before any details of the anterior relationship are worked out.

The amount of increase in VDO that is needed to satisfy an acceptable anterior relationship is usually minimal. Remember that if the VDO is increased, it must include all the teeth. If posterior teeth do not need restorations, look at options for repositioning the anterior teeth by orthodontic or surgical solutions.

Severe Labial Wear of Lower Incisors

When lower incisors wear severely on their labio-incisal surfaces, it is usually a sign of improperly contoured upper lingual restorations (Figure 35-14).

It is a classic example of interference to the envelope of function that generally requires a concave upper lingual contour for noninterference. The thick bulbous lingual contours that are so prevalent in upper anterior restorations must be altered if the problem is to be treated successfully.

Sometimes the restorations can be reshaped to provide a stable stop on the cingulum and a corrected path from the centric stop to the incisal edge (Figure 35-15). Even if this requires remaking the upper restorations, it should be recommended or restoration of the lower worn surfaces will fail. Wear will continue to be a problem as long as tooth structure interferes with functional jaw pathways.

After reshaping the upper lingual surfaces, the lower incisal and labial contours should be perfected in provisional restorations and then copied in the laboratory.

Use of laminates to restore labio-incisal wear on lower anterior teeth

Severe wear of labial surface of lower anterior teeth often combines with lingual wear of the upper anteriors if there are no stable holding contacts. There is a tendency to erupt as wear progresses. Eventually this type of wear often thins the teeth so much that the incisal portions fracture off and the relationship becomes end-to-end because of compression between the tongue and the lips.

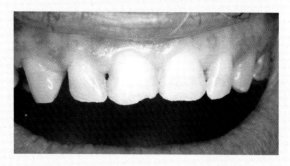

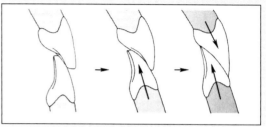

The solution to many unstable anterior wear problems is properly contoured lower incisal edges. A definite labio-incisal line angle is the starting place for stable holding contacts.

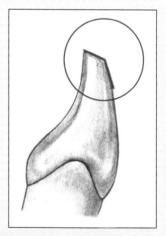

The leading edge of a definite labio-incisal line angle is worn to an angle.

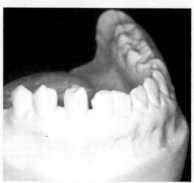

Diagnostic wax-up starts at lower incisal edges.

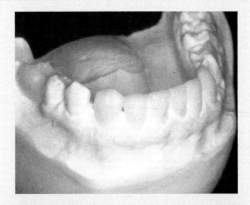

Provisional restorations copy diagnostic wax-up but still need changes in the mouth to relate ideally with upper anterior contacts.

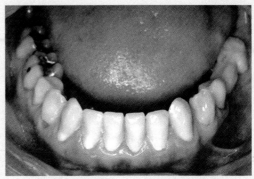

Cast of completed restorations showing definite line angle at leading edge. Stable holding contacts on upper anterior teeth also had to be worked out on the diagnostic casts and refined in the mouth.

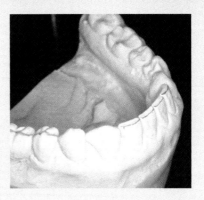

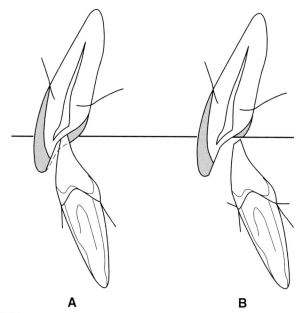

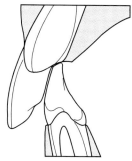

FIGURE 35-17 If the lower teeth erupt up far enough into the worn root surfaces of the upper incisors, the lower segment is too high to correct restoratively. Because the lower incisal plane is so high, it distorts the normal appearance.

A   **B**

FIGURE 35-16 Extreme lingual wear is often the result of posterior incline interferences that deflect the jaw forward. **A,** If the relationship of the teeth is observed in maximal intercuspation, it would appear impossible to restore the worn lingual surfaces without opening the bite. **B,** If posterior interferences to a centric relation closure are eliminated, the jaw is often able to close to the original VDO on a more distal arc of closure. There is then sufficient room to restore the lingual surfaces without increasing the VDO.

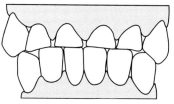

FIGURE 35-18 Lower incisors erupt up with their alveolar process when upper teeth wear severely. This creates one of the most difficult problems to solve because the cementoenamel junctions of the lower incisors are often above the level of the occlusal plane. The resultant reverse smile line is also a difficult esthetic challenge.

Severe Lingual Wear on Upper Anterior Teeth

Excessive wear on upper lingual inclines is most often the result of posterior inclines that deflect the mandible forward. The lower incisal edges are driven forward into the upper lingual surfaces where bruxing patterns may wear the surfaces nearly to the pulp (Figure 35-16, *A*). If we observe the relationship in maximal intercuspation, it will appear impossible to restore lost tooth structure without opening the bite. If the mandible is manipulated into centric relation, however, we will find that it is often posterior to the acquired worn position.

Elimination of centric relation interferences by selective grinding so that the mandible can fully close without forward deflection will often provide room between the lower incisal edges and the upper lingual inclines without increasing the VDO (see Figure 35-16, *B*).

Uneven Wear

Anterior wear is not always equal on both arches. Severe wear may be found on upper teeth with minimal wear on the lower ones. When the enamel is penetrated on one arch, the softer dentin may wear rapidly, permitting the teeth with harder enamel surfaces to erupt up into the more rapidly wearing teeth. Such uneven wear patterns can create very difficult occlusal plane problems (Figure 35-17).

When the upper teeth wear rapidly, the lower anterior segment erupts up to form a severe reverse smile line that is very unattractive (Figure 35-18). Correction is difficult because the eruption of the lower teeth occurs by elongation of the alveolar bone, sometimes making the soft-tissue juncture of the lower teeth too high to correct by restorative procedures alone.

The solution requires lowering of the lower incisal edges to permit a more normal upper smile line. The methods for accomplishing this should be evaluated in the same manner as other programmed treatment planning by consideration of all choices in proper sequence:

1. *Reshaping.* Can the lower incisors be shortened by grinding?
2. *Repositioning.* Is it possible to intrude the lower incisors orthodontically?
3. *Restoring.* Can the lower incisors be shortened restoratively? Can the occlusal plane be improved by an increase in the VDO?
4. *Surgery.* Would a segmental osteotomy be the best way to lower the entire anterior dento-alveolar segment? (Figure 35-19)

The solution to the problem of uneven wear will be more readily determined if a structured approach to analysis takes into consideration all the possible options, or combinations of options. Solutions will be as varied as the problems that

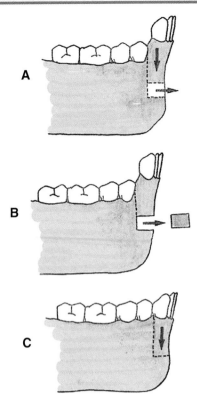

FIGURE 35-19 Segmental osteotomy is a practical approach for inferiorly repositioning the lower anterior dento-alveolar segment when the alveolar process has become elongated. **A,** The gingival margins of the incisors were too high for restorative correction. The alternative of pulp extirpation and crown lengthening surgery is often more radical than osteotomy when the elongation has been severe. **B** and **C,** This procedure permits an esthetically acceptable solution that can also re-establish an effective anterior guidance.

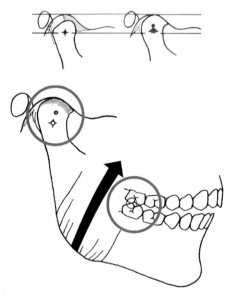

FIGURE 35-20 Molars are subject to attritional wear once the TMJ breaks down.

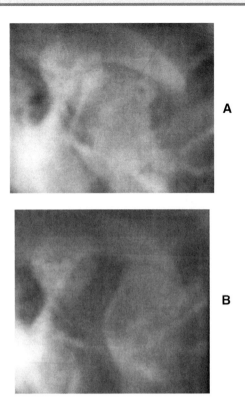

FIGURE 35-21 **A,** Condyle after disk displacement and subsequent osteoarthritic changes in both the condyle and the eminence. **B,** Flattened path of condyle in protrusive.

are presented, but the answers will be found in this orderly process.

Severe Occlusal Wear from TMJ-related Causes

One good reason for developing expertise in disorders of the TMJ is because breakdown of the TMJ can be such an important factor in severe occlusal wear. Any loss of height of the ramus as a result of condylar bone loss or displaced disk has a direct effect on the occlusion. It subjects the posterior molars to excessive overload. Any bruxing or excursive jaw movements put the molars "in the way" and subject them to attritional wear (Figure 35-20).

Displacement of the disk is often followed by perforation of the retrodiskal tissue and subsequent loss of bone on the condyle and the eminentia (Figure 35-21).

This loss of ramus height leads to two progressively damaging effects.

1. Severe wear of posterior teeth that are in direct interference to all functional jaw movements.
2. Severe wear of anterior teeth (Figure 35-22). This results from the need to protrude the jaw to achieve anterior contact. As the condyles move down, the mandible pivots around the last molar to allow the anterior teeth to move up and into interference with the upper anterior teeth.

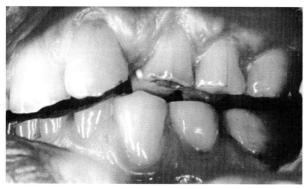

FIGURE 35-22 Pattern of severe wear that is common when ramus height is lost from TMJ breakdown. This is the occlusal relationship when condyles are seated in adapted centric posture.

Treatment planning for severe wear from TMJ breakdown

The type of TMJ intracapsular disorder shown in Figure 35-21 would be classified as Piper Class V b (see Chapter 26). It is almost always associated with excessive attritional wear on the molars. Eventually, if the occlusion is not corrected, the excessive wear will involve the anterior teeth even though it results in an anterior open bite when the joints are seated. This is so because there is a natural tendency to protrude the jaw to achieve anterior contact when ramus height is lost.

The protocol for treatment planning does not change.

1. *Determine the most stable TMJ position.* The bone-to-bone condyle-fossa relationship can be classified as *adapted centric posture* if it can comfortably accept loading. The results of a perfected occlusion can be just as predictably successful as intact joints in centric relation except that the occlusal result will not be as stable. Periodic occlusal adjustments will be necessary from time to time as further loss of the bone occurs on the articulating surfaces. However, the situation is manageable if the occlusion is maintained in a perfected posterior disclusion. Patients should be forewarned of the necessity of doing this.
2. *Do a diagnostic wax-up on mounted casts.* The goal is to determine the best choice of treatment for establishing anterior contact in adapted centric posture. This typically involves reshaping posterior teeth to close the VDO at the anteriors, plus restoring the an-

terior teeth to ideal contact, *then* restoring the posterior teeth to harmony with the seated condyles and the contacting anterior teeth.
3. *Prepare the teeth, and place provisional restorations.* The anterior guidance, lip closure path, phonetics, and esthetics should be worked out in the mouth.
4. *Copy the provisional anterior segments after the patient approves them for comfort, function, and esthetics.* The upper and lower anterior restorations can be completed before the posterior segments are restored to final restorations.
5. *Set up routine recall examinations.* The occlusion should be monitored carefully for new posterior interferences as the condyles slowly lose height. Failure to make the usual minimal corrections when needed activates incoordinated muscle hyperactivity and accelerates further attrition.

Note: In earlier years it was believed that a group function occlusion would slow the wear process by distributing it over more teeth. This actually had a reverse affect of accelerating wear because it activated more muscle forces against the teeth and the TMJs. Several occlusal corrections per year were needed to keep the masticatory musculature in a completely comfortable and peaceful state. When I changed the occlusal pattern to immediate posterior disclusion, the need for follow-up occlusal corrections was dramatically reduced to minimal adjustments about once every 12 to 14 months.

Wear from Extreme Habitual Bruxing

The most problematic wear problem results from *delta-stage* bruxing. Delta-stage bruxers exert almost continuous bruxing through all stages of sleep. They are recognizable by enlarged masticatory musculature and multiple exostoses of alveolar bone. The alveolar bone becomes dense—almost sclerotic. Radiographs show small trabeculae and very dense bone. As the teeth wear down, the alveolar process elongates, leaving limited room to restore without increasing the VDO.

The problems are compounded because compressive forces against the teeth can reach over 900 pounds during repeated clenching. Increasing the VDO can intensify muscle contraction forces. The dense bone around the teeth does not respond as normal alveolar bone does. This is because it is so unyielding, and increases in VDO are not compensated for by regressive remodeling or intrusion.

In this patient, there is no hint of periodontitis, and the TMJs are intact, a common finding in delta-stage bruxers.

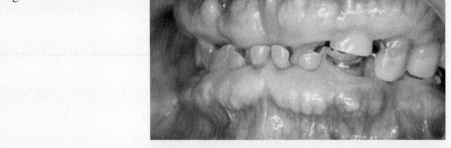

The lower arch was restored with provisional restorations *(bottom)* copied from a diagnostic wax-up.

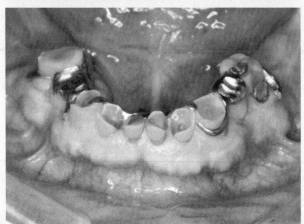

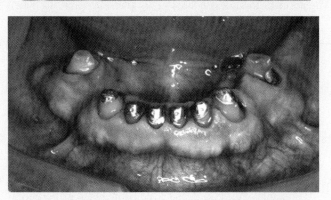

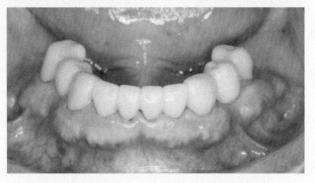

The upper teeth were then restored with provisional restorations, and the occlusion was meticulously adjusted after the patient approved the comfort and appearance of the provisional restorations.

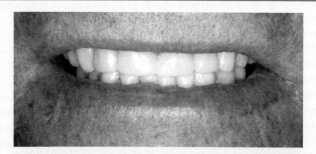

The final restorations duplicated them.

Failed treatment. The obviously successful case above illustrates why early claims of success may not be valid. In spite of complete comfort and function, these porcelain-metal restorations were destroyed within 3½ years. Excessive forces against the anterior guidance destroyed the anterior restorations first, making posterior excursive contact possible. Without posterior disclusion, the posterior restorations were then destroyed. Note the increase in VDO *(final photo)* compared with pre-treatment *(initial photo).*

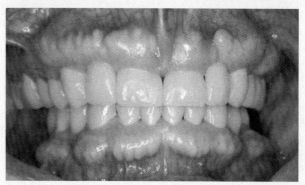

Solving delta-stage bruxing problems

Although an increase in VDO is a good solution for most patients with severe wear, it appears to be detrimental to delta-stage bruxers. Increases in VDO are routinely accommodated for by regressive remodeling of the alveolar process. But when the alveolar process responds to overload by the delta-stage bruxer, it becomes almost sclerotic and it resists the compressive force of the extremely strong musculature rather than accommodating to it. The all too typical result is destroyed restorations or fractured teeth.

The best solution is prevention. If the signs of early delta-stage bruxing are evident (enlarged muscles, severe wear into dentin, dense closely packed trabeculae), *do not wait* until the teeth are worn so badly that there is no room for restorations without increasing the VDO. Crown lengthening is generally contraindicated because of potential healing problems in the condensed bone.

Restoration of wear should be done early enough to achieve as much occlusal thickness of the restorations as possible. Use gold occlusals on posterior teeth. Keep the anterior guidance as flat as possible to avoid interference to the envelope of function. Achieve as much posterior disclusion as possible without increasing the VDO. A nighttime resin appliance may help if it is made at an increased VDO of about 8 mm with anterior contact only. Medication to aid sleep and reduce muscle activity is sometimes appropriate. Educate your patient.

PREVENTING OCCLUSAL WEAR PROBLEMS

Tooth structure that is not in the way of jaw movements will not wear excessively.

There is probably no better reason for advocating functional harmony of the entire masticatory system than for the effect that a peaceful neuromuscular system has on preventing wear problems.

Except for habitual function against abrasive materials, most wear can be prevented. At least it can almost always be reduced to a level whereby the dentition can last a lifetime. The best way to ensure against an excessive occlusal wear problem is by maintaining the optimum harmony possible between the articulation of the teeth and the articulation of the TMJs. This is best accomplished by the following:

1. Preserving the best possible alignment of the condyle-disk assemblies.
2. Observing and correcting any signs of instability in the dentition. It is especially important to maintain a stable anterior guidance.
3. Observing and correcting as much as possible any problems of masticatory muscle hyperactivity.

When a wear problem is noticed, meticulous attention should be given to providing equal-intensity contacts on the maximum number of teeth possible. Occlusal contact should occur in centric relation, and all posterior teeth should disclude the moment the jaw leaves centric relation. The anterior guidance should be nonrestrictive if possible.

Wear problems should be diagnosed early and treated before tooth structure is worn beyond the point of acceptable restoration. Patients also should be advised of the consequences of noxious habits.

References

1. Abrahamsen TC: The worn dentition—pathognomonic patterns of abrasion and erosion. *Int Dent Journal* 4:268-276, 2005.
2. Dzakovich JJ: In vitro reproduction of the non-carious cervical lesion. *Am Acad Rest Dent* February 2006 (in press).

Suggested Readings

Grippo JO, Simring M, Schreiner S: Attrition, abrasion, corrosion and abfraction revisited: a new perspective on tooth surface lesions. *J Am Dent Assoc* 135:1109-1118, 2004.

Miller WD: Experiments and observations on the wasting of tooth tissue variously designated as erosion, abrasion, chemical abrasion, denudation, etc. *The Dental Cosmos* XLIX (1)(2)(3), 1907.

Chapter 36

Solving Deep Overbite Problems

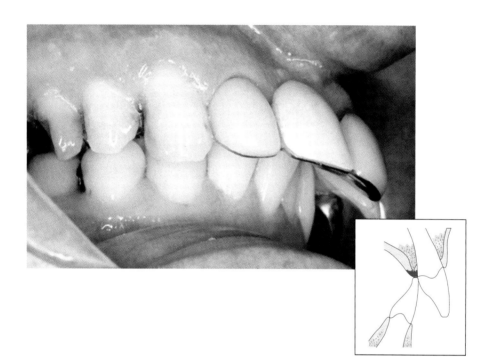

PRINCIPLE

A deep overbite is not a problem if all teeth have stable holding contacts in centric relation.

DEEP ANTERIOR OVERBITE

A deep overbite is not itself a problem. Many patients are treated unnecessarily to "correct" a deep overbite because of a mistaken idea that all deep overbites are unstable. Often the "corrected" anterior relationship is less stable than the deep overbite relationship. Analysis of every deep overbite should always start with observing the relationship of the lower incisal edges to determine if they meet a stable holding contact on the upper anterior teeth. This analysis must be done in centric relation, which means that mounted diagnostic casts are essential whenever maximal intercuspation is not at centric relation. Posterior interferences will have to be eliminated on the casts to see where the lower incisal edges will end up at complete closure to centric relation.

Patients with deep overbite relationships that do not provide centric contacts for the anterior teeth are almost always in trouble. Some form of treatment is indicated in most of these patients. Patients with deep overbite relationships that have stable anterior contact in centric relation are almost never in trouble (from the arch relationship). The key word in the preceding statement is *stable*: Such patients rarely need corrective treatment. Just having anterior contact may not be sufficient if the contact does not serve as a stop to pre-

vent continuous eruption of the lower anterior teeth. Eruption of the lower anterior teeth into the gingival tissues or into the palate is the number-one problem associated with deep overbites. Treatment should always be designed to prevent this from happening or to correct it in a stable fashion if it has already occurred.

Tongue Posture and Deep Overbites

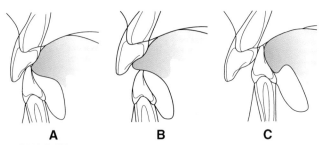

FIGURE 36-1   Tongue position in ideal anterior relationship (**A**), overjet (**B**), and deep overbite (**C**).

One reason why deep overbites that lack stable holding contacts so routinely get into problems is because with a deep overbite there is no room for the tongue to get over the incisal edges to stop eruption. Note the comparison in Figure 36-1 between the tongue position with an ideal anterior relationship versus the position as a substitute for holding contacts in an overjet patient. Then look at the tongue position with a deep overbite and it will be apparent why teeth erupt to the palatal tissue.

Neutral Zone Considerations

Most deep overbites occur in tight neutral zones that dictate a vertical tooth inclination with a very restricted envelope of function, and with little or no horizontal movement. The vertical envelope of function is an advantage because it makes posterior disclusion automatic regardless of the angulation of the condylar path. The tight neutral zone is the primary concern because the vertical inclination of the upper anterior teeth often makes it difficult to align lower incisal edges with a definite stop on the upper cingulums. If the upper incisal edges are moved forward while torquing the roots lingually to achieve lower anterior contact, it can create interference with the lip-closure path and the neutral zone as well as causing problems with phonetics. It does not cause a problem with the envelope of function because it does not restrict it. However, interference with the neutral zone is likely, in time, to result in an unstable relationship, especially for the upper anterior teeth. A better alternative is to maintain the upper incisal edge positions as much as possible while torquing the roots back to achieve a better contact position for the lower incisal edges.

Upper Lingual Contours

A major cause of deep anterior overbite problems is improperly contoured lingual surfaces on upper anterior teeth. If there is no definite holding contact for lower incisors, they will continue to erupt as they slide up the steep lingual contours. As the lower incisors become locked behind the upper anterior teeth, they erupt into the gingival tissue. It is also common for the lower lip to then position itself behind the upper anterior teeth, forcing the incisal edges forward and up. If upper restorations are made with a combination of no holding contact plus incisal edges too far forward, the eventual result is a deep overbite combined with an incisal edge overjet (see Figure 36-1).

APPLYING THE PRINCIPLES

A poorly made anterior fixed bridge with no holding contacts. The lower incisors erupted up to impinge on gingival tissues. The lower lip position is behind the upper incisors because the tight neutral zone prevented the lip from fitting in front for a normal lip seal. The result was very unesthetic as well as unstable.

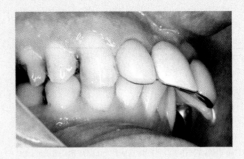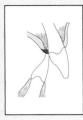

The first goal of treatment is to achieve stable holding contacts on all anterior teeth.

The first treatment option: Reshape

This is one of the most frequent treatment choices in a severe deep overbite. It is often necessary to reshape the lingual of upper restorations to provide a holding contour. It is also necessary to shorten the lower incisors if they have erupted up too far to make contact and if their incisal edges have been worn to a ragged edge, which they often are.

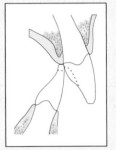

The second treatment option: Reposition

If the upper incisors have been wedged forward, they can be moved back so lower incisor contact can be achieved. This actually changes the neutral zone as the lower lip will be able to slide in front of the labial surfaces to hold them back as the lips seal. It will also improve the esthetics by getting rid of the "buckteeth" appearance.

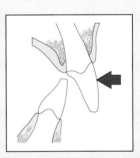

A simple but effective appliance for moving the anterior teeth back into a predetermined position against contoured slots in the palatal part of the appliance. A rubber band directs the teeth into the slots.

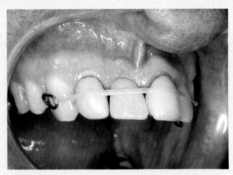

Note the complete lack of holding contacts on the straight lingual contours of the original restoration.

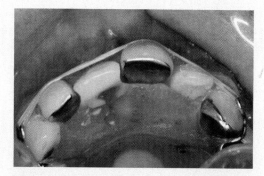

As the anterior teeth are brought lingually, their lingual contour has to be recontoured to permit anterior teeth contact into a stop.

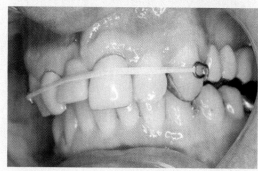

The third treatment option: Restore

After the teeth have been brought into an acceptable alignment by reshaping and repositioning.

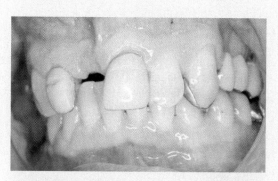

The teeth are prepared and provisional restorations are used to refine the anterior guidance and esthetic concerns.

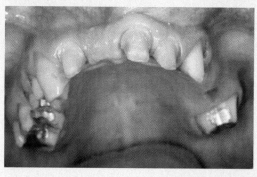

To achieve contact on all lower anterior teeth, it is often necessary to move one or more teeth forward. Any tooth that is not in contact will supraerupt.

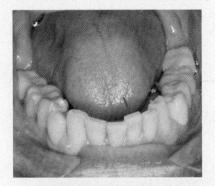
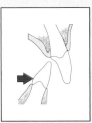

After the teeth have been repositioned for centric relation contact, the final details are worked out in provisional restorations. The patient may wear the provisionals as long as necessary to determine that they are comfortable, functional, and esthetically acceptable.

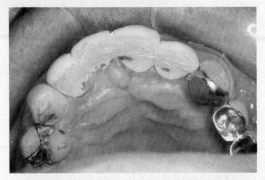

After approval, the details must be communicated precisely to the technician via casts of the approved provisionals mounted in centric relation. A putty silicone index communicates the exact incisal edge positions. A customized anterior guide table communicates the lingual contours, leaving nothing to chance for fabrication of the finished restorations.

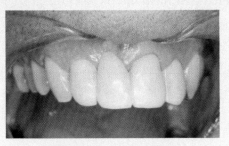
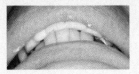

DEEP OVERBITE WITH TISSUE CONTACT

The most common problem with deep overbite alignment is what happens when the lower incisors erupt up into soft tissue lingual to the upper anterior teeth. It is, however, not always a problem. Tissue contact for lower incisors is not a problem if:

1. The upper lingual tissue has been unaffected by the contact (Figures 36-2 and 36-3). This will be determinable by careful observation and history. It is unlikely to be an acceptable stop for the lower incisors in most patients. It is never acceptable if there is a prominent incisive papilla.
2. The contacted tissue is dense, firm, flat, and shows no sign of inflammation.
3. The lower incisor tissue contact is simultaneous with contact against the lingual surface of the cingulums of the upper incisors, making it impossible to move the mandible without immediate separation of the teeth from the tissue. In other words, there must be a vertical envelope of function with no horizontal movement during any excursion.
4. The incisal edges of the lower incisors are smooth with no sharp edges.
5. The incisal plane of the lower anterior teeth is acceptable esthetically and must be in conformity with the rest of the occlusal plane.

DEEP OVERBITE PROBLEMS ASSOCIATED WITH AN ANTERIOR SLIDE

If a deep overbite problem is complicated by posterior interferences that deflect the mandible forward, there is often a tendency to produce extreme wear on the upper anterior lingual surfaces. Sometimes the bruxism effect of the lower incisors carves out the lingual contours and forms a concavity that extends up above the level of the gingival margin. The eruption of the lower incisors keeps pace with the wear on the upper, and the anterior contact ends up in a hole in the upper teeth (Figures 36-4 and 36-5). This type of case sometimes looks unsolvable, but an understanding of what has taken place will serve to simplify the treatment plan.

Such a problem calls for a three-step solution:

1. *We must equilibrate to permit the mandible to close without deflection from posterior teeth.*
2. *We must shorten the lower incisors to position the incisal edges in an optimum relationship to previsualized centric stops on the upper incisors* (Figure 36-6). The lower anterior teeth must always be shortened in such cases either orthodontically or restoratively. Sometimes periodontal surgery is necessary to lower the gingival margin on the mandibular teeth because of eruption of the teeth and corresponding vertical growth of the alveolar bone.
3. *We must restore the upper lingual contours to establish stable centric stops* (Figure 36-7). We must be certain to harmonize the protrusive and lateral excursions after the centric contacts have been determined.

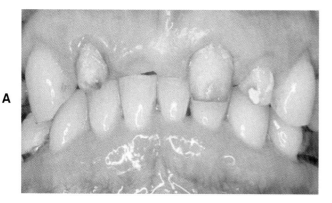

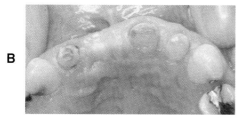

FIGURE 36-2 **A,** Lower incisor tissue contact shows no sign of irritation. **B,** Because of acceptable canine contact and problems of esthetics if lower incisors are intruded or shortened, it is acceptable to maintain tissue contact when new upper restorations are made.

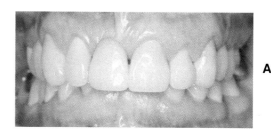

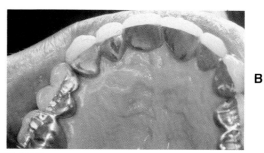

FIGURE 36-3 **A,** Completed restorations made with incisor contact on tissue are shown. Increasing the VDO to accomplish tooth-to-tooth contact would have made the upper anterior teeth too long. By finalizing all details in provisional restorations before proceeding with final labwork, a good result that is acceptable to the patient is assured. **B,** Soft tissue is still healthy one year after completion.

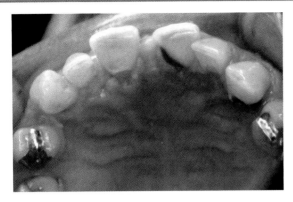

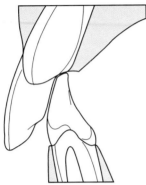

FIGURE 36-4 Apparent deep overbite with severe wear up into roots of upper anterior teeth.

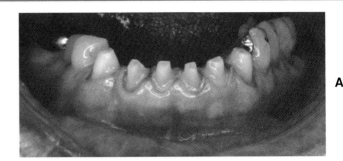

A

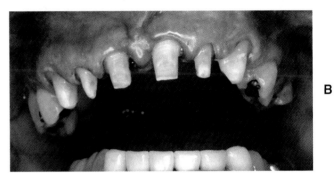

B

FIGURE 36-6 A, Lower anterior teeth are prepared for provisional restorations. B, Lower provisional restorations are placed and upper anterior teeth are prepared for provisionalizaton, so details of occlusal plane can be worked out along with anterior guidance.

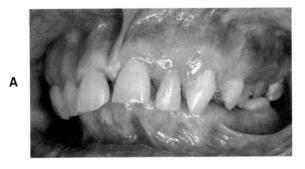

A

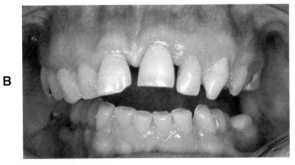

B

FIGURE 36-5 A good example of why all occlusal analysis must start at the temporomandibular joints in centric relation: A, Maximal intercuspation showing severe deep overbite after displacement of the condyles from centric relation. B, The jaw-to-jaw relationship when both condyles were seated in centric relation is shown. Remember that the goal of treatment is always to make the teeth fit the correct jaw-to-jaw relationship, so this is the relationship to which treatment planning must be directed. Follow the same rules for programmed treatment planning in correct sequence to arrive at the best Treatment.

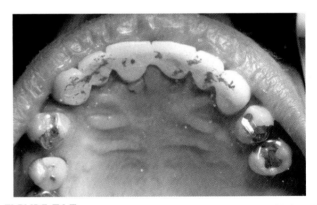

FIGURE 36-7 First set of upper provisional restorations was fabricated from diagnostic wax-up. Here anterior guidance is being worked out after locating an acceptable incisal plane and labial contour. Because of advanced periodontitis, a more permanent provisional restoration was fabricated from guidelines established in this preliminary provisional.

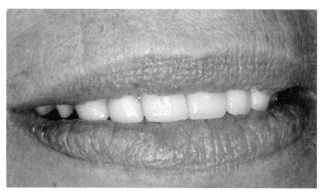

FIGURE 36-8 Provisional restorations fabricated in composite on gold copinged base splinted together. Because periodontal treatment was extensive, both upper and lower provisional restorations were fabricated to hold up for a longer time period than usual.

Special Considerations

The entire success of this treatment plan hinged on getting the back teeth out of the way before the anterior guidance could be determined. The treatment option selected for that was to reshape the posterior teeth to reduce the height enough to achieve anterior contact in centric relation, while simultaneously leveling the occlusal plane (Figure 36-8). Posterior restorations were not attempted until the anterior guidance was worked out to complete satisfaction. Final restorations were completed after periodontal treatment established maintainably healthy supporting tissues.

DEEP OVERBITE WITH SEVERE WEAR

In some deep overbite cases, the upper lingual surfaces are worn severely and are in contact with the entire labial surface of the lower incisors. In some of these cases, elimination of the deflecting posterior interferences is all that is required to provide room for restoring the upper anterior teeth. When they are restored, the centric contact should be moved as much as possible from the labial surface to the lower incisal edge. The labio-incisal edge of the lower should normally be the contact in centric relation, but because of the naturally steep inclines, contact in protrusive and lateral excursions may be almost entirely on the labial surface. There is no harm in such an arrangement as long as the patient is given whatever freedom is needed for "long centric" before the surface-to-surface contact occurs. When needed, even a fraction of a millimeter of "long centric" seems to be the difference in whether patients continue their wear problems or eliminate them.

DEEP OVERBITE PROBLEMS WITH NO DEFLECTIVE INTERFERENCES

Not all deep overbite problems are associated with deflective interferences. One of the most difficult problems to solve is the extremely worn deep overbite that contacts surface to sur-

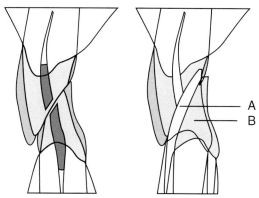

FIGURE 36-9 One of the most difficult deep overbite problems to solve is shown. If there is extreme surface-to-surface wear and no deviation into centric relation, there is no way to provide room for the restorations unless teeth are moved or the VDO is increased. A, Centric relation surface-to-surface contact is shown. B, Position of the teeth at an increased VDO provides the needed room for restoration. The arc of opening directs the teeth back as well as down. If this procedure is used, posterior teeth must also be restored to the new VDO.

face in centric relation (Figure 36-9). Sometimes the upper lingual surfaces have worn almost through the teeth, leaving a sharp, thin incisal edge. If the lower labial surfaces have also worn, the problem is complicated even more.

One may wonder how the problem can be solved without either increasing the vertical dimension of occlusion (VDO) or moving teeth. The answer is that it cannot. Unless either the upper anterior teeth are moved labially or the lower teeth are moved lingually, there is insufficient room to restore the lost surface of either. Increasing the VDO will provide room for the restoration, but this necessarily involves the restoration of posterior teeth also.

It is usually difficult to move the lower teeth lingually, so the orthodontic repositioning most often is confined to the upper anterior teeth. It is not difficult to move these teeth with a removable appliance, but patients with deep overbite generally have tight upper lips. The trick is to keep the teeth forward after the appliance has been removed.

Since the badly worn upper anterior teeth will need to be restored anyway, we can go ahead and prepare them as soon as they are in the desired position and make a plastic provisional splint to serve as a retainer. The temporary splint stabilizes the teeth very well while the bone fills in and the periodontal fibers become realigned. It also introduces the patient to the new overjet, which has been necessarily increased, gives us plenty of time to work out acceptable esthetics and function, and lets the patient adapt to the slightly changed appearance and phonetics.

Neutral Zone Considerations

A point that often is missed is that the neutral zone is *compressive*. This means that as the lingual of the upper anteriors and the labial of the lower teeth wear away, the lips press the upper teeth back by the same amount of the wear in resistance is the forward push from the tongue against the

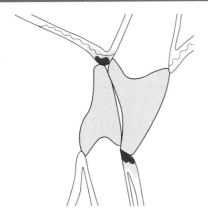

FIGURE 36-10 Deep overbite with lingually inclined anterior teeth almost always ends up in trouble because there are no stops for either upper or lower teeth. Notice impingement of gingival tissue by incisal edge.

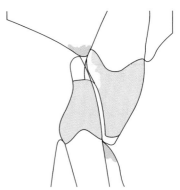

FIGURE 36-11 After shortening both upper and lower anterior teeth, some type of stop must be provided. If the lower teeth can be shortened enough, the stop can usually be added on to the upper lingual surface. Because of intense lip pressure, even orthodontic correction will fail unless stable stops are provided as part of the treatment. If it is possible to move the lower anterior teeth forward, one can often provide the stop by grinding the upper lingual surface to provide a ledge. This does not require movement of the upper teeth, so it does not disturb the balance of the teeth with the pressure of the lips.

lower teeth. This means that we can move the upper anterior teeth forward by the amount of wear off the lingual without interfering with the original neutral zone.

Lingually Inclined Anterior Teeth

Deep overbite problems that result because of unstable centric contact are generally easier to solve if there has not been a great deal of wear because there is usually room to reshape the teeth to establish stability of the centric stops. Given enough time, a relationship that usually ends up in trouble is the deep overbite with lingually inclined anterior teeth (Figure 36-10). When the upper anterior teeth tilt back toward the lingual, there is no convenient stop for the lower teeth. The centric contact is usually made against the lower labial surface by the upper incisal edge. The contact in combination with lip position is usually sufficient to stabilize the upper teeth, but there are no stops to prevent the lower incisors from erupting on up into the palate. Sometimes the combination allows the upper anterior teeth to supraerupt also, so the incisal edges of the upper teeth traumatize the lower labial gingiva while the lower incisal edges injure the palatal side tissues.

The resolution of such problems almost always involves reshaping the upper lingual surfaces and shortening the lower incisors. If the upper teeth impinge on labial tissues, they must be shortened also (Figure 36-11).

To solve the problem, the lower incisal edges must be moved forward into the stable ledge type of centric stops on the upper surfaces, or upper lingual stops must be extended by restoration. The repositioning of the incisal edges may be accomplished either by restoration or by orthodontic movement. If the lower teeth are moved forward, the contour change on the upper surfaces involves selective shaping of the lingual surfaces to provide definite stops. It may or may not require restorative treatment of the ground surfaces, depending on whether the enamel surface is penetrated.

If it is impossible to provide stable centric stops, an alternative may be to do the necessary shortening of supraerupted teeth and then splint the unstable teeth in each direction until we can join to a tooth on each side that has as a stable centric stop. The splinted teeth will be unable to erupt back into tissue contact because they will be held in check by the teeth with the stable stops.

Complete orthodontic resolution of the problem is always the first choice of treatment if it can provide stability. This is particularly so if it would eliminate the need for extensive restorative procedures that would otherwise be unnecessary. However, if orthodontic movement is contemplated on patients with lingually inclined upper and lower anteriors, the factor of an extremely strong buccinator-*orbicularis oris* complex must be considered. The lingual inclination is almost surely associated with a very strong lower band in a high position. A surgical release procedure for lengthening the buccinator muscles may be considered if anterior tooth angulations are to be changed.

DEEP OVERBITE PROBLEMS WITH NO CENTRIC CONTACT

Of all the occlusal relationships observed, the one that will most predictably lead down the path of eventual destruction is the deep overbite relationship when there are no centric stops to prevent the lower anterior teeth from erupting into the soft tissues.

The proximity of the upper and lower teeth in a deep overbite makes it nearly impossible for the tongue to substitute for the missing centric contact. The tongue can rest against the lingual surfaces, but there is not enough room for it to be interposed between the lower incisal edges and the palate. Thus there is nothing to stop the continual eruptive process of the lower anterior teeth until they meet the soft tissues.

Unfortunately, two of the most common approaches to solving this problem are methods that have absolutely no chance of success. In fact, the procedures are harmful. They are as follows:

1. Shortening the lower anterior teeth by grinding
2. Depressing the lower anterior teeth with an anterior bite plane that also allows extrusion of the posterior teeth

Unless the shortened teeth are provided with stable centric stops, they will simply erupt, alveolar process and all, back into the palatal tissue. We have seen lower anterior teeth that have been shortened so many times that they were ground off to the gumline. The elongated alveolar process was then hitting into the palate.

A basic rule to follow when treating deep overbite problems is: *Never shorten the lower anterior teeth unless stable centric stops are provided* or some means of stabilization is effected.

Another popular treatment for deep overbite is even more detrimental: Increasing the vertical height of the posterior teeth to correct a deep overbite problem is absolutely contraindicated unless stable holding contacts are provided for the anterior teeth. In the absence of anterior contact, the lower incisors will erupt, while simultaneously the upper incisors are usually inclined lingually by the lip pressure. The posterior teeth will not maintain the increased VDO, and they will be intruded by an amount equaling the dimension of the vertical increase. The end point of such treatment almost invariably is a stepped occlusal plane along with a worsened problem of anterior guidance disharmony.

Some patients manage to maintain a stable occlusal relationship despite the lack of centric tooth-to-tooth contacts. Patients with wide, smooth incisal edges in contact with dense, resistant palatal tissue may be able to maintain stability if their functional cycle is nearly vertical. Such patients usually have steep canine protection and utilize practically no lateral or protrusive excursions. This, in combination with the type of tooth-tissue contact, is within the resistance range of the tissues, and nothing needs to be done.

SOLVING DEEP OVERBITE PROBLEMS ORTHODONTICALLY

A basic restorative tenet is to avoid unnecessary restorative treatment. If we can avoid restorations by moving the teeth into a correct relationship, orthodontics is the method of choice.

Improved methods of torquing the anterior teeth into stable contact make it possible to correct the unstable deep

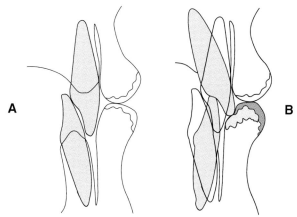

FIGURE 36-12 When teeth are orthodontically repositioned from a deep overbite (**A**) to a position that has an acceptable stop (**B**), care must be taken not to incline the teeth in such a way that the incisal edges interfere with the lip-closure path and the neutral zone. It is usually best to maintain the position of the upper incisal edges as closely as possible while torquing the roots back. The tighter the neutral zone, the more problematic it becomes to interfere with it.

overbite and improve esthetics at the same time. The key to successful orthodontic treatment is the same key used for restorative success: stable centric contacts. The ideal relationship is lower incisal contact against the upper cingulum. In accomplishing this, we must take care to avoid moving the upper incisal edges into the lip-closure path (Figure 36-12). If this cannot be achieved, combining selective grinding with tooth movement is often the practical approach, followed by reshaping the upper lingual surfaces to provide a stable stop and then moving the teeth so that the lower incisal edge fits into the stop. Elongated lower anterior teeth must frequently be shortened to permit correct repositioning.

The orthodontist should be the best judge of the practicality of solving any deep overbite problem by tooth movement. If complex, long-term orthodontic treatment is required, it can be weighed against other methods or combinations of methods. A comparison of advantages and disadvantages can be made, and a logical solution can be determined. In the young patient with healthy virgin teeth, however, all possible steps should be taken to avoid the restorative approach.

It is essential for the treating orthodontist to understand the concepts of anterior guidance. Too many deep overbite problems are actually caused by faulty orthodontic procedures, and many orthodontic attempts at solving deep overbite problems fail because of inadequate understanding of anterior guidance. A strong recommendation may be made to review the principles of anterior guidance (as outlined in Chapter 17) before the treatment plan is finalized.

It has been a pleasure to collaborate on numerous cases during the past few years with enlightened orthodontists who understand the problems and know how to solve them. The methods are available, but they will work only in the hands of those who understand the goals of anterior function and long-term stability.

SOLVING DEEP OVERBITE PROBLEMS BY RESTORATIVE RESHAPING

The preparation of anterior teeth and subsequent reshaping by restorations can accomplish many benefits.

1. Full-coverage restorations on shortened lower anterior teeth can be shaped to move the incisal edges forward. Often this is all that is necessary to provide stable contacts.
2. The lingual surface of upper anterior teeth can be contoured additively toward the lingual to provide holding contacts for the lower anterior teeth (Figure 36-13). The extent of such lingual contouring is strictly limited, however, by the effect that it has on the health of gingival tissues. Under no circumstances should contours that overprotect the gingival margins be permitted. Clinical judgment mixed with common sense must be the deciding factor regarding the limits of the lingual extension.
3. A combination of restoring upper lingual surfaces to provide improved centric stop locations and of restoring lower anterior teeth to provide improved incisal edge location is often a practical approach. It is particularly logical when the anterior teeth require restorations anyway for other reasons.

In a nutshell, restorative procedures can be used to either move lower contacts forward or upper contacts inward. In the process, the contacts can be either raised or lowered. The changes must fall within the limits of acceptable stress direction for each tooth and within contour limitations dictated by requirements for maintainable gingival health.

SOLVING DEEP OVERBITE PROBLEMS BY SPLINTING

In some arch relationships, too much stress would be directed off the long axis if teeth are moved or restored to contact. Teeth that have supraerupted into the palatal tissue can be shortened to relieve the pressure against the soft tissues, but unless they are stabilized in some manner, they will reerupt right back up. Splinting is often the most practical method of stabilizing such lower anterior teeth. By joining the teeth with no stops to a tooth on each side that does have a centric contact, one can stop any further eruption.

The splinting can be accomplished in a variety of ways. If incisal edge reduction has been necessary to the extent of exposing dentin, full coverage would be the method of choice. If esthetic improvement is not needed and the incisal edges are intact, resin bonded lingual restorations for splinting are both conservative and effective.

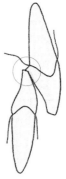

FIGURE 36-13 In some instances, the upper cingulum can be extended slightly to provide a stop for a lower tooth (usually after the lower tooth has been shortened). Care must be taken not to overprotect the gingival tissue from such extensions.

When full coverage is used, centric contact on the "stop" tooth should be in a hard material, preferably porcelain, for its esthetic value as well as its durability. Upper anterior teeth without centric contact are usually kept from supraerupting by the lip contact. They would rarely require splinting for stabilization unless other factors demanded it.

In the absence of posterior teeth, the lower anterior teeth can be stabilized by modifications in partial denture design. Combining continuous clasp splinting of the anterior teeth with replacement of the posterior teeth has the effect of preventing their continuous elongation. Swing-lock design partial dentures accomplish the same results. Although such procedures are effective, they must be considered compromise approaches to the problem because of their esthetic shortcomings. When possible, permanent splinting or night-time appliances are more desired solutions.

MINIMIZING OPERATIVE INTERVENTION THROUGH THE USE OF BITE PLANES TO SOLVE DEEP OVERBITE PROBLEMS

For reasons of age, health, economics, or timing, it is not always practical for some patients to undergo optimum orthodontic or restorative treatment. When a deep overbite problem is causing discomfort from tissue impingement or if future problems are imminent, something must be done to relieve the pain or prevent the problem from worsening or recurring. The least complicated way of preventing supraeruption of the lower anterior teeth is to provide contacts on a removable bite plane. Just wearing the bite plane at night is sufficient to keep the teeth from erupting back into tissue impingement after they have been shortened.

The night guard can also be used as a preventive measure for young adults who have excessive overbite relationships and no holding contacts to prevent supraeruption. It can serve as an interim measure to keep them out of trouble until more definitive measures can be taken when time, cir-

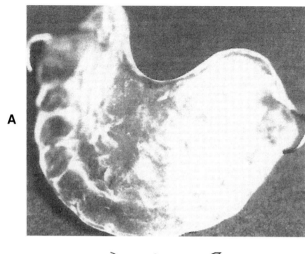

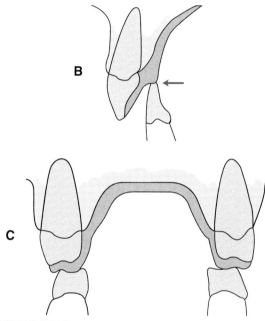

FIGURE 36-14 A night guard appliance is very effective as a compromise procedure for preventing the supraeruption of noncontacting anterior teeth. The appliance (A) is fabricated of clear acrylic resin. Two wrought wire clasps help to stabilize it and provide a simple means of removal. The appliance should be adapted to the palate and should extend to form a continuous smooth contour with the buccal surfaces (B). A stable centric stop should be provided for the lower anterior teeth *(arrow),* and this stop should be in perfect harmony with the posterior occlusal contacts on the appliance (C).

cumstances, or economics permit. Fabrication of the night guard should be carried out on centrically mounted models. The appliance is most esthetically acceptable when it is made of clear acrylic resin. It must provide stable centric contacts for all lower teeth, and it should be equilibrated so that there is no interference to any excursive movement.

The thin palatal coverage should extend up and over all the posterior teeth. It should extend to the bucco-occlusal-line angle to stop as a continuation of the natural buccal contours (Figure 36-14). The occlusal table should be extended

around to allow the lower anterior teeth to contact on the anterior bite plane simultaneously with posterior centric contact. The acrylic appliance should cover the lingual surfaces of the upper anterior teeth, and a comfortable anterior guidance should be worked out in the appliance to provide posterior disclusion.

Wire clasps can extend around the distal of the last molar on each side and engage a slight undercut on the buccal. The clasps are really used more for convenient removal of the appliance than they are for retention. For comfort's sake, the appliance should fit precisely without rock. Patients should be instructed to thoroughly clean their mouths every evening before insertion of the appliance. It should be worn every night. The Biostar technique (described in Chapter 32) is another excellent method for constructing a night guard appliance that usually eliminates any need for clasps.

Patient acceptance of the night guard is surprisingly good. Patients report that it is comfortable to wear, and some patients have worn such appliances for years rather than undergo orthodontic treatment or resort to splinting procedures for stabilization.

The use of a night guard appliance is a compromise solution for keeping deep overbite patients out of trouble, but it is an acceptable compromise if it is properly made and religiously worn.

USING REMOVABLE PARTIAL DENTURES TO SOLVE DEEP OVERBITE PROBLEMS

When an upper partial denture is required, it can sometimes fulfill a double purpose by serving as a contact for the lower anterior teeth. If the palatal bar is designed to cover the tissues behind the upper anterior teeth, the lower anterior teeth may be permitted to contact the palatal bar to prevent supraeruption. The contour of the palatal coverage may be designed to permit protrusive excursions of the lower anterior teeth to slide smoothly from the palatal coverage onto the lingual inclines of the upper anterior teeth.

Although this seems to be the most practical way to solve some unusual deep overbite problems, it should be cautioned that the restorative procedures demand extreme preciseness and perfect occlusal harmony of the removable segment. Too much pressure will cause tissue problems on the lingual gingival area.

Tooth support for the partial, in combination with tissue support, is an absolute requirement.

This procedure is something of a last-resort solution that has its main value in arch relationships that do not have sufficient posterior tooth support. When some tissue support is needed from the upper teeth to enable the lower anterior teeth to actually carry part of the stresses of the lower arch, this procedure has merit. In situations in which the lower anterior teeth are not actually needed to lend support, splinting the anterior teeth to prevent supraeruption will suffice. This procedure is not needed.

SUMMARY

A deep overbite is a problem only when the anterior relationship is not stable. All methods of treating deep overbite problems are designed to either provide stable holding contacts to prevent supraeruption of the lower anterior teeth or to stabilize by other means the teeth that cannot be positioned or restored to contact.

Chapter 37

Solving Anterior Overjet Problems

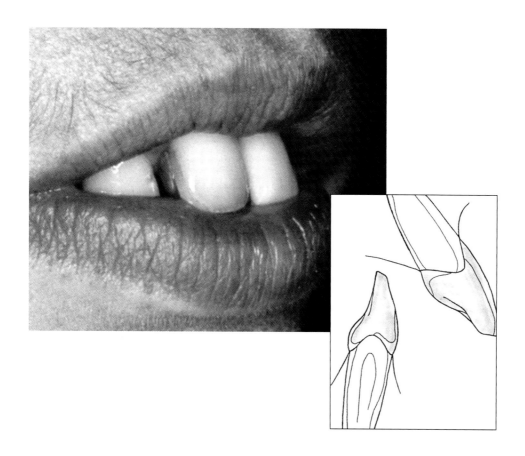

IMPORTANT CONSIDERATIONS

Extreme anterior overjet
1. Overjet patients present the greatest difficulty for providing centric stops on all the teeth.
2. Careful observation is important to make sure the overjet relationship is not stable before attempting to correct it. Examine tongue and lip habits. The lip is often locked behind the upper anterior teeth.
3. The tongue is a common substitute for holding contacts. Evaluate to see if it effectively stabilizes the lower incisors.
4. Evaluate the horizontal component of jaw function before arbitrarily moving anterior teeth.
5. Problems with posterior teeth stability are common with anterior overjet because of the difficulty of providing anterior guidance with posterior disclusion.
6. It is essential to determine whether the overjet is caused by maxillary protrusion, or by mandibular insufficiency before a treatment plan is selected. (Use the nasion perpendicular analysis.)

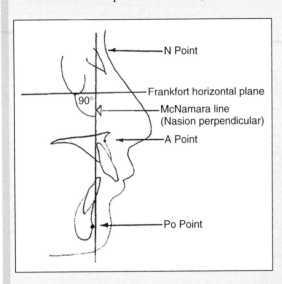

Note the A point is forward of the nasion perpendicular while Po is in correct alignment with the cranial base. The maxilla is the problem.

7. Overjet problems are common in children with airway problems because the tongue must posture forward to permit mouth breathing. Correction of the airway problem is critical to correction of the overjet problem.

Treatment objectives
1. Ensure the stability of lower anterior teeth.
2. Provide the best possible anterior guidance. (It may be necessary to use premolars.)
3. Use posterior group function on the working side to disclude balancing side if the overjet is not corrected.
4. Correct the facial profile when indicated. Esthetics is often the main reason patients seek treatment.

EXTREME ANTERIOR OVERJET TREATMENT CHOICES

1. *Reshape.* Some overjet problems can be corrected by closing the vertical dimension of occlusion (VDO) to permit the arc of closure to move the lower anterior teeth forward into contact with the upper anterior teeth.
2. *Orthodontics.* This is very often the best solution, sometimes in combination with restorative dentistry.
3. *Restorative dentistry* to restore holding contacts or to splint incisors to teeth that have contact in centric relation.
4. *Removable appliances* to provide palatal bar stops for lower incisors.
5. *Surgery* to move the maxilla back or the mandible forward or to reposition the maxillary anteriors back with

an osteotomy. Careful analysis is needed to determine the best option (Figure 37-1).

THE PROBLEMS OF ANTERIOR OVERJET

Patients with excessive overjet have three specific problems, each of which may contribute to accelerated deterioration of the teeth and supporting structures.

Problem 1

In excessive anterior overjet relationships, the lower anterior teeth have no stabilizing contact with the upper teeth, either in centric relation or near centric relation. Hence they have

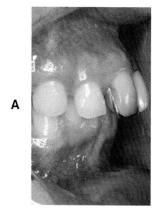
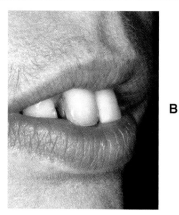
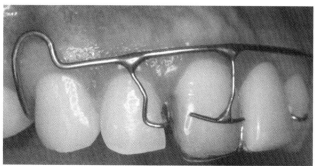

FIGURE 37-1 Overjet problems are often combined with other problems of occlusion because the causes of overjet can also cause anterior splaying (**A**) and neutral zone problems that intensify the overjet such as entrapment of the lower lip (**B**). All options for treatment must be evaluated, as treatment often requires a combination of reshaping, repositioning, and restorative dentistry as shown in **C**. Following the process of programmed treatment planning gives clear direction for choosing the right combination of treatment choices.

a tendency to supraerupt, drift out of alignment, and frequently impinge on the palatal tissues.

Problem 2

Excessive overjet relationships make it difficult or impossible for the anterior guidance to do its job of posterior disclusion.

Problem 3

A third problem that is often associated with excessive anterior overjet is esthetics. The classic bucktooth appearance has long been used by cartoonists to depict stupidity. It is not a pleasant appearance, and it is often the real reason why patients seek treatment.

The resolution of anterior overjet problems involves four considerations:

1. Stabilization of the lower anterior teeth
2. Providing the best possible anterior guidance for posterior disclusion in protrusion
3. Providing the best possible relationship for disclusion of the balancing inclines
4. Improving the position, alignment, or shape of the upper anterior teeth for better esthetics

Although all four of these requirements are interrelated, they can be considered separately for simplicity. It is helpful to keep in mind that anterior overjet problems may result from either maxillary anterior protrusion or mandibular anterior retrusion. Regardless of the cause of the problem, the requirements for stable occlusion do not change.

SOLVING THE PROBLEM OF STABILIZING THE LOWER ANTERIOR TEETH

It is not always necessary to stabilize lower anterior teeth just because they lack contact in centric relation. If the anterior overjet problem is not too severe, the teeth may contact in protrusive and lateral function enough to stabilize them and prevent their supraeruption.

Even in severe overjet problems, the tongue may position itself between the palate and the lower anterior teeth during each swallow. The tongue thus acts as a substitute for the missing tooth contact and serves to stabilize the position of the teeth. There are many patients with healthy mouths who do not have anterior tooth contact in any functional position. There is no need for operative intervention to stabilize teeth that are already stable.

There are other substitutes for anterior tooth contact. The lips sometimes are positioned in ways that serve to stabilize teeth with an apparent anterior overjet problem. Lip biting, sucking in the lower lip, and other habit patterns are very often beneficial because they serve as substitutes for missing tooth contact. Many times such habit patterns are all that is needed to stabilize the position of the teeth and prevent problems. No treatment plan should ever be initiated that does not consider the effect of habit patterns.

In evaluating habit patterns, we must differentiate between habits that stabilize teeth when there is a true interarch malrelationship and habit patterns that cause problems. Some habit patterns are actually responsible for the overjet problem we are trying to resolve. Harmful habit patterns are those that lead to instability of the occlusion.

A major facet of diagnosis is to determine whether there is occlusal instability. If a habit pattern has substituted for missing tooth contacts, the teeth are firm, the patient is comfortable, and in our clinical judgment the stability is maintainable, there would be no need for operative intervention. However, such a relationship should be kept under careful scrutiny because it takes very little to disturb the delicate balance of an occlusion that depends on a habit pattern for its stability.

If a habit pattern is the primary cause of the overjet problem, elimination of the habit is the major aspect of treatment. Limited success has been reported in correction of such occlusal relationships with myofunctional therapy. However, if the habit can be eliminated by any practical means, it would certainly be the treatment of choice.

Some habits result from attempts to cushion the teeth against striking an occlusal interference. Equilibration sometimes eliminates the need for such habit patterns, and when there is no reason to bite the lip or hold the tongue between the teeth, the normalized lip pressures return the upper anterior teeth back to their correct relationship with the lower teeth.

When a habit pattern cannot be broken, we have no choice but to work around it. As an example, it would be folly to restore lower anterior teeth to come into contact in the presence of an unbreakable tongue-thrust swallowing pattern.

In the presence of a habit pattern, attempts at stabilization of the lower anterior teeth should follow this sequence:

1. It should be determined whether the anterior relationship is stable because of a beneficial habit pattern.
2. It should be determined whether a harmful habit pattern is contributing to the problem. If it is, we must evaluate the possibilities of either eliminating the habit through myofunctional therapy, eliminating the cause of the habit, or a combination of both.
3. If the habit is beneficial or if a potentially destructive habit cannot be eliminated, we must design the treatment to cooperate with the habit. In any conflict between the teeth and a habit pattern, the teeth will lose.

Not all overjet problems are related to habit patterns. The majority are interarch relationship problems that require intervention of some type to resolve the instability. Unstable lower anterior teeth can be treated with some of the same options that are used for deep overbite problems. Deep overbite relationships with no anterior contact are also actually problems of overjet. The following five options may be used singly or in combination to solve the problem of supraeruption of the lower anterior teeth in patients with overjet problems.

1. For patients with severe overjet, the *orthodontic approach* often requires some extractions. Orthodontics is usually the first choice of treatment.
2. *Restorative reshaping* to establish holding contacts is usually not possible in patients with severe overjet unless the teeth are repositioned orthodontically first.
3. *Splinting* is often necessary in severe overjet problems to prevent the lower anterior teeth from supraerupting. In very severe overjet problems, it may be necessary to extend the splinting all the way around the arch to stabilize lower posterior teeth that cannot contact ideally. If the contacts cannot be designed to direct the forces down the long axis, splinting may be necessary to counteract the lateral stress.
4. *Night-guard biting planes* may be used as a compromise treatment. They can be used as a Hawley type of retainer also to stabilize upper anterior teeth that have been repositioned lingually. If nighttime use of the appliance is sufficient to stabilize the occlusion, it may serve as a practical alternative to extensive restorative treatment when circumstances rule out more complex approaches. Details for fabrication are in Chapter 32. It is the same type of appliance that may be used in deep overbite problems.

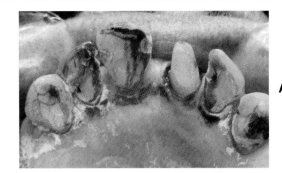

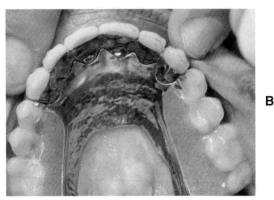

FIGURE 37-2 Overjet with no posterior teeth. **A,** Centric relation contact *(green marks)* are on tissue lingual to the upper anterior teeth. The anterior guidance should be refined in the mouth so it can be copied on a custom anterior guide table. **B,** Centric relation contact on palatal bar is shown. Anterior guidance continues smoothly onto lingual surfaces of anterior restorations. When the holding contacts are on a removable partial denture base, the base must be tooth supported to maintain the relationship between the fixed and removable segments. Care must be taken not to increase the VDO when a removable partial denture base is used. This is because any increase in VDO will have a tendency to compress the partial base into the tissue as the muscles attempt to regain their contracting muscle length.

5. The *use of removable partial dentures* to stabilize the lower anterior teeth may have special adaptation for patients with severe overjet. Sometimes it is the only practical way to achieve stabilizing contact for the lower anterior teeth. The lower anterior teeth can contact the upper palatal bar to provide excellent stabilization (Figure 37-2). In severe arch relationship problems, the saddle area of the partial restoration may also provide contact for lower posterior teeth that are in severe lingual version.

Lower removable appliances may also be used to stabilize teeth. Partial restorations with continuous clasps or swing-lock designs, as well as extended overlay partial dentures, may sometimes be used as compromise treatments.

> The basis for treatment: Lower anterior teeth without stable holding contacts can be prevented from supraerupting if we provide either something for the teeth to contact or something to hold the teeth in place so that they cannot supraerupt.

The five methods of accomplishing this should be reviewed in Chapter 30 for further details.

PROVIDING PROTRUSIVE DISCLUSION OF THE POSTERIOR TEETH

Patients with severe anterior overjet rarely have vertical patterns of function. The vertical "chop chop" biters are mostly confined to those with steep anterior guidances or those who have no need to protrude the mandible. Patients with end-to-end relationships and anterior crossbites have nothing to gain by mandibular protrusion. However, patients with too much anterior overjet have to protrude the mandible to allow the anterior teeth to function. Consequently, their pattern of function is usually quite horizontal. Unless the posterior teeth are discluded in protrusion, they are subjected to excessive stress. Therefore the arch relationship that needs posterior disclusion the most often has no way to provide it because the anterior teeth are not in contact until considerable protrusion has already occurred.

One of the most common problems seen in severe anterior overjet relationships is hypermobility of the posterior teeth with varying degrees of periodontitis. The overjet patient is particularly susceptible to traumatogenic periodontal breakdown unless the treatment plan can provide some means of discluding the posterior teeth when the mandible is protruded. The rule to follow for protrusive disclusion is: *When the anterior teeth cannot provide the guidance to disclude the posterior teeth in protrusion, the job should be assigned to the most anteriorly positioned tooth on each side that can.*

The canines can usually be shaped to provide a protrusive guidance, but it is sometimes necessary for the upper first premolars to assume this role. In really severe overjet conditions, the job may even be given to the upper second premolars. Which teeth serve as the protrusive guidance is not too important as long as the guiding tooth on each side discludes all of the teeth distal to it. If a first premolar is in the best position to serve as the guidance but is not strong enough to assume the role, it should be strengthened by splinting to whatever degree is needed to provide the necessary stabilization.

Even a pontic may serve as the protrusive guidance. It is position that is important. The stress diminishes as the distance from the condylar fulcrum increases, so the farther forward the guidance can be positioned, the less stress is exerted on the guiding tooth (or the bridge abutments if the guide tooth is a pontic). Contouring the guidance tooth for protrusive disclusion is accomplished the same way that the protrusive pathway of any anterior guidance is worked out.

PROVIDING DISCLUSION OF THE NONFUNCTIONING INCLINES

In severe anterior overjet relationships, the anterior teeth may not be able to contact in lateral excursions. In such cases, disclusion of the nonfunctioning inclines must be accomplished by posterior teeth on the working side. When only posterior teeth contact in working excursions, the lateral anterior guidance must be established on the contacting tooth that is farthest forward. From that point back, varying degrees of group function can be worked out to distribute the lateral stresses.

It is usually preferable to have all of the posterior teeth in group function when they do not get help from the anterior teeth, but this is not an unbreakable rule. The distribution of lateral stresses must always be worked out according to the resistance capabilities of the teeth sharing the occlusal forces.

Unlike the anterior teeth, posterior teeth in eccentric contact do not have the capacity for shutting off elevator muscle contraction, so premolars are not generally capable of resisting the same forces that the canines can. Premolar roots are usually much shorter than the average canine root, and premolars do not have the benefit of the dense bone of the canine eminence. Deep flutes or bifurcations make the premolars more susceptible to irreversible periodontitis than the single-rooted canine. Finally, premolars, being closer to the condylar fulcrum, are in a position of greater stress than the canine. For all of these reasons, a single premolar should rarely serve as the lateral anterior guidance.

When excessive overjet prohibits the anterior teeth from contact in lateral excursions, the balancing inclines should be discluded by group function of all or most of the posterior teeth on the opposite side. When posterior group function must occur without any help from anterior teeth, the working inclines must be perfectly harmonized to make sure the lateral stresses are evenly distributed. Functional inclines should never be steeper than the patient's normal functional pathways. To accomplish this in posterior restorative cases, we should correct the lingual inclines of the most forward guiding tooth, following the same rules that are applicable for harmonizing any lateral guidance. All teeth distal to the guiding teeth should then be harmonized to the guiding tooth. Functional path procedures work well to accomplish this harmony. It can also be done with several different instrument approaches. If restorations are not needed, inclines must be corrected by equilibration until group function is achieved.

IMPROVING THE POSITION OR SHAPE OF UPPER ANTERIOR TEETH WITH EXCESSIVE OVERJET

Improving the esthetics of buckteeth is one of the most stimulating challenges a dentist can face. The improvement in appearance is especially gratifying when it also helps to stabilize the occlusion, reverse destructive tendencies, and provide better comfort. These are all achievable goals that can be fulfilled if the treatment plan is carefully designed for optimum results rather than for expediency.

Too often the correction of maxillary anterior protrusion is attempted by simple reshaping of the teeth with full-coverage restorations. Many cases can be solved in this manner, but better results can be achieved for most patients with problem overjet if the upper anterior teeth are moved into better alignment before any restorative reshaping is finalized.

Correcting Upper Anterior Tooth Position Orthodontically

Circumstances permitting, complete orthodontic treatment is the method of choice if it eliminates the need for extensive restorative procedures. But if extensive restorative treatment is needed anyway, minor tooth movement procedures are still beneficial in a large percentage of the cases we treat. Furthermore, minor tooth movement is often simplified when it is combined with a restorative approach. Teeth can be narrowed or shortened to provide direct access to their corrected position. Esthetic temporary bridges can sometimes be used to hold teeth in position after they are moved, and provisional restorations can sometimes serve the same purpose as orthodontic bands.

One of the most practical methods for repositioning upper anterior teeth is to use a removable upper appliance with an anterior bite plane to keep the lower anterior teeth from supraerupting during treatment. A rubber band extends around the labial surfaces of the upper anterior teeth to apply pressure lingually. The palatal acrylic appliance contacts the lingual surface of each tooth.

The appliance is activated when the acrylic splint is cut back for whatever amount of movement is desired. Cutting it back a little at a time prevents the movement from occurring too rapidly and serves as the control for the amount of movement. Guides can be cut into the acrylic splint to direct teeth laterally or to rotate them. Teeth that are in correct position can be stabilized by the lingual acrylic bite plane while others are selectively moved. The rubber band is not too obtrusive and very few patients ever object to its appearance.

Narrowing the upper anterior teeth is often necessary to permit sufficient lingual movement. The stripping procedures can be accomplished a little at a time as the teeth are moved. Movement can be accomplished by activated wires or by rubber bands.

Applying the principles

The problem shown is an overjet with lower incisor contact on palatal tissue. There are also esthetic concerns.

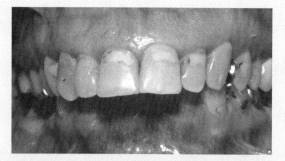

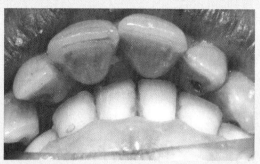

The lower lip locks behind the upper anterior teeth, affecting speech and causing exposure to unesthetic drying of the incisors'[1] labial surfaces.

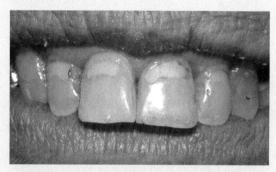

First treatment option: *Reshape*. Analysis on mounted casts showed the need to narrow the incisors to make room for moving the incisor segment lingually.

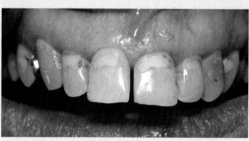

Second treatment option: *Reposition*. After narrowing the incisors to a predetermined width, an appliance is made with a lingual plate contoured to receive the teeth into their predetermined position as they are moved lingually.

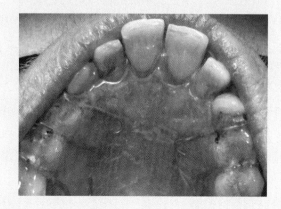

A rubber band attaches to the appliance to move the teeth into the contoured slots in the lingual plate. Use of such appliances is a simple way to achieve dramatic results, but alternative methods using bands or brackets must always be considered if final positioning requires horizontal bodily movement of roots.

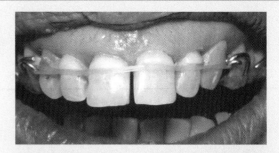

Results of repositioning show an improved incisal plane as incisal edges move down as they are pulled back into a position that permits contact with the lower incisors. *Note:* The appliance increases the VDO to allow room to move the upper teeth back. The lingual contours are then reshaped to ideal contact with lower incisors.

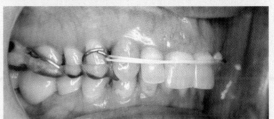

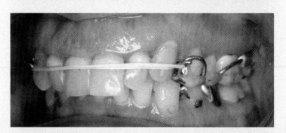

Third treatment option: *Restore.* Teeth are prepared, and a provisional restoration is made as a copy of the diagnostic wax-up. The provisional restorations are refined in the mouth following the guidelines explained in Chapter 16. The restorations are tested for a smooth functioning anterior guidance, making sure that immediate disclusion of the posterior teeth is achieved. This may require some reshaping of posterior surfaces.

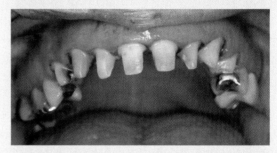

Note: All of the procedures described above were done to determine the exact end result desired. The next step is to communicate every detail to the technician.

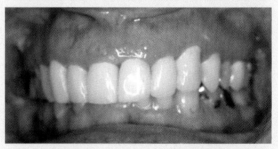

Communication. The mounted cast of approved provisionals provides exact details to the technician. The putty silicone index communicates incisal edge position and contour. The custom anterior guide table communicates the exact lingual contours.

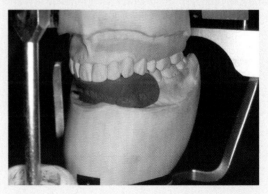

Final restorations copy all of the details. Nothing is left to chance.

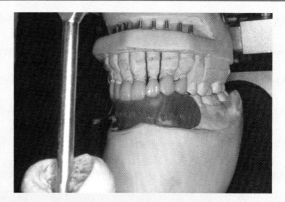

Finished restorations (far right) showing improved relationship to smile line. The lip-closure path now permits the lower lip to pass in front of the upper anterior teeth, which has the effect of changing the neutral zone from the original relationship shown.

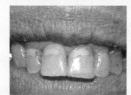
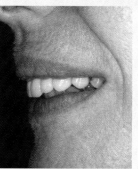

This relationship illustrates incisal edge contact on the inner incline of the lower lip during pronunciation of *V*. Total comfort and function were assured in the final restorations because they copied all of the details worked out in the provisional restorations.

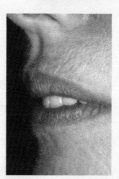

Post-op stabilization. Because teeth were repositioned, a period of post-op stabilization is indicated. This can be easily accomplished with a simple Biostar appliance made of flexible vinyl. It requires no clasps because it snaps over the teeth and engages the undercuts for retention.

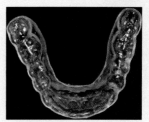
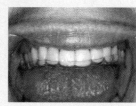

The appliance is adjusted for equal intensity centric relation contacts. It is also contoured to establish an anterior guide ramp for immediate posterior disclusion *(not shown)*. Patients are instructed to wear the appliance at night for three months. If the teeth remain stable after removal, it is no longer needed. Teeth that are in a correct neutral zone position do not need continuous stabilization.

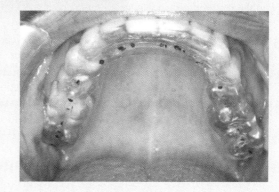

As the upper anterior teeth are being moved back into a better alignment, their relationship with the lower incisors should be repeatedly checked with the appliance removed. It is usually necessary to reshape the upper lingual surfaces after they are moved to provide stable holding contacts for the lower anterior teeth. The reshaping can wait until the teeth are in their final position, though, because the bite plane prevents the lower teeth from interfering. The shaping should be done immediately after the appliance is removed.

When anterior contact has been established, the appliance can be modified to permit all the teeth to contact. The rubber band should then be replaced by a labial retainer wire to stabilize the teeth in their new position for a few weeks.

If the anterior teeth are to be restored, preparations can be made for making a provisional splint to serve as a retainer. The temporary splint can also be used to refine the anterior guidance and resolve any esthetic problems.

Reshaping the Anterior Teeth with Restorations

Any time a major change is made in the shape of anterior teeth, it should be made first in temporary restorations. The changes should be worked out on mounted study models so that the result can be visualized before treatment is started. When the teeth are prepared and the preplanned temporary restorations are placed, the anterior guidance can be refined for minimal stress and optimum comfort. Modifications can be made to achieve the best esthetics and phonetics. Complete patient approval can be secured before the final restorations are fabricated.

The methods described in Chapter 36 are also applicable for patients with overjet problems. There are some special considerations, though, that should be noted:

1. Malposed teeth should not be restored until they have been moved into the best possible position. "Warping" the labial surface of malposed teeth back into alignment can sometimes produce a round, very unnatural appearance. When the root goes one way and the crown goes another, the appearance is unpleasant and artificial. As far as practical, the root should be aligned to the restored crown. This also produces better stress direction.

2. The restored lingual contours should not be allowed to overprotect the gingival tissues. Sometimes our attempt to achieve centric contact results in too much lingual extension. If the contours are not compatible with maintainable tissue health, they are not acceptable. Alternatives to centric contact will have to be considered.

3. We must be certain to provide sufficient "long centric." Some patients with excessive overjet develop a protruded "jaw set" to compensate for the malrelationship. It becomes such a definite part of their functional movements that any interference to it is annoying. Even though the "new look" is a great esthetic improvement, such patients may complain constantly that the upper anterior teeth have been "pulled in too far." Fortunately, such patients are in the definite minority, but the potential problem should always be considered. The most likely cause for such a feeling is an actual interference to the centric relation arc of closure. Be certain that during closure to centric relation the lower teeth do not strike the lingual inclines of the upper anterior teeth before complete closure to centric relation. If the final restorations are not fabricated until the relationship has been approved in the temporary restoration, such a problem is extremely rare.

EQUILIBRATING THE OVERJET PROBLEM

Some patients with excessive overjet have anterior contact only in their protruded, acquired occlusal position. The following inquiry is often made: What will happen if I equilibrate such a patient and permit closure back into centric relation? The anterior contact in the acquired position would be lost. Wouldn't equilibration be contraindicated in such cases?

The answer has many facets to it. Proper equilibration is rarely contraindicated. If a patient is comfortable and has no sign of any problem or any potential for accelerated deterioration, there would be no reason to equilibrate. But as this text has already pointed out, patients with malocclusion and no problems are rare. Patients with excessive overjet with occlusal interferences and no problems are extremely rare. We should correct any problem that has a damaging effect on the long-term health of the teeth and supporting structures. Each case demands clinical judgment in this regard.

Equilibrating such patients does not usually create a problem. Most often, what appears to be a long slide is really a minimal protrusive deviation. The difference between centric relation and centric occlusion is usually a fraction of a millimeter when the interferences are eliminated. If anterior contact occurred in the acquired position before equilibration, it has been my clinical experience that most patients will have enough contact in excursive function to maintain the position of the lower anterior teeth after equilibration.

If any forward movement of the upper anterior teeth has resulted from the protrusive deviation, lip pressures will probably bring the upper anterior teeth back in after the interferences are removed and the mandible stops deviating forward. Lower anterior teeth frequently erupt on into contact if arch relationships permit.

If loss of anterior contact does cause a problem as a result of equilibration, the problem is treated the same as any other overjet problem. The options for solving the problem are the same. However, if there was contact in maximal intercuspation before equilibration, it should take a minimum of minor tooth movement to regain the contact in centric relation. Removable appliances can usually be used most effectively to solve the problem with very little difficulty.

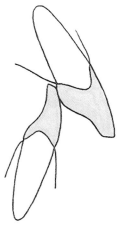

FIGURE 37-3 Upper anterior overjet. Anterior teeth are flared out from lower incisor contact against the lingual slope of the cingulum. This problem frequently occurs from loss of posterior support. A special treatment problem is created because of loss of posterior tooth anchorage for moving the incisors back. The upper incisors are also blocked by the lower incisors.

SOLVING OVERJET PROBLEMS WHEN THERE IS INSUFFICIENT POSTERIOR ANCHORAGE

When upper anterior teeth have flared labially because of lost posterior tooth support, a twofold problem is created. There is a loss of vertical stops by the posterior teeth. This loss allows the lower anterior teeth to close too far on a forwardly directed arc; thus the lingual movement of the upper anterior teeth is blocked (Figure 37-3). The problem is compounded by insufficient posterior anchorage for providing a stable base for moving the anterior teeth. Since movement of the anterior teeth is usually required to reposition them in a more favorable relationship, it is essential to find acceptable anchorage. There are four ways of accomplishing this, as follows.

Extraoral Anchorage

The use of headgear provides sufficient anchorage, but for adult patients such headgear is usually unacceptable.

Intraoral Tissue-Supported Base

A tissue-supported base with posterior teeth can provide the increased VDO to unlock the lower anterior teeth from upper lingual contact. But tissue support makes poor anchorage and often results in soft-tissue irritation from moving the base rather than the teeth. This problem can usually be solved by the application of pressure to move only one tooth at a time while the other anterior teeth are used as anchorage for the partial. Movement can be controlled by removal of acrylic material on the lingual of one tooth and waiting until that tooth is moved to contact it. Then some acrylic resin

is removed on a different tooth. By alternating with one tooth at a time, we can make the fit of the partial base in the palatal vault serve as resistance without creating too much pressure on the soft tissues. The higher the vault, the better this method works. Very flat ridges do not provide sufficient anchorage to utilize this method.

Implant Anchorage

If there is sufficient bone in the posterior ridge areas to place an osseointegrated implant on each side, the implants can serve as anchorage for moving the anterior teeth. It will still be necessary to open the VDO enough to disengage the lower anterior teeth from the upper lingual surfaces.

Anchorage from the Lower Arch

If there are a sufficient number of lower posterior teeth, they may be banded for added stabilization and used as anchorage for elastics attached to the upper anterior teeth.

SURGICAL CORRECTION

In severe arch malrelationships, the treatment of choice may be orthognathic surgery. Before any surgical approach is selected, a careful evaluation should determine whether the overjet problem is the result of maxillary protrusion, mandibular retrusion, or a combination of both. The rule to follow always is: *Leave what is right; change only what is wrong.*

Cephalometric analysis is a helpful diagnostic method, but it must be used in combination with neutral zone analysis and esthetic profile observation. Please read Chapters 43 and 44 for more information regarding cephalometric determinations and surgical methods for correcting severe arch malrelationships.

Suggested Readings

Burstone CJ: Lip posture and its significance in treatment planning. *Am J Orthod* 53:262-284, 1967.

Geiger A, Hirschfel L: *Minor tooth movement in general practice,* ed 3. St Louis, 1974, Mosby.

Goldstein MC: Orthodontics in crown and bridge and periodontal therapy. *Dent Clin North Am* July:449-459, 1964.

Graber TM, Vanarsdall RL, Vig KWL: *Orthodontics: Current principles and techniques,* ed 4, St Louis, 2005, Mosby.

Hinds EC, Kent JN: *Surgical treatment of developmental jaw deformities.* St Louis, 1972, Mosby.

Isaacson KG, Reed MT, Muir JD: Removable orthodontic appliances. Oxford, 2002, Butterworth Heinemann.

MacIntosh RB: Orthodontic surgery: Comments on diagnostic modalities. *J Oral Surg* 28:149-159, 1970.

Proffit WT, White RP: Treatment of severe malocclusion by correlated orthodontic surgical procedures, *Angle Orthodont* 40:1-10, 1970.

Willison BD, Warunek SP: *Practical guide to orthodontic appliances.* Buffalo, NY, 2004, Great Lakes Orthodontics, Ltd.

Solving Anterior Open Bite Problems

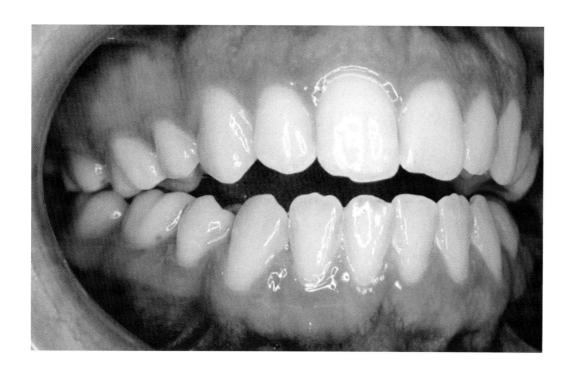

PRINCIPLE

The first determination is what caused the open bite.

IMPORTANT CONSIDERATIONS

Anterior open bite
1. If there is an open bite, something will be filling the space. Teeth always erupt unless something stops the eruption. It can be a tongue, lips, cheeks, a thumb, a pipe, an occlusal splint, or anything that consistently prevents the teeth from erupting. Before closing a bite, it is important to know if the cause of the open bite is correctable on a continuing basis.
2. The most important determination is what caused the open bite.
3. Always evaluate the condition of the temporomandibular joints (TMJs). Loss of condylar height usually causes progressive anterior separation.
4. If a habit pattern caused the open bite, correction will be unsuccessful unless the habit is eliminated.
5. Skeletal malrelationships can usually be successfully treated.
6. There are many degrees of open bite depending on tongue or lip habits that intrude teeth or prevent their eruption.
7. Many anterior open bites are stable.
8. A major problem of anterior open bite is trauma to posterior teeth.
9. A second major problem is lack of an anterior guidance for posterior disclusion.

Treatment objectives
1. Maximize the number of equal-intensity occlusal contacts on both sides of the arch.
2. Correct a "reverse smile line" on upper anteriors when indicated for esthetic improvement.
3. If only one arch is malaligned, close the anterior relationship by correcting the arch that is wrong. Do not alter a correctly aligned arch to conform to one that is malrelated.
4. If a habit pattern cannot be broken, the occlusion must conform to the habit.
5. Achieve posterior disclusion in protrusive by determining the anterior guidance as far forward as possible.
6. If anterior guidance cannot be achieved for disclusion of the balancing side, use group function of the working side posterior teeth.
7. If condylar breakdown is progressive, correction of the occlusion must keep up with it.

FINDING THE CAUSE

Treatment planning for anterior open bites requires that the cause of the open bite be considered. If the cause of the separation is still an active factor, closure of the opening will be unsuccessful unless that factor can be altered along with the changes in occlusion.

An important decision that must be made in solving an anterior open bite problem is to determine whether it is really a problem that needs solving. Since many anterior open bite problems are the result of habit patterns, the habit must be eliminated or treatment must be planned to work with the habit if it is unbreakable.

The major causes of anterior open bite in order of probable frequency are as follows:

1. Forces that result from thumb or finger sucking, or use of pacifiers.
2. Crowding. If anterior teeth are rotated forward off their basal bone, the forward inclination causes separation.
3. Airway obstruction:
   a. Inadequate nasal airway creating the need for an oral airway (mouth breather)
   b. Allergies
   c. Septum problems and blockage from turbinates
   d. Enlarged adenoids or tonsils
4. Lip and tongue habits
5. Intracapsular TMJ deformations
6. Neurologic problems (such as cerebral palsy) lead to tongue posture problems
7. Skeletal growth abnormalities, probably resulting from the above problems as well as from pure skeletal growth asymmetries.

There are varying degrees of habit-caused anterior open bites (Figure 38-1). Since the degree of anterior separation is usually a clue to the habit that caused it, this is where the analysis should start. It should be understood that noticing the amount of anterior separation is, at best, empiric. It is not meant to be a precise criterion. Even such generalized evaluations, however, can serve as helpful starting points from which to evaluate the cause of problems and formulate practical treatment approaches.

> Remember: *All occlusal analysis starts at the TMJs.* This is especially important when analyzing anterior open bite problems (Figure 38-2).

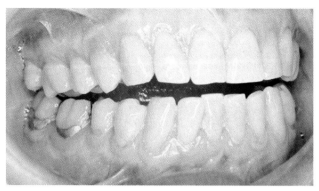

FIGURE 38-1 Progressive anterior open bite is almost always an indication of loss of condylar height. Note the matching wear facets on the anterior teeth, a certain indication that the teeth were once able to contact.

APPLYING THE PRINCIPLES

Before Treating, Determine the Cause of the Open Bite

Try to determine if a tongue habit *caused* the open bite or if the tongue position is the *result* of the open bite. If the tongue is the cause of the open bite and the tongue habit cannot be eliminated, we must work with the tongue habit. There are many anterior open bite patients with stable dentitions. If teeth are moved or restored into a conflict with the tongue position, the tongue will win. The teeth will be intruded or moved until the tongue regains its original space (Figure 38-3).

Protective Tongue-Biting Habits

Many patients position the tongue between the teeth to protect a prematurely contacting tooth. They are not aware of the habit, and the habit usually disappears when the occlusion is corrected. The correct treatment approach is to equilibrate the occlusion if it can achieve maximal contact without mutilation. If the cause of the tongue thrust was a protective response, the tongue will stay out of the way so the teeth can then erupt back into contact.

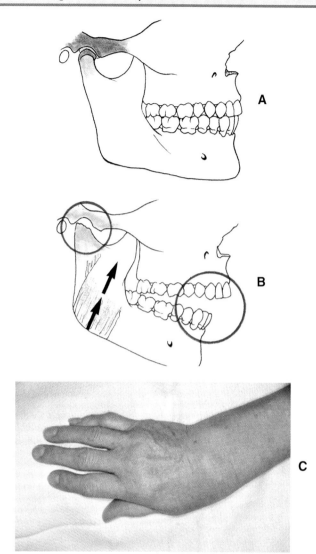

FIGURE 38-2 **A,** Intact TMJs with perfected occlusion. **B,** The same occlusion when condylar height is lost. **C,** Signs of rheumatoid arthritis show up early in the wrist and finger joints. It almost invariably leads to condylar breakdown and anterior open bite (see Figure 38-1).

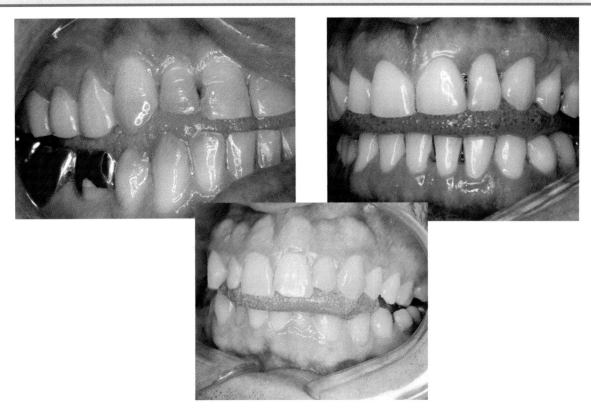

FIGURE 38-3 Three anterior open bite patients with unbreakable tongue-biting habits. The *upper-left* dentition was originally restored to complete occlusal contact. The tongue resumed its original position between the teeth and returned the open bite space to its original dimension and contour. The reopening occurs without discomfort to the patient within 10 to 12 months. It does not seem to cause any problems with supporting tissues. The key to observing when an open bite should be left as is: The teeth are stable, and the patient is comfortable. Oddly enough, these patients are not generally concerned about the appearance of their smile, as it is usually not a problem. If you must restore, be considerate of the tongue position.

Anterior open bite in a patient with occluso-muscle pain. Deflective interferences on molars created a slide to maximal intercuspation. At maximal intercuspation, no contact was possible for the anterior teeth.

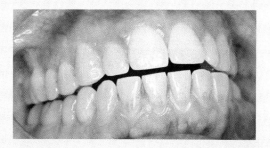

Tongue posture at maximal intercuspation.

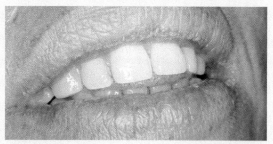

Maximal intercuspation after occlusal correction by equilibration. Anterior teeth still could not contact opposing teeth.

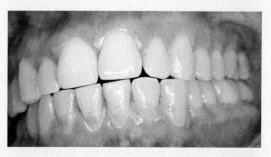

Position of teeth after 10 months. No orthodontic treatment or any other attempt was made to close the anterior open bite. The teeth erupted to contact because the tongue no longer maintained a posture to cushion the bite for protection of the deflective premature contact.

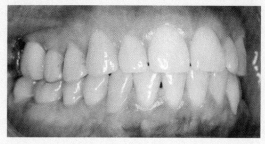

MINIMAL ANTERIOR OPENING

An anterior separation of approximately 1 mm is usually caused by a lip-sucking habit. The patient develops a negative pressure and sucks the mucosal tissues between the front teeth. The inner part of the lower lip at or below the vermillion border is involved, and so the habit is not readily apparent.

This habit is usually developed as a protective device to avoid a posterior interference. Perfecting the posterior occlusion through selective grinding eliminates the need for the habit and it usually ceases after equilibration. When the habit is eliminated, the anterior teeth move into contact and no further treatment is needed.

The time required for the teeth to reposition themselves after the cause of the habit is eliminated varies. I have seen complete self-correction of the anterior relationship occur within two to three weeks, and in other patients it requires months. If the arch relationship permits anterior contact and there is nothing interposed between the teeth to prevent eruption, the lower anterior teeth will erupt and the upper anterior teeth will find their balance with lip pressures.

If the anterior teeth do not require restorations for other reasons, we must not become impatient if we do not see immediate results. We should keep the posterior occlusion refined as perfectly as possible and let nature take its course. Very few patients will fail to respond.

Some patients will not break the lip-sucking habit regardless of how perfect the posterior occlusion is. We have

no choice but to work around the habit, and this can be done very effectively (Figure 38-4).

If anterior teeth must be restored in the presence of an unbreakable habit, the restored surfaces must be positioned the same as the natural surfaces were. Some minor esthetic corrections can usually be made, but the labial and lingual surfaces must be positioned the same.

Preparing every other anterior tooth is the most practical approach. By doing that, both labial and lingual contours can be duplicated according to the adjacent unprepared teeth. Incisal edge positions can be precisely duplicated, and the restored teeth will fit right into the position that the unbreakable habit pattern dictates.

We can easily diagnose separations caused by holding objects between the teeth by asking questions or by observing. Open spaces should not be closed unless the patient is willing to stop the habit. If a pipe stem is the cause of the separation, the separation should be duplicated in any restorations of the area if the patient plans to continue the pipe smoking (Figure 38-5). Pencil biting, nail holding, or other occupation-related habits should be treated similarly.

It should be determined whether a moderate anterior opening is really a problem. If the canine guidance is not disturbed by the separation of the incisors, the potential for stability of the occlusion is good (Figure 38-6). The occlusion should be checked carefully to make sure that there are no balancing-side interferences, and posterior teeth should be discluded in protrusion by the most forward teeth that can do the job. When posterior occlusal harmony is perfected, it

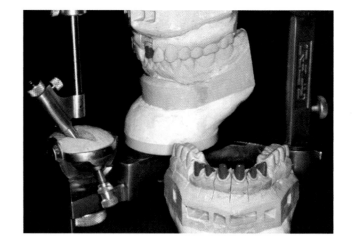

FIGURE 38-4 Minimal open bite as a result of an unbreakable tongue or lip habit. The relationship of the teeth to the lips or tongue is maintained by working with a cast of every other anterior tooth prepared. The patterns on the E/O (every/other) cast are transferred to the master cast so exact copies of the lingual contour can be made. Final restorations will be stable and completely comfortable.

Comment: If a space from an unbreakable lip or tongue habit is filled, the tongue or lip will reposition between the restored teeth and force them apart and into a more forward position in the arch. If the habit cannot be broken, it is better to maintain the open bite and balance the teeth with the habit.

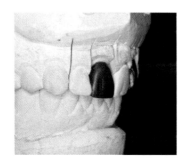
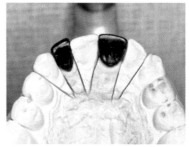
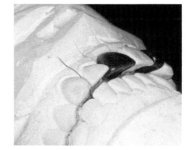

is surprising how often the anterior opening closes down, but even if it does not, there will be no harm caused if the stresses can be distributed over most of the posterior teeth.

SEVERE ANTERIOR OPEN BITES (5 mm OR GREATER SEPARATION)

Although it appears certain that abnormal deglutition and other tongue-thrust patterns play some role in all severe anterior open bites, it is also apparent in most instances that there is a vertical dysplasia within the bone system itself. In many anterior open bites, the anterior teeth are actually supraerupted in their unsuccessful attempt to close the open space. It is doubtful that such supraeruption would result from a depressive type of tongue habit. We must differentiate between such skeletal malrelationships and those that were caused primarily by habits that have depressed the anterior teeth.

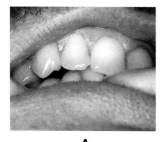 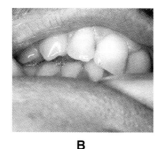

A   B

FIGURE 38-5 A, A small opening at the canine as a result of holding a pipe stem. B, When the pipe smoking habit was stopped, the tongue was forced into the space to maintain it. To prevent biting the tongue, closure of this space would require surgical removal of the protuberance on the tongue that has expanded into the space.

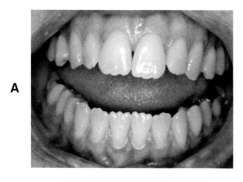

A

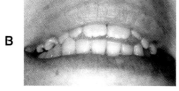

B

FIGURE 38-6 A, Mamelons still present on a 42-year old patient. Tongue posture prevented any contact. The occlusion was stable and in harmony with centric relation. B, Note the canine contact at maximal closure.

Very often, severe open bite problems are the result of habits that were caused by other habits. The anterior open bite that results from a thumb-sucking habit is often perpetuated by a tongue-thrust swallowing habit. The tongue thrust results from an attempt to seal off the anterior opening to develop the negative pressure for the swallow.

Combining occlusal correction with myofunctional therapy has the capability of solving the problem if the patient can cooperate, but it has an uncertain prognosis because it is difficult to predict patient cooperation in changing such a set swallowing pattern. Our results with myofunctional therapy have not been successful over an extended time period.

If the problem is habit caused, orthodontic procedures can almost always be used successfully to realign the anterior teeth. The only problem is keeping them there after they are moved.

Solving the problem of achieving a stable anterior relationship may require a three-pronged attack:

1. Orthodontic correction of anterior tooth relationships
2. Occlusal equilibration to eliminate the need for protective tongue or lip habits
3. Use of a retainer at night

Fixed Splinting for Stabilization

A fourth approach to maintaining teeth in a stable relationship is sometimes tried when tongue pressures are a problem. Its effect is rarely long lasting. Remember the adage that *"When teeth and muscle war, muscle never loses."* It doesn't matter if the teeth are splinted. If they are in the way of where the tongue wants to be, it will move the entire segment of splinted teeth to re-establish the anterior open bite.

Stabilization by a removable retainer used at night can work in some patients if it can do two things in addition to a good fit in a high vault (Figure 38-7).

1. Increase the vertical dimension of occlusion (VDO) to make more room for the tongue. Contact should be on anterior teeth only.
2. Redirect the tongue so it can't push on the lingual surfaces of the teeth to flare them forward.

If none of the above plans can stabilize the teeth, there are surgical solutions that may be considered such as enlarging the vault space or reducing the size of the tongue. Such decisions beg for caution.

Closure of Anterior Open Bite

Based on nothing more than clinical observation of many patients over a long time period, I have observed two characteristics of anterior open bites that are based on the contour of the separation. By using these characteristics (Figures 38-8, 38-9, and 38-10) as a simple visual guideline, the treatment results have been consistent. I feel safe in recommending its use with an invitation for further study of its rationale.

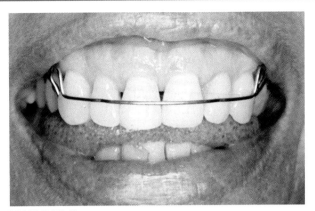

FIGURE 38-7 An example of an oversize tongue. Use of a retainer at night was able to maintain the anterior teeth in position because of a high palatal vault that helped to stabilize the retainer. Failure to wear the retainer resulted in flaring of the upper anterior teeth in a short time. No other treatment was necessary.

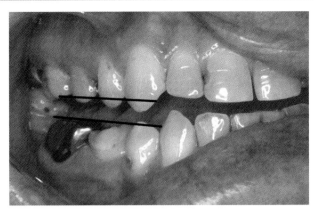

FIGURE 38-9 If the opening is more parallel at the posterior teeth, there is almost no chance of closing the space and having it stay closed. The tongue finds its way between the teeth and reopens the space. This dentition may be as stable as a normal occlusion, as compression against the tongue holds the teeth in an open bite.

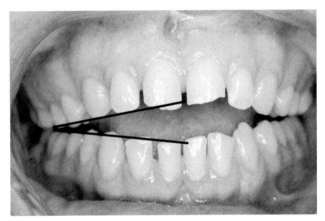

FIGURE 38-8 When the opening is progressive from back to front, resembling a *V* laid on its side, we have never had a problem closing the VDO to achieve anterior contact. With this configuration, the tongue does not have a tendency to reopen the bite. Closure of the open bite may require a combination of reduction on the posterior teeth and moving or restoring the anterior teeth.

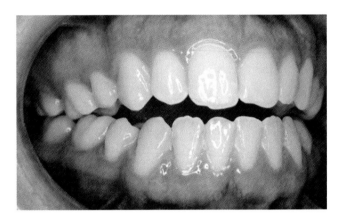

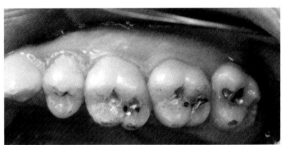

FIGURE 38-10 First option for treatment: *Reshape*. By selective reshaping, the centric relation contact on one molar was expanded to contact on three molars on each side. This did not achieve complete closure of the anterior space, but it made the occlusion comfortable and stable. The tongue substituted for the teeth that could not contact in centric relation.

Applying the principles

Anterior open bite. Contact in centric relation is only on second molars. Esthetics is a major concern of the patient. Objective: anterior contact.

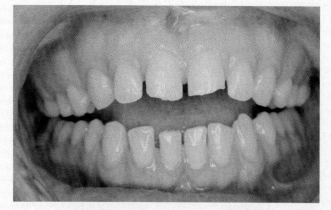

First treatment option: *Reshape.* Contour of space indicates that the tongue will not be a problem if the space is closed. The question to ask: How much closure can we get by reduction of the posterior teeth? This can be determined on the mounted casts.

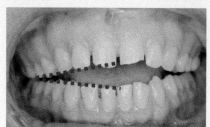

Analysis of mounted casts indicates that it is practical to shorten the molars to gain anterior contact. Adjustment on the casts shows that contact in the canines could be achieved by judicious reshaping of the molars to close the bite. Remember that 1 mm of reduction of the second molar results in 3 mm of closure at the anterior teeth. After equilibration of the casts, a tentative wax-up of the upper anterior teeth is performed and an acrylic resin overlay is made that can slip right over the fractured teeth.

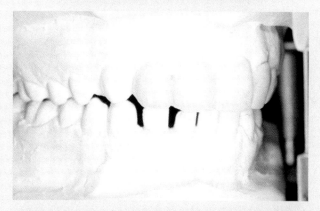

This overlay can then be shaped in the mouth to show the patient in advance what a change in the incisal plane would do for the smile.

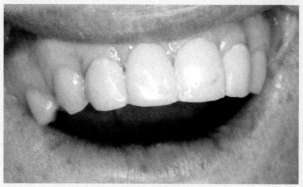

Completed restorations. Contact in centric relation establishes an anterior guide with immediate posterior disclusion and long-term stability of the dentition. By closing the VDO, an attractive smile can be achieved without anterior teeth that are too long.

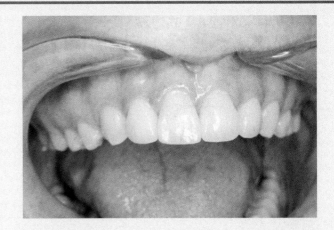

Surgical option

Inclination of opening toward the front suggests that a successful result can be achieved by closing the vertical space between the anterior teeth. The first treatment option of reshaping could only achieve this much closure without mutilating the molar teeth. This leads to evaluation of repositioning the teeth but it would have to involve the dento-alveolar process to achieve an acceptable esthetic result.

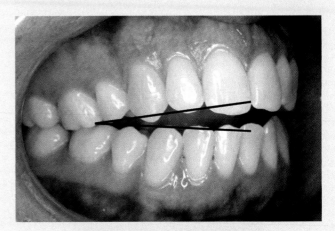

Important rule: *Don't change what is right to fit what is wrong.* Analysis shows that the height of the lower incisal plane is correct.

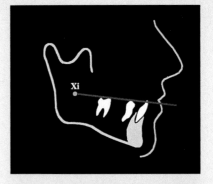

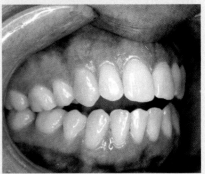

Thus, the upper dento-alveolar segment should be repositioned down to close the space and gain contact with the lower teeth.

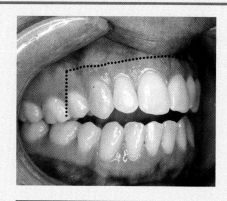

Final result achieves a pleasant esthetic result as well as a functional anterior guidance. The steep guidance was acceptable because the envelope of function was very vertical (as it is on most anterior open bites).

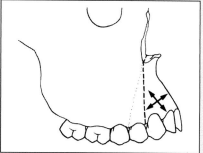

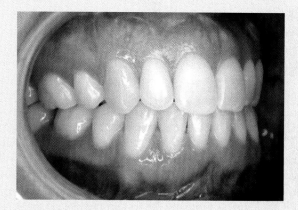

TREATING PROTRUSIVE LATERAL TONGUE-THRUST PROBLEMS

In a protrusive lateral tongue thrust, the tongue is spread out and held between all the anterior and posterior teeth except the most distal teeth on each side (see Figure 38-9). Often the only teeth in contact are the second or third molars. Unlike the straight protrusive tongue thrust with its progressively much larger anterior opening, the lateral tongue habit usually produces a fairly even separation of all noncontacting teeth. Although it usually occurs with a slightly prognathic mandible, it can occur with any arch relationship.

Correction of the occlusal separation appears very simple. Shortening one or two opposing teeth on each side that have contact usually closes the VDO enough to bring most of the other teeth into contact. If the arch relationship permits, the occlusion may sometimes be corrected by selective grinding at the closed VDO. Most often, though, occlusal reconstruction is necessary to provide cusp-tip–to–fossa relationships with stable form.

When full occlusion is restored to a patient with lateral tongue thrust, the patient will be comfortable, will function well, and will generally be pleased with the good result. There is only one big problem: The good occlusal relationship will almost never stay that way. Unless the lateral tongue habit can be broken, the original separation will recur. I have found it virtually impossible to permanently break severe lateral tongue habits if the anterior teeth were included in the open bite separation.

It is not impossible to break the habit. We have actually achieved occlusal contact on previously separated teeth with no treatment other than retraining the patient to swallow properly. Results have been achieved for up to a year and slightly longer. Eventually the pattern returns and the separation recurs without the patient even being aware of it. It should be emphasized that our clinical experience should not be interpreted as meaning there are no permanent solutions. It is just honest reporting that we have not been able to maintain long-term occlusal contact with any method we have used up to now. Myofunctional techniques have not provided the answer.

Just because we cannot predict long-term maintenance of occlusal contact does not mean we cannot achieve an acceptable degree of occlusal stability. By working with the habit, we can let the tongue stay interposed between the teeth and can improve the occlusion of the teeth that do contact, so that stress direction is made as ideal as possible on the occluding teeth. Achieving a harmony between tooth contact may seem hard to imagine, but it can be achieved rather easily because the tongue serves as its own positioner. The teeth merely adapt to whatever pressures it provides.

It is a mystery how patients with so little occlusal contact can function, but it does not seem to be a problem as far as they are concerned. Patients can maintain comfort, function, and a surprising degree of stability with the protrusive lateral tongue-thrust habit. Before attempting to correct such a relationship, we must be certain there is a real need for change.

There is no way for the noncontacting anterior teeth to provide any anterior guidance, but this is not a problem because protrusive lateral tongue thrusters are usually vertical "chop choppers." They do not as a rule protrude the mandible or use lateral jaw movements.

If this combination of procedures does not produce the desired occlusal stability, a fourth procedure may be necessary. Splinting may be required to hold the anterior teeth in their corrected position. Unless anterior restorations are required for other reasons, however, permanent splinting should not be considered until it has been positively determined that it is needed. Stabilization by removable retainers should be tried first. After a suitable time for reorganization of the supporting tissues, the retainer should be removed a day at a time. If no tooth movement occurs, it should be left out for gradually longer periods. Splinting should be considered only as a last resort when maintainable stability cannot be achieved without it. Then it should be used with careful discretion. Even splinted teeth can be moved out of alignment if a strong habit pattern is still present.

If the tongue habit resulted from an initial thumb-sucking habit, the prognosis is better than if the anterior open bite is hereditary. Our success record in correcting anterior tooth position in hereditary skeletal anterior open bites is poor, but the potential for achieving stability of the dentition is good, even without complete correction of the anterior position.

Severe anterior open bite relationships present the following problems:

1. Poor anterior esthetics. This is often the only reason the patient seeks help.
2. The anterior guidance cannot do its job. Posterior disclusion in protrusive and balancing excursions cannot be accomplished by the anterior teeth.
3. The posterior teeth are overstressed. The teeth nearest the condylar fulcrum usually receive the greatest stress with no help from the anterior teeth.

With no anterior guidance, elevator muscle hyperactivity is increased, so the potential for overload on the contacting molars is increased (Figure 38-11). However, if the teeth that do contact in centric relation can be made to simultaneously contact on both sides with equal intensity, there does not seem to be a problem with maintaining them in a stable relationship. The vertical contracted length of elevator muscles establishes a set dimension between the mandible and the maxilla at the position of the muscle origin or attachment. The teeth erupt into that set space until they meet an opposing force equal to the eruptive force. If the tongue takes up part of that space, it becomes the stop for eruption. It does not appear that the teeth that contact opposing teeth receive any more load than the teeth that contact the tongue.

I have followed many patients with anterior open bite for many years, and if the contacting teeth are adjusted for

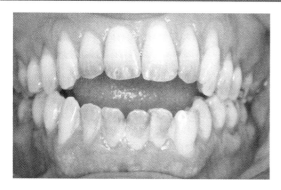

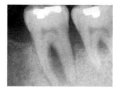

FIGURE 38-11 Mouth with extensive plaque, though the only teeth with advanced bone loss are the teeth that have deflective, premature contacts.

equal-intensity loading against vertically directed stops, these dentitions stay just as stable as those with full occlusal contact.

Before treatment is initiated, we should determine whether the anterior open bite is the result of a skeletal malrelationship. Cephalometric evaluation can be used to determine whether the problem is skeletal or is the direct result of habit-caused depression of the anterior teeth. If the skeletal relationship is good and the tongue habit is generally limited to protrusive thrusting, the prognosis is good for realigning the anterior teeth.

If a skeletal relationship is the primary cause of the anterior open bite and the skeletal bone is too far separated to permit correction within the dento-alveolar process, the prognosis for realigning the anterior teeth conservatively is poor. But if the tongue thrust is limited to protrusive thrusting, the potential for achieving good stability of the entire dentition is excellent. The nonsurgical treatment of choice for this specific problem is to close the VDO by reducing the height of the posterior teeth. This can be done by selective grinding or by orthodontic intrusion.

The greater the reduction of posterior tooth height, the greater will be the reduction of the anterior opening. In most cases, the posterior teeth can be shortened enough to bring the canines into contact. The distribution of stresses onto more teeth can usually be further improved by reshaping the centric contacts at the closed VDO and establishing working-side group function for disclusion of the balancing inclines. If such reshaping exposes dentin, cast restorations should be placed to protect the occlusal surfaces.

The closure of the anterior opening that results from the decreased VDO produces a greatly improved appearance. Even though the space may not be completely closed, any reduction of the anterior opening results in a noticeable esthetic improvement that is gratifying to the patient.

Even though the closed vertical appears stable, there is growing evidence that the actual mandible-to-maxilla relationship does not stay at the new closed dimension. It appears that elongation of the alveolar bone matches the amount of tooth reduction so that the loss of vertical is temporary. Unless, however, the tongue is interposed back between the arches after correction, the corrected occlusal relationship will stay surprisingly stable, and the increased dimension of alveolar bone will go unnoticed.

The preceding results are achievable in skeletal malrelationships if the tongue thrust is primarily a protrusive thrust. The tongue seems to readily adapt to the closed vertical without disrupting the changed alignment. The protrusive thrust in this type of problem was not the cause of the open bite, so it can easily conform to a more closed relationship.

If the protrusive tongue habit also includes a *lateral* tongue thrust, however, the prospects for stable correction by closing the VDO are practically nonexistent. This is true regardless of whether the lateral tongue thrust occurs with or without a skeletal malrelationship.

Lateral stresses on the contacting posterior teeth should be minimized as much as possible by flattening of cusp inclines.

If a patient with protrusive tongue thrust requires extensive restoration of the posterior teeth because of caries or general breakdown of existing restorations, there may be nothing wrong with making an attempt at occlusal correction in the new restoration. A relapse of the corrected occlusion does not seem to cause any discomfort or injury, so it may be worth the try. I would, however, draw the line at restoring occlusions to contact that had no other reason to be restored, unless there was positive evidence that the habit could be eliminated and that the restorative procedures were needed to preserve the remaining teeth.

The more predictive approach to treatment, however, is to first determine if the occlusion is stable by checking for signs of hypermobility or change of tooth position. If there is no instability problem, we can restore the occlusal surfaces to the same relationship with the tongue by preparing every other posterior tooth and taking an impression before completing the rest of the preparations. The resulting cast can be used to guide the technician to the precisely correct contours, and the stable relationship with the tongue can remain unchanged.

Rheumatoid Arthritis

The deformity of the TMJs that occurs in rheumatoid arthritis may cause a separation of the anterior teeth, and the separation may continue to enlarge as the deterioration of the joints progresses.

Attempts to restore or reposition the anterior teeth back to contact are contraindicated. The patient should be kept comfortable by maintenance of the best possible occlusal relationship on the teeth that contact. Selective grinding can usually be used to eliminate any deflective contacts and to reshape any interfering inclines up to a point. If the loss of condylar height progresses, it may be necessary to remove the last molar to allow the condyles to seat.

If a pain-dysfunction disorder should develop in a patient with rheumatoid arthritis, the degree of joint deformity will have no effect on the resolution of the pain aspects of the syndrome. With rare exceptions, these patients respond just as quickly and just as predictably to occlusal therapy as patients with normal joints.

Even though the disk is destroyed in the rheumatoid joint, there can still be a bone-to-bone stop for the condyle that does not require lateral pterygoid muscle resistance to the elevator muscles. Although the nature of this uppermost position is tenuous, patients can be kept reasonably free of muscle pain in the joint region by correction of occlusal interferences on the posterior teeth that strike.

ORTHODONTIC CORRECTION OF ANTERIOR OPEN BITES

It appears that conventional intraoral orthodontic techniques would be successful only in patients who have tooth derangements without a severe skeletal malrelationship. If the morphology of the mandible itself must be changed, it appears rather logical that extraoral orthopedic appliances would be needed. Graber[1] has pointed out that such orthopedic appliances can effect a change in a relatively short period of time *if the treatment is accomplished during a period of fairly rapid growth.*

Dentists have the obligation to their young patients to notice any open bite tendencies because of such skeletal malrelationships. Patients should be referred for orthodontic evaluation early enough for the orthodontists to take advantage of the growth periods.

In adult patients, it is easier to shorten teeth than to depress them. Shortening a second molar 1 mm produces as much as 3 mm of anterior closure; so the best approach for

resolving severe anterior open bite problems appears to be a combined effort between the restorative dentist and the orthodontist.

The VDO should be closed as much as possible by reduction of the height of the posterior teeth. Severe shortening will require restoration of the occlusion. There should be orthodontic alignment of the anterior teeth into the best relationship possible after they have been brought as close together as possible by the vertical closure.

Surgical correction of anterior open bite problems has become more and more a logical choice of treatment. Very often the correction can be done better and faster by surgery, and the facial profile may be improved at the same time.

Reference

1. Graber TM: Physiologic principles of functional appliances. St. Louis, 1985, Mosby.

Suggested Readings

Akin E, Sayin MO, Karacay S, et al: Real-time balanced turbo field echo cine-magnetic resonance imaging evaluation of tongue movements during deglutition in subjects with anterior open bite. *Am J Orthod Dentofacial Orthop* 129:24-28, 2006.

Alimere HC, Thomazinho A, de Felicio CM: Anterior open bite: a formula for the differential diagnosis. *Pro Forno* 17:367-374, 2005.

Chen YJ, Shih TT, Wang JS, et al: Magnetic resonance images of the temporomandibular joints of patients with acquired open bite. *Oral Surg Oral Med Oral Pathol Oral Radiol Endod* 99:734-742, 2005.

Clark WJ: Twin block functional therapy: applications in dentofacial orthopedics, ed 2, London, 2002, Mosby.

Guray E, Karaman AI: Effects of adenoidectomy on dentofacial structures: A 6-year longitudinal study. *World J Orthod* 3:73-81, 2002.

Gurton AV, Akin E, Karacay S: Initial intrusion of the molars in the treatment of anterior open bit malocclusions in growing patients. *Angle Orthod* 74:454-464, 2004.

Ricketts RM: Respiratory obstruction syndrome. *Am J Orthod* 54:495-507, 1968.

Solow RA: Equilibration of a progressive anterior open occlusal relationship: A clinical report. *Cranio* 23:229-238, 2005.

Treating End-to-End Occlusions

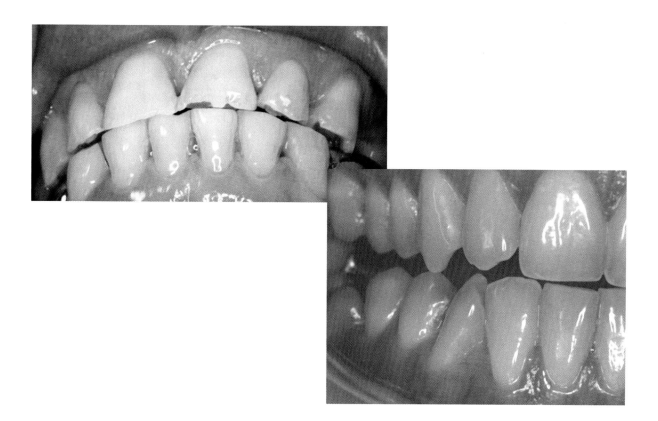

ANTERIOR END-TO-END RELATIONSHIPS

IMPORTANT CONSIDERATIONS

1. Anterior end-to-end relationships may be very stable if they are in harmony with centric relation. These patients typically do not protrude past anterior contact if it is properly designed. Lateral anterior guidance is achieved by sliding sideways against the flat incisal edges.

2. Condylar guidance can usually combine with flat anterior guidance to disclude all posterior teeth.

3. The principal problem that often occurs with a flat anterior guidance is failure to disclude the posterior teeth in excursions, so care must be taken to make sure the occlusal plane and fossae contours are correctly related for disclusion by the condylar path on the balancing side (Figure 39-1). This typically requires flatter occlusal contours for disclusion on the working side because working side disclusion is achieved solely by the lateral anterior guidance.

4. Changing an anterior end-to-end occlusion to an overlap relationship steepens the anterior guidance and will probably cause a bruxing wear problem on the anterior teeth. When such changes are made, the patient should be warned about probability of wear. It is, however, sometimes a necessary compromise that is manageable.

5. A nighttime bruxing appliance is in order whenever the envelope of function is restricted. Changing a flat end-to-end anterior guidance to a more restricted overlapped anterior relationship almost invariably results in wear, hypermobility, or movement of the upper anterior teeth. The nighttime appliance should be designed as a retainer to reduce these problems, and patients should be informed of the potential problems.

6. Even though restriction of the anterior guidance causes wear, etc., it is not usually uncomfortable for the patient as long as there are no interferences to centric relation closure.

7. The ideal solution is to maintain the anterior guidance as flat as possible if esthetic goals can be met without an anterior overbite relationship.

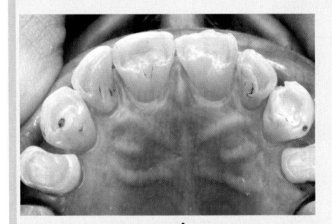 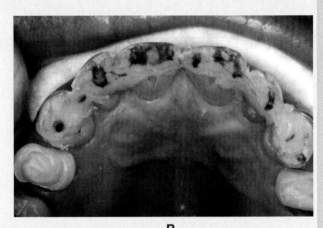

| A | B |

FIGURE 39-1 **A,** When working out anterior guidance for an end-to-end anterior relationship, all posterior interferences must be eliminated first. The anterior guidance can then be determined directly on the teeth, or if the incisal edges must be restored, the guidance can be worked out on composite or acrylic resin attached to the teeth **(B),** to be copied then from a cast of the corrected contour.

RESTORING END-TO-END ANTERIOR TEETH

If restorations are a necessity on end-to-end anterior teeth, their anterior guidance function can be improved greatly with subtle changes in contours.

Minimal changes in incisal edge position can effect gross improvements in anterior function. Moving the upper incisal edges forward and the lower incisal edges inward can extend the protrusive contact by a couple millimeters or more

(Figure 39-2). In combination with the downward movement of the protruding condyles, this 2 mm to 3 mm of added anterior guidance should be sufficient to disclude the posterior teeth if the posterior occlusal form is correspondingly contoured to be discluded by a flat anterior guidance.

A strong warning should be noted here against steepening end-to-end anterior guidance angles. The guidance should remain nearly flat. Improvement should be made in the form of extending anterior guidance contact, not steepening it. Most dentists are surprised to find how effective a

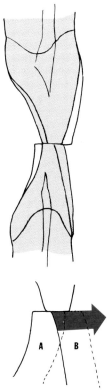

FIGURE 39-2 *Anterior end-to-end (shaded); relationships do not generally present a difficult problem. Notice how little change is needed to provide a flat anterior guidance of several millimeters. In addition to the added protrusive contact (arrow in lower illustration), the anterior contact can also be maintained until the lingual incisal line angle of the lower reaches the labioincisal line angle of the upper. Position A represents centric relation. Position B represents the most protruded relationship possible without loss of anterior contact. The changes in incisal edge relationship can be accomplished either restoratively or orthodontically, depending on individual factors in each case.*

perfectly flat anterior guidance can be, but even a horizontal zero-degree guidance can fulfill all the disclusive needs of the posterior teeth if occlusal contours are also kept flat enough and the occlusal plane is correct.

Restorative recontouring of teeth in an end-to-end bite can cause special problems if the stresses are moved off the direction of the long axis. In a long-standing end-to-end relationship, the stresses are so confined to the long axis that the periodontal fibers and the bone trabeculae are not aligned to resist lateral stress. Suddenly changing a tooth's contour to subject it to lateral forces may produce unwanted effects of tenderness or hypermobility until the fibers realign and the bone becomes more resistant to the lateral forces. Great care should be taken to avoid contours that will direct the stresses off the long axis. If it is absolutely essential to restore an incisal edge off the long axis too far, it may be necessary to stabilize the tooth in that position by splinting. Fortunately, this is a rare requirement because in most cases it would be better to move the tooth orthodontically rather than restore it to a stressful contour.

End-to-End Relationships With Extreme Wear

When anterior teeth have undergone extreme wear, an end-to-end relationship presents a special problem. This is especially true if the wear has penetrated near pulpal exposures on both upper and lower anterior teeth.

The worn incisal edges must be covered with a thickness of restorative metal or porcelain, or both, but the teeth cannot be reduced further without exposure of the pulps. The choice that must be made is between increasing the vertical dimension of occlusion (VDO) or endodontically treating the teeth and maintaining the VDO.

Since eruption of the teeth and vertical growth of the alveolar bone do not normally allow loss of VDO, even in extreme wear situations, the addition of restorative materials over the incisal edges must be considered as an increased VDO. In end-to-end problems like the preceding, however, increasing the VDO is usually the lesser of evils. When it can be done without too much disruption of muscle balance, it is a better choice of treatment than multiple root canals.

CAUTION: The VDO should be increased no more than is necessary to provide room for the restorative materials on the incisal edges. A 1½-mm increase should usually provide the needed space. As with any increase in VDO, the occlusion should be checked periodically for several months after the restorations are placed.

Special Considerations

An end-to-end occlusion is very often treated as a malocclusion simply because it does not conform to the requirements of a Class I relationship. That is not an acceptable reason for altering any occlusion. Instead, the decision to alter the occlusal relationship should be based on a careful evaluation of the following factors.

Stability
Whether an end-to-end occlusion is stable depends principally on two factors:

1. Harmony with the neutral zone
2. Noninterference with the envelope of function

Harmony with the neutral zone can occur with a variety of tooth-to-tooth relationships because strong tongue, cheek, and lip pressures can stabilize teeth just as effectively as perfected intercuspal relationships. In fact, neutral zone conformance is more important to stability than the intercuspal alignment because there is no intercuspal relationship that will remain stable if it is not in harmony with muscular forces.

Occlusal analysis on end-to-end relationships is incomplete unless it includes a careful search for specific signs of instability. If there is no evidence of hypermobility, excessive wear, or migration of teeth, the end-to-end relationship can be considered stable from an occlusal perspective. This stability would not occur with nonconformity to either the neutral zone or the envelope of function.

Function

It is rare for a patient with a stable end-to-end relationship to complain of inadequate function. I know of almost no instances in which such patients even complained of any degree of impairment in function. If there is a sufficient number of stable holding contacts that are coordinated with centric relation, loss of function does not appear to be a problem for the patient with an end-to-end occlusion.

Esthetics

The irony of an anterior end-to-end occlusion is that although many dentists believe it should be "corrected," most patients believe it is the ideal relationship. I have had many patients with a normal overbite relationship complain that their teeth were not "correctly" aligned end to end. But I do not remember a single patient with skeletal end-to-end occlusion ever complaining that he or she wanted his or her teeth to overlap. In the absence of noxious habit patterns that destroy the incisal plane relationship, an anterior end-to-end occlusion often results in a beautiful smile. It rarely needs to be altered for esthetic reasons.

Skeletofacial profile

There can be several different causes of anterior end-to-end relationships. The effect on facial profile is often a major consideration, and in a notable percentage of patients who seek treatment the chief complaint is more likely to be related to facial profile than it is to the actual occlusal relationship.

Evaluation of skeletofacial profile problems requires cephalometric analysis as well as mounted diagnostic casts. The purpose of the cephalometric evaluation is to determine whether the end-to-end relationship is caused by an underdeveloped maxilla or an overdeveloped mandible, or some combination of both. We can rather easily make this decision by observing the relationship of both arches to one or more of the standard facial planes that can be plotted on a lateral cephalometric radiograph.

The use of McNamara's plane provides an easily used reference for this determination (see Chapter 44).

Neutral zone

If an end-to-end relationship occurs posterior to the facial plane or the McNamara plane, it results in a "pushed-in" appearance as a manifestation of bimaxillary deficiency (Figure 39-3). This type of occlusal relationship should be treated with caution because it is usually accompanied by a very strong buccinator-*orbicularis oris* limitation on arch size. If muscular limitation is a factor in restricting arch size,

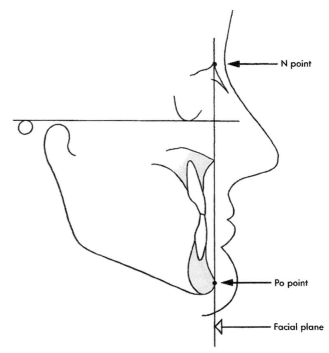

FIGURE 39-3 An end-to-end relationship of incisors occurs posterior to the facial plane, indicating a bimaxillary deficiency. Thinner than normal soft tissue and deep cleft indicate a strong perioral muscle pressure against the anterior teeth. This would normally mean a strong stabilizing influence from the neutral zone where the teeth are now. This type of relationship also occurs with a small orifice.

the soft-tissue thickness as shown on the cephalometric radiograph will be thinner than normal, especially in the lower lip. If this is observed, any attempts at advancement of maxillary or mandibular segments should be preceded by an analysis of the musculature and possible alteration of the position or length of the muscle itself.

If an end-to-end relationship occurs anterior to the McNamara plane, it indicates a bimaxillary protrusion. In some patients, this procumbency creates a very attractive facial profile, especially when combined with high cheekbones. This relationship probably never occurs in combination with a strong or restrictive buccinator-orbicularis oris complex. Examination of soft-tissue thickness on the lateral cephalometric radiograph will normally reveal a thicker than normal dimension. If surgical correction of either arch length is considered, it should be planned to achieve the best profile. This can normally be accomplished with a predictably good prognosis because there is rarely a conflict with the neutral zone. The exception is evidenced by the finding of an oversized tongue, but this does not usually occur in end-to-end occlusions that have anterior tooth contact in centric relation.

POSTERIOR END-TO-END RELATIONSHIPS

IMPORTANT CONSIDERATIONS

1. Are all teeth stable or unstable? (Look for wear or hypermobility.)
2. Can the anterior guidance disclude the posteriors? If so, an end-to-end occlusion is not a problem.
3. If anterior guidance cannot disclude the posterior teeth in lateral excursions, correct the posterior relationship by the best choice of:
   - reshaping
   - repositioning
   - restoring (with centralized cusps)
   - surgery

   Evaluate each method and select the most practical way to fulfill the requirements for stability. The goal is posterior disclusion of the balancing side either by the anterior guidance or by the posterior teeth on the working side.
4. Anterior guidance can sometimes be steepened if it is not steeper than the lateral path originally found during excursions dictated by posterior teeth (Figure 39-4).

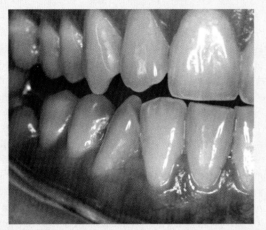
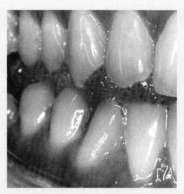

FIGURE 39-4 An end-to-end occlusion is not necessarily unstable. All occlusions should be evaluated for compliance with the requirements for stability, recognizing that the tongue can often substitute for holding contacts. Look for signs of stability or instability before altering an occlusion. This occlusion is stable; therefore no treatment is needed.

RESTORING END-TO-END POSTERIOR TEETH

In posterior cusp-tip–to–cusp-tip relationships, centric relation interferences should be relieved by flattening of the upper cusp tip and, if needed, selective shaping of the lower cusp tip. The goal is to provide as much stability as possible in centric relation and as much relief as possible in excursions (Figure 39-5).

When a lower cusp tip is positioned against an upper surface that is flat, the downward movement of the orbiting condyle is sufficient to disclude the balancing side, even in the presence of a horizontal anterior guidance and a flat working side, if the occlusal plane is correct. Since the teeth in end-to-end relationships are usually in rather good balance with the tongue and cheeks and the direction of force

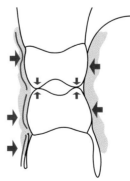

FIGURE 39-5 Stability is not totally dependent on cusp-fossa alignment. End-to-end contact can be stable if stops can prevent eruption in a strong neutral zone.

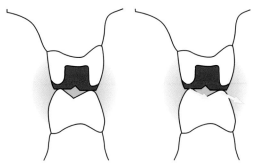

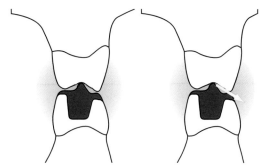

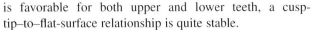

FIGURE 39-6 A lower-cusp-tip–to–upper-flat-surface relationship. This type of end-to-end relationship can provide good stability as long as lateral function contact is not needed.

FIGURE 39-7 The centralized lower cusps can contact in working excursion to disclude the balancing side. Contours can be made to look quite natural.

is favorable for both upper and lower teeth, a cusp-tip–to–flat-surface relationship is quite stable.

If the posterior teeth must be restored, the same decision regarding contour may be made. We have several options for restorative contouring of posterior end-to-end relationships. Which type of occlusal form is selected should depend to a large degree on the answer to the following question: *Can the anterior guidance function as a discluder of protrusive and balancing inclines?* In the presence of a functioning anterior guidance, flat occlusal morphology can be used. Stable centric stops can be provided in several ways. Each type should be evaluated from several standpoints.

Lower Cusp Tip to Upper Flat Surface

This relationship (Figure 39-6) can provide almost normal lower posterior occlusal form, with slight modifications to flatten and broaden upper cusp tips to serve as stops for the more rounded lower cusps. Enough overjet can be provided to hold the cheek away from the contacts. This type of occlusal form is adequate as long as the teeth are positioned in harmony with the cheeks and tongue and as long as posterior disclusion is permissible in all eccentric positions.

Centralization of the Lower Cusps

By converging the lower buccal and lingual cusps into single centralized cusps, it is practical to place them in the central fossae of the upper teeth (Figure 39-7). Stress direction is ideal for both upper and lower teeth, and function is excellent. With centralized lower cusps, the upper working inclines can be used to disclude the balancing inclines on the opposite side, and it can be accomplished within the limits of the normal neutral zone.

Even though it is a departure from normal occlusal anatomy, lower centralized cusps are an innovative way to solve unilateral end-to-end problems. There are no real disadvantages to the procedure, and even the esthetic difference from normal contours is not noticeable. It permits normal buccal and lingual contours at the gingival level for both upper and lower teeth, and the stress direction can be made so ideal that stability is usually not a problem.

The alternative of warping cusps and relocating fossae works fine if the arch relationship is slightly off line, but a true end-to-end occlusion requires too much warping to consider it as a practical approach. The resultant stress directions are too unfavorable.

Warped Posterior Contours

The practice of "warping" posterior contours to move lower cusps in and upper cusps out is probably overdone. It often results in stresses that are directed off the long axis. It is done in an attempt to position cusp tips into fossae, but if stability can be achieved in other ways, there is no need to place cusp tips in fossae if the fossae inclines are not needed in lateral excursive contact. In normal arch relationships, cusp-tip–to–fossa contact is a natural, practical way to achieve stability, but directing the forces off the long axis just to reproduce textbook anatomy is not practical. Rather than thinking in terms of preconceived ideas of contours, it is wise to develop concepts of stress direction and then locate the directional contacts in a manner that provides the best possibilities for stability. Every occlusal contour should be evaluated in this manner, and this is particularly so when arch relationships are not ideal.

In posterior end-to-end relationships, if it is possible to warp a lower cusp in lingually to an improved fossa location, stress direction can usually be maintained through the long axis of both upper and lower teeth. But warping upper cusps out buccally is usually stress-producing. Warping is not practical if it creates buccal or lingual contours that overprotect the gingival margins.

Warping of the buccal or lingual contours may also create a latent problem of stability that is often overlooked in treatment planning. Particularly in patients with strong tongue or buccinator pressures, such contour alterations result in nonconformity to a limited neutral zone. The result is a continuous horizontal migration of the restored teeth until their position between the opposing muscular forces is neutralized. For this reason, it is not uncommon for posterior teeth that have been restored with warped contours to require multiple occlusal adjustments after insertion of the restorations. This phenomenon is most noticeable in the molar region where the wider, stronger part of the tongue versus the stronger part of the buccinator muscle creates a firm pressure against any tooth surface that is extended outside its neutral zone position.

Warping cusp tips and repositioning fossae is good restorative technique if it can be accomplished within limits of correct stress-directioning, adequate stability, and contouring for tissue maintenance.

UNILATERAL END-TO-END RELATIONSHIPS

If one side of the arch is in an end-to-end relationship but the other side is in a cusp-fossa relationship, there is a definite potential for causing harm to the side that occludes correctly.

The correctly occluding side is capable of discluding the balancing inclines on the end-to-end side, but the end-to-end side has no fossa wall contact to disclude the opposite balancing inclines of the intercuspated teeth. If the anterior teeth are in end-to-end relationships also, they may not be capable of providing the lift that is needed to disengage the balancing inclines of the intercuspated side either. There are at least three practical solutions for unilateral end-to-end problems:

Orthodontics

Repositioning the end-to-end side into a correct intercuspation will enable it to assume the job of discluding the opposite-side balancing inclines.

Flattening of the Balancing Inclines on the Intercuspated Side

If the balancing inclines are made flat enough, they will be discluded by even a horizontal working-side pathway. The downward path of the orbiting condyle will help in the disclusive effort.

End-to-End Relationship of the Anterior Teeth

An end-to-end relationship of the anterior teeth can serve quite well as a lateral anterior guidance because the lower incisors maintain contact as they pass laterally across the upper incisal edges. The distance traveled in anterior contact is enough to disclude flattened balancing inclines. When end-to-end canines disengage laterally, the incisors are still in contact. This is sufficient to protect the posterior teeth from balancing-side interferences if the balancing inclines are made flat enough and the occlusal plane is correct.

Working inclines should normally be flattened also, just to provide symmetry of function, as long as all balancing inclines are discluded. However, it is not imperative that working-side inclines be the same on both sides.

Chapter 40

Treating Splayed or Separated Anterior Teeth

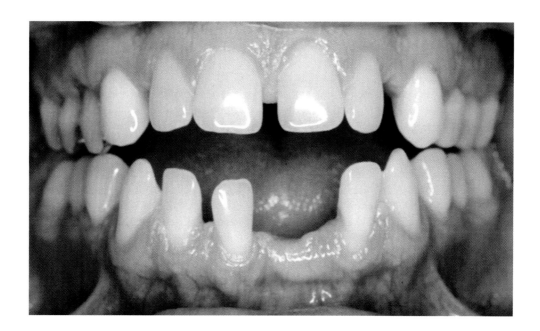

PRINCIPLE

Respect the neutral zone corridor.

IMPORTANT CONSIDERATIONS

Splayed anterior teeth

Some splayed anterior teeth with spaces are healthy and have stable holding contacts. Always determine if the spacing has been that way or has resulted from shifting of the teeth. If the teeth are stable and the supporting structures are healthy, the decision is based on the patient's esthetic desires.

1. Why are teeth splayed? Find the cause.
2. Can the spaces be closed by constricting the arch without interference to the anterior guidance?
3. Will constricting the arch size interfere with the tongue? Usually it will.
4. Can the teeth be moved together if the lingual contours are reshaped to make new holding contacts?
5. If the teeth have stable holding contacts, can the spaces be closed restoratively or with bonding?
6. Is the problem related to an arch size discrepancy?

Observation

Splayed anterior teeth are usually in a definite neutral zone corridor. They can be moved or reshaped within that corridor, but movement toward either the tongue or the lips usually results in interference with the musculature and eventual instability.

> Splayed anterior teeth are those that incline outwardly from strong tongue pressure. The labial inclination results in spaces between the teeth.

Uneven spacing between teeth can also be caused by disharmony between the size of the teeth and the size of the arch. Regardless of the reason for the spacing, individual teeth without proximal contact will always migrate to a neutral zone position between tongue and lip pressures. Unless there are some overriding reasons for altering the arch form, any restorative or orthodontic treatment should maintain the existing curvature of the arch. It is acceptable to close spaces between the teeth either by restoration or by lateral movement to improve spacing within the arch form. The best esthetics is usually achieved by a combination of lateral tooth movement to improve spacing combined with restorative procedures for reshaping teeth or adding pontics if the space requires.

As with any other alteration of anterior teeth, provisional restorations should be used to determine and verify the correct incisal edge positions and tooth contours before completion of the final restorative treatment. Spacing requirements should be worked out on mounted casts before initiating any orthodontic treatment, and a full wax-up should be completed. It is often surprising how effectively a good result can be worked out with a minimum or no lateral movement of teeth when shaping teeth is explored via the wax-up. It is sometimes necessary to add an extra incisor if the spaces cannot be filled with normal-shaped teeth. The goal is to end up with incisal edges with consistent widths and normal tooth size.

If the splaying effect has created an unacceptable arch form that must be changed for esthetic or functional reasons, the neutral zone must be changed also. Thus treatment planning must be based on a determination of how the existing neutral zone was established. The same arch configuration may result from different lip or tongue variations, some of which are easily altered, whereas others require more complex solutions.

The most common neutral zone configuration found with splayed lower anterior teeth is the effect of a strong forward tongue posture combined with a strong lower band of the buccinator that is positioned low. The tongue pushes the incisal edges forward while the buccinator-*orbicularis oris* band of muscle holds the roots back lingually. Attempts at changing tooth position by alteration of the arch form in the presence of strong neutral zone confinement will predictably fail. If arch form is to be altered, the excessive pressure either from the tongue or from the perioral musculature must be reduced, or stabilization must be increased.

Even loose teeth will passively relate to their neutral zone position. If hypermobility occurs coincident with splaying, the hypermobility will almost certainly be related in some way with tooth interference to some functional jaw movements. Varying degrees of periodontal breakdown may be noted, but they may have little relevance to the splaying effect.

Splaying of lower anterior teeth is rarely caused by occlusal interferences. It is almost always a neutral zone phenomenon. An exception to this observation, however, can be noted occasionally in relation to mandibular prognathism. If the upper incisors interfere with the centric relation arc of closure so that the lingual surfaces of the lower incisors strike them, the mandible is forced into a protrusive displacement that also loads the lower incisors in a labial direction. In most cases, the mandible accommodates to the displacement, but in some patients the lower incisors do the accommodating by flaring out labially into a crossbite with splayed incisors.

There are generally no neutral zone problems associated with correction of this type of arch-form problem. It can be treated by use of the same guidelines as are recommended for other anterior crossbite problems.

Changing the Neutral Zone

If only the upper anterior teeth are splayed, changes in the neutral zone relationship can often be achieved so that lip pressures are reversed. When the lower anterior teeth are upright but the upper teeth are splayed, the lower lip will usually be found substantially lingual to the upper anterior teeth during swallowing. This lip posture forces the lower anterior teeth lingually and upper anterior teeth labially. The lower teeth have tongue-pressure resistance against the lower lip, so they may actually be stable, but the lower lip is an outward force against the upper anterior teeth that is added to the forward tongue pressure, and this cumulative force easily overpowers the upper lip. The more the upper teeth splay, the less resistance can be applied by the upper lip against the angled labial surfaces.

The treatment approach for splayed upper anterior teeth is often aimed at repositioning of the teeth back into a more upright position. When the incisal edges are moved lingually, the lower lip can slide in front of the upper teeth for a more normal lip seal during swallowing. As soon as the lower lip is postured labially to the upper anterior teeth, the neutral zone is changed. The lower lip assumes an inward resistance role to outward tongue pressure rather than being an additive outward force.

Because the lower incisors generally supraerupt when upper anterior teeth splay, it is often necessary to shorten them to make room for proper upper tooth alignment. It may also be necessary to alter the shape of the upper lingual surfaces to provide stable holding contacts. Remember that vertical stability of both anterior segments is an essential goal of treatment. It may be provided orthodontically or restoratively if simple reshaping cannot achieve an acceptable result. If holding contacts cannot be provided, the treatment plan should consider whether stabilization with splinting is needed or whether a bite plane type of substitute is necessary.

Many patients with splayed anterior teeth also have an anterior open bite because of a strong tongue posture, but this would never be the case with supraeruption of lower anterior teeth. When such supraeruption has occurred, stable holding contacts must be provided or the teeth must be vertically stabilized by some other treatment approach.

Severe bone loss in the anterior segments may result in splaying of both upper and lower anterior teeth in the absence of posterior tooth support, but this may still be related to strong tongue pressure. Nevertheless, it is often possible to realign the teeth to a more vertical position if stable holding contacts are provided. The prognosis is improved whenever a more normalized lip seal can be facilitated by the better tooth alignment.

SPLAYING AS A RESULT OF AN ENLARGED TONGUE

An oversized tongue may be the sole causative factor in some splayed dentitions. In some patients, the tongue force can be overcome by nighttime use of a retainer. If the dentition is healthy and the patient does not object to wearing the retainer, it is a logical treatment approach for some patients. It will not work if the tongue size is too large to be counter-resisted.

Surgical techniques for decreasing the size of the tongue have improved and can be considered in selected patients.

Regardless of the treatment approach used for splayed anterior teeth, conformity with the neutral zone should be the first consideration before any treatment plan can be finalized.

APPLYING THE PRINCIPLES

Splayed teeth are almost always positioned within a strong neutral zone corridor. Upper anterior teeth are sometimes in a splayed relationship because of deflective posterior interferences that force the mandible forward. As the lower anterior teeth are forced forward into the upper anterior teeth, they move them forward and in the process cause them to separate. It is important to determine if the splayed upper anterior teeth are in a stable relationship before any restorative corrections are made to close the spaces or move the teeth. The following case by Dr. Dewitt Wilkerson is an excellent example of adhering to the principles that are critical to long-term stability and function.

The patient presented with the primary concern of improving the esthetics of his smile. The teeth were splayed, separated, and inclined forward. All teeth were firm with no sign of wear or fremitus.

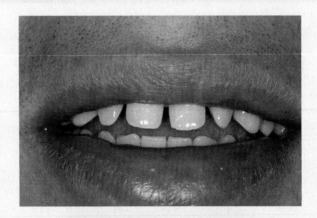

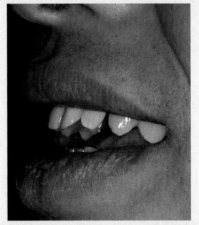

Maximal intercuspation. There is a long slide from the first contact at the most closed position. It is important to determine if the slide forward is the cause of the anterior teeth being flared and separated. The observation that the anterior teeth are tight with no hint of fremitus puts this theory in doubt.

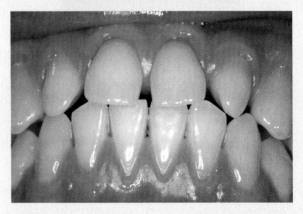

Centric relation. The jaw-to-jaw relationship at the first posterior tooth contact in centric relation. It is essential to determine what the anterior relationship would be if the posterior interferences are removed. The true arc of closure to anterior contact in centric relation can then be determined on mounted casts.

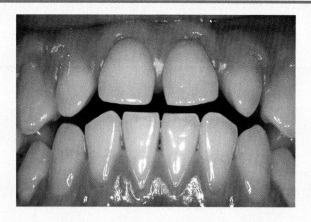

If the anterior teeth can contact after a deflective slide to maximal intercuspation, it is okay to achieve contact in centric relation. If anterior contact cannot be achieved at the most closed position, it indicates that there is a tongue- or lip-biting habit that is responsible for the separation. Before deciding on anterior contact in centric relation, *it is necessary to eliminate a habit pattern that is a primary cause of the splaying and open bite. If the tongue- or lip-biting habit cannot be stopped, you must work with the ongoing habit pattern and maintain the anterior open bite. In the analysis of this patient, anterior contact occurs at the most closed position, so contact should be the goal in the finished restorations.*

Equilibration of casts. It is apparent from this step that posterior deflective interferences can be eliminated without mutilating the posterior teeth. It is possible to achieve anterior contact in centric relation. The only way this decision can be made with assurance of accuracy is on mounted diagnostic casts.

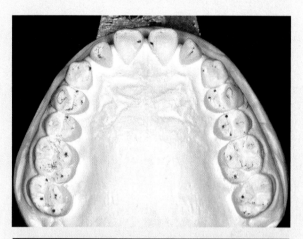

Anterior guidance. This important step can only be achieved after all interferences to centric relation closure have been eliminated. Now it is apparent that an acceptable anterior guidance can be maintained on the central incisors and canines, so laminate restorations will be the ideal restorations. It will be necessary to restore the lateral incisors with full coverage to achieve contact in centric relation.

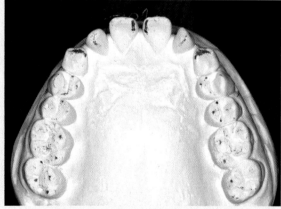

Diagnostic wax-up. This step has several purposes, not the least of which is to decide on the best contours for each of the teeth to be restored. Modifications may be needed when the provisional restorations are placed, but this is the "best guess" to be copied in the provisional restorations.

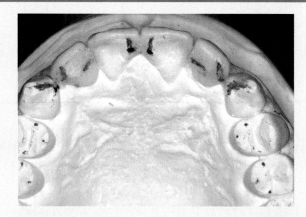

Neutral zone considerations. Splayed anterior teeth are usually in the most balanced relationship between tongue and lip pressures. Thus, it is important to maintain their neutral zone position. The lines on the central incisors mark the forward part of contour that should not be violated when laminate restorations are made.

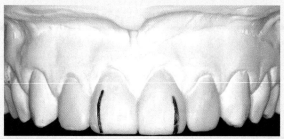

The diagnostic wax-up completed. This is the best guess for what the final contours should be. This is an ideal visual aid in presenting treatment to the patient. It is also the contours that are copied for fabricating provisional restorations as well as a preparation guide for how much tooth structure to remove.

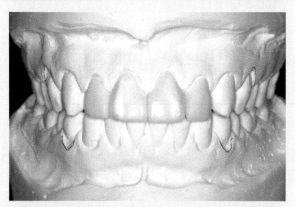

Prepared teeth. Note centric relation contact on centrals and canines.

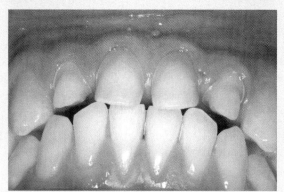

Matrix used as reduction guide and for direct fabrication of provisional restorations.

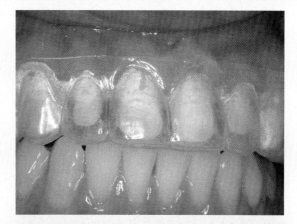

Provisional restorations in place.

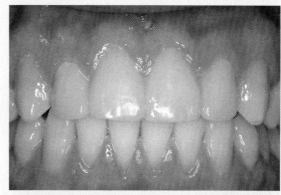

Patient can test the provisionals to be sure that appearance, phonetics, and function are all acceptable.

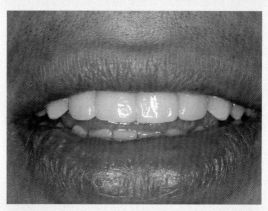

Functional esthetics. Mounted cast of the approved provisional restorations eliminates all guesswork for the technician.

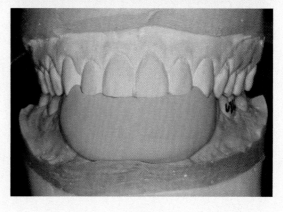

The putty silicone index precisely communicates the incisal edge position and contour that can then be copied in the wax-up on the master die model.

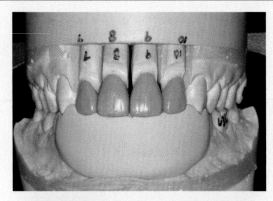

A customized anterior guide table dictates the exact configuration of the lingual contours. The wax patterns will be used to process the restorations in the IPS Empress® Esthetic (Ivoclar Vivadent Inc., Amherst, NY).

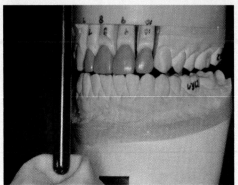

Precise doctor/technician communication yields precise results. The finished restorations follow the exact guidelines that were worked out in the mouth and tested in function. The putty matrix simplifies communication in a way that is verifiable by both the technician and the dentist.

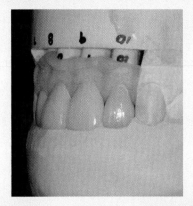

Lingual contours on the restorations match what was worked out in the mouth and communicated via the customized anterior guide table.

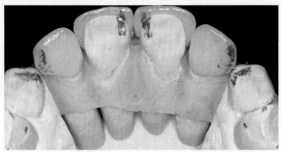

Note the precise duplication in the mouth of the anterior guidance on the articulator. This eliminates almost all the need for adjustments in the mouth when the restorations are placed.

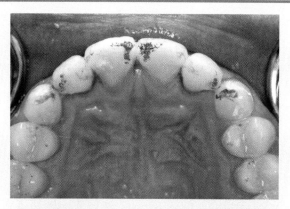

Finished restorations with a predictably successful outcome because the process that guarantees it was followed faithfully.

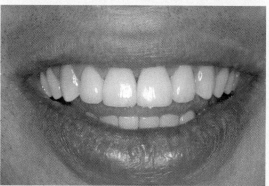

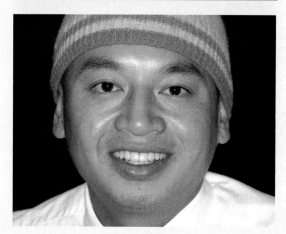

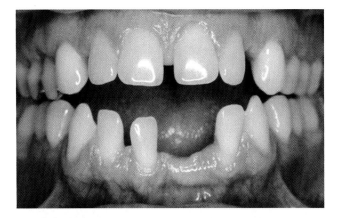

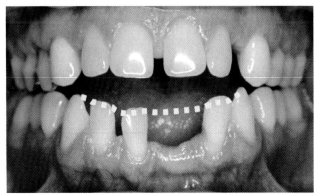

FIGURE 40-1 Teeth can be moved, rotated, or restored with long-term stable results as long as they stay within the neutral zone corridor *(yellow line)*.

NEUTRAL ZONE CONSIDERATIONS

The splayed upper and lower anterior teeth in Figure 40-1 are in a strong neutral zone relationship that cannot be violated. There is also a vertical relationship established by an unbreakable tongue thrust. Any interference to the tongue or lip pressures will result in movement of the teeth after restoration. It should be apparent that individual teeth that are in a stable relationship are exactly where the combination of lip and tongue pressures wants them to be. There is a simple rule to follow:

> Do not attempt to move or restore teeth outside of a strong neutral zone corridor. Teeth that are moved outside of their neutral zone will in time be moved back to where opposing muscle forces are equalized.

See Figure 40-2 for treatment of this dentition.

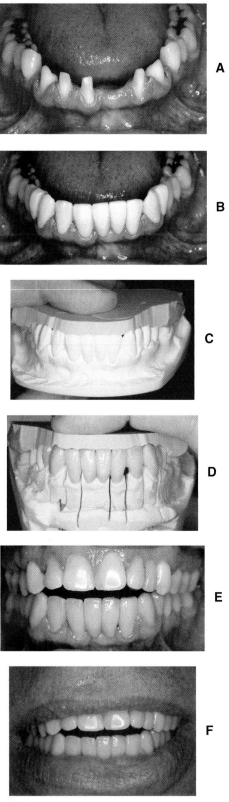

FIGURE 40-2 **A,** Lower anterior teeth prepared. **B,** Provisional restorations copied from a diagnostic wax-up that maintained tooth positions within the neutral corridor. **C,** Index on cast of approved provisionals. **D,** Index used to complete final restorations. **E,** Upper restored within its neutral zone required an extra lateral incisor to maintain arch form. **F,** Note vertical opening for strong tongue position.

USE OF LAMINATES TO CLOSE SPACE

The restoration of splayed or separated anterior teeth often results in some of the most dramatic improvements in appearance (Figure 40-3). If the importance of the neutral zone is understood, it simplifies treatment. The diagnostic wax-up is extremely valuable in deciding on the best treatment option, because in some patients it is necessary to move teeth in order to maintain acceptable size balance of the teeth. This is usually apparent when working with the diagnostic casts.

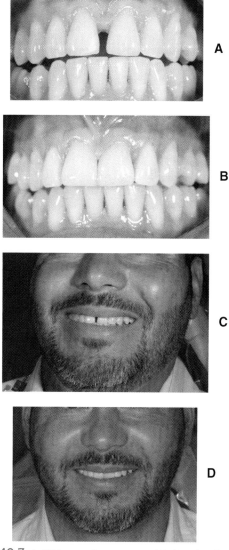

FIGURE 40-3 **A,** Wide space between central incisors is solved without interfering with the neutral zone corridor. **B,** Laminates bonded to the mesial surface of each central incisor result in an excellent esthetic result. Note complete closure of the interproximal space all the way to the interdental papilla. Acceptability of wider centrals was tested with composite. It resolved the esthetic problem without moving any teeth (**C** and **D**). (*Case provided courtesy of Dr. Glenn DuPont.*)

Chapter 41

Treating the Crossbite Patient

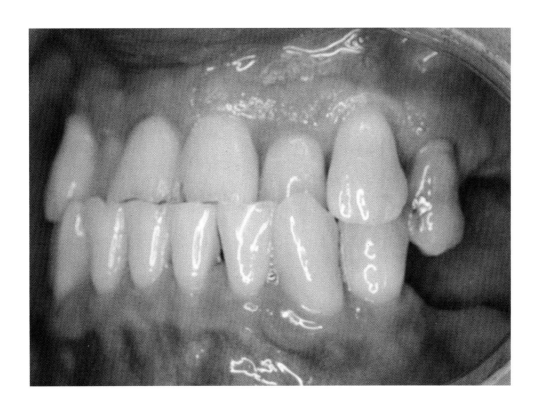

PRINCIPLE

Don't change what is right to fix what is wrong.

Probably no other type of occlusal problem is treated improperly so routinely as the crossbite relationship. Far too often, the treatment accomplished to "correct" a crossbite is significantly more harmful than the crossbite itself. This is particularly unfortunate because when properly treated, crossbite relationships can be among the most stable, most predictably maintainable occlusions.

Crossbite problems should be divided into two categories: anterior crossbite and posterior crossbite. Anterior crossbite presents an entirely different set of problems and considerations from posterior crossbite. Although they may or may not occur together, they should be considered separately because each segment is judged by a different set of criteria.

ANTERIOR CROSSBITE

IMPORTANT CONSIDERATIONS

Never treat an anterior crossbite without first analyzing the tooth-to-tooth relationships at the selected vertical dimension in centric relation.

1. Is the anterior crossbite the result of mandibular prognathism or maxillary deficiency?

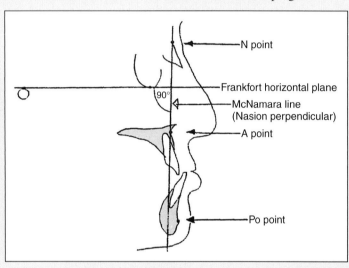

Note in this analysis the Po point is forward of the nasion perpendicular. The A point is on the line indicating that the prognathic mandible is the problem.

2. What is the anterior relationship in centric relation? If it is end to end in centric relation, how much vertical displacement of the condyles is there in maximal intercuspation?
3. Do the anterior teeth need to be restored because of wear or appearance?
4. Is the crossbite an esthetic problem? Can the anterior teeth be restored end to end?
5. The importance of vertical dimension in crossbite problems is critical. Class III patients often respond unfavorably to increasing the vertical dimension of occlusion (VDO).
6. Anterior guidance is not a problem, as anterior crossbite patients do not protrude. They have vertical envelopes of function.
7. Disclusion of the balancing side should be achieved by group function of the working-side posterior teeth.
8. Orthognathic surgery is often the treatment of choice for correction of facial profile problems and can result in good occlusal relationships.

ANALYSIS OF ANTERIOR CROSSBITE

If there are no centric relation interferences, Class III occlusions are among the most trouble-free, stable occlusions. Thus the most common reason for correction is unacceptable esthetics.

Mandibular prognathism results from a true basal jaw dysplasia. The horizontal growth of the mandible exceeds the horizontal development of the maxilla, and the lower an-

terior teeth end up in front of the upper anterior teeth. Anterior crossbite can also result from underdevelopment of the maxilla (maxillary retrognathism).

Because mandibular prognathism is primarily a skeletal malrelationship, it is more practical to prevent it than it is to correct it after it has happened. As with other skeletal deformities, it is amenable to treatment by extraoral orthopedic traction if treatment is started early enough to intercept the mandibular growth and manage it through the growth years.

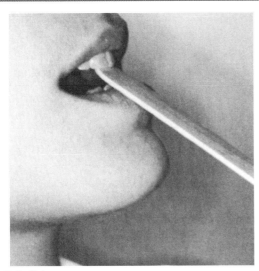

FIGURE 41-1 Anterior crossbite in children can often be corrected by pressure from a tongue depressor blade several times a day. A dental nurse illustrates the position of the blade.

At the first sign of an anterior crossbite, even the youngest patient should be referred to a competent orthodontist. Graber reports successful resolution of anterior crossbites in three to four months using extraoral appliances worn only at night by children two to six years of age.

Most orthodontists agree that once an anterior crossbite relation is established, it will get progressively worse with each growth spurt. It makes little difference in the young child whether the crossbite is a true skeletal malrelationship or a pseudocrossbite caused by faulty tooth position; if the lower anterior teeth get in front of the upper anterior teeth before growth has been completed, the tendency will be toward excessive horizontal growth of the mandible. Thus pseudocrossbites in young children usually become true skeletal crossbites in adults.

For early crossbite analysis, computerized cephalometric growth predictions can be useful. Ricketts has set up parameters of comparison regarding growth direction and degree that can guide the diagnostician in selecting the proper course of treatment.

Simple crossbites from tooth malposition can often be corrected in young children by pressure applied several times a day with a tongue blade (Figure 41-1). As soon as the upper teeth establish an overlap on the lower ones, the exercise can be stopped. They will be guided into position from that point by their own inclines.

After the last of the pubertal growth spurts has finalized the shape of the mandible (about 12 years of age in females and 18 years in males), any treatment of anterior crossbites becomes corrective rather than preventive. What are the problems associated with anterior crossbite that need correction? As with other types of skeletal dysplasias, the "problems" are often more apparent than real. Patients with anterior crossbite can commonly substitute for unfulfilled occlusal criteria, or they may eliminate the need for some of the usual requirements for stability. Before changes are initiated, each criterion for maintainable occlusion should be carefully analyzed to see whether it is needed.

Problems With Anterior Crossbites

The problems or potential problems that are commonly associated with anterior crossbites are as follows.

Esthetics
The most common reason, by far, that patients seek treatment is to improve their appearance. Elimination of the "bulldog look" of prognathism can be accomplished in several ways, but surgery seems to be the only practical method if the prognathism is severe.

No centric contact on anterior teeth
In many crossbites, the patients do have anterior contact, but it is reversed so that the incisal edges of the upper teeth contact the cingulum of the lower teeth. In more severe malrelationships, there is no anterior contact. The usual problem associated with lack of centric contact is supraeruption of the teeth. This is rarely a problem with anterior crossbites because the upper lip substitutes for the contact and holds the lower anterior teeth in place. The tongue prevents the upper teeth from supraerupting. If supraeruption is a problem, it can be solved by provision of centric contact through surgical correction of the arch relationship, by orthodontic repositioning of the teeth, by restorative reshaping, or by splinting to teeth that have centric contact. Combinations of these treatment modes may also be employed.

No anterior guidance
Anterior crossbites cannot provide anterior guidance for either protrusive or lateral excursions. It does not, however, constitute a problem. Prognathic patients do not use protrusive movements, so there is no need to provide disclusion of the posterior teeth in protrusion. When a prognathic patient protrudes, it makes the problem worse, so there is no tendency to include such movements in function.

Most prognathic patients limit their function to vertical "chop chop" movements, but it is wise to provide balancing incline disclusion anyway. The necessary lift can usually be provided by the working-side inclines. Since there is no anterior guidance to help the posterior teeth, group function of the working inclines is usually the occlusion of choice.

Pseudoprognathism

Some anterior crossbites are not the result of a true mandibular prognathism. The pseudoprognathism results from tooth interferences that force the mandible forward or simply give the appearance of protrusion because of the inverted anterior relationship.

If the upper anterior teeth slant lingually to permit the lower anterior teeth to close in front of them, the prognosis is usually favorable. It is often just a matter of moving the upper anterior teeth forward and jumping them over the lower ones. The rest of the alignment is routine.

It is almost always necessary to open the bite during the correction because the upper teeth must be free to move forward. This can be accomplished with a removable lower appliance that provides a steep incline plane to wedge the upper anterior teeth forward past the lower incisal edges (Figure 41-2). Such appliances must be worn continuously to be effective and should be removed only for cleaning. They usually accomplish the "crossover" in a matter of weeks. Once the upper anterior teeth are in front of the lower

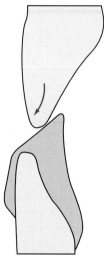

FIGURE 41-2 Fabrication of a steep incline plane is often effective in correcting some crossbites. The acrylic appliance must be worn almost continuously until the upper teeth "jump over" the lower ones. The appliance is no longer necessary when the crossover occurs.

ones, conventional removable appliances may be used to align and refine the anterior relationship if necessary.

Any time the bite must be held open to move teeth, it can take up to several months for the teeth to settle back to their correct VDO. We should not rush any restorative treatment after the use of such appliances. We must make certain that the occlusion has stabilized first.

If extensive restoration of all the anterior teeth is required, it may permit a simplified combination approach to correction of the crossbite. By shortening the anterior teeth enough to permit the upper anterior teeth to pass forward of the lower ones, removable appliances that do not require any bite opening can be used. The upper anterior teeth are free to be moved forward, and the lower anterior teeth can be moved inward (Figures 41-3 and 41-4). As soon as the teeth are in an acceptable relationship, the preparations can be completed and provisional plastic bridges can be made to serve as retainers. Permanent restorations should not be started for at least two months after completion of the tooth movement.

Two important considerations should be kept in mind when we are moving linguoversion upper anterior teeth forward. First, we must make sure that there is sufficient alveolar bone labially. Teeth should not be moved so far or so fast that they create dehiscence in the labial plate. Second, when linguoversion upper anterior teeth are moved labial to the lower teeth, the stresses exerted on the teeth are reversed. It takes time for the bone and the periodontal ligaments to realign to these new stresses. The teeth may be tender to function until this realignment takes place.

Some anterior crossbites that appear severe may be false manifestations of occlusal interferences. All such occlusal problems should be evaluated on diagnostic casts *that have been mounted with a facebow record in centric relation.*

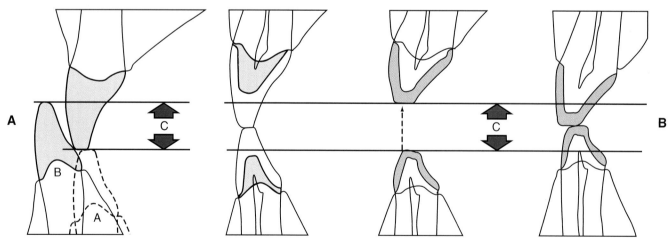

FIGURE 41-3 How to get in trouble. Analysis of casts that are unmounted or on Galetti-type articulators that do not duplicate the correct condylar axis. **A,** Deep overbite in maximal intercuspation *(B)* after contacting end-to-end in centric relation *(A).* Note the difference in the VDO *(C)* between the first contact in centric relation (end-to-end) shown in **B** compared with a much more closed VDO after the anterior goes into a crossbite relationship *(A).* In order to achieve complete tooth contact on posterior teeth, it might appear that the anterior teeth could be shortened and restored at that position to provide an end-to-end anterior result at maximal intercuspation. That would be a serious misjudgment because the arc of closure is quite different when the mandible closes on the true condylar axis.

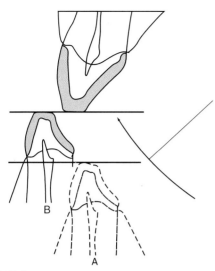

FIGURE 41-4 What really happens if the anterior teeth are shortened *(A)* and the VDO is closed *(B)*. The arc of closure always positions the lower anterior teeth forward as the jaw closes to achieve posterior contact.

Without such an analysis, serious mistakes in treatment planning can be made. I have seen patients who were scheduled for surgical reduction to correct a prognathism but who actually required only selective occlusal grinding to permit the mandible to close back in centric relation. Minor orthodontic procedures at the correct jaw position then replaced the "need" for the extensive surgery.

Incorrect analysis more often tends to *oversimplify* anterior crossbite problems, however. Even correctly mounted casts are invitations to trouble if they are not interpreted correctly.

Mounting diagnostic casts with a facebow is critical. Serious mistakes in treatment planning can be made if the condylar axis is not the same on the articulator as it is in the patient, so the use of Galetti-type articulators is invitation to major problems. Unmounted casts have no place in analysis of crossbite problems for the same reason: There is no way to evaluate the horizontal position of incisal edges unless the casts are related to the correct condylar axis.

Improvement of anterior alignment in a crossbite always requires an increase in VDO . . . never a decrease.

Why Increasing the VDO Works

Increasing the VDO is often the best treatment plan for anterior crossbites (Figures 41-5 and 41-6) for the following reasons:

1. If the increased VDO at the anterior teeth is offset by upward movement of the condyles from maximal intercuspation to centric relation, the interference with elevator muscle contracted length may be minimal or none. Thus converting an anterior crossbite to an end-to-end relationship may result in a stable occlusion.

2. Even if increasing the VDO cannot be offset completely by upward condylar repositioning, the increased VDO can be well tolerated as the muscles return it to their original contracted length. If all teeth are in contact in centric relation, the corrected occlusion will be maintained with minimal adjustments required (see Chapter 13).

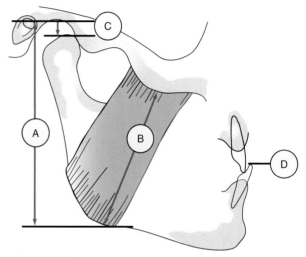

FIGURE 41-5 Note the length of the masseter muscle **(B)** as it relates to the ramus height **(A)** when the condyles are displaced down to the eminentiae at maximal intercuspation. The anterior teeth are in a crossbite relationship at this protruded jaw position **(D).**

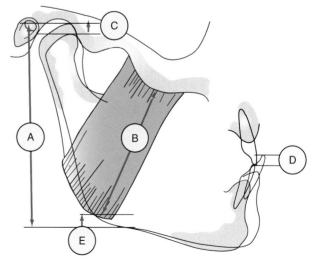

FIGURE 41-6 Note that the length of the masseter muscle **(B)** would be shortened as the condyle moves up **(C)** to shorten the ramus height **(E).** As the anterior VDO is increased **(D),** it is compensated for by the upward movement of the condyles **(C)** to maintain muscle length **(B)** without needing to lengthen it.

Applying the principles

Anterior crossbite at maximal closure. At this most closed position, the condyles are displaced down and forward.

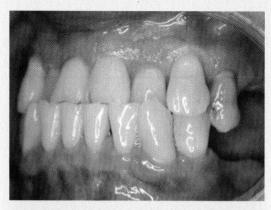

The end-to-end relationship occurs in centric relation when the condyles have moved up their eminentiae.

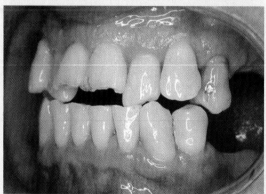

An existing removable partial denture was used to increase the VDO at the anterior end-to-end relationship. Analysis on the articulator showed that the increase in VDO was nearly matched by upward movement of the condyles, so no increase in muscle length was needed to restore the anterior teeth to an end-to-end relationship.

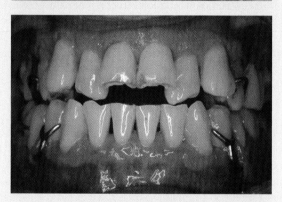

Based on the analysis on the mounted casts, the anterior teeth were narrowed a predetermined amount to facilitate moving them into a better alignment that was pre-established on the diagnostic wax-up.

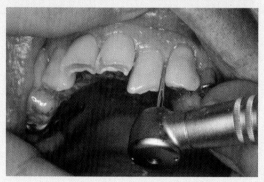

A continuous clasp was cast to fit the repositioned teeth on the diagnostic wax-up.

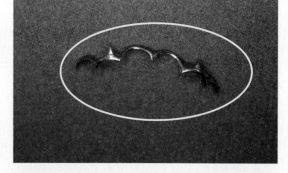

The clasp is bonded to the canines on each side. The canines and central incisors are in the neutral zone and will not be moved. The appliance is a simple way to move the lateral incisors into a predetermined position.

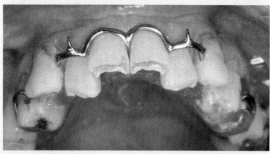

Small rubber bands are used to pull the lateral incisors into the slots designed to receive them.

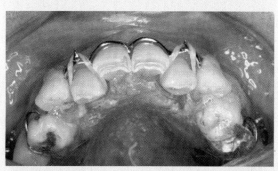

Alignment of the teeth progresses.

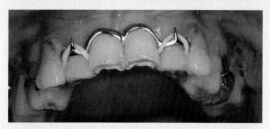

After the lateral incisors are aligned, direct composite build-up is used to develop contacts and contours. When the preliminary contour is worked out, it is copied in provisional restorations that serve as a retainer until final preparation and completion.

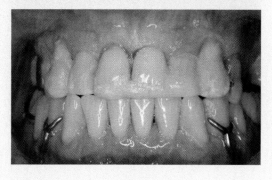

As the anterior teeth are shortened and the mandible arcs closed, the lower anterior teeth follow an arc around the condylar axis that is in a forward direction. The lower anterior teeth do not follow a vertical upward path of closure. The only way to know the correct path is by studying diagnostic casts mounted with an open centric relation bite record on an instrument that correctly records the condylar axis. A facebow is essential.

Furthermore, it will be necessary to eliminate occlusal interferences on the casts to permit closure of the diagnostic models to the same VDO as the acquired position. This is the only sure way of knowing the correct location of the lower anterior teeth when the mandible is closed to the proper VDO without deviation. We may evaluate various options for improving the anterior relationship only when we know the precise position of the teeth *at the vertical dimension of the complete occlusal changes.*

Of all the occlusal relationships we may be called on to treat, the necessity for complete preoperative analysis is probably the greatest in anterior crossbite problems. Not only should casts be equilibrated, but a complete wax-up of all anterior teeth should also be accomplished. The wax-up should represent the final contours and tooth position. These finalized goals should then be evaluated to make certain they are attainable, and a step-by-step treatment plan should be outlined to achieve them.

Until an accurate model of the projected result can be fabricated and its practicality verified, it is extremely poor judgment to proceed with any irreversible operative procedures.

It would seem unnecessary to comment any further on the need for correct facebow mountings, but we never cease to be amazed at how often this requirement is ignored. The use of Galetti or Crescent articulators is an open invitation to trouble. The axis of closure is so erroneous on instruments of this type that preplanning is totally inaccurate. It is far too common a mistake to plan a treatment and sell the patient on a beautiful result that cannot be delivered.

Most "hit and slide into" crossbites that appear to be pseudocrossbites are not false at all. They are most often true prognathic skeletal malrelationships. The interfering tooth contacts are usually interferences more to the arcing path of closure than to the final position at full closure.

Many patients who hit end-to-end in centric relation need only a slight reduction of the upper labial surfaces or a minimal reshaping of the lower lingual surfaces to provide a nondeviating path of closure to the correct VDO (Figure 41-7). Although the interference may produce an extremely long and devious slide, the length of the slide does not necessarily represent the amount of displacement at the closed position. In other words, we may have a long slide with minimal protrusive deviation.

To determine the true horizontal displacement of the mandible at the acquired occlusal position, we note the distance of the articulator condyle from its centric stop position. The distance of the ball from the stop is representative of how far back the lower incisal edges will be moved when centric interferences are eliminated.

If an analysis of the mounted casts indicates that restorative reshaping of the anterior teeth is not feasible, the patient must be told the facts. Temporomandibular joint (TMJ) pain can be relieved by selective elimination of interferences to centric relation closure, but we can make no improvement in the patient's appearance without resorting to more radical methods.

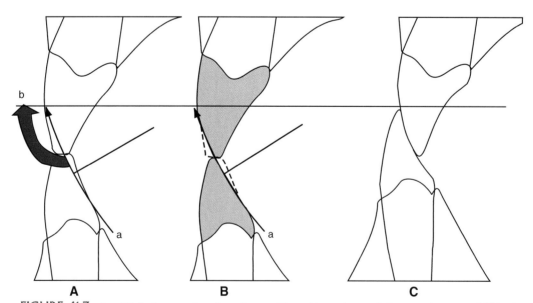

FIGURE 41-7   **A** and **B,** In the correction of anterior crossbite problems, the arc of closure, *a,* is an essential bit of information. Although the slide into the acquired position, *b,* may look severe, the deviation from centric relation is often correctable when the labial surface of the upper teeth and the lingual surface of the lower ones are shaved off. **C** represents the undeviated centric relation position of the teeth after correction. The crossbite is still present, but there is no deviation. This is the treatment of choice for solving TMJ problems in many crossbite patients with centric interferences if the contour changes are minimal. It may be wise in some patients to add a stop on the lingual of the lower incisors.

Often, selective shaping of incisal edges improves the appearance noticeably. Orthodontic evaluation would also be in order to see whether tooth position approximately within the skeletal framework can practically be improved.

In a nutshell, the conservative approaches for resolving anterior crossbite problems can be summarized as follows:

1. Selective shaping and occlusal equilibration
2. Orthodontic repositioning of the teeth within the present bone framework
3. Restorative reshaping
4. A combination of the above procedures

It is almost always possible to provide comfort, function, and stability to anterior crossbite relations with one or more of the above procedures. But it is not always possible to satisfy the esthetic requirements of some patients.

Fortunately, one of the most important aspects of an esthetic smile is not related to the upper-to-lower alignment. Rather it is how the upper incisal plane is viewed when the teeth are apart. Normally only the upper anterior teeth show when smiling, so a pleasant arrangement of the upper incisal edges is not generally affected by the position of the lower teeth except in severe mandibular prognathism. On the other hand, the lower incisal edges show when speaking, so a nicely ordered lower incisal plane can be attractive, even in crossbite.

A combination of reshaping and restoring is the method I have found to be preferred for the majority of anterior crossbites that can contact end to end in centric relation. The combination approach usually involves some increase in VDO to hold the posterior contacts at the anterior end-to-end position, so this method is best reserved for when posterior restorations are needed.

Increasing the VDO causes the lower incisors to arc back more in line with the upper anterior teeth. It also separates the lower teeth from the interfering upper labial inclines that force the mandible forward, so the occlusion can be reconstructed into a centric relation harmony.

If the increased VDO is established with equal-intensity centric contacts on all teeth, there will be a favorable prognosis. However, some occlusal adjustments may be necessary for a period of months while the muscles reorder the VDO to conform to their contracted length.

Despite an increased VDO, many patients I have treated in the above manner have remained completely stable and have required little or no posttreatment equilibration. The probable explanation for this is related to the horizontal displacement of the condyles when the crossbite directed the mandible forward. To displace the mandible forward, the condyles had to move down the eminentiae. When the mandible was moved back to centric relation, even though the VDO was increased at the incisors, it was decreased at the angle of the mandible where the elevator muscles attach (see Figure 41-6). This is so because the condyles were allowed to move up as the mandible moved back.

The above option of opening the bite is a logical choice if:

1. An acceptable end-to-end relationship can be achieved at the incisors in harmony with centric relation.
2. The required increase in VDO is acceptable.
3. The posterior segments require restoration for other reasons.

If conservative procedures fall short of optimum esthetics, the patient must make an important decision. There seem to be only two practical choices:

1. Live with the prognathism with fairly good assurances that the dentition can be maintained.
2. Select a surgical correction.

Surgical Correction of Anterior Crossbite

There are three methods for correcting an anterior crossbite surgically that seem to be universally accepted as safe, practical solutions:

1. Resection through the ramus so that the body of the mandible can be moved distally into alignment with the maxilla.
2. Horizontal resection of the maxilla so that it can be moved forward into alignment with the mandible.
3. Sectional osteotomies so that an anterior segment can be repositioned. This is not ideal if there is a severe skeletal discrepancy.

At one time, surgical correction was believed to be a radical procedure to be avoided except as a last resort. Advancements in surgical methods have changed this. When indicated, a surgical correction may require far less time and discomfort for the patient than more complex treatments that will not achieve a comparable result.

CAUTION: Before surgery is attempted, the TMJs must be in optimum position and alignment, and the occlusal relationship must be predetermined in relation to a verifiable centric relation. If the surgical result is to be considered a success, the lower arch must be aligned with the upper arch when the condyles are in centric relation. Failure to achieve this relationship has been the most common shortcoming of surgical results we have seen. Planning for surgery requires that casts must be mounted with a facebow in centric relation, and any changes in arch position must be related to that three-dimensional alignment.

Temporomandibular Disorders and Anterior Crossbite

The resolution of TMJ pain is accomplished in the same way for anterior crossbite patients as it is for other arch relationships. Interferences to centric relation must be eliminated to permit the muscles to relax from their state of spasm.

In anterior crossbite relationships, the interfering inclines are usually found on the anterior teeth. Most often, equilibration can be accomplished by shaving off part of the labial surfaces of the upper anterior teeth or the lingual surfaces of the lower anterior teeth, or both surfaces. Some occlusal adjustment may also be needed on the posterior teeth, but selective grinding should follow the usual rules of procedure.

On rare occasions, we may be required to resolve a severely painful occluso-muscle problem on a patient with crossbite who cannot be equilibrated without destruction of the anterior teeth. If the lower teeth are locked forward of the upper teeth and it is not possible to correct the problem with selective grinding, the most likely alternative is surgical correction. If that is not possible, a compromise treatment utilizing an occlusal centric relation splint at increased VDO may be the only practical approach to getting the patient out of pain.

POSTERIOR CROSSBITE

IMPORTANT CONSIDERATIONS

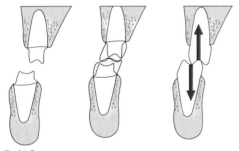

Three questions to ask before "correcting" a posterior crossbite:
1. Are the teeth ideally situated in the alveolar process?
2. Would a change in tooth position benefit tooth-to-muscle harmony, or is the relationship in harmony with the tongue and the perioral musculature?
3. Can the lower posterior teeth disclude as they move toward the tongue (balancing-side disclusion)?
   Determining the best treatment choice for posterior crossbite. In most instances, it is "leave it alone" unless there are interferences to centric relation or excursions.
   Analyzing cusp/fossae relationships in crossbite cases. The lower lingual cusp and the upper buccal cusp become the stamp cusps.
   The most common treatment mistake in crossbites: Confusing balancing side disclusion. Regardless of the arch-to-arch relationship, the lower posterior teeth should never contact while moving toward the tongue.

Treatment objective
Crossbite occlusions follow the same rules as normal occlusions with regard to the requirements for stability. They just use different cusps for holding contacts.

FIGURE 41-8 Warping cusps to change a crossbite into a "normal" occlusion is a bad idea. It creates unnecessary lateral forces on the teeth and alters the neutral zone relations. A crossbite relationship is the correct relationship for ideal axial forces if the skeletal base is larger on the mandible.

It is difficult to understand why posterior crossbite is so routinely treated as something that must be "corrected." Actually, a posterior crossbite relationship can be every bit as stable, functional, comfortable, and esthetic as its more normal counterpart. Yet it is quite common to see such stable relationships warped out of proportion into contours that overprotect the gingival tissues and invite stresses to be directed off the long axes to a damaging degree, all under the guise of "correcting" a crossbite (Figure 41-8).

Evaluating Posterior Crossbites

Most posterior crossbites are the direct result of basal bone relationships. The posterior teeth are usually positioned properly within their own alveolar process, but the mandibular bony arch is proportionately wider than the maxillary bony arch. When the teeth assume the most stable relationship within the bone, the tooth-to-tooth relationship is reversed from what is normally considered "correct." But is such a crossbite relationship incorrect? It is not if it fulfills the necessary criteria for maintainable occlusion. Most often this relationship is more correct than it would be if the teeth were changed to the normal form of intercuspation.

In evaluating the acceptability of a posterior crossbite relationship, the following observations should be made.

Tooth-to-bone relationship in the same arch
Are the teeth ideally situated in the alveolar process? Would the tooth-to-bone relationship be improved if the mandibular teeth are moved lingually or the maxillary teeth buccally? If the teeth are properly positioned within their alveolar bone, which in turn is harmoniously aligned with its basal bone, the usual indication would be to maintain this tooth-to-bone balance. There would have to be some very

compelling reasons for disturbing such a relationship before any change in tooth position should be considered.

Relationship of the teeth to the tongue and cheeks

Are the teeth in harmony with normal tongue and cheek pressures, or have they been moved into the crossbite relationship by abnormal muscle patterns or habits? If deviate tongue or cheek patterns have moved the teeth into a malrelationship, is it possible to correct the abnormal habit pattern? Would a change in tooth position or contour benefit the tooth-to-muscle harmony or the overall stability?

Occlusal relationship

Upper-to-lower tooth relationships should be evaluated for direction of stresses, distribution of stresses, and stability. If the occlusal relationship causes stresses to be directed favorably up or down the long axes, the first requirement of stability has been fulfilled. If the occlusal contours permit favorable distribution of lateral forces in excursive movements, the second requirement of stability can be fulfilled.

When both of these requirements have been satisfied, neither stability nor function needs to be slighted. Optimum function with excellent stability is just as practically attained in a posterior crossbite relationship as it is with normal intercuspation.

If the posterior teeth are in harmony with their supporting bone, if tooth alignment does not interfere with muscle activity, and if occlusal contours are correctly related to the optimum direction and distribution of stresses, there is no occlusal relationship that is more stable than a posterior crossbite.

Restoring Posterior Crossbite

One of the most common mistakes we will see is balancing incline interference in a posterior crossbite that has been restored. We should take a careful look at the next few crossbite patients who have had occlusal restoration of the posterior teeth. In my experience, most of the patients examined were functioning on the lingual inclines of the lower buccal cusps in mediotrusion (Figure 41-9). It is a prevalent fallacy that when teeth are in a crossbite relationship the balancing inclines should be reversed from what they normally are. This is a serious error that is extremely stress-producing.

Upper inclines that face the cheek or lower inclines that face the tongue should never contact in lateral excursions. This rule should be followed regardless of the arch relationship. A helpful way to remember the preceding rule is to learn another rule: *When the lower posterior teeth move toward the tongue, they must disclude.* The side that moves toward the tongue is always the orbiting, condyle side, and all posterior tooth contact should be eliminated on this side because the condyle is unbraced. There is no way to harmonize the occlusion to all degrees of muscle contraction on the unbraced condyle side. Crossbites are no exception. All inclines should disclude when the lower teeth move toward the tongue.

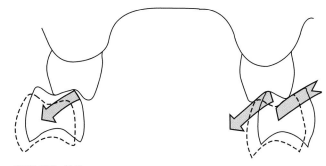

FIGURE 41-9 The most common mistake in treating posterior crossbite relationships is to build the balancing inclines into function. This is a very stressful relationship.

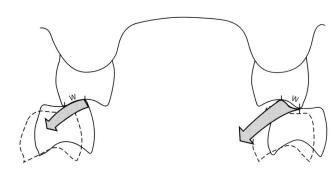

FIGURE 41-10 The correct crossbite relationship. When teeth move toward the tongue, they should never be in contact. The relationship illustrated here is just as functional and just as stable as a normal arch relationship. The working side *(W)* discludes the balancing side in lateral excursions. The centric stops are stable.

When posterior crossbites are being restored, the *lower lingual cusps* become the functioning cusps. They fit into the same upper fossae and function against the same inclines as the lower buccal cusps do in a normal relationship (Figure 41-10). If posterior group function is desired, the lower lingual cusps contact the lingual inclines of the *upper buccal cusps* in working excursions (laterotrusion). This working incline contact can be used very effectively to disclude the opposite-side balancing inclines.

The *lower buccal cusp* is a nonfunctioning cusp in crossbite relationship, and its lingual inclines should never contact; so it should be shortened slightly from the normal contours so that it does not interfere in balancing excursions (mediotrusion). In patients with a more pronounced curve of Spee, the lower buccal cusps will need to be progressively flatter as we proceed posteriorly.

In establishing the occlusal plane on posterior crossbite relationships, it is best to keep the plane on the low side in back. Nothing is lost if the occlusal plane is lower than necessary on the distal (as long as both upper and lower crown-to-root ratios are considered). However, an occlusal plane that is too high distally could make it impractical to provide centric stops that would be free of protrusive or balancing interferences from the upper lingual cusps and the lower buccal cusp in crossbite.

If the lower teeth are tilted lingually and the upper teeth are fairly vertical, the buccal incline of the lower lingual cusp can serve as the functioning incline for working excursions.

It is difficult to evaluate whether lateral stresses would be resisted any better or worse on the lower lingual cusp incline or the upper buccal cusp. It is doubtful that it would matter too much whether there is a slight stress difference because whichever incline is used must be in harmony with the lateral anterior guidance and the condylar movements. Furthermore, most crossbite patients do not use lateral functional movements to the usual extent. Their function very often follows a more vertical pattern.

If the anterior guidance is capable of resisting all of the lateral stresses without help from the posterior teeth, there are no contraindications to posterior disclusion in all eccentric positions.

The *upper lingual cusp* is a nonfunctioning, noncontacting cusp in crossbite relationships. It should be designed to hold the tongue out of the way and to serve as a gripper of fibrous foods without ever coming into contact with the lower tooth. It can come close to contact, but it should never touch.

Fossa contours

There are no differences in the principles of fossa design whether or not the teeth are in crossbite. Lower fossae must be contoured to receive the upper buccal cusps in a stable centric relation contact. Fossae walls must be harmonized so that they are not steeper than the lateral anterior guidance to permit the cusps to pass in and out of the fossae without interference.

The use of the fossa-contour guide as explained in Chapter 21 is just as practical for crossbite relationships as it is for normal occlusions. If the contours of the lower fossae are correctly harmonized, the upper posterior teeth may be restored by several different approaches, including functionally generated path techniques.

Some dentists believe that in crossbite situations the upper teeth should be restored first and the functionally generated path technique should be used on the lower teeth. This is certainly not necessary if lower cusp tip placement and fossa contours are correct. It is far more practical to restore the lower posterior teeth first and then use the functional path procedures on the upper teeth where it is easier to stabilize the base for the functional wax.

With a correct anterior guidance, posterior crossbites can be restored one arch at a time as long as some method of providing correct fossa contours is used.

Equilibrating Posterior Crossbites

If the lower lingual cusp is to serve as the functioning cusp, it is treated in the same manner as a lower buccal cusp in normal intercuspation. All upper inclines are treated in the usual way. Upper working inclines are either harmonized to whatever degree of group function is indicated, or they are ground out of contact if disclusion is preferred.

The buccal inclines of the upper lingual cusps are balancing inclines that should always be ground out of all contact in any eccentric jaw position. The only variation in selective grinding of the upper lingual cusp is that the cusp tip can be shortened. It will not be a functioning cusp, so it can be shaped without regard for maintaining contact of any kind.

In crossbite, the tip of the upper buccal cusp takes on a new importance because, when possible, we want it to serve as a holding contact. Consequently it should never be shortened unless it interferes in both centric and lateral excursions. It is better to shape the upper buccal cusps when necessary to improve the bucco-lingual position in the lower fossae and then do most of the selective grinding on the lower fossa walls and cusp inclines.

If the lingual inclines of the upper buccal cusps are to serve as the working inclines, the lower fossae can be opened out. There is no need to provide lower working incline contact if it is present on the upper teeth. Conversely, if the buccal inclines of the lower lingual cusps are to serve as the working incline contact, there is no need to provide upper working incline contact. Walls of the upper fossae can be opened out, and all upper inclines become nonfunctional.

There is no harm in providing functional incline contact on both upper and lower teeth simultaneously, but there do not appear to be any observable benefits from doing it. There would be no reason, however, to grind functioning inclines away if they are already present and functioning correctly.

The equilibration of crossbite relationships, as with other relationships, should provide noninterfering closure into centric relation. Determining which cusps should function against which inclines should be based on a tooth-to-tooth appraisal of what will provide the most stability with the least lateral stress.

Suggested Readings

Berliner A: *Ligatures, splints, bite planes and pyramids,* Philadelphia, 1964, JB Lippincott.

Graber TM, Vanarsdall RL, Vig KWL: *Orthodontics: Current principles and techniques,* ed 4, St Louis, 2005, Mosby.

Isaacson KG, Reed MT, Muir JD: *Removable orthodontic appliances.* Oxford, 2002, Butterworth Heinemann.

Proffit WR, White RP: Treatment of severe malocclusions by correlated orthodontic, surgical procedures, *Angle Orthod* 40:1-10, 1970.

Ricketts RM, Roth RH, Chaconas, SJ, et al: *Orthodontic diagnosis and planning,* vol 1-2. Denver, 1982, Rocky Mountain Orthodontics.

Subtelny JD: Cephalometric diagnosis, growth and treatment: Something old, something new? *Am J Orthod* 57(3):262-286, 1970.

Chapter 42

Treating Crowded, Irregular, or Interlocking Anterior Teeth

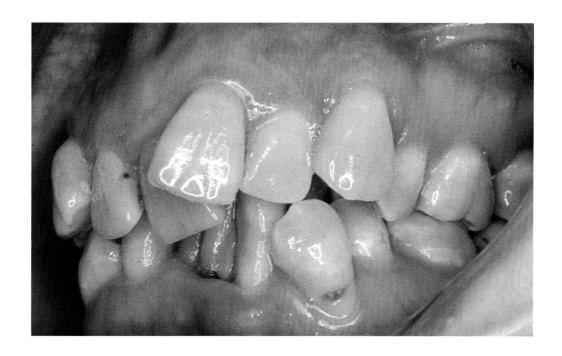

PRINCIPLE
Don't start any treatment until you can visualize the end result and determine the steps to achieve it.

IMPORTANT CONSIDERATIONS

1. Where to start . . . can the temporomandibular joints (TMJs) seat comfortably in centric relation?
2. Is load testing negative? If positive, find out why before continuing.
3. Determine if the occlusion is stable.
   a. Are the anterior teeth stable?
   b. Are the posterior teeth stable?
   c. Always check all teeth for signs of stability or instability (see Chapter 29).
4. If the teeth are stable
   a. Is esthetics a problem that needs correction?
   b. Is function a problem?
   c. Is cleanability a problem (from crowding)?
5. If the occlusion is unstable or if correction is required for other reasons
   a. Is there room in the arch for correction?
   b. Is there a discrepancy between tooth size and arch size?
   c. Honor the neutral zone. Don't try to keep teeth in the arch if it would require over-expansion or interference with the lip-closure path.
6. Can the alignment of the anterior teeth be corrected without major changes to the posterior occlusion?
7. Do the posterior teeth interfere with complete closure to anterior contact in centric relation? If so, determine the best treatment choice for getting the back teeth out of the way so the front teeth can contact in centric relation (see Chapter 30).
   a. Do the anterior teeth contact in maximal intercuspation?
   b. If not, determine if a tongue or lip habit is the reason.
   c. Can the tongue or lip habit be broken?
   d. Will it be necessary to work with the habit?
8. On mounted diagnostic casts, analyze all five options for
   a. Getting the back teeth out of the way
   b. Correcting anterior tooth alignment and position
   c. Establishing stable holding contacts on anterior teeth
   d. Establishing stable holding contacts on posterior teeth
   e. Posterior disclusion

ANALYSIS OF CROWDED, IRREGULAR, OR INTERLOCKING ANTERIOR TEETH

Irregularities in anterior teeth alignment may occur in combination with a variety of other occlusal problems. Crowded incisors may be seen in deep overbites, crossbites, open bites, or almost any other type of arch malrelationship. The anterior misalignment may be the result of an arch malrelationship, or it may be a contributing cause. It may occur in combination with an ideal posterior intercuspation, or the posterior teeth may also be misaligned.

Although anterior teeth must be precisely coordinated with the posterior occlusion, the anterior segments should be evaluated as a separate functional unit. The importance of the anterior guidance as a determinant of posterior occlusion requires that anterior tooth position and alignment have priority over occlusal analysis for the posterior segments. Correction of anterior irregularities must result in a stable relationship that is capable of discluding the posterior teeth in eccentric excursions. At the same time, any changes to anterior alignment must relate to the lip-closure path, phonetic function, and neutral zone harmony.

After a lecture on the importance of anterior guidance, a dentist proceeded to convince one of his 47-year-old patients that she would lose her teeth if she did not have the irregular interlocked anterior bite corrected. Even though the appearance was not particularly noticeable and of no concern to the patient, she agreed to proceed with the extensive plan of orthodontics and restorative reshaping because she did not wish to have her teeth become loose and develop periodontal problems from her malocclusion.

Fortunately, the dentist had second thoughts about his treatment plan when he realized that the lady had no sign of hypermobility, wear facets, or even beginning periodontitis. He reasoned that at 47 years of age she would surely have had some signs of deterioration if causative factors of destruction had been present. The patient gratefully accepted his changed diagnosis and continued to live happily with her irregular but healthy dentition.

Unfortunately, all patients are not that lucky because all dentists are not goal-oriented to maintainable health. Some are oriented to preconceived ideas of what an occlusion must look like rather than how particular occlusal relationships exert their stresses.

Every occlusion must be evaluated on the basis of its potential for destruction, but such an evaluation must consider how the patient functions with a given relationship. An irregular anterior bite is potentially destructive only if:

1. It is uncleanable.
2. It is unstable.
3. It interferes with the patient's functional movements.
4. It fails to provide the necessary disclusive effect for the posterior teeth.

Any one or more of the above problems is reason enough to warrant some type of intervention by the dentist. If none of these problems is being manifested by the irregularity, the only other reason for initiating corrective treatment is to improve the esthetics.

Irregular anterior teeth can present a formidable esthetic problem, but in the absence of destructive tendencies it should be the patient's decision to improve the appearance or leave it as it is. However, when the irregularities are definitely contributing to an accelerated deterioration of the teeth or the supporting structures, it is the duty of the dentist to report this to the patient and to suggest ways of solving the problem.

In the absence of any esthetic concern, irregular anterior teeth should be evaluated in each of the potential problem areas.

Cleanability

If the irregularity is great enough, it may be difficult to clean between crowded anterior teeth. Sometimes three teeth may bunch up to form a funnel-like opening between them. If the teeth are not cleanable, they are not maintainable. Lack of cleanability is reason enough to recommend correction of the irregularity.

Stability

Irregular anterior teeth are often unstable because of a lack of centric holding contacts. Teeth that do not have an antagonistic stop will supraerupt unless something substitutes for the missing contact. Cutting off individual elongated teeth to align their incisal edges is a common practice that does not work. Shortened teeth will simply erupt right back out of alignment unless a stop is provided or some form of stabilization is utilized.

Substitutes for centric contact can be provided in several ways. Any noncontacting tooth that does not supraerupt has something that is preventing the eruption. It can always be determined clinically what the substitute is. Some things to look for are as follows.

Eccentric function
If the tooth contacts enough in function, it may not need centric contact to keep it from supraerupting.

Ankylosis
Ankylosed roots will keep the tooth from erupting further.

Overlapped cingulum
If adjacent contacting teeth lap over the cingulum of a noncontacting tooth, they can lock the tooth into position and prevent any further eruption.

Tongue or lip habits
Habitually interposing the tongue or the lips between the teeth will prevent noncontacting teeth from erupting.

If none of the above stabilizers is found, irregular anterior teeth with no contact will supraerupt. This predictable instability is a definite indication for correcting the irregularity, at least to a point of maintainable stability.

Functional interferences

It would appear that the anterior teeth in an interlocking bite would be subjected to abnormal lateral stresses. In most cases, the mandible cannot move forward or laterally without direct interference from some of the malposed anterior teeth. Yet it is common to find patients in their later years with firm, healthy interlocking teeth. The reason is clear. For teeth to be stressed laterally, the mandible must move laterally. Since the interlocking bite restricts lateral movement, the patient develops functional patterns of movement that have no horizontal component. Strictly vertical patterns of movement seem to be the rule in interlocked bite relationships.

If the bite is interlocked in centric relation, there is rarely a problem with lateral stress on either the anterior or posterior teeth. It is not uncommon to find interlocked bites with no deviation from a terminal hinge closure into maximum occlusal contact.

If the bite is interlocked in a deviated jaw position, it would be unusual not to find severe wear facets, some degree of periodontitis, hypermobile teeth, or some related TMJ symptoms.

Centric interferences can usually be eliminated with selective grinding, but tooth movement may be necessary to resolve other problems. If stable centric relation stops are established, most patients will still maintain the vertical functional stroke in the new occlusal position if the interlocking bite is still present. There is usually no need to provide lateral or protrusive guidances in such cases, but this decision must not be taken lightly. Each case must be carefully evaluated regarding the relationship of the teeth to the envelope of function.

Existing Periodontal Problems

If periodontal destruction is already noticeable, it is certainly an indication that causative factors are present. A very careful evaluation of the tooth arrangement should be made to determine (1) whether it is contributing to the periodontitis and (2) whether correction of the irregularity is necessary for the resolution of the periodontal problem. If extensive restorative procedures are needed for any reason, it would usually be advantageous to correct the irregularity as a matter of practicality. It depends, however, on the severity of the irregularity and its potential for causing future harm.

METHODS OF CORRECTING ANTERIOR INTERLOCKING BITES

It is very easy to oversimplify the treatment for correction of anterior interlocking bite problems. Some problems are simple to solve. Others may be extremely complex. Cases with interlocked anterior teeth can be divided into two categories:

1. Cases that have sufficient room in the arch to accommodate the anterior teeth when they are properly aligned
2. Cases that have insufficient room for the anterior teeth to be aligned without changing posterior arch form

The first category is easy to solve. It involves primarily the labial or lingual realignment of teeth into spaces that are wide enough to accept them (Figure 42-1). There is no need for arch expansion in such cases, and excellent results can usually be obtained with removable appliances and minor tooth-movement procedures.

When there is insufficient room to align the anterior teeth, the problem becomes more complex. We can no longer simply move the anterior teeth forward or backward into alignment because the teeth are too wide to fit into the space that is available at the position of correct incisal edge alignment.

In general terms, we have at least five possible ways of solving the space problem:

1. We can narrow the teeth so that they will fit into the available space.
2. We can widen the space by reshaping the adjacent teeth.
3. We can reduce the number of teeth that must fit into a given space.

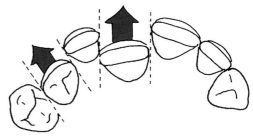

FIGURE 42-1 Irregularly arranged anterior teeth that have room in the anterior segment to accommodate the teeth if they are realigned. This is the simplest alignment to correct.

4. We can increase the space by changing the shape of the arch.
5. We can change the axial inclination of the anterior teeth.

The preceding treatment approaches may still be oversimplified because of arch-to-arch relationships. It may be a simple matter to align the teeth in each arch individually, but the resultant arch-to-arch relationship may then be incompatible. It may be necessary to narrow one arch and expand the other.

Orthodontists have excellent methods for evaluating such problems, and any patient who cannot be successfully treated with a simplified approach should be referred to a competent orthodontist.

It should be obvious that properly mounted study casts are a necessary part of any treatment planning. No corrective procedures should be started unless the finished result can be clearly visualized and the corrections worked out in detail on the casts.

Applying the principles

The upper-left central incisor was locked behind the lower incisors. Because the incisal third of the tooth was fractured, it was just shortened further so it could be moved forward without having to open the bite temporarily to move it past the lower incisal edges.

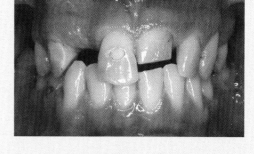

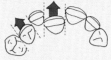

A simple removable appliance was used with a finger spring to push the tooth forward until it was positioned in alignment with the other upper anterior teeth.

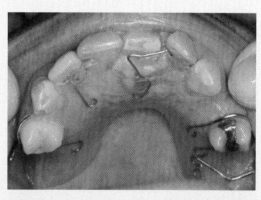

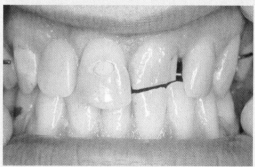

After the tooth was in position, it was prepared for provisional restorations.

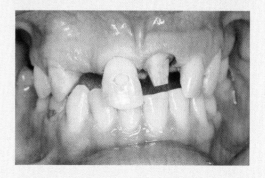

The anterior guidance was refined so a cast could be made and mounted in centric relation to fabricate a custom anterior guide table.

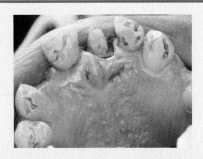

Preparations were then completed.

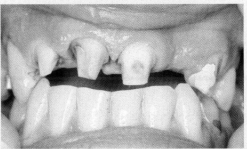

A provisional restoration was copied from the diagnostic wax-up. This will serve as a retainer until the bone stabilizes. After approval, permanent restorations will copy it.

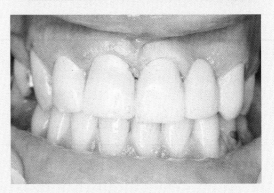

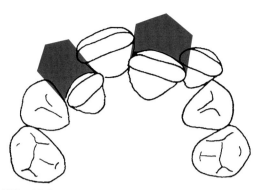

FIGURE 42-2 Irregularly arranged anterior teeth with insufficient room for realignment.

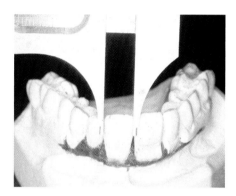

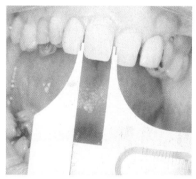

FIGURE 42-3 First treatment option: *Reshape.* Many dentitions with crowded anterior teeth have stable posterior teeth that can be equilibrated to a perfected centric relation. If there is not enough room in the anterior segment to reposition the teeth to establish holding contacts in centric relation, it is often possible to narrow the anterior teeth enough to make room for them without changing the posterior occlusion. By working out the details on mounted casts, the teeth can be narrowed a predetermined amount before moving them into a good alignment.

Narrowing Crowded Teeth to Permit Alignment

Teeth cannot be moved into correct alignment without altering either the width of the space or the width of the teeth (Figure 42-2). If, on mounted models, the crowded anterior teeth are individually separated and removed from the model, they can then be repositioned back on the cast and tacked with wax in the corrected alignment (Figure 42-3). Since the space will not be sufficient to accommodate all the

teeth in the new alignment, the last tooth is left off. The space that is left is measured and subtracted from the width of the unplaced tooth. The difference will be the total reduction in width that must be distributed over all the anterior teeth in that arch. By dividing that figure by the number of anterior teeth involved, we will know how much each tooth must be reduced in width to fit into the correct alignment.

Teeth in the anterior segment can be narrowed up to a combined total of 6 mm without the enamel being penetrated. Radiographs of each tooth should be studied to determine the thickness of the enamel before any width reduction is started. The enamel is usually thickest on the distal of the central and lateral incisors, and considerable reduction can be done on either the mesial or distal of the canines. If necessary, the mesial of the first premolars can be reduced.

Width reduction is commonly referred to as "stripping." It is accomplished with thin separating disks and abrasive strips, or a mechanical stripper. Ground surfaces should be rounded and polished with sandpaper strips and disks.

After the teeth have been narrowed to the proper width, there are several techniques that can be used for moving them into their predetermined correct position in the arch.

Finger pressure
It is surprising how quickly some teeth can be moved into alignment by having the patient exert finger pressure several times a day in the right direction, once room has been provided.

Ligatures and rubber bands
Elastic ligature material or rubber bands can often be used to align anterior teeth. They can be used alone in some cases but frequently should be combined with arch wires to preserve the arch form. Arch wires can sometimes be incorporated into cemented temporary restorations.

Removable appliances
Very often the simplest approach is to use a removable appliance. The methods of providing directed pressure to the teeth are limited only by the imagination. Tooth movement can be effected by finger springs, rubber bands, spring-loaded devices, and pressurized arch bars.

Bands
Uncontrolled tipping forces against an incisor crown have the tendency to torque the tooth around a rotational axis located near the center of the root. Removable appliances that are designed to move the crown lingually usually produce a concurrent labial movement of the root. Conversely, labial crown movement produces lingual root movement. It is frequently necessary to exert greater control over the axial inclination of anterior teeth than is practical with removable appliances. Bonded brackets or bands permit controlled movement of both the crown and the root. There are several methods for exerting the torque effect on the bracket. Square-edged wire that is twisted and then seated into the bracket slot may be used to apply continuous torquing force

on the bracket walls as it tries to untwist itself. Twin wires may also be used to accomplish the torquing effect, or light wires may be bent to serve as springs that attach to the brackets. There are many variations in how the force is applied, but the net effect is accomplished through controlling the force through the bracket. The arch wire may exert direct pressure and torque at the same time, so the control over specific tooth movement can be very precise.

Although almost any desired tooth movement may be possible with innovative removable appliances, the use of bands is very often the most practical and expeditious method when control of torque is critical.

Cemented brackets

The advantages of bracket control can be achieved without the disadvantages of bands. With directly cemented brackets, the thickness of the bands is eliminated between the teeth, and the esthetic problems associated with bands are minimized.

The potential variations in using directly cemented brackets are exciting.

Vinyl repositioners

For minor tooth movement, a soft vinyl appliance may be worn. Teeth are cut off and repositioned on a stone model, and the vinyl appliance is fabricated over the corrected model. It is worn much like an athlete's mouth guard, and it has the effect of exerting gentle pressure on selected teeth until they are moved into the predetermined position. It then serves to hold them in place as long as the appliance is worn.

If tooth repositioning is followed by occlusal correction to harmonize the teeth to the new position, stabilization is enhanced, but some form of retention is also necessary until the bone and ligaments realign to the new position.

Invisible retainers

The use of vinyl overlay materials for moving teeth has become more popular as techniques have been improved. The process involves cutting out and repositioning teeth on the cast. An appliance is then fabricated from a flexible ethylene vinyl acetate (EVA) polymer joined to a semirigid polycarbonate material. The appliance is formed on the cast by use of a Biostar. The flexible appliance moves up to four teeth at a time for small incremental movements. Further movement requires a new retainer made on a cast with further corrections of tooth positioning until the teeth are aligned in their final position. By mounting the casts in centric relation, tooth movement can be directed to an idealized predetermined position.

Invisalign®

Invisalign® is a commercial process that has much promise if used with an understanding of occlusal harmony. It utilizes a series of computer-generated sequences for tooth movement to achieve an ideal alignment of teeth in both arches. For each step in the sequence a clear overlay of a flexible matrix is made that includes slight changes in tooth position. The flexible overlays guide the tooth movement step-by-step toward a predetermined occlusal relationship. As movement is completed for each overlay, the next overlay is placed to achieve the next movement until the finished result is achieved.

Dr. Jeff Scott has developed a process for producing an acceptable occlusal relationship using Invisalign®. The process is shown in the following steps.

Patient with upper-left lateral and canine locked behind lower teeth. The upper-right lateral and canine are lingually inclined to create a poor esthetic alignment.

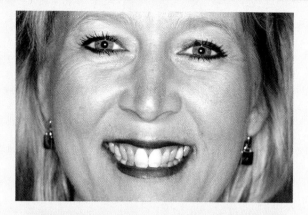

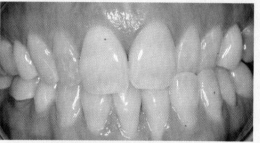

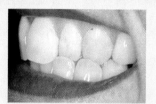

A centric relation bite is made using bilateral manipulation with load testing to verify centric relation.

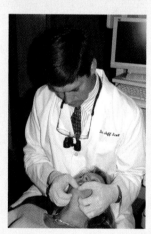

Continued

PROCEDURE   Producing acceptable occlusal relationship using Invisalign®—cont'd

Casts are mounted in centric relation with an earbow for location of centric relation condylar axis.

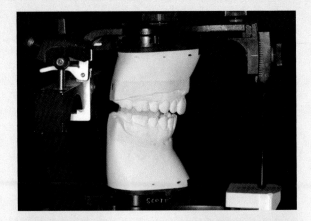

A silicone index is made to relate the casts to centric relation at first point of tooth contact.

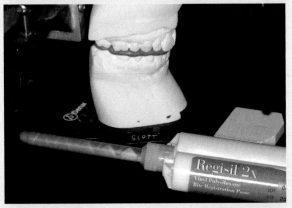

The index is used in the computer-generated jaw relationship to which the teeth will be aligned. This corrects for discrepancies inherent in unmounted casts related to maximum intercuspation.

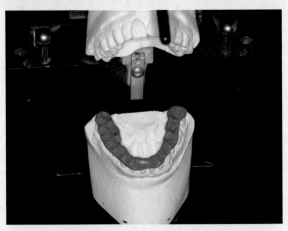

Series of Invisalign® overlays to be used in sequence.

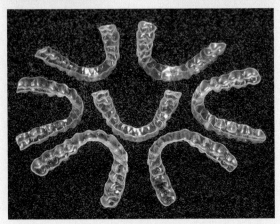

PROCEDURE   Producing acceptable occlusal relationship using Invisalign®—cont'd

Computer-generated image of starting point.

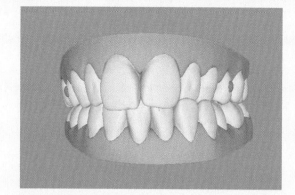

Image of projected treatment goal. The treatment goal for this patient includes the use of laminates for the initial determination of where the teeth needed to be positioned to facilitate an esthetic and functional result.

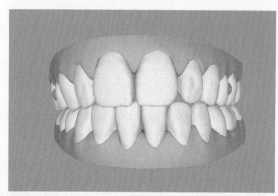

Teeth after movement to the predetermined treatment goal. Planning included use of laminates for final esthetic position and contour on right and left laterals and canines.

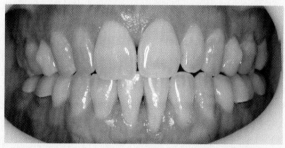

Teeth prepared for laminates.

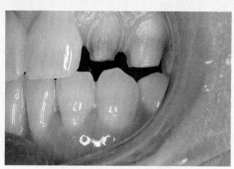

Laminates in place on left side where anterior crossbite was before treatment. Contours on these teeth would have been severely compromised without the orthodontic repositioning.

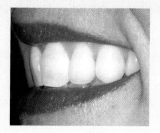

Continued

Finished result of very conservative treatment. Central incisors were bleached to lighten color, avoiding any need for restorations on them. Note the uniform occlusal contact in centric relation, made possible by aligning the teeth to a correct maxillo-mandibular relationship.

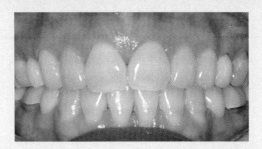

CORRECTING ANTERIOR IRREGULARITY WITH SELECTIVE EXTRACTION

In the presence of a stable posterior occlusion, the selective extraction of a single lower incisor is sometimes a practical step in resolving the problem of crowded lower anterior teeth. If the combined width of the remaining three incisors equals the space available in the arch and if stable centric holding contacts can be provided for each tooth, there are no real contraindications to the extraction approach.

The fact that there are only three teeth occupying the space that normally has four is not noticeable. It creates no problems of esthetics, function, or stability as long as the teeth that remain can be brought into correct anterior function.

If there is a slight size variation between the three remaining teeth and the available space in the arch, one can usually resolve the problem by stripping the contact area to further narrow the tooth width, or selected teeth can be crowned or bonded if more width is needed.

Bands or directly cemented brackets should usually be used if much repositioning of lower incisors is required after a selected tooth is extracted. The brackets permit lateral movement of the root along with the crown so that the teeth may maintain a stable upright position rather than merely tilting them into contact. If the lower incisors are to be included in a restorative splint, the axial relationship of the root is less important. Stabilization will be achieved by the splint.

Extracting All Lower Incisors

Certain circumstances justify the extraction of all lower incisors when they are crowded. Lower incisors can be replaced with a fixed bridge about as successfully as they can be restored. If periodontitis has resulted in considerable bone loss around the lower incisors, it is difficult to restore the long-exposed root surfaces with full-coverage restorations unless the axial alignment is near perfect. Maintenance of gingival health is sometimes complicated by the retention

of such teeth, especially if root surfaces are close together or if the level of alveolar bone is irregular.

Extraction of crowded lower incisors is indicated under the following conditions:

1. If extensive restorative procedures are indicated that necessarily include the lower incisors whether they are retained or not, and if retention of the lower incisors would not lend any advantage to the remaining teeth
2. If retention of the lower incisors would create problems of maintenance
3. If retention of the lower incisors would require unnecessary complication of the treatment plan without yielding a commensurate value to the plan

Much time, effort, and expense can be wasted trying to save lower incisors that could be restored more effectively with a fixed bridge. The difficulty of cleaning between splinted lower incisors is almost reason enough to recommend a fixed bridge when extensive periodontitis is a problem. If the realigned lower incisors would be cleanable and would have the potential for lending support to other teeth, they should be saved.

Extracting Upper Anterior Teeth

Selective extraction of upper anterior teeth is rarely indicated because of the problems it creates esthetically. However, each case must be evaluated individually. It is sometimes possible to extract both lateral teeth to provide a good alignment, but if extractions are necessary, it is almost always better to extract the first bicuspids to provide room for the correct alignment of all six upper anterior teeth.

Combining selective extraction with restorative reshaping may have great merit for severely crowded anterior teeth if the posterior occlusion is stable. Sometimes the extractions permit narrower restorations than could be achieved otherwise. As an example, extremely wide lateral incisors could be replaced with narrower pontics. Additional room can be gained when the central incisors are narrowed and the mesial of the canines is reduced.

Such measures should be used only when complete orthodontic correction must be ruled out for good reason. Combined extraction and restorative techniques should almost never be used on very young patients. They should be reserved for mouths that can benefit in other ways from the restorative procedures. The decision to extract any tooth is a major one that should be made only when the benefits outweigh the disadvantages.

COMBINING RESTORATIVE PROCEDURES WITH ORTHODONTICS

Restorative reshaping of any tooth should not be considered if the restoration can be avoided by moving the tooth into a better alignment. However, when the need for restoration is evident, the combination of restorative reshaping and orthodontics can often be used to great advantage.

Being able to narrow teeth or shorten them often facilitates their movement through or into spaces that would otherwise not accommodate them. Once in position, they can be restored back to proper contact and occlusion.

Crowded anterior teeth with stable posterior teeth

If the posterior teeth are stable with good holding contacts in centric relation, there is no reason to move them if the anterior teeth can be aligned without disturbing the posterior occlusion. Analysis on mounted diagnostic casts clarified a treatment plan that required stripping to narrow the incisors and then repositioning them into stable centric relation contact.

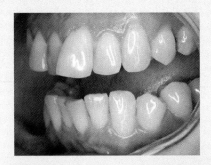

An appliance was constructed to open the vertical dimension of occlusion (VDO) to make room to move the upper incisors into position without interference from the lower incisors. Space was opened to make room to move the laterals to open space for the centrals.

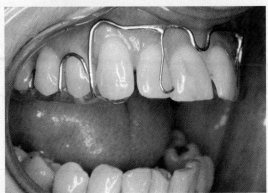

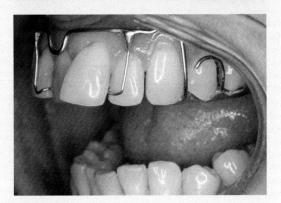

High labial appliances work very well for aligning anterior teeth. "Putters" can be used to move the laterals distally and for rotating the centrals into alignment while moving them into the space.

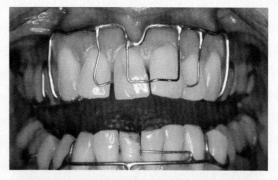

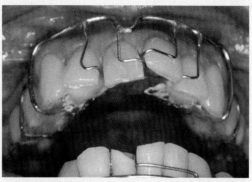

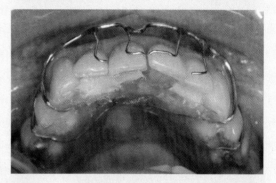

Lower incisors were stripped to make room for the malpositioned incisors to be moved into its slot. Note how the upper-left central is being rotated as it is moved into alignment.

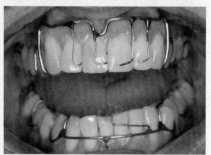

Teeth aligned can now be restored with ideal contours.

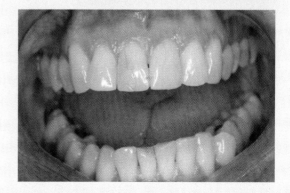

Crowded anterior teeth with severe posterior interferences

When severe anterior crowding is combined with severe interferences to centric relation, it is all the more important to follow the most critical rule for problem solving:

> All occlusal analysis starts at the TMJs.

This patient came to the office for esthetic restoration of the anterior teeth. Her former dentist had recommended upper and lower six-unit anterior bridges. She came in for a second opinion, primarily concerned about getting the best esthetic result. The former dentist had never mounted casts or checked her TMJs.

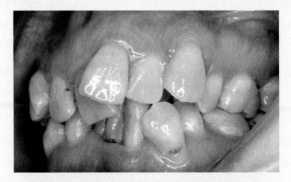

The jaw-to-jaw relationship at the first tooth contact in centric relation. Examination revealed that her TMJs were intact but she suffered severe occluso-muscle pain with daily headaches and sore posterior teeth.

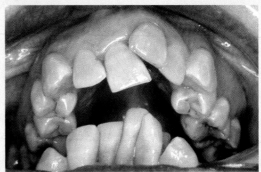

Because of advanced periodontal lesions with deep intrabony involvement in the anterior segment, several teeth were not savable. Following the recommended *programmed treatment planning* process, teeth that are not savable were marked with an *X* to be extracted. By removing those teeth from the casts, the planning was simplified but the problem of the posterior interferences required major decisions in order to get the back teeth out of the way enough to achieve anterior contact in centric relation. It would have been impossible to plan properly without mounted diagnostic casts.

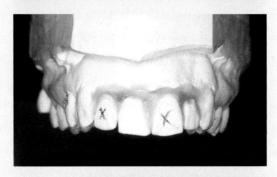

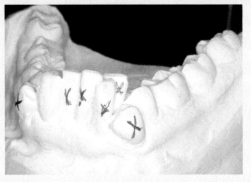

Extraction of unsalvageable teeth (**A**) was followed with immediate placement of a removable appliance (**B**) for replacing the lost teeth and also fitted with finger springs for moving the teeth to a predetermined position (**C**).

By planning the entire treatment on casts mounted in centric relation, the options for getting the back teeth out of the way could be evaluated to accomplish enough closure to achieve anterior contact in centric relation.

The VDO for achieving anterior contact could also be determined so alignment of the anterior teeth could proceed.

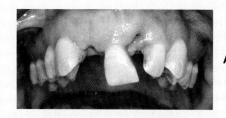

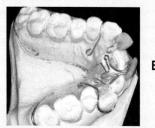

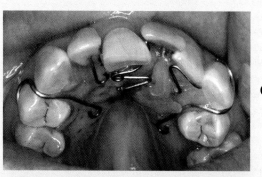

A temporary immediate replacement could be fabricated for replacing the missing teeth.

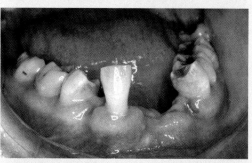

A finger spring could be added for moving the canine into a predetermined position.

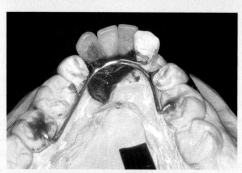

The orthodontic mechanism could be waxed in and processed to fabricate the immediate appliance.

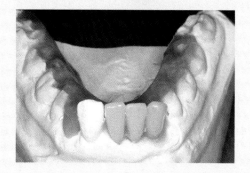

After the teeth were positioned in their planned alignment, they were held in retention for two months, during which time reduction of the posterior teeth was carried out to close the VDO enough to achieve anterior contact. The rubber band retainer is a simple nonobtrusive way to hold the teeth against a lingual plate of acrylic resin.

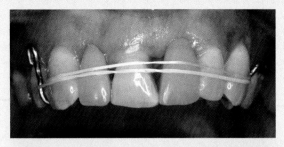

As soon as the teeth were stable enough to prepare, both upper and lower anterior teeth were prepared for provisionalization.

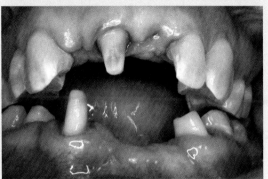

All final details of incisal plane and anterior guidance were then worked out on the provisional restorations.

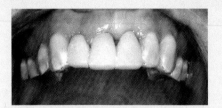

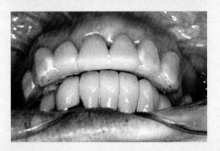

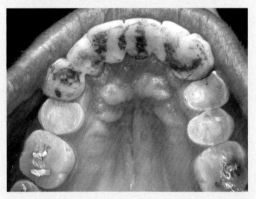

Upper and lower impressions of the approved provisionals were mounted. A customized anterior guide was made so the exact configuration of the anterior guidance could be duplicated in the final restorations.

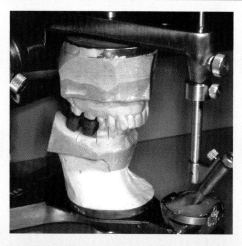

Finished restorations showing how flat the anterior guidance had to be to avoid excessive reduction of the molars. Because the details were first worked out in the provisionals and accepted by the patient, a good result was assured. All occluso-muscle discomfort was eliminated and the headaches disappeared.

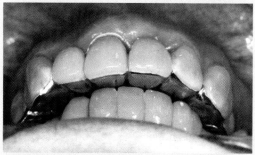

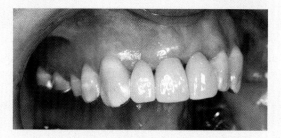

Restorative reshaping combined with orthodontics is not generally used to advantage as often as it could be, especially in adult orthodontics.

The advantages do not stop with easier movement of teeth. Temporary acrylic restorations can be fabricated to serve as orthodontic appliances to take the place of bands. They may serve as anchorage, as guides to direct teeth into better position, and finally as extremely good retainers to hold the teeth in place while the supporting tissues reorganize.

RELATIONSHIP OF ANTERIOR TEETH TO POSTERIOR TEETH

I frequently see patients undergo extensive orthodontic treatment involving premolar extractions when a more esthetic result could be achieved without extractions, in a fraction of the treatment time and frequently without even using bands or brackets. This should not be misinterpreted as a blanket condemnation of premolar extraction. There are arch relationships that are served best by selective extractions (as has already been pointed out). There are some cases, however, that might be treated differently.

If the posterior occlusion is stable but the anterior teeth are crowded, it should not be considered an automatic extraction case. If stripping procedures or restorative reshaping can provide the room for aligning the anterior teeth into an acceptable anterior guidance relationship, there is often no reason to involve the posterior teeth, even when they are not in a Class I relationship.

There are two technique-oriented concepts of orthodontic treatment that might make the above suggestion hard to accept. These concepts are (1) that certain posterior cusps must fit in certain corresponding fossae and (2) that a deep overbite relationship is always bad.

Neither concept is valid. Posterior teeth can be maintainably stable in dozens of different relationships from the classic Class I cusp-tip–to–fossa relationship to an end-to-end bite or even a crossbite. Stability depends on the direction of stress and the distribution of centric holding contacts, not on specific cusp-tip–to–fossa relationships. The Class I relationship is ideal, but it is not necessary for stability.

In regard to the anterior relationship, there is absolutely nothing wrong with a deep overbite, provided that there are stable centric contacts and the inclines can be harmonized to function (see Chapter 36). Given stable centric contacts and functional inclines, deep overbites are just as maintainable as any other anterior relationship, *and the esthetic result is often far superior to the "pushed-in" face of the incorrectly diagnosed extraction case.*

Many patients are far more handsome or beautiful with prominent anterior teeth and a smile line that complements their lip line. Although this may still be accomplished in selected cases with extractions, such a decision should be made on the basis of treating the face instead of merely letting the anterior teeth fall victim to some technique concept of cusp-tip location and incisal edge relationship.

If the anterior alignment can be corrected without involvement of the posterior teeth, that's fine! If arch expansion will improve the relationship, that is fine too. If the problem cannot be solved without extractions, we must take out teeth. But we must not get out the forceps until it has been positively determined that:

1. The facial contours, lip support, smile line, and general esthetics will be better with extractions than without.
2. The occlusion cannot be stabilized for the long term without extractions.
3. The posterior relationship must be changed to correct the anterior relationship; simple expansion of the arch will not suffice or is not practical.
4. The above decisions are based on a tooth-by-tooth determination of stress direction and stability of existing centric contacts or potential contacts that might be achieved through reshaping or needed restorations.

It is probably worth repeating that it is easy to oversimplify the correction of irregular anterior teeth. Mounted diagnostic models enable treatment decisions to be tested on models before any conclusion is finalized. This is a highly recommended procedure.

GROWTH PROBLEMS AND CROWDED LOWER ANTERIOR TEETH

In young patients who have completed successful orthodontic alignment of the anterior teeth, the result is often spoiled later by a delayed crowding of the lower anterior teeth. The same crowding effect may be seen in young patients who have had naturally well-arranged teeth until their middle or late teens.

Some orthodontic authorities believe that the crowding results from civilized man's failure to wear the anterior teeth into an edge-to-edge relationship. Because of this failure, the anterior teeth supposedly continue to erupt while the posterior teeth do not. The continued eruption is said to cause crowding of the lower anterior teeth as the overbite deepens. This concept is based on studies of Stone Age man's dentition. Some orthodontists still attempt to produce the edge-to-edge bite of severely worn Stone Age dentitions, even in young adults. Hopefully such a stereotyped "orthodontic look" will become a thing of the past as more orthodontists are learning that moderate procumbency is often a desired esthetic trait and that anterior teeth need not be edge to edge to be stable. Even deep overbites can be stable if adequate centric stops are provided.

The problem results from a growth spurt during which the mandible grows faster than the maxilla. The lower anterior teeth are simply caught in the squeeze and crowd up behind the upper anterior teeth, which are held in place by pressure from the lip.

A careful analysis of growth pattern through cephalometrics may enable the astute orthodontist to predict the problem in some cases, but all growing children should be continuously observed for any beginning sign of lower anterior crowding, since it is not uncommon for mandibular growth to continue after maxillary growth has ceased.

The problem is sometimes preventable by use of a simple lingual arch bar bonded or joined to bands on each lower canine. The bar prevents the lower incisors from collapsing inward and forces the upper anterior teeth to keep pace with the lower growth spurt. It may have some effect on limiting the growth spurt also, but regardless of how it works, the net effect is to hold the lower anterior teeth in good alignment during the period when mandibular growth occurs at a faster rate than maxillary growth.

CAUTION: Before placing such an appliance, be certain that the neutral zone is not violated for the anterior teeth.

Other than minor occlusal adjustment by selective grinding, no other treatment is required except in unusual cases of excessive mandibular development. Once the growth of the mandible has ceased, there is no further need for the appliance. If proper centric contacts are provided and the anterior guidance is in harmony with the envelope of function, there will be no problem of maintaining the relationship indefinitely.

If lower anterior crowding develops after the growth years, it is virtually always caused either by a posterior occlusal interference that drives the mandible forward into the upper anterior teeth or by failure to provide adequate centric contact for the lower incisors. Supraeruption and subsequent crowding can occur easily if stable centric stops are not present.

Suggested Readings

Altemus LA: Mechanotherapy for minor orthodontic problems, *Dent Clin North Am* July:303-312, 1968.

Geiger A, Hirschfeld L: *Minor tooth movement in general practice,* ed 3, St Louis, 1974, Mosby.

Goldstein MC: Adult orthodontics and the general practitioner, *J Can Dent Assoc* 24:261, 1958.

Goldstein MC: Orthodontics in crown and bridge and periodontal therapy, *Dent Clin North Am* July:449-459, 1964.

Goldstein MC: Seminar at L.D. Pankey Institute, Miami, Florida, October 1973.

Graber TM, Vanarsdall RL, Vig KWL: *Orthodontics: Current principles and techniques,* ed 4, St Louis, 2005, Mosby.

Isaacson KG, Reed MT, Muir JD: *Removable orthodontic appliances.* Oxford, 2002, Butterworth Heinemann.

McCreary CF: Personal communication, St Petersburg, Florida, 1973.

Schlossberg A: The removable orthodontic appliance, *Dent Clin North Am* 1972 July:487-495.

Wank GS: The use of grassline ligature in periodontal therapy, *Dent Clin North Am* July:473-486, 1972.

Wellison BD, Warunck SP: *Practical guide to orthodontic appliances.* Great Lakes Orthodontics, Ltd, Buffalo, NY, 2004.*

*This practical guide to orthodontic appliances gives details on fabrication and usage of many different types of appliances, as well as other useful information regarding the use of brackets and invisible retainers.

Chapter 43

Solving Severe Arch Malrelationship Problems

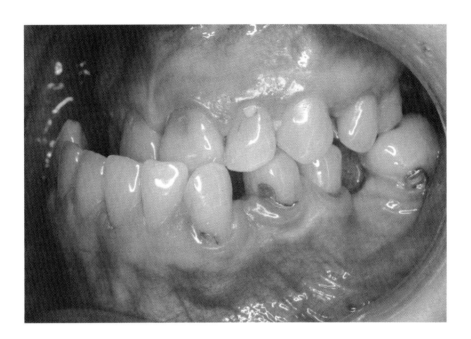

> **PRINCIPLE**
>
> The fundamentals of programmed treatment planning are consistent even for the most complex, multidisciplinary occlusal problem.

IMPORTANT CONSIDERATIONS

Severe arch malrelationship

1. Determine if the arch malrelationship is unstable. Look for signs. If it is unstable, mount casts in centric relation and start the evaluation by determining the best choice of treatment for establishing centric relation stops.
2. Determine if the arch malrelationship is an esthetic problem for the patient. If so, do diagnostic work-up on casts to serve as a starting point for fabrication of the provisional restorations that will then be refined in the mouth.
3. Establish centric relation stops on anterior teeth if possible. Determine the best treatment option for eliminating posterior interferences to anterior contact in centric relation.
4. Don't proceed with final posterior restorations until anterior relationship is accepted.
5. Correction often requires a multidisciplinary approach. Evaluate all five options. Choose the best option.

Treatment objectives

1. If the relationship is unstable or requires treatment for improved function or esthetics, the first objective is to provide stable holding contacts. Evaluate each treatment modality (reshape, reposition, restore, surgery). Determine the best method for solving each problem, consistent with the patient's needs or desires.
2. If surgical correction is indicated, be sure to determine which arch is in best harmony with the system so corrections can be made on the arch that is malrelated. Both arches may require correction for best results.

No matter how complex or complicated a severe arch malrelationship may appear, the process of programmed treatment planning does not change. What may appear as a baffling problem to solve is dramatically simplified, at least in regard to treatment selection, if the following rules are consistently adhered to:

1. *Get the mouth healthy.* If extensive treatment is to be performed, it is all the more important that the supporting tissues are maintainably healthy. This should be a "no compromise" rule. Rule out teeth that cannot be saved.
2. *Get the temporomandibular joints (TMJs) stable.* Regardless of how disordered the arch-to-arch relationship may be, the starting point will still be to verify that the joints are stable and can accept loading. Until the condition and position of the TMJs is known, you are only guessing at the correct jaw-to-jaw relationship.
3. *Follow the correct sequence.* The complexity of the problem does not change the sequence of treatment-planning decisions.
4. *The requirements for stability guide the process.* Each requirement must be fulfilled in correct order. Always evaluate for signs of stability if any requirement has not been fulfilled. Before making changes, determine if any unfulfilled requirements for stability have been substituted for.
5. *Evaluate all five treatment options.* This rule applies for each requirement for stability. Don't make snap treatment decisions without considering the pros and cons of other options. Choose the best option only after comparing.

ANALYSIS OF SEVERE ARCH MALRELATIONSHIPS

Arch malrelationship problems fall into two general categories:

1. Those that result from malposition of the teeth in relation to an acceptably aligned skeletal base
2. Those that result from a malrelationship of the skeletal base

Although many arch relationships can be corrected by orthodontic treatment alone, some occlusal problems are too severe to be treated successfully without a combined approach that may involve the expertise of several different specialists. The prosthodontist, the maxillofacial surgeon, and the orthodontist may need to work as a team to solve certain severe malrelationships. When this is necessary, the treatment must be coordinated so that each specialist can perform without constraints that result from lack of understanding by the other specialists regarding the final goals of treatment. Unfortunately, even a team approach can fall short of an optimum result if some member of the team does not direct the treatment toward a final goal of harmonious occlusion.

For an ideal goal-oriented result, the logical specialist to coordinate the direction of treatment should be the specialist who has the final responsibility for the completion of treatment.

If the orthodontist will have the final responsibility, the orthodontist should direct the surgeon or the prosthodontist regarding the preparation for a finished orthodontic result. If the prosthodontist has the ultimate responsibility for a complete prosthetic result, input from that specialist should clearly outline what is needed from the surgeon or orthodontist. It is terribly discouraging to attempt an acceptable prosthetic treatment plan after surgical or orthodontic treatment has been completed with no consideration for the result. This can be avoided if the last person to be responsible for the result is involved in treatment decisions related to preparing the patient for the final treatment result.

Just as with other types of occlusal problems, the treatment of complex arch malrelationships cannot be solely directed toward a single textbook version of Class I occlusion, not because it isn't a worthwhile goal in some or even most patients, but rather because it is not a necessary or even acceptable goal in some patients. There are many options for treating arch malrelationships, and the prudent diagnostician will evaluate all options before recommending treatment. There are many considerations that only the patient can evaluate, and the patient is entitled to know if there is more than one way to achieve a result that would be acceptable. As long as the inviolate goal of optimum oral health is not compromised, the treatment approach that best suits the patient's total needs is the one that should be considered.

The analysis of severe arch malrelationships should result in a treatment plan that accomplishes four specific goals:

1. Optimum oral health
2. Occlusal stability
3. Comfortable function
4. An esthetic result that is acceptable to the patient

Because it may be possible to accomplish the first three goals without satisfying the fourth, severe arch malrelationships should always be analyzed to determine which segments, if any, are properly related to the cranial base and the skeletofacial profile. With improved surgical techniques, realignment of the skeletal base can be accomplished with such predictive results that it should at least be considered as an option to be evaluated before a final treatment plan is determined. Regardless of the mode of treatment selected, the segments of the occlusion that are correctly related should not be altered to conform to the segments that are malpositioned. Thus a careful analysis is in order so that treatment is directed to maintain what is correct and change only what needs to be changed. The process for making such decisions requires an orderly sequence.

The first step in planning treatment for complex arch malrelationships is an interview with the patient to find out from these basic questions what the patient's perception is:

1. Are you uncomfortable?
2. Can you function satisfactorily?
3. How do you feel about your appearance?

There are many arch malrelationships that do not need treatment. If there are no signs of instability, no discomfort, and no complaint about function or appearance, there is no need for intervention. A personal example may help to illustrate this point: A 72-year-old surgeon in excellent health was referred for correction of a severe arch malrelationship. His entire lower arch was completely buccal to his upper arch. He did not have holding contacts on any teeth. There was no anterior guidance, and only the balancing side came into contact in lateral excursion. Upon questioning, he reported no discomfort and no problems of any kind with mastication, and he had 32 firm teeth with no excessive wear. His supporting tissues were completely healthy. When asked about his appearance, he laughed that his prominent lower jaw had never been any concern to him. In fact, he considered it one of his strong features and wouldn't change it, even if he could. No treatment was needed, and none was wanted.

The above patient had a stable occlusion. The tongue and the cheeks substituted for the missing holding contacts, and a vertical pattern of function eliminated the need for anterior guidance or lateral disclusion. The lack of any sign of instability confirmed that diagnosis.

But would the same conclusion be drawn if the patient had been 32 years of age instead of 72?

The answer is yes. The diagnosis would be the same because regardless of the age of a mature adult, the complete lack of any sign of instability along with an explanation of why the occlusion is stable is proof enough that treatment is not needed at that time.

The critical element in diagnosis however is the thorough examination. The decision that no treatment is needed can only be made after a careful determination that there are no causes or effects of instability. If tooth positions are changing or if teeth are loose or are wearing excessively, some interception of causative factors should be delineated and explained to the patient regardless of how comfortable or how functional the occlusion feels. Patients cannot make an informed decision unless they are aware of all the facts. Patients cannot know the facts unless a thorough examination determines them.

The value of cephalometrics in restorative dentistry has not been well understood, and consequently it has not been used to full advantage. In determining any treatment plan, all practical methods of treatment should be evaluated and compared. The patient should be made aware of the various options and should have a reasonable explanation of why a particular treatment approach is favored. When there are obvious facial profile problems related to the arch malrelationship, cephalometric radiographs are very helpful in the initial stage of diagnosis because an analysis of those films helps us to determine which segments are correct and which segments need to be altered. This is valuable information for determining treatment approaches because each treatment potential can then be analyzed in relation to a correct goal.

With background information from the patient interview, a sequence of analyses can be used to develop all viable options for treatment. Thoroughness requires the following:

1. A complete intraoral examination, including periodontal examination
2. Screening examination and history to determine the condition of the TMJs; a more intensive TMJ exam when indicated
3. Correctly mounted diagnostic casts in centric relation
4. Complete radiographic series of the teeth and jaws; panoramic films routinely included
5. Cephalometric radiographs if facial profile is a problem or if any alteration of the skeletal base is contemplated
6. Completed medical history

Special tests or specialty examination information may also be required for specific problems, and a conference with other specialists who have treated the patient may be in order.

DESIGNING TREATMENT WHEN THE SKELETAL BASE IS ACCEPTABLY ALIGNED

In severe arch malrelationships, the skeletal base is rarely in perfect alignment, but if the skeletal profile appears acceptable and careful interviewing of the patient determines that it is not an esthetic concern, a treatment plan approach is initiated for the purpose of correcting tooth relationships without altering the existing skeletal base. Since the alveolar bone can be made to move with the teeth, it may be effectively altered orthodontically within the context of this approach.

If the skeletal base is not to be changed, diagnostic procedures are aimed at determining where the teeth must be positioned for a stable occlusal relationship. This determination is best organized by use of correctly mounted diagnostic casts. Correct mounting requires verified centric relation bite records and the use of a facebow.

Analysis of the mounted casts must be related to the requirements for stability described in Chapter 29. Each requirement for stability is analyzed in sequence, starting with the first requirement of stable holding contacts for each tooth. If we divide our analysis into separate treatment objectives, it greatly simplifies the treatment planning.

First Treatment Objective: Stable Holding Contacts

The first focus should be on establishing stable holding contacts on the anterior teeth. The most common occlusal problem at this stage is interfering contacts on posterior teeth that prevent anterior contact in centric relation. If this is so, lock the condyles in centric relation and determine the best choice of treatment for getting the back teeth out of the way so the jaw can close all the way to maximal intercuspation without displacing the condyles.

Four treatment options should be analyzed in sequence to determine which option, or combination of options, would best fulfill this objective. The option choices are as follows:

1. Selective grinding/reshaping
2. Orthodontics/repositioning
3. Restoration
4. Surgery

Analysis of first treatment option: selective grinding

On duplicated casts that are also mounted, the first step is to determine how much correction can be accomplished with selective grinding. When all interferences are eliminated so that the casts can close to maximum occlusal contact in centric relation, the results are sometimes surprising. What appears to be a severe occlusal problem may not be severe at all when the occlusal relationship is evaluated in centric relation at the correct vertical dimension.

It is often not possible to completely achieve holding contacts on the anterior teeth by selecting grinding of the posterior teeth. If this is the case, determine if conservative occlusal equilibration will improve the relationship enough to minimize the need for other treatment choices to achieve anterior contact in centric relation.

It is amazing how far out of alignment the mandible can be driven by occlusal interferences. Severe facial asymmetries can result from deviation around malposed teeth. Pseudoprognathism can result to a degree that surgical correction might be contemplated if centrically mounted casts were not studied first at the correct vertical dimension of occlusion (VDO). The only effective way to determine the true tooth-to-tooth relationship at the correct VDO is to equilibrate the casts until the articulator can close to the same VDO as maximum occlusal contact. The closure must be confined to the centric relation axis.

The casts can be poured with dowel pins so that the posterior segments can be removed. This permits a quick analysis of the anterior relationship on a centric relation arc. But it does not permit analysis of the tooth-to-tooth relationships of the posterior teeth.

In my practice I have seen several patients with apparent severe arch malrelationships who were scheduled for corrective surgery. But when casts were mounted in centric relation with an open bite record and the interferences to the centric relation arc of closure were cleared, the severe deviation of the mandible was eliminated. Even apparently severe prognathic patients may have acceptable profiles if the mandible is not forced into protrusion by occlusal interferences.

There is no acceptable substitute for centrically mounted diagnostic casts in the diagnosis of arch malrelationships. The casts should be equilibrated to the patient's most closed VDO in centric relation before any further decisions regarding treatment selection are made. A second set of casts should be preserved in their original relationship so that a comparison can be made at any point of treatment.

The decision to use selective grinding should be based on three factors:

1. Amount of tooth reshaping needed
2. Condition of teeth to be reshaped
3. Comparative analysis with other methods of treatment

If gross reshaping is needed on teeth that require restorative procedures for other reasons, even severe reshaping can often be used to advantage. If alternative treatments would be severely complicated or prohibitive for one reason or another from the patient's standpoint, reshaping, even extensive reshaping in some cases, may be the treatment option of choice.

If only minor reshaping is required to achieve an acceptable result, equilibration would generally be the option of choice.

If the problem cannot be resolved by selective grinding, the second step in the sequence should be pursued—orthodontic evaluation.

Analysis of second treatment option: orthodontics

The purpose of this analysis is to determine how much can be accomplished by orthodontics toward moving the teeth into an acceptable relationship. By working with both the original casts and the equilibrated casts, the orthodontist can determine whether it is possible to move teeth within the existing skeletal base into an acceptable alignment or whether it is possible to alter the arch alignment orthopedically to resolve the malrelationship without surgery. A cephalometric evaluation is an important part of this diagnostic procedure.

By working with both the equilibrated casts and the unchanged casts, we can also comparatively evaluate a combination approach whereby reshaping and repositioning procedures are both utilized.

If the problem is too severe to be solved with orthodontics or a combination of orthodontics and selective grinding, the third step in the sequence should be followed—restorative evaluation.

Analysis of third treatment option: restoration

Restorative procedures can be used in a variety of ways to resolve arch malrelationship problems. Restorative options include the following:

1. Restorative reshaping to provide holding contacts.
2. Fixed/removable prostheses for substituting for missing occlusal contacts.

It is possible to recontour teeth restoratively into unlimited shapes, but unless the recontoured crown form complies with factors of stress direction and tissue health, it may create a bigger problem than it solves. Restorative reshaping should be limited to crown contours that result in axially aligned loading in centric relation. The health of the supporting tissues should never be compromised by overprotection of the gingival tissue regardless of what other advan-

tages may be gained from it. In the evaluation of restorative solutions to arch relationship problems, periodontal considerations are often the limiting factor that determines the logical extent of the reshaping.

If holding contacts cannot be provided by restorative recontouring, or some combination of restoring, reshaping, and repositioning, the next treatment approach to consider is to see if the need for holding contacts can be eliminated by splinting. If teeth without contact can be joined to teeth that have good occlusal stops, their vertical position in the arch can be stabilized. The decision to splint is sometimes the logical treatment of choice when the teeth to be splinted are also useful as abutments for fixed replacement of missing teeth, or when restorations are needed for other reasons.

But the disadvantages of splinting make its use a secondary choice if it is practical to provide holding contacts by other means.

Fixed/removable prostheses are often an excellent treatment choice when there are edentulous segments that require removable appliances. The combination of tooth and tissue support can often be used effectively to substitute holding contacts on the removable appliance when stable stops cannot be provided on the teeth themselves. As a compromise treatment, a well-made bite plane can often provide stable holding contacts around an arch that would otherwise require major, complex treatment approaches. I have maintained numerous patients for many years with such appliances who could not afford the more costly surgical and restorative treatment (Figures 43-1 to 43-4).

Analysis of fourth treatment option: surgery

If the arch malrelationship problem cannot be solved satisfactorily by some combination of reshaping, repositioning, and restorative procedures, it will be apparent on the mounted diagnostic casts. When tooth movement alone, even with recontoured teeth, cannot provide an acceptable occlusal relationship, consideration should be given to surgical repositioning of segments of the dento-alveolar structures on an unchanged skeletal base.

If skeletal base relationships are acceptable and facial profile is not a problem, we can often correct the occlusal malrelationship by shifting a section of the dentition on an unchanged skeletal base. There are many ways in which sectional osteotomy methods can be used to great advantage. As better surgical techniques have been developed, this procedure has become more useful. Several basic types of sectional osteotomy procedures are illustrated at the end of this chapter along with other surgical methods to show some of the basic methods for surgically correcting each type of arch malrelationship.

The surgical method selected depends on a sequence of diagnostic analyses to determine first the best method, or combination of methods, for establishing stable holding contacts on all the teeth. From that point on, determination of the correct anterior guidance can proceed.

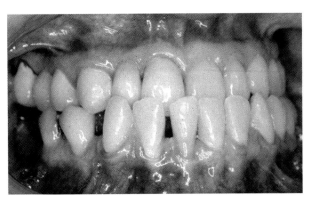

FIGURE 43-1 Maximal intercuspation in a patient with a severe arch malrelationship. The patient had intolerable discomfort that had been diagnosed previously as temporomandibular disorder (TMD). Empty-mouth clench caused severe discomfort.

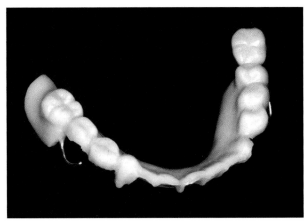

FIGURE 43-3 An occlusal splint fabricated on a cast metal base with cured composite allowed maximal occlusal contact in centric relation.

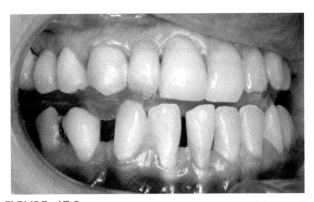

FIGURE 43-2 Arch-to-arch relationship when the condyles were in centric relation. Load testing, Doppler, and other tests indicated that joints were intact and not a source of pain. In this relationship, the patient could clench with maximal muscle contraction with no discomfort. Muscle palpation produced discomfort in all elevator muscles and severe tenderness in the medial pterygoid muscle. The diagnosis was "occluso-muscle pain" from severe displacement of the TMJs during maximal intercuspation. Treatment planning analysis indicated surgical correction as the best treatment option. The patient's health and finances ruled that out.

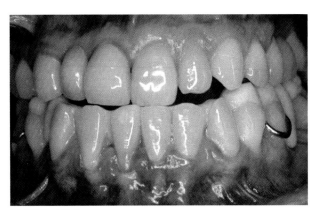

FIGURE 43-4 The occlusal splint in place resulted in complete comfort for the patient even during firm clenching. The compromised treatment was enthusiastically accepted by the patient. The splint is worn 24/7.

PROCEDURE   Analysis and treatment using a combination of specialists

In the following arch malrelationship, the restorative dentist was the coordinator of treatment because he had the final responsibility for an extensive restorative result. In other cases, the oral surgeon or the orthodontist may determine the goals of treatment. Regardless of who leads the team approach, it is essential that a very clear model of the finished result should be constructed in advance of treatment.

No irreversible treatment (other than for an emergency) should be started until the finished result can be clearly visualized and all steps are outlined for the complete treatment.

A severe arch malrelationship resulted from multiple fractures of the maxilla and mandible. The skeletal base is acceptable. The dento-alveolar process is misaligned.

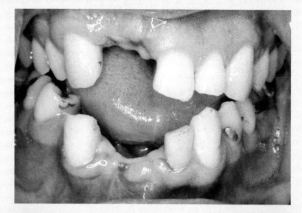

Mounted diagnostic casts at centric relation indicate an anterior open bite and a Class III anterior relationship. The treatment goal will be to determine how to best achieve anterior contact in centric relation. In spite of the severity of the arch malrelationship, the sequence of treatment choice analysis doesn't change.

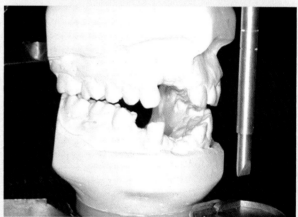

First treatment option: Reshape. Analysis should be done on casts to see how much correction can be accomplished by reshaping. Some improvement can be made for posterior teeth. Because of multiple fracture lines, onlays are indicated for all posterior teeth regardless of reshaping needs, and so gross reshaping is a logical step to improve the arch relationship. Even though it will not completely resolve the goal of anterior tooth contact, note that it does help toward that goal.

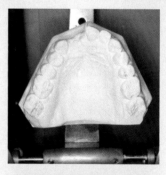

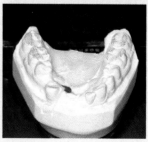

Continued

PROCEDURE   Analysis and treatment using a combination of specialists—cont'd

Second treatment option: Reposition. Move the teeth on the cast to a position that would allow anterior contact. A diagnostic wax-up on the repositioned teeth will demonstrate what could be accomplished if it is possible to move teeth this far. Consultation with an orthodontist reveals that the need for tooth movement is more than can be accomplished by orthodontics.

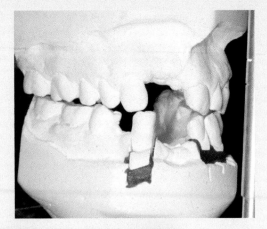

Third treatment option: Restore. A rough wax-up is done to evaluate potential for establishing contact with restorations if teeth could be moved to a better position more aligned with the upper anterior teeth. Because the teeth cannot be moved that far orthodontically, the next treatment option is brought into consideration.

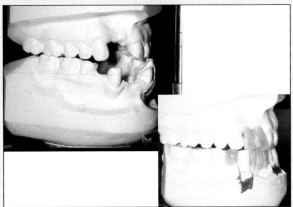

Fourth treatment option: Surgery. By removing a segment of the alveolar process between the canine and the second premolar, the anterior dento-alveolar segment can be moved back into a position that will permit alignment with the upper anterior teeth. After the segment is placed into an acceptable position on the casts, an index is made to guide the surgeon in placing the segment into the predetermined position.

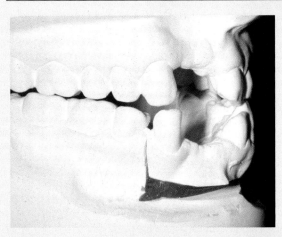

The patient after surgery. Before surgery, the reductive shaping of the posterior teeth brought the anterior segments close enough to achieve contact after surgical alignment. Now new casts are made and mounted in centric relation.

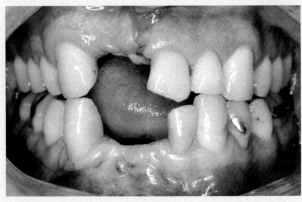

PROCEDURE   Analysis and treatment using a combination of specialists—cont'd

A new diagnostic wax-up is made after the surgical repositioning of the lower segment. This wax-up is then used to form a matrix for forming the provisional restorations after the teeth are prepared.

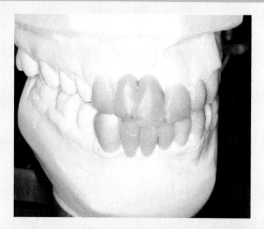

Because there are no guidelines remaining for precise contouring and alignment of the anterior teeth, both upper and lower anterior teeth are prepared (**A**) and provisional restorations are placed (**B**). Remember that a diagnostic wax-up for anterior teeth is only a best guess. Final contours and incisal plane must be established in the mouth.

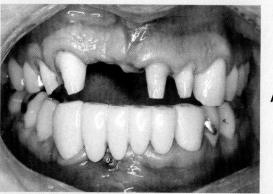

A

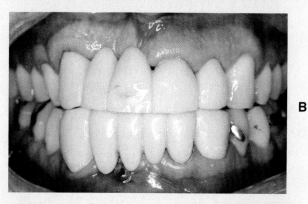

B

After refinement of the provisional restorations in the mouth, the original waxed-up contours had to be reshaped because of a tight neutral zone and a vertical lip-closure path. This required considerable reduction of the labial contours on the provisional restorations to conform to a correct functional matrix. New labial embrasure contours can now be formed on this surface.

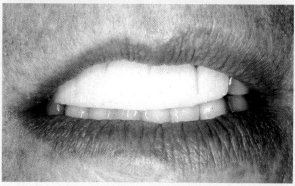

Continued

Reshaped provisional restorations reflecting the correct inclination, incisal edge positions, and labial matrix form established in the mouth.

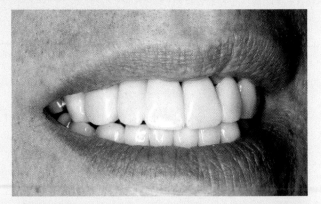

Finished anterior restorations copy the provisional restorations as explained in Chapter 16. Remember that the functional contours of the anterior guidance cannot be accurately determined until all posterior interferences to centric relation have been removed.

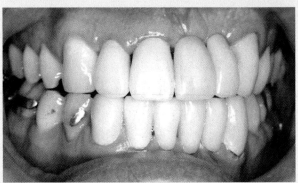

After the anterior guidance has been finalized, the lower posterior teeth can then be restored (A). Note that the fossa guide ensures that lower fossa inclines will be flatter than the lateral anterior guidance to ensure posterior disclusion in excursions (B). You can review that process in Chapter 21.

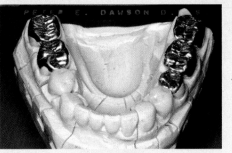

A

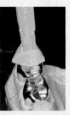

B

The upper posterior restorations can then be completed on an articulator. The key to accuracy now is a perfected centric relation mounting and condylar paths set flatter than the patient's. If the posterior teeth are made to contact in centric relation, and disclude in all excursions on the articulator, the same result will be automatically achieved in the mouth.

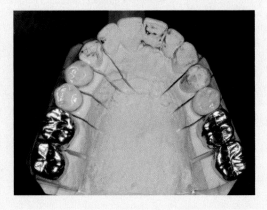

PROCEDURE   Analysis and treatment using a combination of specialists—cont'd

Completed restorations **(A)** compared with original arch malrelationship **(B)**. The process of programmed treatment planning provided an orderly step-by-step format leading to a predictable end result.

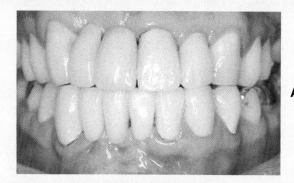

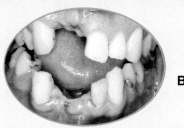

DESIGNING TREATMENT WHEN THE SKELETAL BASE IS NOT ACCEPTABLY ALIGNED

It is not the purpose of this text to outline all of the details of surgical treatment for orthognathic deformities. There are, however, some underlying principles of treatment planning that relate to what constitutes an acceptable occlusal relationship. And there are some basic surgical objectives that must relate to those goals for good occlusion. By comparing some of the methods with the objectives, we can develop a frame of reference as a basis for communication between the specialties involved.

Starting Point for Analysis

The starting point for analysis of any severe arch malrelationship must be a determination of the arch relationship when both condyles are in centric relation. If there are any problems of health, position, or alignment of the condyle-disk assemblies, they should be resolved to an acceptable level before orthognathic surgery is attempted. Unless the condyle-disk assemblies are in a healthy, physiologically correct relationship, any surgical alignment of the dentition will be misaligned in relation to correct joint position. For that reason, mounted diagnostic casts articulated in a verified centric relation are essential.

Cephalometric analysis should be used with diagnostic casts and a clinical examination to determine the specific parts that need alteration. A review of Chapter 44 is useful to explain some of the ways in which cephalometric analysis is used to guide the determinations.

General practitioners as well as prosthodontists and orthodontists should familiarize themselves with the following basic methods for correcting severe arch malrelationships. In many instances, a surgical correction is less traumatic and more readily tolerated than long and extensive orthodontic or prosthodontic treatment, and the results of treatment may be superior. It is an important tenet of restorative dentistry that contour depends on position. Even when extensive restorative treatment is needed, we can often greatly improve it by first correcting the alignment of malrelated arches.

The following surgical methods are illustrated to show how some of the most common arch malrelationships can be corrected (Figures 43-5 to 43-11).

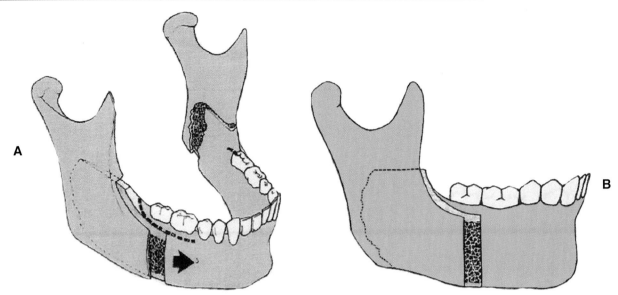

FIGURE 43-5 Sagittal split osteotomy *for advancement of the mandible.* This procedure results in a stable forward repositioning (**B**) with little or no relapse because the entire lower band of the buccinator muscle is moved forward with the segment, thus eliminating abnormal pullback from a stretched muscle. Notice how the cut is positioned to avoid the origin of the buccinator muscle. *Heavy dotted line* in **A** shows the origin of the muscle.

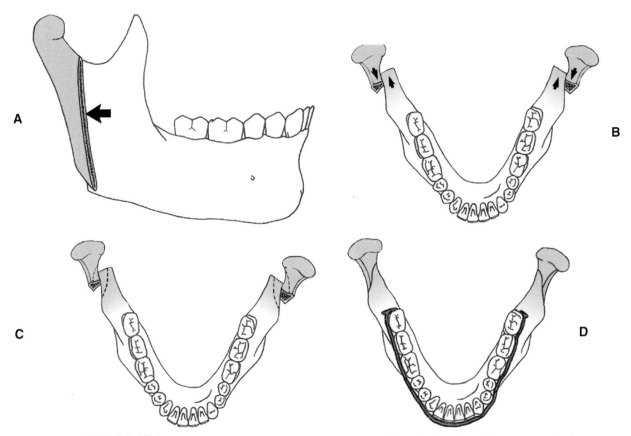

FIGURE 43-6 Vertical ramus osteotomy *for mandibular retraction.* **A,** A vertical cut through the ramus permits the anterior segment to be moved back. The overlap that results (**B**) is reduced to create a better juncture of the segments (**C**). Notice that the buccinator muscle (**D**) is unaffected by the repositioning because it is moved in its entirety with the retracted segment.

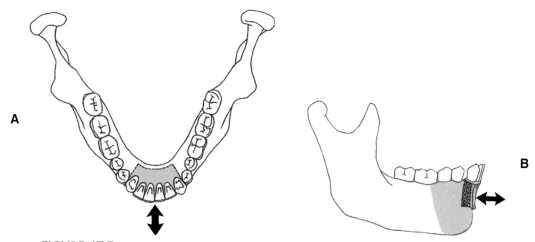

FIGURE 43-7 Anterior segmental osteotomy (mandibular) *for repositioning the anterior segment.* This procedure is used to reposition the anterior dento-alveolar segment without altering the skeletal base. It can be employed to change the inclination of the anterior segment or to level the occlusal plane. **A,** Normal pattern of the cut. **B,** Potential for repositioning. If the section is to be lowered, its height is reduced on the lower border.

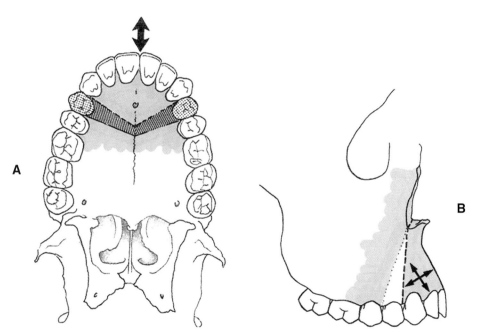

FIGURE 43-8 Segmental osteotomy (maxillary) *for repositioning anterior segment.* The anterior segment can be sectioned and repositioned to move the maxillary anterior dento-alveolar segment horizontally, change the inclination of the entire segment, or alter the segment's vertical position. **A,** It can be combined with removal of a segment. **B** shows how the inclination can be altered.

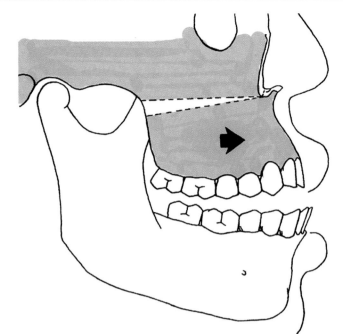

FIGURE 43-9 Full maxillary osteotomy *for maxillary advancement.* The maxilla can be sectioned above the roots and the entire dentition advanced forward to correct a skeletal maxillary retrusion.

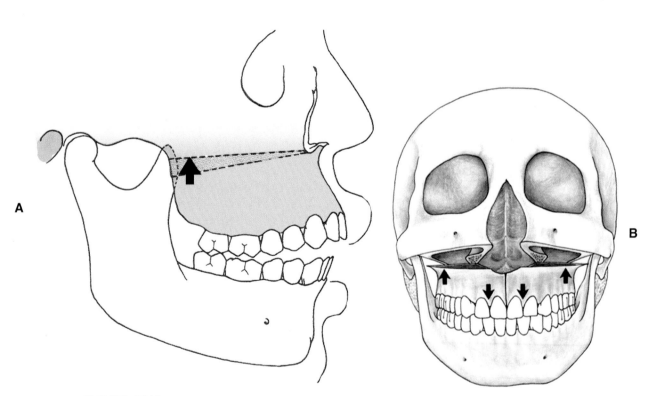

FIGURE 43-10 Full maxillary osteotomy *for closing anterior open bite.* **A,** By removing a segment from the posterior maxilla, one can elevate the posterior dento-alveolar segment to permit the anterior open bite to be closed. This upfracture procedure does not interfere with contracted elevator muscle lengths, so it provides a very stable result with little or no relapse. **B,** A full osteotomy permits a repositioning of the maxilla from several dimensions.

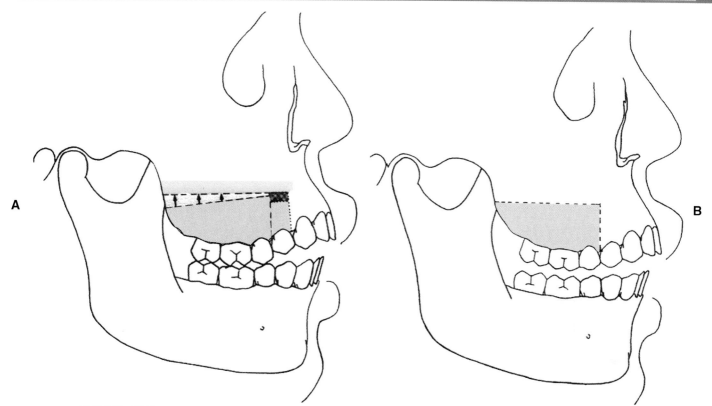

FIGURE 43-11 Segmental osteotomy with ostectomy *to level occlusal plane in posterior segments.* **A** and **B,** By removing a section of bone, one can elevate a segment of the maxillary dento-alveolar process without moving the anterior segment. This procedure could be combined with removal of the first premolar for horizontal repositioning if needed in addition to the change of VDO. This procedure does not interfere with elevator muscle contraction lengths, so it results in good stability.

NONSURGICAL TECHNIQUES FOR STABILIZING SKELETAL MALRELATIONSHIPS

Despite advances in surgical technique, a large percentage of arch malrelationships will still be treated by nonsurgical methods. It is possible to stabilize some arch-size discrepancies simply by providing stable holding contacts to prevent supraeruption.

Treating the Complete Lingual-Version Lower Arch

When all lower teeth are completely lingual to the teeth in the upper arch, there will almost invariably be a skeletal mismatch that is not correctable by orthodontics because there are no occlusal stops. Both arches erupt into a side-by-side relationship (Figure 43-12). Such relationships may be stable if tongue and cheeks substitute for the missing occlusal stops. If continued eruption is a problem, it can be corrected when holding contacts on the lingual surfaces of the upper teeth are provided and the cusp height on the lower teeth is shortened (see Figure 43-12, *B* and *C*).

If the lower arch can be expanded even slightly to engage the new stops, that is all that will be required to estab-

lish stability. There are no concerns about anterior guidance or balancing-side interferences because such patients have vertical patterns of function and have a strong neutral zone horizontally because of the added width between the outward and inward muscle action. In some patients, it may be possible to establish stops by simply reshaping tooth surfaces, but it will more often require restorations to provide the holding contacts (Figure 43-13). There are many configurations that can benefit from this treatment approach, including unilateral arch discrepancies.

Treatment Choices When the Lower Arch Is Too Wide for the Upper Arch

If the lower teeth are completely buccal to the upper arch, the nonsurgical approach is the same as the treatment for lingual-version lower arches, except that the position of the holding contacts is reversed (Figure 43-14). There is still no concern about lateral excursions because the steep locked-in occlusion produces a vertical envelope of function.

The decision of how to treat locked-in occlusions depends on how the occlusion got that way. If the malrelationship occurred as a result of a congenital arch-size discrepancy, problems with stability will generally be solved when we merely provide centric holding contacts. But if the arch discrepancy resulted from an accidental injury or a poor prosthetic or surgical correction, the locked-in occlusion may not conform with a pre-established pattern of function, and stress may result. If any signs of instability are present or if masticatory dysfunction is causing discomfort or breakdown, a conservative treatment approach may not be acceptable.

If the occlusion appears stable and if the patient is not bothered by esthetics or lack of function, it would generally be in order leaving it as it is. I have observed patients who have relationships like the ones just described who have maintained stable, healthy dentitions for many years with no sign of accelerated deterioration.

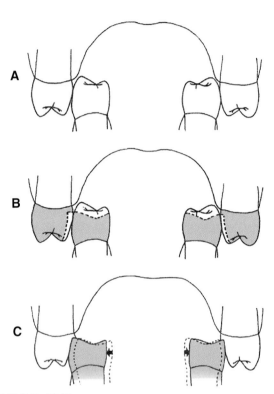

FIGURE 43-12 **A,** When the lower arch is in complete lingual version to the upper arch, supraeruption of the unopposed lower teeth is a potential problem. If the tongue does not substitute for the missing contact, centric holding contacts must be provided. This involves shortening of the lower supraerupted teeth and contouring of the upper lingual surfaces to provide holding contacts. **B,** After contouring is completed, the lower arch is expanded into position for contact in centric relation. This relationship is usually all that is necessary for maintenance of the occlusion. Splinting may be required in some cases. Functional working excursions can be worked out on the upper inclines. **C,** If lower teeth in a lingual-version relationship have supraerupted all the way to tissue contact, the correction is accomplished in the same manner except that the centric stop on the upper teeth may be right at or near the gingival margin. A shallow notch may be all that is necessary to provide a stable centric holding contact. The working excursion in this type of problem is extremely steep, but it does not present a problem because functional movements are almost always vertical.

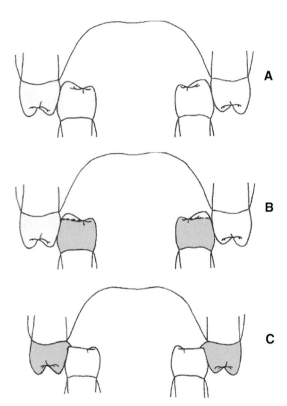

FIGURE 43-13 **A,** Because of a strong horizontal neutral zone (due to the double thickness of teeth), stability problems are often limited to vertical control of eruption. **B,** Shortening the contact cusp and providing a restored stop close to the gumline (**C**) is often all that is needed. Functional movements are limited to vertical, so excursive pathways are of no concern.

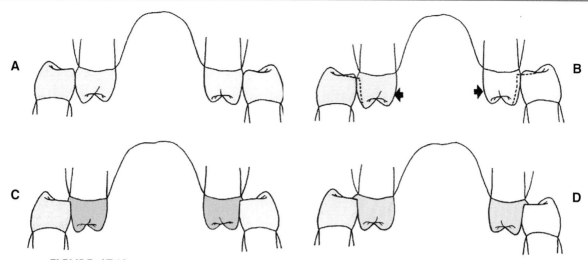

FIGURE 43-14 **A,** When the mandibular teeth are in complete buccal version to uppers, the supraeruption of both arches is the principal problem to solve. **B,** Stable stops can be established when the lower lingual cusps are shortened and the upper buccal surfaces are reshaped to establish a stop. **C,** The upper arch is then expanded enough to engage the stops. **D,** An alternative method is to provide a stop near the gingival margin by restoration.

Chapter 44

Using Cephalometrics for Occlusal Analysis

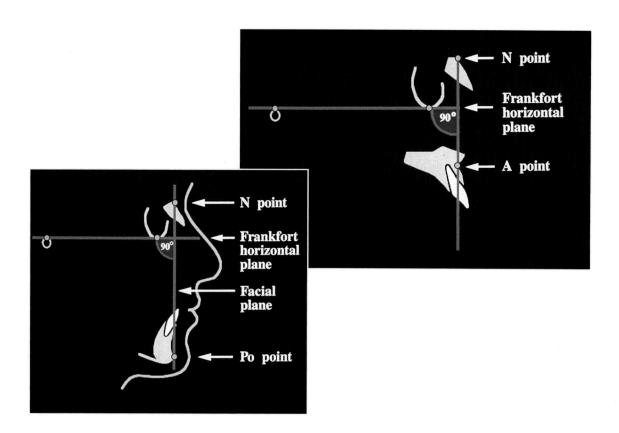

PRINCIPLE

The primary goal of orthodontics should be to make correct occlusal relationships harmonious with correct skeletal jaw relationships.

LIMITS OF CEPHALOMETRICS

Because cephalometrics has been so closely related to predicting growth in children, it has not received the attention it deserves as an aid to treatment planning for adult occlusal problems. Furthermore, the complexity of growth analysis has unnecessarily complicated attempts to simplify cephalometrics for use by general and restorative dentists. It does, however, have great value in occlusal problem analysis for adults, and because growth analysis is unnecessary for mature patients, the use of cephalometrics can be simplified.

Total adherence to cephalometric "norms" does not provide enough information for making a final treatment judgment. Its use must be combined with an analysis of neutral zone factors and established patterns of function. The goal of treatment should be anatomic and functional harmony for individuals who do not always fit cephalometric averages, but the averages can be used as guidelines in combination with other relevant information to tip off the examiner to which segments are in normal relationships and which ones are not. If a dento-alveolar segment that appears normal cephalometrically also appears normal to profile analysis and functional relationships, it should not be changed to conform to a malrelated part. A basic rule in treatment planning is to preserve what is right and change what is wrong.

Cephalometric analysis is an aid to making that decision.

ELEMENTS OF CEPHALOMETRICS

There are two basic elements forming the entire system that must be learned to make cephalometric analysis understandable:

1. Points
2. Planes

Points are precisely located spots that relate to specific bony landmarks. They are the first thing that is located on a tracing of a cephalometric radiograph. Points can also be recorded on soft-tissue landmarks and as intersecting points where two planes cross.

Planes are determined by joining two points with a straight line.

Points

Bony landmarks

There are 11 bony landmarks (on lateral cephalometric analysis) that can be easily learned as a beginning foundation for occlusal analysis (Figure 44-1).

1. *P point* (portion) is located at the most superior convexity of the external auditory meatus.
2. *O point* (orbital) is located at the most inferior convexity of the external border of the orbital cavity. It is the anterior landmark for determining the Frankfort plane.

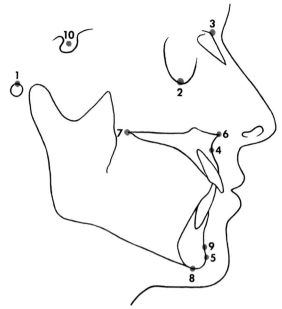

FIGURE 44-1 Bony landmarks on lateral cephalogram.

3. *Na point* (nasion) is located at the most forward point of the nasofrontal suture. It is the upper point for determining the facial plane.
4. *A point* (subspinale) is located at the deepest point of concavity on the labial surface of the maxilla between the anterior nasal spine and the alveolus. It is the upper landmark for the A-Po plane. It also signifies the juncture of the basal bone with the alveolar process.
5. *Po point* (pogonion) is the most anterior point on the symphysis. It is the lower landmark for both the facial plane and the A-Po plane.
6. *ANS point* is the anterior tip of the nasal spine.
7. *PNS point* is the posterior tip of the nasal spine.
8. *M point* (menton) is the most inferior point on the symphysis of the mandible.
9. *PM point* (protuberantia mentalis) is a point above the pogonion where the profile changes from convex to concave.
10. *S point* (sella turcica) is the center of the sella turcica.
11. *Xi point* is the geometric center of the mandibular ramus (Figure 44-2).

Soft-tissue landmarks (Figure 44-3)
1. *Pn point* (pronasale) is the most anterior point of the nose.
2. *Po' point* (soft-tissue pogonion) is the most anterior point on the soft tissue of the chin.

Planes (Related to Lateral Cephalometric Analysis)

For a general appraisal of skeletal, occlusal, and profile relationships, we can generate a considerable amount of helpful information by observing two sets of five planes on a lateral cephalometric analysis:

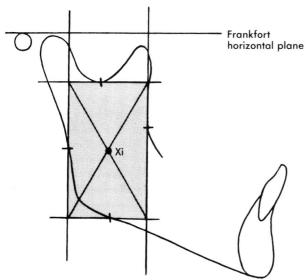

FIGURE 44-2 Xi point. A rectangle is formed with the top and bottom parallel to the Frankfort horizontal plane and the sides perpendicular. Each line is drawn to tangent to points on the borders of the ramus to form the rectangle. The Xi point is located at the intersection of diagonals and represents the geometric center of the ramus.

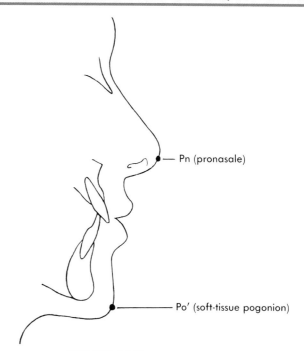

FIGURE 44-3 Soft-tissue landmarks.

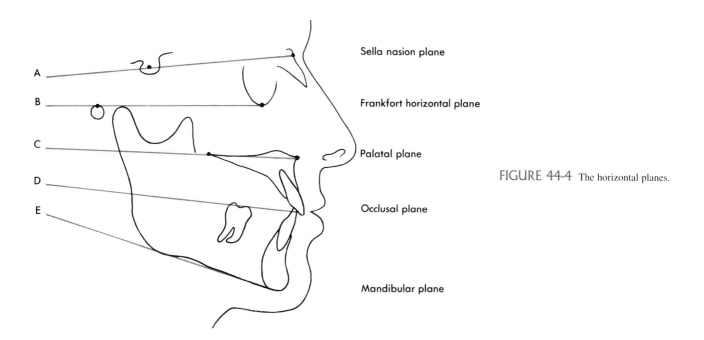

FIGURE 44-4 The horizontal planes.

1. Horizontal planes (Figure 44-4)
   a. Sella nasion plane (S Na)
   b. Frankfort horizontal plane (FH)
   c. Palatal plane (ANS to PNS)
   d. Occlusal plane (OP)
   e. Mandibular plane (MP)

2. Vertical planes
   a. N-A line (connecting nasion with A point)
   b. Facial plane (Na to Po)
   c. A-Po plane
   d. Esthetic plane (Pn to Po')
   e. McNamara line (nasion perpendicular)

HOW THE PLANES ARE USED FOR OCCLUSAL PROBLEM ANALYSIS

From a lateral viewpoint, the cephalometric planes are an aid for determining five essential relationships that are keys to diagnosis and treatment planning.

1. Anteroposterior relationship of maxilla to cranial base.
2. Anteroposterior relationship of mandible to cranial base.
3. Relationship of upper teeth to maxilla.
4. Relationship of lower teeth to mandible.
5. Vertical relationships of mandible and maxilla to cranial base and to each other.

As stated, a cephalometric analysis is never relied on as the sole determinant of treatment. Rather it is one part of a diagnostic triad that includes the following:

1. Cephalometric analysis
2. Mounted diagnostic casts
3. Clinical examination and evaluation

If all three parts of the analysis are in agreement, the diagnosis can be made with assurance. If any one of the above evaluations does not agree with the others, it should be considered a red flag. Blind dependence on certain cephalometric norms can destroy an attractive facial profile, but this can be avoided when the analysis is combined with clinical observation that includes evaluation of every patient for occlusal stability as part of a total examination. Regardless of the relationship to the norms, a dentition is stable if there are no signs of tooth hypermobility, excessive wear, or migration. When a stable occlusion is found in combination with an abnormal cephalometric analysis, the reasons for the stability should be determined before any changes are contemplated. The dentition may be stabilized by unbreakable habit patterns or strong neutral zone relationships. Similarly, a unique profile may be attractive and stable, even though it is not "normal."

The significance of skeletal norms must be adjusted for age, sex, and race, but the following evaluations make the most usable analysis as applied to adult white males.

Evaluating the Horizontal Position of the Maxilla

Maxillary depth refers to the anteroposterior relationship of the maxilla to the cranial base. It is determined by the degree of angulation of the N-A line in relation to the Frankfort horizontal plane (FH) (Figure 44-5). This reference determines whether a Class II or Class III malocclusion is attributable to the maxilla.

Norm: A 90-degree angulation indicates that the maxilla is in a normal relationship.

Maxillary protrusion is indicated by an angulation greater than 90 degrees. The higher the angle, the greater is the horizontal excess of the maxilla.

Maxillary retrusion: Inadequate growth of the maxilla in an anterior direction is indicated by an angulation less than 90 degrees. The lower the value, the greater is the deficiency.

Evaluating the Horizontal Position of the Mandible

Mandibular depth refers to the anteroposterior position of the mandible to the cranial base. It is determined by the degree of angulation of the N-Po line in relation to the Frankfort horizontal plane (FH) (Figure 44-6). This reference determines whether a Class II or Class III malocclusion is attributable to the mandible.

Norm: A 90-degree angulation indicates that the mandible is in a normal relationship horizontally.

Mandibular prognathism is indicated by an angulation greater than 90 degrees. The higher the angle, the greater is the mandibular excess in an anterior direction.

The *retrognathic mandible* is indicated by an angulation of less than 90 degrees. The lower the angle value, the greater is the mandibular deficiency. A severe deficiency produces an "Andy Gump" type of deformity.

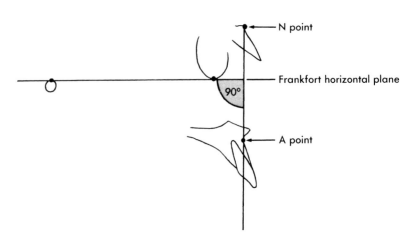

FIGURE 44-5 Maxillary depth analysis for "normal" anteroposterior relationship of the maxilla to the cranial base. An angle greater than 90 degrees indicates maxillary protrusion. An angle less than 90 degrees indicates retrusion. This analysis indicates whether the maxilla is responsible for a Class II or Class III malocclusion.

Evaluating the A-P Relationship of the Maxilla to the Mandible

In a normal patient with a straight profile, the A point falls on the facial plane. This indicates a harmonious relationship between the maxilla and the mandible. This relationship is the easiest to treat and is consistent with a pleasant profile.

The relationship of the A point to the facial plane determines the amount of convexity of the profile. If the A point is anterior to the facial plane, the patient's profile will be convex (Figure 44-7).

If the A point is posterior to the facial plane, the profile will be concave (Figure 44-8).

The convexity analysis relates the maxilla to the mandible. It indicates a retrognathic relationship with a plus dimension of the A point and indicates a prognathic relationship when the A point is posterior to the facial plane. The convexity analysis, however, does not specify which

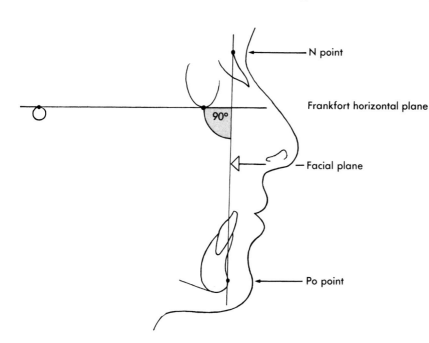

FIGURE 44-6 Mandibular depth analysis for "normal" anteroposterior relationship of the mandible to the cranial base. An angle greater than 90 degrees indicates mandibular protrusion. An angle less than 90 degrees indicates retrusion, though a slight reduction in value is considered acceptable.

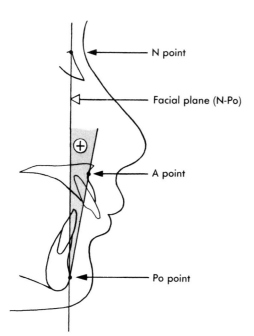

FIGURE 44-7 Convexity analysis. The A point is anterior to the facial plane, an indication of a convex facial profile. This analysis by itself does not show which jaw is at fault because a convex profile can result from either a protruded maxilla or a retruded mandible.

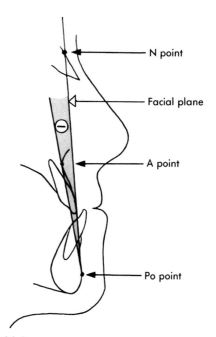

FIGURE 44-8 The concave profile is indicated by convexity analysis because the A point is posterior to the facial plane. In this patient, the Class II occlusion is caused by a protruded mandible, but that conclusion is not determinable by this analysis alone. This analysis relates one jaw to the other but does not relate either jaw to the cranial base to determine which jaw is at fault.

jaw is at fault. Thus convexity analysis should be used with individual analysis of mandibular depth and maxillary depth to determine where corrections should be made. A quick reference relationship of either or both arches can be analyzed in relation to the McNamara line.

The McNamara line is a reference plane that relates the anteroposterior positioning of both jaws to each other as well as to cranial components. The McNamara line is also referred to as a "nasion perpendicular" because it is con-structed by extending a vertical line downward from the nasion, and perpendicular to the Frankfort horizontal plane (Figure 44-9).

The construction of a true vertical facial line provides a simple, quick assessment for identification of discrepancies in the horizontal plane that more clearly defines the problem, such as mandibular skeletal protrusion or a maxillary skeletal retrusion (Figure 44-10) instead of a simplistic diagnosis of Class III malocclusion. It will

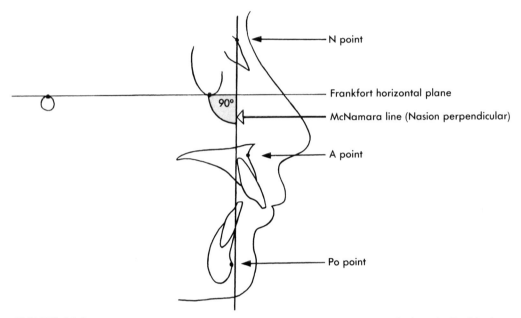

FIGURE 44-9 The McNamara line (nasion perpendicular) is drawn from N point perpendicular to the Frankfort horizontal plane. With this analysis, both the maxilla and mandible can be related to a "true" vertical expression of the anterior facial plane. Both jaws can thus be related to the cranial base in one analysis. In the analysis above, it is obvious that the cause of the Class II relationship is a protruded maxilla because the A point is in front of the nasion perpendicular, whereas the mandible is slightly behind the line and within a normal distance.

FIGURE 44-10 Clinical example of how cephalometric analysis can aid a prosthodontic treatment plan: This patient was treated unsuccessfully by four different dentists with attempts to prosthetically build out an upper edentulous area to align upper teeth with the lower incisors. This is an example of changing what is right to fit what is wrong. Analysis shows that the maxilla is in correct anteroposterior relationship (A point is on the line). The mandible, however, is severely prognathic (Po point is far anterior to the line). An acceptable result in this patient is not possible without surgical reduction of mandibular length.

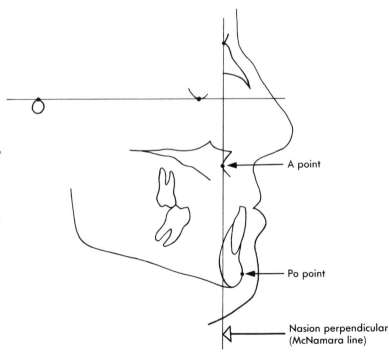

also indicate when both arches are either protruded or retruded.

The analysis relates the maxilla and mandible to the nasion perpendicular in linear (millimeter) rather than angular (degree) measurements. So the position of the maxilla in relation to the "true" vertical plane is measured in millimeters. In a normal, attractive profile, point A lies on or slightly ahead of the McNamara line.

The relationship of the mandible to the cranial base is also measured in millimeters from the nasion perpendicular, so it is not influenced by any maxillary reference points. Thus, it is a true representation of the chin position in relation to the cranial base. In a growing child with a mixed dentition, the Po point lies normally 6 mm to 8 mm posterior to the nasion perpendicular. Mandibular growth increases the value approximately 0.5 mm per year until it reaches a normal relationship range of –2 mm to –4 mm posterior to the McNamara line.

Relating Teeth to Skeletal Bases

One of the advantages of using the A point is that it is a skeletal relationship that can be evaluated whether or not teeth are present. Thus, it can be a helpful determination to make in the analysis of where to relate teeth on a denture.

The *A-Po plane* is the reference plane that relates the denture bases (Figure 44-11). The A-Po plane is also referred to as the *maxillomandibular line,* and it is an easy reference to which both upper and lower teeth can be related to the maxilla and the mandible. That reference, in turn, can be related to the facial plane.

The *upper incisor protrusion* is measured in millimeters from the A-Po line. The norm is ±3.5 mm, with a deviation of ±2.3 mm. Upper incisor inclination is measured by degrees of angulation with the A-Po line. The norm is 28 degrees, with a deviation of ±4 degrees.

The *lower incisor protrusion* has a norm of +1 mm from the A-Po line, with a deviation of ±2.3 mm.

The *lower incisor inclination* has a norm of 22 degrees, with a deviation of ±4 degrees.

The *interincisal angle* relates the long axes of the incisors to each other (Figure 44-12). The norm is 130 degrees. Clinical deviation is 6 degrees. Lower angles indicate protrusion. Higher angles tend toward a deep overbite.

The relationship of the teeth to the skeletal bases is far more dependent on neutral zone factors than on any form of arbitrary positioning based on averages. There is probably no other part of the dentition that is so critically dependent on being in harmony with the musculature. Any malalignment of the teeth with the muscular forces of the tongue or the lips and the perioral musculature will lead to instability. Furthermore, it is not necessary to have the anterior teeth conform to any set angulation or even range of angulations. As long as the anterior teeth are in harmony with jaw function and have definite holding contacts to stop their eruption, they can be stable regardless of their interincisal angle.

Many patients with deep overbites and even some lingual inclination (greater than 180 degrees) can be kept completely stable if definite holding contacts are in place (Figure 44-13).

Lingual inclination of anterior teeth is not uncommon in patients with short upper lips because during swallowing the lower lip must stretch to seal with the upper lip. This creates greater lower lip pressure against the upper labial surfaces, moving the incisal edge toward the lingual. In severely tight-lipped patients, it may be necessary to add holding contacts on the upper teeth to prevent supraeruption. However, with stable centric stops even lingually inclined anterior teeth can be vertically and horizontally stable. When teeth are related to a naturally tight neutral zone, the lip-closure path is not interfered with, and phonetic relationships are preserved between the lips and the incisal edges. Even though the incisor inclinations do not fall within normal values, both esthetics and function may be better served.

Cephalometric norms do not necessarily relate to these important factors, so the clinical evaluation should have primary importance in diagnosis and treatment planning for anterior tooth inclinations. There seems to be a growing con-

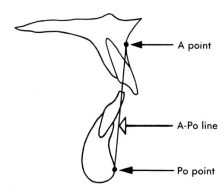

FIGURE 44-11 The A-Po line is the reference plane for the denture bases. It does not relate to the cranial base, but with the addition of the facial plane or the nasion perpendicular, the maxillomandibular relationship can be put into perspective with total facial profile. Inclination or protrusion of the anterior teeth relates to this line.

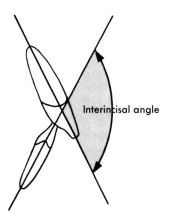

FIGURE 44-12 The interincisal angle relates the long axis of upper and lower incisors to each other. The norm is 130 degrees, but we put very little importance on this angulation, preferring instead to establish the interincisor angle from functional relationships that vary considerably, even among "normal" dentitions.

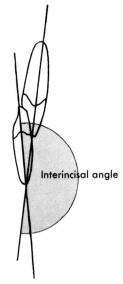

Interincisal angle

FIGURE 44-13 Lingually inclined anteriors with an interincisal angle greater than 180 degrees may be completely stable if they have stable holding stops and if they are in harmony with neutral zone factors and functional jaw movements. If a change in inclination is contemplated for teeth in this relationship, care should be taken to maintain the upper incisal edge position in harmony with the lip-closure path and a very tight lip relationship.

sensus among top orthodontists that cephalometric norms can be used as a quick reference for average anterior tooth inclinations, but clinical evaluation is far more reliable for this particular relationship.

Evaluating Vertical Skeletal Relationships

Evaluation of the *mandibular plane angle* is one of the most effective ways of determining if an anterior open bite is a skeletal malrelationship. This is an important determination because the treatment of a skeletal open bite is often quite different from that for an open bite caused by a habit pattern.

The mandibular plane angle relates the mandibular plane to the Frankfort horizontal plane (Figure 44-14).

Norm: 25 degrees.

Anterior skeletal open bite: A high angulation indicates that the open bite is a skeletal malrelationship caused by the mandible.

Deep overbite: A low angulation indicates that the deep bite is skeletal and is caused by the mandible.

Lower facial height: Another measurement that relates to the divergence of the maxillomandibular angulation. Ricketts has shown that in normal growth this angle stays constant with age. The measurement is made at the intersection of lines from ANS (anterior nasal spine) to Xi and from PM (protuberantia mentalis) to Xi (Figure 44-15).

Norm: 47 degrees, with a clinical deviation of 4 degrees.

The higher the angle, the more likely there is a skeletal open bite. The lower the angle, the more there is a tendency for deep overbite.

Evaluating the Occlusal Plane

The functional occlusal plane is a plane that relates to the occlusal surfaces of the molars and premolars (Figure 44-16).

The purpose of analyzing the occlusal plane cephalometrically is to determine its correct vertical position in both the anterior and posterior segments. An esthetically pleasing occlusal plane is close to the center of the ramus (Xi point) at the posterior and slightly below the lip embrasure at the anterior. The lower incisal edges are normally slightly above the level of the functional occlusal plane.

Vertical maxillary excess

If the occlusal plane is too far below the lip embrasure, it indicates a vertical maxillary excess. This refers to the typical "gummy smile." The occlusion may appear normal in every other respect, but when the lips are at rest, the entire labial surface and part of the gingival tissues may be exposed. Periodontal health may be affected because of continuous exposure of the gingival tissues to the air. The patient may show lip strain from trying to keep the teeth covered.

When treating a vertical excess problem in the maxilla, it is important to consider the full occlusal plane and the importance of maintaining a correct anterior guidance. The problem is usually solved surgically.

Vertical maxillary deficiency

A high occlusal plane anteriorly may indicate hidden upper incisors and an excessive visibility of the lower anterior teeth. This creates a "bulldog" appearance to the smile, which is unesthetic. With age and a loss of tissue resiliency, the upper lip elongates to a lower level at rest, and so it is a normal occurrence for older patients to expose less of the upper teeth when smiling.

Although cephalometric analysis may relate the level of the anterior occlusal plane to the lip line, it should be remembered that variations in lip length and phonetic function may be more critical determinants. The relationship of the upper incisal edges to the lower-lip smile line can be determined clinically, and the precise incisal edge position can be determined from observation during lip-closure path and lip contact at the *f* and *v* position. In edentulous patients, these guidelines can be determined from wax esthetic controls, and then the denture teeth can be set to those guidelines. My experience would indicate that both esthetics and function can be adversely affected by variations in incisal edge position that are so minute that careful clinical observation and testing are required to determine these guidelines accurately. Cephalometrics can be helpful as a reference, but it is doubtful that it should ever override decisions based on clinical analysis of functional relationships, at least as far as the anterior teeth are concerned.

The posterior level of the occlusal plane should approach the level of Xi point. Problems occur particularly when the posterior occlusal plane is too high because it interferes with protrusive disclusion. The level of the posterior occlusal plane can be so effectively determined on mounted diagnos-

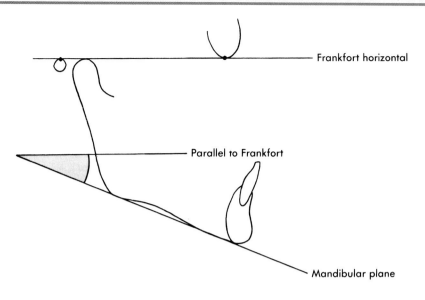

FIGURE 44-14 Mandibular plane angle.

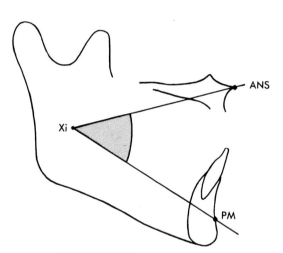

FIGURE 44-15 Lower facial height.

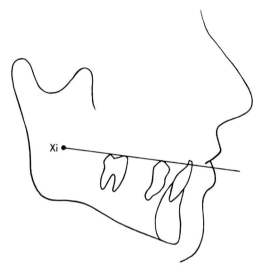

FIGURE 44-16 The functional occlusal plane relates to the occlusal surfaces of the molars and premolars. It does not bisect the incisors. It is close to the Xi point in the back and aligns slightly below the lip embrasure in the front.

tic casts that it is doubtful that cephalometric analysis is necessary from an occlusal analysis viewpoint. The advantage of mounted casts is that the posterior occlusion can be related to the disclusive effect of the condylar path and the anterior guidance, two very critical factors in determining the acceptability of any occlusal plane.

The use of a Broadrick flag or a simplified occlusal plane analyzer (SOPA) as advocated in Chapter 20 effectively relates the posterior occlusal plane to the Xi point on mounted diagnostic casts. This is the result achieved, however, only if the condyle is used as the posterior survey point in determining the occlusal plane. The use of the Broadrick flag or SOPA is not applicable for nonrestorative cases, however, so occlusal plane analysis cephalometrically does have real value for orthodontic and surgical analysis if it is used with clinical evaluation.

The superior surface of the retromolar pad is also an effective clinical landmark for locating the posterior level of the occlusal plane. It is especially useful when the posterior ridges are edentulous.

Evaluating the Soft-Tissue Profile

The relationship of the lips to the nose and the chin can be evaluated by analysis of the esthetic plane (Figure 44-17). This plane connects the tip of the nose (Pn point) with the soft-tissue pogonion (Po′).

For the most pleasing appearance, the ideal position of the lower lip is close to the esthetic plane. In edentulous patients, the resorption of alveolar ridges allows the lips to sink back. If denture teeth can be positioned to support the lips closer to the esthetic plane, the appearance will be improved.

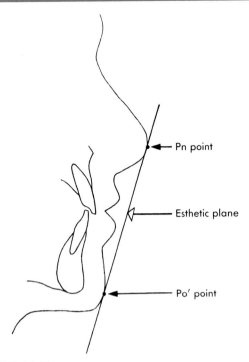

FIGURE 44-17 The esthetic plane. There are no standards for lip position that are applicable for all patients. However, the generally accepted norm is for the lower lip to be within approximately 2 mm from the esthetic plane. This is quite variable in different races and is affected by nose and chin prominence. One can make this analysis clinically by laying a flat ruler against the nose and chin.

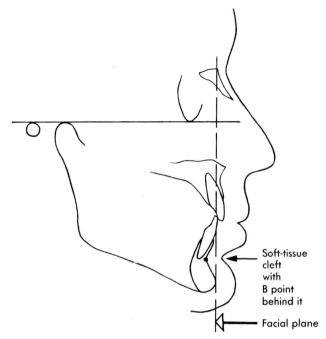

FIGURE 44-18 The B point is the mandibular counterpart to the A point in the maxilla. It is the deepest part of the concavity between the lower incisor and the bony chin. When it is located too posterior to the facial plane, it indicates the probability of a strong buccinator band limitation on the growth of the dento-alveolar process at the level of the roots. A soft-tissue cleft and button chin are classic profile evidence of this restriction. It may be in combination with normal anteroposterior growth of the skeletal chin.

There are three considerations related to the esthetic plane, as follows.

Size of the nose or prominence of the chin

Excess of either nose or chin may cause the upper and lower lips and teeth to appear retruded. Evaluating the position of the teeth in relation to the nasion perpendicular will give a different perspective in determining whether a profile problem is caused by a normal relationship of the teeth to an abnormal esthetic plane, or vice versa.

Inclination of upper incisors

Protrusion of the upper incisors has a tendency to fold the lower lip and push it forward, creating an unpleasant profile. Changing the neutral zone by inclining the upper incisors back not only improves the esthetics, but also allows the lip to seal more effectively and helps to stabilize the teeth in the more upright position.

Strength and position of perioral musculature

A protruded, button chin with a deep cleft above it forms a very characteristic profile that may be an indication of a strong lower band of the buccinator compressing the underling mentalis muscle. It is often associated with vertical or even lingually inclined incisors because of an exceptionally strong neutral zone effect. The upper band of the buccinator may also be restrictive, creating a retrusion of the upper

dento-alveolar process in relation to a normal chin and nose. The restrictive effect of the musculature may also be predominantly directed at the roots and the alveolar process while the tongue exerts a strong forward pressure to incline the crowns forward. The skeletal base may continue to grow while forward growth of the alveolar processes is limited by the tight band of muscle. Cephalometric evidence that this has occurred may be found in a soft-tissue profile with a cleft and a button chin and possibly a B point (supramentale) that is considerably behind the facial plane (Figure 44-18).

CONCERNS ABOUT THE USE OF CEPHALOMETRICS

One of the most important benefits of cephalometric analysis is the information it provides for determining the anteroposterior relationship of the mandible to the cranial base. This is determined angularly by the relationship of the facial plane (N-Po) to the Frankfort horizontal plane, or it may be determined linearly by relating the Po point to the nasion perpendicular (McNamara line). Either method provides valuable information in determining whether or not the mandible is at fault in a Class II or Class III malocclusion.

The accuracy of the above determinations is totally dependent on the condyles being in centric relation when the lateral cephalogram is made. A significant error is possible if the cephalogram is made in the maximum intercuspal relationship because the mandible can be displaced several millimeters forward of centric relation. This would completely invalidate the relationship of the Po point to the facial plane or the accuracy of the angle formed with the FH plane. Despite this obvious error, there seems to be very limited willingness to change the practice. The errors in diagnosis are very real and are common. In my own practice, I have seen numerous patients who have been treatment planned for major corrections that were not needed, including recommendations for surgery where only minimal occlusal correction was required, and the errors in diagnosis were made from inaccurate cephalograms.

Two simple procedures can eliminate the mistakes in diagnosis from cephalometric analysis of displaced mandibles:

1. The use of centrically mounted diagnostic casts as an essential part of occlusal diagnosis.
2. The use of centric relation bite record to hold the mandible at the seated position of the condyles during the radiographic procedure. From that position, the mandible can be closed on the tracing when the condylar axis is maintained near the center of the condyle.

Slavicek[1] has developed a method for correcting the position of the mandible when the cephalometric tracings are made so that the mandible is correctly related to the cranial base in centric relation. These corrections are made by transferal of information from centrically mounted casts so that the position of the mandible on the tracing is correct.

Williamson[2] has consistently emphasized the importance of seated condyles to an accurate cephalometric analysis and utilizes mounted diagnostic casts as an important part of orthodontic treatment planning. Numerous other orthodontists are in agreement and are now including mounted diagnostic casts as an essential part of diagnosis.

It is true that an astute diagnostician and master dentist could correct most occlusions without using either mounted casts or cephalometrics just as a master builder could build a house without plans. The question is, "Why would one want to?" Planning from an accurate base of information eliminates trial-and-error treatment and prevents mistakes. Cephalometric analysis can be used to improve the odds. Mounted diagnostic casts and clinical observation, however, are a necessary part of a reasonable occlusal diagnosis.

The second major concern about too much dependence on cephalometric analysis is related to the inclination of the anterior teeth. The success or failure of the anterior relationship depends so much on harmony with the musculature and the surrounding soft tissues; it is not a reliable practice to position these teeth arbitrarily according to averages. It is probable that most postorthodontic instability problems are caused by failure to position the anterior teeth precisely enough in the neutral zone, which is not determinable from cephalometric analysis. Furthermore, the ranges of lip movement during function vary so much, even among "normal" faces, that it would seem unlikely that the static analysis of centric relation would be accurate enough to use exclusively, as a definite guideline.

Just as we are unable to precisely determine anterior relationships from mounted diagnostic casts, which are three-dimensional, it would be impossible to determine those relationships from two-dimensional cephalograms. Both, however, provide helpful information, but the final "fine-tuning" of anterior teeth inclinations, anterior guidance, and functional relationships can be made accurately only by clinical observation of the dynamic relationship of the soft tissues with the teeth during function.

References

1. Slavicek R, Mack H: Model analysis with articulator related grid in an occlusal registration instrument (ORI). *Inf Orthrod Kieferorthops* 14(1):77-81, 1982.
2. Williamson EH, Caves SA, Edenfield RJ, et al: Cephalometric analysis: comparisons between maximum intercuspation and centric relation. *Am J Orthod* 74(6):672-677, 1978.

Suggested Readings

Bishara SE: *Textbook of orthodontics.* Philadelphia, Saunders, 2001.

Chaconas SJ, Gonidis D: A cephalometric technique for prosthodontic diagnosis and treatment planning, *J Prosthet Dent* 56(5):567-574, 1986.

Di Pietro GJ, Moergeli JR: Significance of the Frankfort mandibular plane angle to prosthodontics, *J Prosthet Dent* 36:624, 1976.

Graber TM, Vanarsdall RL Jr, Vig WL: *Orthodontics: Current principles and techniques,* ed 4, St. Louis, 2005, Mosby.

Ricketts RM: Role of cephalometrics in prosthetic diagnosis, *J Prosthet Dent* 6:488, 1956.

Skafidas TM: *Cephalometric analysis manual,* Atlanta, Georgia, 1987, Department of Orthodontics, Emory University School of Dentistry.

Wallen T, Bloomquist D: The clinical examination: Is it more important than cephalometric analysis in surgical orthodontics? *Int J Adult Orthodont Orthognath Surg* 1(3):179-191, 1986.

Chapter 45

Postoperative Care of Occlusal Therapy Patients

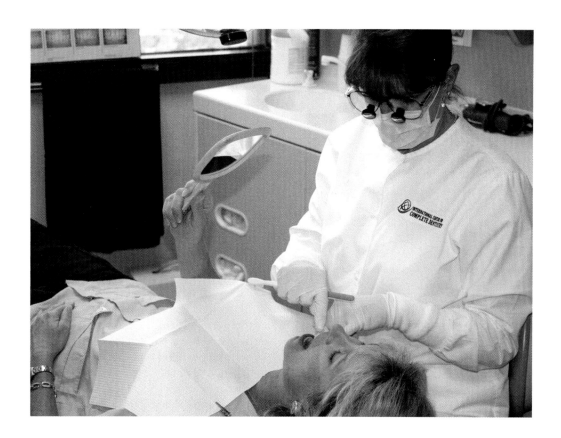

PRINCIPLE

The goal of complete dentistry is long-term health of the total masticatory system.

A GOOD EXAMPLE OF POSTOPERATIVE CARE

Dr. Daulton Keith, a periodontist in Charleston, South Carolina, has one of the most effective programs for keeping his patients healthy for life, even after extensive periodontal treatment. His postoperative maintenance does not wait until treatment has been completed. It starts with a discussion with each patient before he even examines the mouth at the first appointment.

At that first appointment, Dr. Keith outlines the treatment goals that must be achieved if long-term health and stability are to be expected. He starts by explaining what will be expected of the patient during and after treatment. This initial discussion is then given credibility by explaining with actual examples the consequences of falling short on any of his stated goals.

Dr. Keith begins his instructions to the patient with three "no's":

1. *No smoking.* He points out the restrictive effect of smoking on the capillary blood supply to the periodontal tissues and explains why it is so difficult to achieve long-term health of the necessary supporting structures unless the patient agrees to stop. He also clarifies smoking's other risks to general health.
2. *No hard candy.* A habit of sucking on hard candies can be devastating to the teeth, especially at the cementoenamel junction where decay can cause so many problems.
3. *No more than two soda drinks per week.* The corrosive effect of high-acid carbonated drinks is too well documented to be ignored. We now recognize the damage they do to the occlusal surfaces.

The patient then learns what must be accomplished by the doctor if long-term health of the dentition is to be achieved.

1. *Cleanability.* Every tooth surface must be made cleanable all the way to the gingival attachment.
2. *Cleanliness.* The patient must be taught how to keep all tooth surfaces clean, and must be motivated to do it.
3. *Occlusal stability.* A perfected occlusion is necessary for distribution of forces to the teeth and their supporting tissues.
4. *Temporomandibular joint (TMJ) stability.* It is not possible to maintain a stable occlusion in a mouth with unstable TMJs.

By understanding the plan for getting a mouth healthy enough to be maintained and also understanding what the patients' responsibilities are for their own health, postoperative care becomes part of the total treatment rather than an afterthought. Patients can be continuously educated and helped with their compliance from the start of treatment. The principles behind this highly successful program are applicable to all patients including occlusal therapy patients. There is a sound principle that underlies the concept:

Principle

Optimum oral health must be the goal of the complete dentist. That means maintainable health of all the structures of the masticatory system.

Occlusal therapy cannot be isolated from all of the other requirements for long-term maintenance of oral health. It does, however, require special consideration for different conditions.

OCCLUSAL THERAPY FOLLOW-UP

When the active treatment phase has been completed for a patient with an occlusally related problem, a program of postoperative care should be planned that gives the patient the best long-term prognosis.

This plan must be related to the condition of the various parts of the masticatory system after occlusal therapy has been completed. There are seven major considerations that should influence the program of postoperative care:

1. Condition of the connective tissue of the TMJ
2. Presence or absence of an acceptable disk
3. Condition of supporting structures of teeth
4. Degree of fulfillment of all requirements for occlusal stability
5. Presence of habit patterns or nocturnal bruxism
6. Ability or willingness to follow a meticulous oral hygiene program
7. Dietary patterns or general health problems

Abnormalities in any of the above factors may be a reason for special postoperative counseling. If damage to the connective tissues of the joint has weakened the ligaments, or if surgery has been used to correct such problems, it may be necessary to follow up with physical therapy or a soft diet for a period of months. An excellent help for patients during this reparative stage is *The I-Can't-Chew Cookbook* by Randy Wilson.[1] Connective tissue heals slowly, and patients must be educated regarding what they must do or not do to prevent damage.

If the disk is absent or irreparably displaced, patients should be counseled about the importance of maintaining a perfected occlusion. Especially important is the need to correct any posterior occlusal interferences as they may occur because of their trigger effect on muscle hyperactivity. It is also important to advise patients that there is a probability of gradual loss of height of the condyle when the disk is not in place. The occlusion must be checked at each recall appointment to see if the last molar is hitting prematurely, since this is the obvious result of the degenerative joint disease that routinely occurs on the surface of a diskless condyle.

Patients with compromised support for the teeth should be advised of any special requirements for maintenance and may require a closer recall schedule. Mobility patterns should be monitored and recorded for comparison at subsequent appointments. Recordings of sulcular depth should be compared at reasonable intervals.

When any compromise has been made with fulfilling all requirements for occlusal stability, the dentition will be in jeopardy. It should be specifically monitored to make sure that signs of instability are not allowed to reach an irreversible level without the patient being advised of what should be done. It should be noted in the patient's record that the problem was explained and treatment recommended. If patients choose not to follow the advice, they should be told what special measures they should take in home care to at least slow down the expected damage.

Habit patterns can be destructive, or they may have a stabilizing effect on a malrelated occlusion. Any habit pattern should be noted, and effects of such habits monitored for any changes. If the effects of bruxism are progressive, steps should be recommended for reducing the damage. At each recall appointment, patients should be informed about the status of any effects resulting from habit patterns.

Different patients respond in different ways to attempts at getting them to follow proper home care procedures. Patients with poor hygiene should be constantly encouraged in a helpful way. Stern lectures and criticism rarely work, so they may as well be avoided. A record should, however, be kept of each patient's personal oral hygiene, and the patient should always be informed of the effects he or she can expect if procedures are not followed.

Patients who are unable or unwilling to follow hygiene recommendations should be encouraged to come in for more frequent recalls. Dietary counseling should be a part of any recall appointment if effects that customarily result from an inadequate or imbalanced diet are noted.

The recall appointment for patients with special problems should not be treated in a perfunctory manner as if the problems were normal. That appointment should always be used to help the patient overcome whatever special problems are present so that the destructive effects can be prevented or at least reduced.

Fortunately, most of my patients who accept complete treatment end up with maintainably healthy masticatory systems. The postoperative care for uncompromised patients who have been effectively treated to fulfill all the requirements for occlusal stability must still be tailored to suit each patient, but I have found great benefit in a technique I refer to as "prodding." Patients are asked to find any disharmonies in a completed occlusal restoration.

In my office, it has been the standard policy for years to encourage patients to try to find fault with their occlusal result. It is a policy that eventually leads to excellence in patient comfort because it forces the dentist to accept nothing short of an optimum occlusal result.

Telling patients to critically evaluate their occlusions, to "be fussy about how it feels," is the opposite of what is often implied at the completion of treatment: "This is it. Now you must learn to live with it." Many dental patients end up stressed emotionally because they believe that they have no recourse but to live with their uncomfortable dentistry. Patients truly appreciate the opportunity to point out areas of

discomfort. It has been my experience that when given this opportunity they will rarely abuse it. Patients almost always try to be fair to any dentist who is obviously committed to their best interests. Just letting patients know they have the right to expect comfort takes away almost all the urgency and fearfulness about the completed treatment. The dentist can and should systematically evaluate any problem and try to find a solution for it. Such an approach may sound impractical, but it will pay unexpected dividends for both the patient and the dentist (if the dentist is competent enough to correct the problems).

For best long-term maintainability, patients should be instructed in how to evaluate occlusal problems. Early correction of a newly developed interference is usually simple and not very time-consuming. Patients should be told to report any of the following indications of occlusal disharmony:

1. Any discomfort in the teeth when chewing
2. Any indication of a "high" tooth or any sign that one or more teeth contact before the rest when closing; any tooth that can be made to hurt by biting on it
3. Any sign of tooth hypermobility
4. Any discomfort in the TMJ area
5. Any limitation of function

Any one of these signs or symptoms is an indication that the occlusal relationship is producing excessive stress. Each problem is correctable and should be resolved to prevent accelerated deterioration.

Signs of bruxism should also be observed to see if they are related to occlusal interferences. If the bruxing cannot be stopped, it is all the more important to maintain occlusal harmony or to take steps to reduce the damage.

Since no restorative technique can guarantee 100 percent permanent occlusal harmony, the logical approach to long-term maintainability is to correct occlusal discrepancies whenever they occur and whenever they have the potential for causing breakdown. Enlisting the patients' aid in reporting such problems is just as practical as asking them to report bleeding gums or hypersensitivity.

Unless instructions are given regarding what to look for and unless patients are encouraged to be critical about their occlusions, they tend to accept discomfort as part of the normal "breaking-in" experience. Unfortunately, such self-adjustment of an incorrect occlusion usually occurs by getting the stressed teeth loose enough to accommodate the interfering inclines.

In the absence of an injury, abscess, or severe bone loss, hypermobility is almost always a sign of excessive occlusal stress. It is one of the first detectable signs of periodontal breakdown, and it is almost always completely reversible if corrected early enough. For that reason, no postoperative follow-up appointment is complete without each tooth being checked for hypermobility. Dental hygienists should be trained to examine for hypermobility just as thoroughly as they examine for caries. All postoperative checkups should include such an examination. If any hypermobility is noticed, the occlusal cause of the problem should be located and corrected without delay.

POSTTREATMENT USE OF OCCLUSAL APPLIANCES

It is my opinion that the use of posttreatment occlusal splints is overdone. Patients with a perfected occlusion rarely need to wear an occlusal splint even at night. Even patients who brux or clench tend in most cases to stop damaging the occlusal surfaces if there are no interferences to centric relation and if the anterior guidance is noninterfering with the envelope of function.

Any signs of attritional wear on posterior teeth are indicative of occlusal interferences to complete seating of the jaw joints into centric relation, or interference to excursive movement of the mandible. It should be a sign that initiates correction of the occlusion rather than construction of an occlusal device. Remember that it is impossible to create attritional wear on teeth that are not in the way. If posterior disclusion is effective, even a bruxer cannot wear posterior teeth.

Wear can occur on the anterior teeth, however, if there is any interference to the envelope of function, so posttreatment examination should always look for wear on the anterior guidance surfaces. If it occurs, posterior interferences can then develop.

Nighttime Occlusal Appliance Use

Nighttime occlusal appliance use is indicated whenever the envelope of function must be restricted to achieve an improved esthetic result. This is often necessary when a long-term bruxing habit has flattened the anterior guidance. Changing the horizontal pattern of parafunction to a more vertical (restricted) pattern almost always results in attritional wear or fremitus on the anterior teeth. A nighttime appliance is indicated to reduce the wear on the anterior teeth and to stabilize the occlusion.

Careful observation of wear patterns can clearly indicate whether there are posterior interferences that should be corrected or anterior wear in the absence of posterior interferences. Such anterior wear should be protected by appliance use at night.

In mouths in which TMJ structural disorders or other considerations make it impossible to achieve a perfected occlusion, protective occlusal appliances may be indicated. As long as it is recognized that a perfected occlusion is the preferred treatment whenever possible, use of occlusal splints can be a reasonable choice when signs of wear are evident in mouths that require a compromised treatment. Posttreatment vigilance is always important.

POSTOPERATIVE PERIODONTAL MAINTENANCE

Although there is much evidence that occlusal trauma contributes to many aspects of periodontal breakdown, it is a mistake to believe that it is the only factor. Until scientific research can provide conclusive proof of singular causes for specific effects, occlusal therapy must be considered as only part of any treatment plan. It should also be regarded as only part of any postoperative follow-up observation.

Even though certain clinical observations may be suggestive of occlusal trauma as the probable cause, all other possible causes should also be considered in a multitreatment approach toward the restoration of optimum health.

An illustrative example is the postoperative formation of gingival clefts. Although there is clinical evidence to associate gingival clefts with occlusal trauma, we know they can also be caused by improper toothbrushing, improperly contoured restorations, or postorthodontic pressure from the buccinator-*orbicularis oris* muscle. Each of these causative factors should be evaluated along with the occlusal factors, and each should be corrected when it is found to be a contributing irritant.

Inadequate or improper oral hygiene is a factor that must be considered in every patient we treat. For the occlusal therapist, it is just as important to evaluate, educate, and postoperatively appraise each patient's mouth hygiene as it is to check the occlusion. One of the saddest situations I see is the completely restored patient who has never been taught how to care for his or her investment in extensive dentistry.

Each postoperative checkup appointment should include a careful examination of the periodontal tissues. Either substantial problems should be corrected or the patient should be referred to a competent periodontal specialist.

THE HEALTHY MOUTH: DENTISTRY'S GOAL

Modern dental treatment is designed to focus on one predominant goal: optimally maintainable oral health. Any factor that lessens the maintainability of any oral tissue is a factor that must be isolated and corrected. To do less is to fail the task entrusted to us. Dentists who are dedicated to the concept of optimum oral health will not be able to treat one problem while ignoring others. They will search out and correct all factors that contribute to accelerated deterioration.

The role of occlusal stress will never be ignored by any dentist who believes that his or her patients are entitled to a healthy mouth. But such a goal-oriented dentist will not be guilty of tunnel vision either. Analysis and correction of occlusal problems will fit in perspective into a total plan of treatment designed to provide and maintain the healthiest mouth possible for each patient treated. The competent dentist of today must be the physician of the masticatory system. There is no other specialty of medicine in which one is adequately trained to assume that role. The modern standard of dental practice should reflect that obligation.

Reference

1. Wilson JR: *The I-can't-chew cookbook.* Alameda, California, 2003, Hunter House.

Chapter 46

The Technological Future
for Occlusal Restoration
Lee Culp, CDT

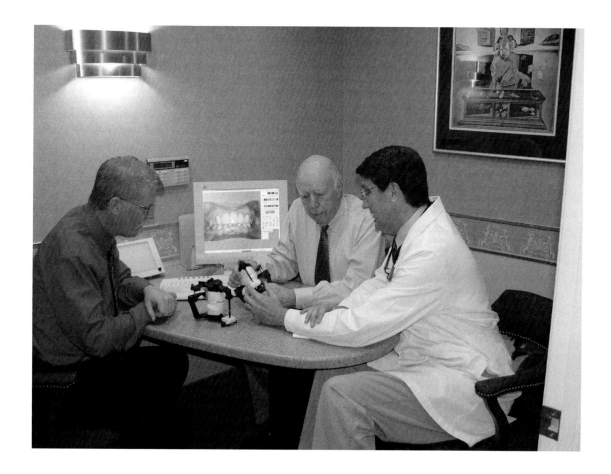

PRINCIPLE

Be not the first to embrace the new, or the last to lay the old aside.

A Paradigm Shift in Dental Technology

My fifty-plus years in dentistry have enabled me to see changes that could not even be imagined in my early years of practice. In every aspect of practice, the changes have been monumental, and with each change has come opportunities for improving the quality of care. Many of the changes in materials and technologies have been frustrating in the early stages, but with time, improvements have been made. In order to present the most current information on our technological future, I've asked Lee Culp, CDT to contribute this chapter. Lee's expertise is internationally recognized, and as a contributing member of the Dawson Center Think Tank and faculty he has earned our trust in the accuracy of his analysis.

The paradigm shift has already occurred, and many of the old ways of producing occlusal restorations have become outdated. The one thing that has not become outmoded is the absolute necessity of a close doctor/technician relationship.

—Peter E. Dawson, DDS

COMPUTERIZED OCCLUSION IN THE LABORATORY

The laboratory technician's primary role in restorative dentistry is to perfectly copy all functional and esthetic parameters that have been defined by the dentist into a restorative solution. It is an architect/builder relationship. Throughout the entire restorative process, from the initial consultation through treatment planning, provisionalization, and final placement, the communication routes between the dentist and the technician require a complete transfer of existing, desired, and realistic situations and expectations to and from the clinical environment. Functional components, occlusal parameters, phonetics, and esthetic information (shade and contour) are just some of the essential information that is required by the technician to complete the fabrication of successful, functional, and esthetic restorations.

Communication of Occlusion

Historically, the transfer of occlusal and functional information from the clinical environment to the laboratory has been somewhat limited. There was little, if any, direct communication of the functional requirements for a case beyond the dentist providing an opposing model and an impression and sometimes an interocclusal record with the shade preferences. With limited guidance, the technician would mount and articulate the case (most often on a hinge articulator) and restore the case by filling spaces and trying to mimic the existing dentition using his or her own interpretation and experience. The result was a close approximation of what the technician hoped would meet or exceed the dentist's and patient's expectations. In situations like this, the dentist ex-

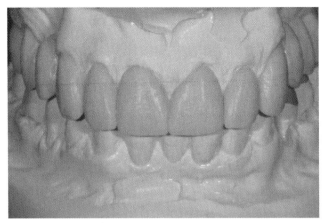

FIGURE 46-1 Diagnostic wax-up.

pected to spend considerable chair time seating a case, adjusting the occlusion, and recontouring restorations. The results were often a complete removal of anatomy and occlusal form, and sometimes an esthetic and functional compromise of the final restoration.

There were of course dentists and technicians that desired more predictable results and sought a solution through advanced continued education courses that encouraged a dentist and technician team approach and also sought out the combination of restorative and functional requirements. This group was introduced to the concept of comprehensive dentistry, which took into account optimum oral health, anatomic and functional harmony, and occlusal stability[1] rather than singling in on just the restoration of aspect/tooth. To accomplish this, the dentist/technician partnership became a "diagnostic team" with the dentist and technician both participating in a complete understanding of the cause-and-effect relationship of the problems, prior to initiating treatment.

Following diagnosis, the first step of confirmation of treatment goals was to design the case in wax, producing a diagnostic wax-up. This diagnostic wax-up was based upon the functional and esthetic desires of the patient and team and also took into account a complete awareness and understanding of any clinical limitations. This approved diagnostic wax-up then became the first three-dimensional blueprint of the case and the map for the course of treatment (Figure 46-1). Once the treatment was initiated, the additional information exchanged between the dentist and technician included the use of anatomic articulators, facebows, transferbows, and rigid interocclusal records, in addition to more detailed prescriptions and photographs (Figure 46-2). The initial three-dimensional blueprint was also followed to fabricate provisional restorations in acrylic, which became the clinical prototypes used to finalize functional, phonetic, and esthetic parameters based upon in vivo results. Impressions of the final provisional design were made, and matrixes were then used to record, transfer, and verify preferred tooth positioning and contouring so that the final restorations were an exact replica of the functionally successful and confirmed

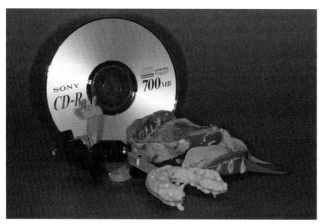

FIGURE 46-2 Dental laboratory communication tools, impressions, digital photos, and facebow transfer.

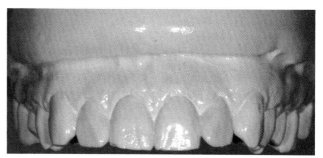

FIGURE 46-3 Preoperative models.

interim restorations. The result of this concept of complete dentistry and a teamwork approach provides predictable, functional, and successful restorations and avoids much of the time-consuming intraoral functional and phonetic adjustment, and esthetic surprises (Figures 46-3 to 46-6).

Unfortunately, today, even with the advanced communication tools, increased knowledge of functional requirements, and the increased patient expectations for esthetic success, the majority of cases are still designed, fabricated, and placed using an exchange of partial or inadequate information, which results in less-than-ideal results for everyone involved.

In addition to the communication tools and the increased partnership between the dentist and technician, materials and fabrication techniques have advanced and allowed technicians to more consistently and effectively duplicate the diagnostic wax-ups using esthetic materials. The introduction of *pressed* ceramics (IPS Empress®, 1987) allowed the "lost wax technique" to be used, taking a diagnostic wax-up directly to a final all-ceramic restoration (Figures 46-7 and 46-8).

COMPUTERIZED DESIGN AND FABRICATION

The first successful introduction of computer-assisted design and computer-assisted manufacturing (CAD/CAM) into dentistry was the chairside CEREC 1 System (Sirona, 1987). The fundamental principle of this concept was to electronically capture a preparation's image and then use software to interpolate the information and create a digital preparation. A virtual restoration design would be suggested and after user-defined parameters were set, the restoration design would be milled from a ceramic block and seated all in one appointment.

Subsequent software and hardware upgrades with the introduction of CEREC 2 and 3 primarily focused on im-

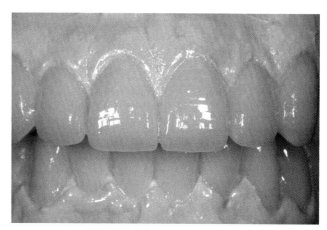

FIGURE 46-4 Diagnostic wax-up.

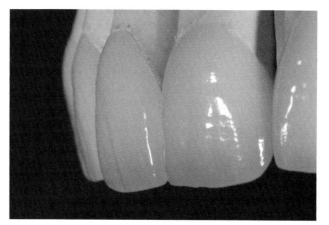

FIGURE 46-5 Final restorations, on model.

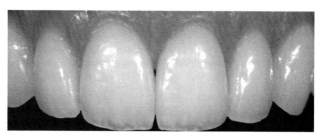

FIGURE 46-6 Final restorations, intraoral.

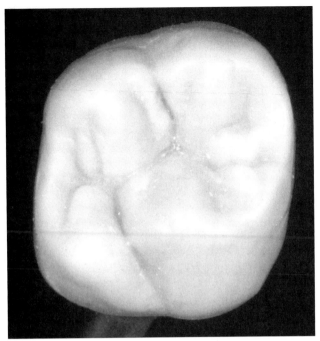

FIGURE 46-7 Wax-up for Empress® restorations.

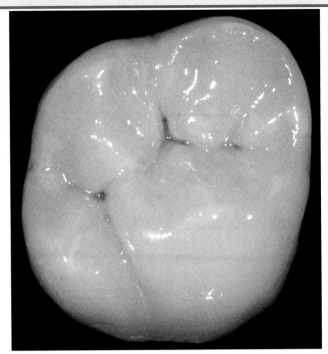

FIGURE 46-8 Finished Empress® ceramic restoration.

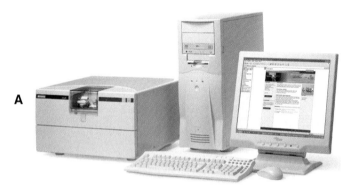

A

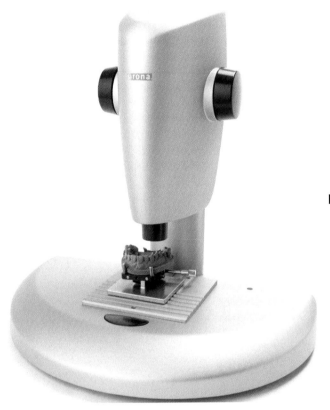

B

FIGURE 46-9 **A** and **B,** Sirona inLab CAD/CAM system. *(Images provided courtesy Sirona Dental Systems, LLC, Charlotte, North Carolina.)*

provements on user friendliness, accuracy, and material milling options.

The introduction of CEREC 3D in 2004 (Figure 46-9) and its accompanying software upgrades and libraries became the first computerized model to accurately present a virtual model and take into consideration the occlusal effect of an opposing (antagonistic) occlusion. It essentially took complex occlusal schemes and parameters and condensed the information and display into an intuitive format that allowed anyone with basic knowledge of dental anatomy and occlusion to make dental restorations on a consistent functional basis (Figure 46-10). For the laboratory, this technol-

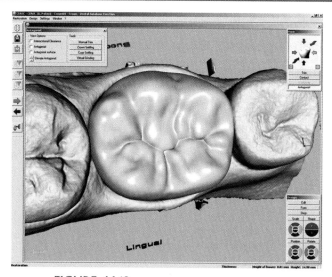

FIGURE 46-10 Computer-designed virtual crown.

ogy effectively automated some of the more mechanical and labor-intensive procedures (waxing, investing, burnout, casting, and pressing) involved in the conventional fabrication of a dental restoration. The CEREC 3D also has chairside applications for the clinician that provide capture and milling of a restoration in just one appointment; however, this discussion will focus and demonstrate the utilization of the CEREC 3D for laboratory applications.

As with any conventional laboratory-prescribed restorative process, this procedure begins the same; the clinician prepares the case according to the appropriate preparation guidelines, impressions the case, and sends all critical communication aspects to the laboratory.

Once the laboratory receives all of the materials, the impressions are poured, the models are mounted, and the dies are trimmed. A bite registration is taken using the mounted models and is used in a subsequent step.

At this time, the procedure moves to the computerized world for scanning and fabrication.

PROCEDURE   Computerized scanning and fabrication of restorations

Step 1: File creation. A file is created within the software for each individual case. Here the operator inputs the patient's name, case number, dentists' name, date, and tooth numbers(s) and type of restoration desired (full crown, veneer, inlay/onlay, or framework [coping]). Additional preferences can be set either globally for all cases from an individual clinician or specifically based upon the individual case. These options include contact tightness preferred, occlusal contact intensity, and the virtual die space that defines the internal fit of the final restoration to the die/preparation. Once all of this information is input, the computer can begin its search among the tooth database libraries to acquire the correct tooth form.

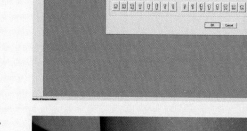

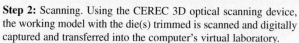

Step 2: Scanning. Using the CEREC 3D optical scanning device, the working model with the die(s) trimmed is scanned and digitally captured and transferred into the computer's virtual laboratory.

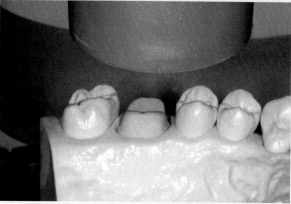

Continued

While the working model is in the same position under the scanner, the bite registration taken from the mounted casts is placed onto the working model. This is also scanned, and the computer can digitally reproduce and virtually create the opposing (antagonist) quadrant using a negative of the image.

The computer now has all of the information it needs to work with the working model—the preparation and the occlusion parameters (from the antagonistic image). This entire capture process takes approximately one minute.

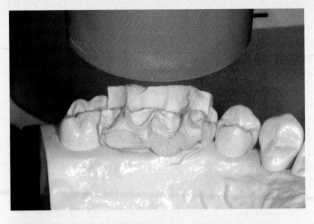

Step 3: Virtual model. The 3D virtual model is then presented to the viewer on-screen and can be rotated and viewed from any perspective.

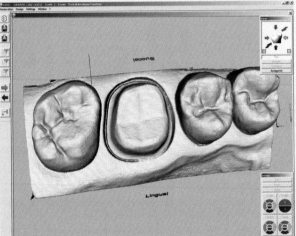

Step 4: Design. The first step in design of the restoration is to virtually section the model and remove the die. Now the parameters and borders of the final restoration are defined using the antagonist information, the adjacent teeth and contact areas, and finally the gingival margins of the preparation.

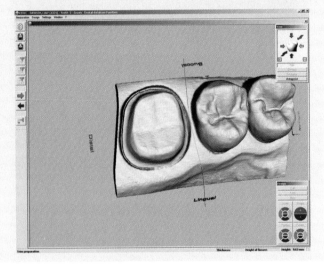

PROCEDURE   Computerized scanning and fabrication of restorations—cont'd

The desired contact areas are marked electronically on the adjacent teeth, and the preparation margins are identified and outlined, greatly assisted by the computer.

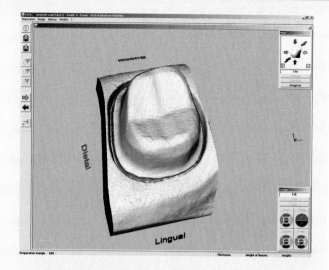

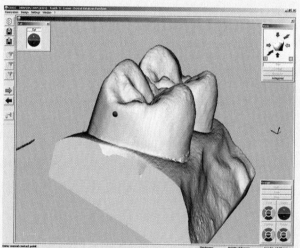

Step 5: Database selection. The computer will now present a database menu that will allow the operatory to select the relative age of the tooth's desired design by examining the surrounding dentition. The operator has a choice between a) 20–young, b) 40–middle, and c) 60–worn dentition anatomy to select from.

From this information and the parameters defined, the computer will now propose a restoration and restoration position over the preparation and within the arch.

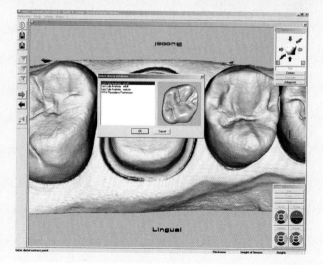

Continued

PROCEDURE   Computerized scanning and fabrication of restorations—cont'd

Step 6: Virtual placement. The computer has placed the restoration in the most appropriate position, based upon all input. However, now the operator's experience and knowledge of form and function are needed to manually position and contour the restoration to the dentally-preferred location.

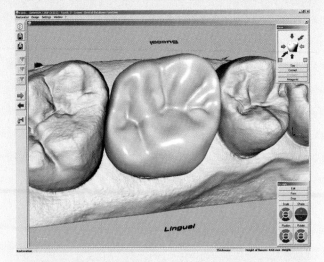

With a few simple mouse-clicks, the position and rotation of the crown can be altered as desired, and the software's "Cusp Settling" application will automatically readjust each individual cusp tip, triangular ridge, the restoration's contours, contacts, and marginal ridges based upon the preferences and antagonistic information according to the newly desired position and rotation. This restoration is in "heavy" occlusion with the initial proposal.

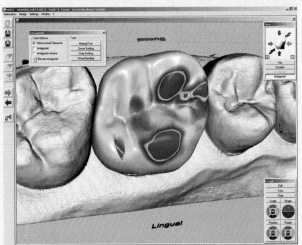

The virtual restoration responds after automatic occlusion adjustment has been selected and adapts all parameters immediately as they relate to the new position.

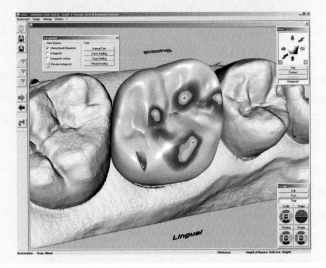

PROCEDURE   Computerized scanning and fabrication of restorations—cont'd

Step 7: Occlusion confirmation. An automated function of the software is that it is designed to propose fossa-point contacts on the appropriate triangular ridges.

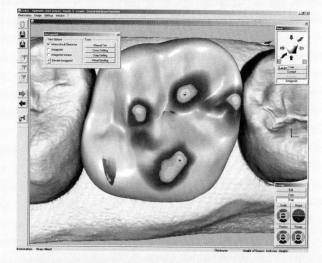

Using the virtual grinding tool, this can be easily modified to provide a Dawson-type "mortar-pestle" arrangement of occlusal-fossa contacts with broad flat holding areas for the opposing cusp tips. The position and intensity of each contact point are graphically demonstrated and color-mapped immediately on the screen and can be adjusted easily pending operator and clinical preference.

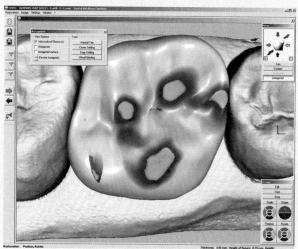

Step 8: Anatomic customization. Customized aspects and artistic creativity are also possible through an array of virtual carving and waxing tools. These can be used to manipulate occlusal anatomy, contours, and occlusal preferences, mimicking the actual laboratory methods and armamentarium. Each step is immediately updated on-screen so the operator can see the effect of any changes.

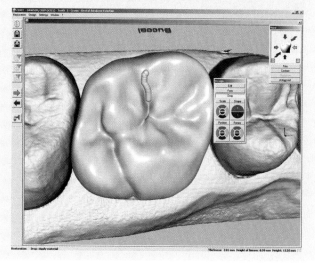

Continued

PROCEDURE   Computerized scanning and fabrication of restorations—cont'd

Step 9: Milling. Once the final virtual restoration has been designed *(top)*, it is simply a matter of loading a chamber with the predetermined shade and size of ceramic or composite block *(middle)*, pressing an on-screen button, and in approximately 15 minutes an exact replica of design is reproduced in ceramic *(bottom)*.

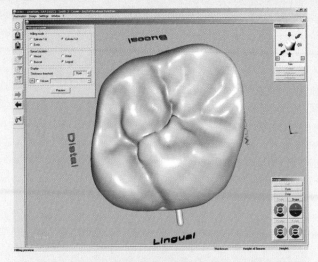

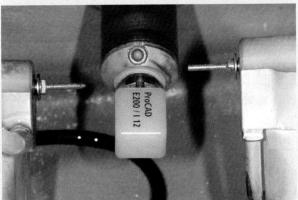

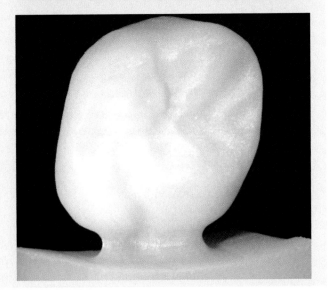

PROCEDURE   Computerized scanning and fabrication of restorations—cont'd

Step 10: Finishing and polishing. The milled restoration can then be customized conventionally using staining and glazing techniques appropriate for the ceramic selected.

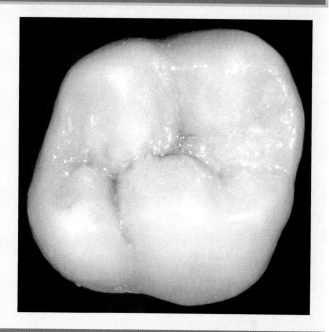

Essentially, the CEREC 3D laboratory system provides greater consistency and efficiency throughout the entire fabrication process by replacing many of the most labor-intensive and variable steps in the procedures. For the clinician, the diagnosis, treatment planning, preparation, and recording steps are all the same as with conventional techniques.

Cynovad

A slightly different and unique approach to computerized design and manufacturing of dental restorations is made available by Cynovad: Neo™ CAD/CAM system (Figure 46-11). This approach primarily focuses on the design and fabrication of a customized wax pattern that is then brought into the conventional fabrication process. The wax is three-dimensionally spray-printed onto a die, using a similar approach that inkjet printers use, however in three dimensions. The primary advantage of this approach is that it is not limited to single or small multiple unit spans, but can take into account full-mouth restoration through a truly comprehensive system. Cynovad's Neo™ CAD/CAM system virtually mounts scanned cases into a fully adjustable *virtual* articulator (Figure 46-12). Using this system, the operator can input all variables of anatomic importance (angles, shifts, curve of Wilson, curve of Spee) and take the virtually mounted models through all possible jaw movements during design. This feature allows unlimited access to any viewing perspective during simulated function and provides an unrestricted view and recording of the function of any restoration's movements. While the CEREC system fab-

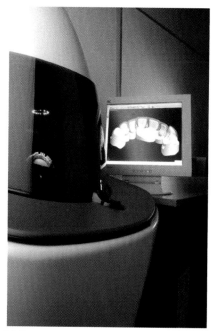

FIGURE 46-11 Cynovad's Neo™ CAD/CAM system. *(Image courtesy Cynovad, Quebec, Canada, http://www.cynovad.com)*

ricates restorations in a virtual centric occlusion pattern, Cynovad's virtual articulator, a feature of the NeoDesign software, can simulate all functional paths including protrusive and excursive movements.

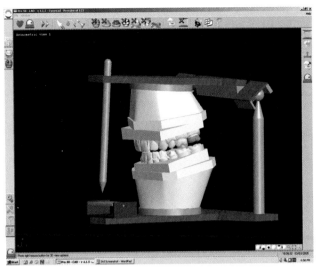

FIGURE 46-12 Scanned models mounted on virtual articulator.

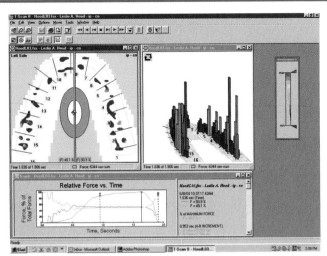

FIGURE 46-14 Digital readout of computer-analyzed occlusal contacts *(Courtesy Tekscan, Boston, Massachusetts.)*

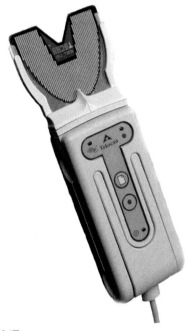

FIGURE 46-13 T-Scan® II occlusal analysis system. *(Courtesy Tekscan, Boston, Massachusetts.)*

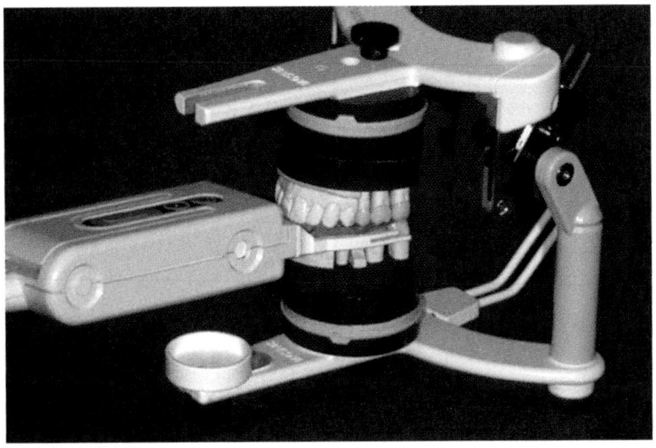

FIGURE 46-15 Tekscan used in laboratory to verify occlusal harmony. *(Courtesy Tekscan, Boston, Massachusetts.)*

COMPUTERIZED OCCLUSAL VERIFICATION

While the profession (both clinically and technically) has welcomed new technology for the diagnosis, fabrication, and delivery of comprehensive dentistry, still the most common method of confirmation and verification of the process is the use of simple articulating paper and the "tap, tap, tap" method. Although this method of functional verification with paper serves a vital purpose and gives immediate feedback, the adjunct use of a computerized system can more objectively assist in the evaluation and verification process.

The T-Scan® II (Tekscan, Boston, Massachusetts) is an electronic occlusal measurement device that can quickly measure individual contact intensity and display the results graphically on a computer screen (Figures 46-13 and 46-14). Because T-Scan II measures individual contact intensity and can relate it over time, it is possible to view jaw or model movements in excursive. In the laboratory, the T-Scan II can be used to verify paper and visual observations to ensure even distribution of occlusal contacts and detect posterior interference in protrusive and lateral movements (Figure 46-15). Clinically, the T-Scan II is used in much the same way as articulating paper, but can quantify and display much more accurate and relevant data, providing the clinician with critical information for integration of the restoration into the functioning environment.

SUMMARY

The successful incorporation of computerization and new technology into the dental laboratory will continue to provide more efficient methods of communication and fabrication while at the same time retaining the individual creativity and artistry of the skilled dental technician. The utilization of new technology will be enhanced by a close cooperation and working relationship of the dentist/technician team.

The philosophy, technique, and procedures that have been outlined in this book are fundamental principles of restorative dentistry. New technologies in dentistry will only be successful if they are combined with a complete understanding of basic comprehensive dentistry. While new technology and computerization can make procedures more efficient, less labor-intensive, and more consistent, they will not replace education, practical experience, and clinical/technical judgment.

Reference

1. Dawson PE: *Evaluation, diagnosis, and treatment of occlusal problems,* ed 2, St Louis, 1989, Mosby.

Chapter 47

Criteria for Success of Occlusal Treatment

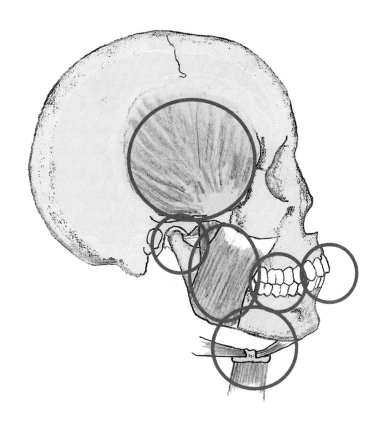

PRINCIPLE

Without specific treatment goals, treatment success cannot be measured.

MEASURING SUCCESS OBJECTIVELY

All occlusal treatment should have specific goals. We often hear claims of success, but we rarely hear how success is measured objectively. Having specific criteria for measuring the results of occlusal treatment is the only way any claim of success can be validated. In addition, specific goals are the only way treatment can be planned with the end in mind. Criteria for success are an essential requirement for achieving successful complete dentistry because they:

1. Define a desired end point for treatment
2. Are an objective measurement for treatment success, partial success, or failure
3. Are a guide for whether treatment has been performed correctly
4. Are a guide for determining if treatment has been completed
5. Are a guide for evaluating different clinical approaches

The following criteria for occlusal treatment success have stood the test of time in clinical practice. Every clinical result should be evaluated on the basis of these criteria. But the criteria are also the basis for diagnosis. These same criteria should be used in evaluating new patients or in re-evaluation of patients of record. If any criterion is not satisfied, it is indicative of a problem that needs to be diagnosed.

Let's look at each criterion for success. Understand the rationale for why it is a valid standard for judging, and learn how each criterion is tested.

In addition to occlusal success, there is always the primary requirement for periodontal health. It should go without saying that the most perfected occlusal result falls short if the supporting structures are not optimally healthy.

IMPORTANT CONSIDERATIONS

Testing for success

Whether treatment has been successfully completed can be ascertained by the following seven criteria:

1. Load test is negative. This means complete absence of any sign of tension or tenderness in either temporomandibular joint (TMJ) when joints are firmly loaded.
2. Clench test is negative. This means complete absence of any discomfort in either TMJ or in any tooth when the patient clenches with maximal muscle contraction (empty mouth).
3. Grinding test: No posterior interferences. This test is to verify that all excursive contact is on the anterior guidance only. Posterior teeth must separate the moment the mandible moves from centric relation.
4. Fremitus test is negative. This test is to ensure that there is no sign of fremitus on any anterior tooth during firm tapping or grinding excursions.
5. Stability test is positive. This test is to verify that there are no signs of instability in either TMJ, in any tooth, or within the total occlusal relationship.
6. Comfort test is inclusive. The patient should have complete comfort of the teeth, lips, face, masticatory musculature, and speech.
7. Esthetics test is inclusive. Both the patient and the dentist should be completely happy with the appearance of the smile and its relationship to the functional matrix.

It is not always a realistic expectation to achieve 100 percent success in all of these goals. The problems in some patients have progressed too far to expect complete correction. When this happens, there should be a reasonable explanation for the compromised treatment result.

Criterion #1: Load Test Is Negative

A long-term successful result requires the fulfillment of this criterion. It is the first criterion for success because complete fulfillment of all the other criteria is dependent on satisfying this first criterion.

If the TMJs cannot comfortably accept firm loading, it indicates that either the condyles are braced by the lateral pterygoid muscles (an unacceptable positioning for the TMJs that leads to muscle incoordination and potential hyperactivity of the masticatory musculature) or there is an intracapsular disorder that has a probability of instability of the TMJs.

Treatment that does not end up with complete comfort of the TMJs during maximal loading by the elevator muscles cannot be considered a completely successful treatment.

A negative load testing result indicates that the TMJs can be successfully positioned into a verifiable centric relation or adapted centric posture, the essential starting point for successful treatment.

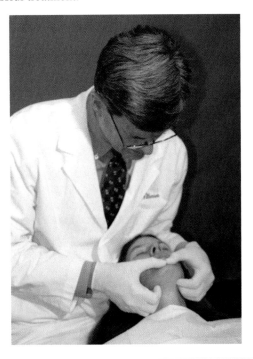

It cannot be considered a successful occlusal result if the TMJs are unstable or uncomfortable.

Criterion #2: Clench Test Is Negative

One of the simplest yet most effective tests for determining if occlusal interference is a factor in orofacial pain is to have the patient close and squeeze the teeth together (empty-mouth clench). Ask the question, "Do you feel any sign of discomfort in any tooth or in either TMJ when you squeeze hard?" A patient with perfected occlusion cannot cause any sign of discomfort in any tooth or in either joint regardless of how hard he or she bites. Discomfort in a tooth is a cer-

tain sign that at least one tooth has a premature or deflective contact. If the clench test also produces discomfort in the masticatory musculature, it is a positive indication for an occluso-muscle disorder, and it cannot be considered a successful occlusal treatment result.

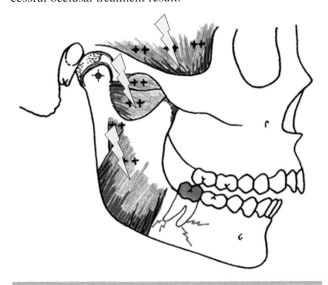

If occlusal treatment is completely successful, maximal clenching pressure should produce no discomfort in either TMJ or in any tooth.

Criterion #3: Grinding Test: No Posterior Interferences

This is another simple test to do, but a very reliable one for determining if there are posterior interferences. If the patient can feel contact on any posterior tooth while grinding the teeth through any or all excursions, it is a positive indication that posterior disclusion has not been achieved, and the result falls short of optimal success.

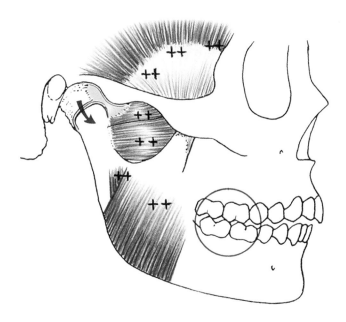

Remember that posterior interferences hyperactivate the muscles while posterior disclusion shuts off all the elevator muscles except the anterior temporal motor units.

This test has great importance for long-term stability of the occlusion because excessive wear of the posterior teeth can only occur if they interfere in excursive jaw movements.

This test must be modified in certain occlusions that do not have anterior contact in centric relation. In such cases, posterior group function on the working side may be necessary. In such cases, firm grinding should not cause discomfort in any posterior tooth.

> If posterior teeth interfere with the anterior guidance, the result is incoordinated, hyperactive musculature and potential attritional wear. It cannot be considered successful treatment.

Criterion #4: Fremitus Test Is Negative

Lightly contact the labial surface of each upper anterior tooth using the edge of your fingernail. Have the patient tap the teeth together lightly, then firmly. Then grind in all directions. Any movement of any anterior tooth is an indication that the tooth is in interference. The interference can occur from a restrictive envelope of function or failure to provide a needed "long centric." The most common cause, however, is a deflective posterior incline that forces the mandible forward into hard contact with the anterior teeth, which is an unacceptable occlusal result.

Harmonious contact through the full range of anterior guidance is critical for long-term stability of the dentition because interferences to the anterior guidance affect the neuromuscular harmony and cause overload on the anterior teeth. The result is excessive wear, hypermobility, or movement of the anterior teeth.

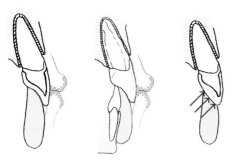

> A perfected occlusion produces no sign of fremitus on any anterior tooth, even with firm clenching or grinding.

Criterion #5: Stability Test Is Positive

The criterion that is often missed or ignored is this test for stability. This refers to stable TMJs and stable dentition. If both the joints and the teeth are stable, there should be no need for readjustment of the occlusion for a period of at least three months (Figure 47-1).

It often takes awhile to achieve occlusal stability because of the rebound of the teeth and/or remodeling of the TMJ structures following occlusal correction. In some structural TMJ deformation, we may not be able to completely satisfy the stability test because the damage to the joint has progressed too far. That must be considered a compromised result. The treatment goal then becomes one of "manageable stability." Bone-to-bone TMJ contact that results from osteo-arthritic breakdown of the condyle and eminence is a classic example. The occlusion cannot be made completely stable, but if all other requirements for a perfected occlusion can be achieved, the stability of the dentition is "manageable."

Signs of instability in the dentition:

1. Excessive wear of teeth
2. Hypermobility
3. Shifting of tooth position

If any of these conditions persist after treatment, the treatment result must be considered as less than optimal success. When there is doubt about the stability of the TMJs, reversible treatment utilizing a full occlusal splint can test for joint stability. Until the occlusion on the splint is stable for three months or more, there can be no claim for a completely successful result. Final treatment should produce the same result without the splint.

Note that long-term stability is not always dependent on a Class I textbook occlusion. There are "physiologic malocclusions" that are stable. Even though they do not look like the ideal, they can still pass all the tests for stability. Unless there are esthetic concerns, treatment is not necessary.

> Every occlusion should be evaluated for stability at regular intervals.

Criterion #6: Comfort Test

The patient should have complete comfort of the teeth, the lips, and the face. Speech should be comfortable and not cause tiredness in the facial and masticatory muscles.

A perfected occlusion results in a peaceful neuromuscular system (Figure 47-2). That is the goal of all occlusal therapy. The masticatory system is also the organ of speech. Disharmony within the system can affect speech in different ways. If changes in the occlusion result in speech changes or lead to muscle fatigue when speaking, the occlusion should be carefully re-examined including the position and contour of the anterior teeth.

It is important for the clinician to prod the patient regarding the comfort issues. I routinely asked every patient to be "very fussy" about the total comfort of the face, lips, and teeth and to let me know if there were any problems with speech. I instructed patients that if the restored teeth did not feel completely natural it would be an indication that some further adjustment would be necessary. This is a

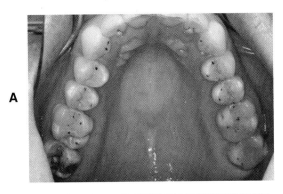

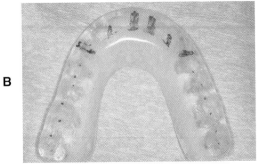

FIGURE 47-1 A, A perfected occlusion that fulfills all the criteria for success is amazingly stable and may require only minimal adjustments over many years. B, If anterior contact is not achieved, the nighttime use of an appliance can effectively substitute for the unfulfilled criteria. A correctly made splint should also be stable.

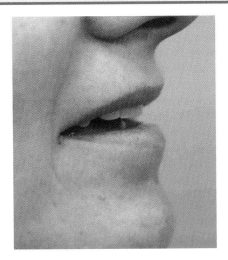

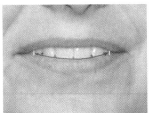

FIGURE 47-2 The comfort test should include comfortable, unstrained speech, the mark of correctly placed incisal edges, and harmony with the neutral zone.

practical approach if all the details are refined in provisional restorations whenever changes are made. Final restorations should not be completed until the provisional restorations can pass all the tests described here.

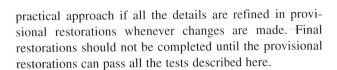

A perfected occlusion results in a peaceful, comfortable neuromusculature.

Criterion #7: Esthetics Test

The patient should be happy with the appearance of the smile. It is a consistent finding that functional harmony is dependent on anatomic harmony. When functional harmony is achieved, the result will also produce the most natural beautiful smile design. That is why we designed and teach the concept of the anterior functional matrix. This matrix defines the outer contours of anterior teeth and makes every esthetic decision an objective decision.

It is important to recognize that patients are not trained in what makes a smile naturally beautiful. They will generally accept results that improve their appearance but fall far short of an achievable ideal result. Thus it is important for the dentist to also approve every restorative result only after a critical appraisal of all esthetic guidelines. This should include the relationship of all tooth contours to the outline form es-

tablished by the matrix of functional anatomy for anterior teeth (see Chapter 16). It is also important to realize that some patients have a biased expectation for an appearance that is not conformative with natural beauty. This is why it is essential to require approval of provisional restorations before proceeding with final restorations. It is during the provisional stage that the clinician can resolve misdirected expectations if they conflict with functional requirements.

The most naturally beautiful esthetics is in conformation with anatomic and functional harmony.

The Goal: *Functional* Esthetics

If all of the criteria for success are fulfilled, the result will be an esthetic result that is also functional, comfortable, and stable. The results shown in Figures 47-3 to 47-7 are examples of functional esthetics achieved by faculty members at the Dawson Center for Advanced Dental Study. Each of these cases fulfills every criterion for success including the complete, long-lasting, and appreciative response from the patient. These results are achievable by any dentist who commits to understanding the principles, develops the skills, and avoids shortcuts: true examples of *complete dentistry.*

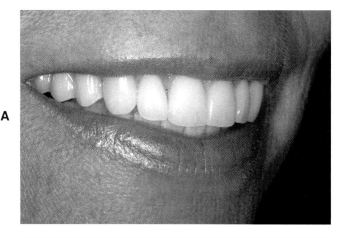

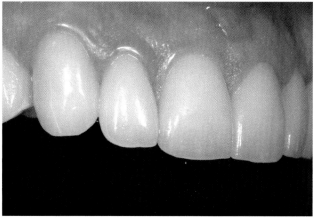

FIGURE 47-3 **A,** A complete reconstruction by Dr. Michael Sesemann. Note how perfectly the teeth relate to an unstrained lip function. **B,** Contour and inclination of the anterior teeth conform ideally to a functional matrix that puts the teeth in perfect functional harmony with no requirements for guesswork.

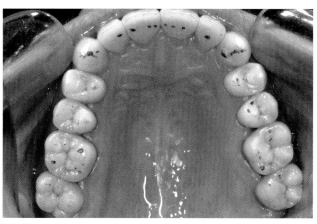

FIGURE 47-4 By perfecting the relationship of the centric relation contacts and precisely determining a correct anterior guidance, the result is equal-intensity, simultaneous contact of all teeth plus immediate disclusion of all posterior teeth in excursions, thereby making it impossible for the patient to wear out the posterior occlusion by attrition. Perfect comfort is the net result.

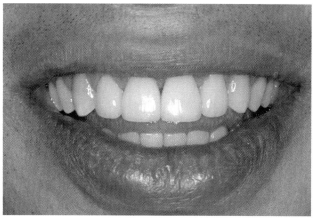

FIGURE 47-5 A conservative reconstruction by Dr. Dewitt Wilkerson that included equilibration to establish stable holding contacts before restoring only the teeth that needed it, using bonded laminate restorations. These anterior teeth are stable because they are in perfect harmony with a tight neutral zone and lip-closure path, a formula that also results in the most natural smile.

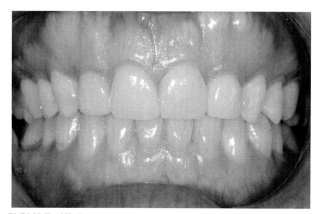

FIGURE 47-6 A complete reconstruction by Dr. Glenn DuPont that changed a very uncomfortable, unesthetic dentition into a perfectly comfortable, stable, and functional smile. All criteria for success were fulfilled in this beautiful smile.

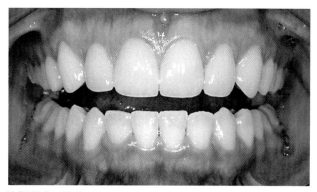

FIGURE 47-7 An excellent esthetic result achieved by Dr. John Cranham using a combination of bonded laminate restorations and full coverage where needed. This natural smile result is also functional and stable because all rules were followed to maintain teeth in a correct neutral zone, perfected anterior guidance, and equal-intensity centric relation contact for all the teeth.

SUMMARY

Dentists have never been better equipped to serve their patients with the highest level of quality and predictability. If that ultimate level of master quality dentistry is to be achieved, dentists must truly become physicians of the total masticatory system. This cannot happen without a comprehensive understanding of the role of occlusion and its dependency on total masticatory system harmony.

The rules are clear. The goals are understandable and their fulfillment is achievable if treatment planning always starts with the end in mind.

Any dentist who commits to learning the rules and developing the necessary skills for achieving each specific criterion for success will have the most essential foundation for an exceptional dental practice and a very fulfilling life.

Index

Note: Page numbers followed by "f" refer to illustrations; page numbers followed by "t" refer to tables; page numbers followed by "b" refer to boxes.